Practical Applications of Prostaglandins and their Synthesis Inhibitors

Advances in Prostaglandin Research

Practical Applications of Prostaglandins and their Synthesis Inhibitors

Edited by

S. M. M. Karim
Research Professor in Obstetrics and Gynaecology
University of Singapore

MTP PRESS LIMITED
International Medical Publishers

Published by
MTP Press Limited
Falcon House
Lancaster, England

Softcover reprint of the hardcover 1st edition 1979

British Library Cataloguing in Publication Data

Advances in prostaglandin research.
The practical applications of prostaglandins and their synthesis inhibitors
1. Prostaglandins
I. Karim, Sultan Magan Mawji
II. Practical applications of prostaglandins and their synthesis inhibitors
612'.405 QP801.P68

ISBN 978-94-011-7845-7 ISBN 978-94-011-7843-3 (eBook)
DOI 10.1007/978-94-011-7843-3

Contents

LIST OF CONTRIBUTORS

S. C. Ng
Department of Obstetrics and Gynaecology,
University of Singapore,
Kandang Kerbau Hospital, Singapore

P. M. Olley
Associate Professor,
Department of Paediatrics,
University of Toronto
Senior Staff Cardiologist,
Hospital for Sick Children,
Toronto, Canada

A. G. Olsson
King Gustaf V Research Institute and
Department of Internal Medicine,
Karolinska Hospital,
Stockholm, Sweden

R. N. V. Prasad
Department of Obstetrics and Gynaecology,
University of Singapore,
Kandang Kerbau Hospital, Singapore

J. M. Rabey
Department of Neurology,
Municipal Government Medical Center,
Ichilov Hospital,
University Medical School,
Tel-Aviv, Israel

S. S. Ratnam
Professor and Head,
Department of Obstetrics and Gynaecology,
University of Singapore,
Kandang Kerbau Hospital, Singapore

A. Robert
Department of Experimental Biology,
The Upjohn Company,
Kalamazoo,
Michigan 49001, USA

R. H. Schultz
ICI Americas, Inc.,
Animal Health Department,
Wilmington,
Delaware 19897, USA

M. Streifler
Department of Neurology,
Municipal Government Medical Center,
Ichilov Hospital,
University Medical School,
Tel-Aviv, Israel

M. Thiery
Professor and Head,
Division of Obstetrics,
Academisch Ziekenhuis,
Rijsuniversiteit Gent,
De Pintelaan 135,
B-9000 Ghent, Belgium

M. Toppozada
Department of Obstetrics and Gynaecology,
Alexandria University,
Egypt

J. Vardi
Department of Neurology,
Municipal Government Medical Center,
Ichilov Hospital,
University Medical School,
Tel-Aviv, Israel

N. Wiqvist
Department of Obstetrics and Gynaecology,
University of Götenborg,
Sweden

H. Zuckerman
Senior Lecturer and Head,
Department of Obstetrics and Gynaecology
Central Emek Hospital,
Afula, Israel

List of Contributors

P. G. Adaikan
Department of Obstetrics and Gynaecology,
University of Singapore,
Kandang Kerbau Hospital, Singapore

J.-J. Amy
Attending Gynaecologist and Obstetrician,
Academisch Ziekenhuis,
Vrije Universiteit Brussel,
Laarbeeklaan 101,
B-1090 Brussels, Belgium

A. Bennett
Professor of Pharmacology,
Department of Surgery,
King's College Hospital Medical School,
Denmark Hill, London SE5 8RX

M. Bygdeman
Department of Obstetrics and Gynaecology,
Karolinska Hospital,
Stockholm, Sweden

A. A. Calder
University Department of Obstetrics and Gynaecology,
Glasgow Royal Maternity Hospital,
Glasgow G4 0NA

L. A. Carlson
King Gustaf V Research Institute and Department of Internal Medicine,
Karolinska Hospital,
Stockholm, Sweden

F. Coceani
Research Institute,
The Hospital for Sick Children,
555 University Avenue,
Toronto M5G 1XB,
Ontario, Canada

M. J. Cooper
44 Jacks Lane,
Marchington,
Uttoxeter, Staffordshire

M. P. Fichman
Clinical Professor of Medicine,
USC School of Medicine,
2025 Zonal Avenue,
Los Angeles,
California 90033, USA

D. Hammond
ICI Pharmaceuticals Division,
Alderley Park,
Macclesfield, Cheshire

S. Harpaz-Kerpel
Lecturer,
Head of Endocrinological Unit,
Central Emek Hospital,
Afula, Israel

K. Hillier
Senior Lecturer in Pharmacology,
Faculty of Medicine,
The University of Southampton,
Southampton SO9 3TU

S. M. M. Karim
Department of Obstetrics and Gynaecology,
University of Singapore,
Kandang Kerbau Hospital, Singapore

N. Kunaratnam
ENT Department,
Singapore General Hospital,
Singapore

D. Legge
Consultant Radiologist,
Mater Misericordiae Hospital,
Dublin 7, Ireland

Preface

This is the fourth in a series of books on *Advances in Prostaglandin Research* published by MTP Press. From laboratory and animal studies a large number of practical applications of prostaglandins have been identified. In some areas clinical trials have also been carried out. There is usually a long time interval between identifying practical applications of new drugs and clinical trials. Most of the information on practical applications of prostaglandins is scattered in different journals.

Although a number of books dealing with prostaglandin research have been published (including some on practical applications in specific areas, e.g. reproduction) there is no single volume dealing with all areas of practical applications of these substances. This book aims at filling this gap and should be of interest to clinicians as well as to medical and basic scientists in academic institutions and in the pharmaceutical industry.

In some areas, exciting potential applications of prostaglandins have been identified from basic research but clinical trials have so far not been carried out. Such areas of practical applications are covered in a separate introductory chapter.

All contributors to the volume are scientists and clinicians actively engaged in prostaglandin research and most are recognized authorities in specific areas. The need for rapid publication in a fast-expanding field is obvious. Attempts have been made to cover work published until the end of 1978 (admittedly, some omissions are inevitable) and publication date set for June 1979. This has only been possible as a result of the co-operation of the contributors in submitting their manuscripts on time and the efforts of the publishers in bringing the book out within 3 months of receiving the manuscripts. Because of the tight schedule involved, all proof checking was carried out by the Editor and his staff. I would like to apologize to the contributors and to readers for any inadvertent errors.

Tables and figures previously published are, in general, acknowledged by a reference in the legends and I am grateful to the respective authors, editors, and publishers for their permission.

PREFACE

My thanks are due to my various colleagues, particularly Professor S. S. Ratnam, Mr P. G. Adaikan, Professor S. R. Kottegoda, Professor Cheah Jin Seng, Professor R. L. Tambyraja, Dr T. MaCarthy, Dr Law Hai Yang, Miss Serene Lai, Mr A. Loganath and Dr Ashim Roy for discussion and advice on the subject matter of some of the chapters and to Miss Tai Mei Yoon, Miss Leong Mei Mei, Miss Wang Gek Choo, Miss Heng Seoh Gek and Miss Sei Mei Fong for assistance in cross-checking journal references and proof-reading. I should also like to thank Miss Lily Koh for expert secretarial help.

Singapore
February, 1979

Sultan M. M. Karim

1 General Introduction and Practical Implications of some Pharmacological Actions of Prostaglandins, Thromboxanes and their Synthesis Inhibitors

K. HILLIER and S. M. M. KARIM

1.1 INTRODUCTION

In almost every branch of medicine there is an intense interest in the prostaglandins (PG), thromboxanes (TX) and inhibitors of their actions or biosynthesis. The study of these substances has already significantly advanced our understanding of several biological processes.

The hope that prostaglandins will further provide the missing link in hitherto unknown biological mechanisms is overwhelming amongst scientists working in the field as is the prospect of valuable therapeutic agents or diagnostic tools resulting from their investigation.

Several practical applications of prostaglandins and their synthesis inhibitors have already been identified. In some of these areas clinical trials have also been conducted. These are reviewed in individual chapters that follow. The purpose of this section is to provide an introduction to the biosynthesis of prostaglandins and thromboxanes and to review potential practical applications of prostaglandins not covered in individual chapters.

1.2 BIOSYNTHESIS OF PROSTAGLANDINS AND THROMBOXANES

A selective introduction to the synthesis of prostaglandins and thromboxanes and the actions of their inhibitors is necessary to an understanding of their therapeutic usefulness and drawbacks (Figure 1.1). A more detailed treatment has been published elsewhere (Hillier, 1978; Vane, 1978).

No tissue stores prostaglandins or thromboxanes as far as we know; they are synthesized upon acceptance of a suitable physiological, pharmacological or pathological signal. The enzymes only act upon free polyunsaturated fatty acids such as arachidonic acid to form prostaglandins and thromboxanes. Therefore, a prior requirement is the former's release from phospholipids, triglycerides and cholesteryl esters, where it is in a bound form and unusable as a substrate for prostaglandin-forming enzymes. In some tissues the availability of free fatty acid is the rate-limiting step in synthesis and an appropriate trigger mechanism would be the activation of phospholipase to

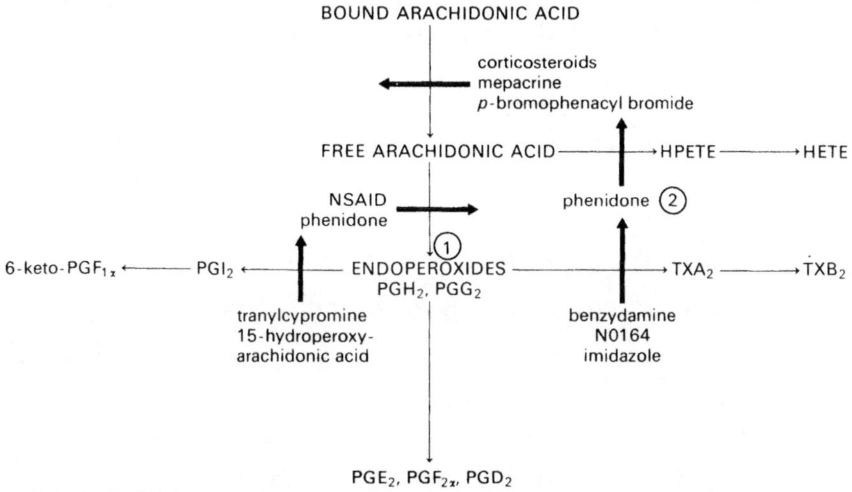

Figure 1.1 Inhibitors of the metabolism of arachidonic acid via the cyclo-oxygenase (1) and lipoxygenase (2) pathways.

1-phenyl-3-pyrazolidone, phenidone (Blackwell and Flower, 1978) inhibits arachidonic acid metabolism by both pathways. References for other inhibitors: corticosteroids (Nijkamp *et al.*, 1976), mepacrine (Vargaftig and Dao Hai, 1972), *p*-bromophenacyl bromide (Mitchell *et al.*, 1977), NSAID (Flower, 1974), tranylcypromine (Gryglewski *et al.*, 1976; Myatt and Elder, 1977), imidazole (Nijkamp *et al.*, 1977), benzydamine (Moncada *et al.*, 1976), N0164 (Eakins and Kulkarni, 1977), 15-hydroperoxy-arachidonic acid (Moncada *et al.*, 1976). Substrate analogues will also inhibit pathway (1) (Lands and Rome, 1976)

NSAID: non-steroidal anti-inflammatory drugs
HPETE: 12-hydroperoxy-arachidonic acid
HETE: 12-hydroxy-arachidonic acid

liberate the free fatty acid from a phospholipid when it can be acted upon by appropriate synthetase enzymes. Availability of appropriate enzymes may also limit prostaglandin formation but this is generally considered to be less important.

The type of precursor fatty acid present determines the prostaglandin formed. The majority of investigators have studied arachidonic acid which is converted to PGE_2, $PGF_{2\alpha}$, PGG_2, PGH_2, TXA_2, TXB_2 and PGI_2. However, it should be noted that arachidonic acid is obtained by desaturation of dihomo-γ-linolenic acid (Figure 1.2). This relative of arachidonic acid can be converted to form different prostaglandin and thromboxane end-products which may have very altered properties from those formed from arachidonic acid. The types of tissue prostaglandins and thromboxanes formed may be modified by dietary intake of different types of polyunsaturated fatty acids.

The next vital step in prostaglandin synthesis is the formation of the common intermediate endoperoxides, PGG_2 and PGH_2. These are unstable but do possess biological activity. They can, for example, stimulate renin release from kidney slices *in vitro* (Weber *et al.*, 1976) and contract vascular and bronchial smooth muscle (Wassermann, 1976).

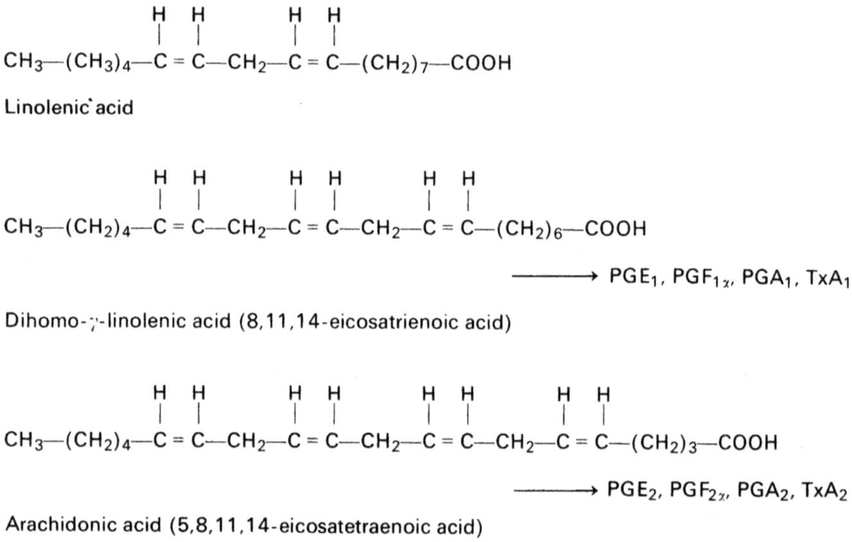

Figure 1.2 Prostaglandins and thromboxanes formed from unsaturated precursor fatty acids

A wide variety of tissues possess the ability to synthesize prostaglandins from arachidonic acid (Christ and van Dorp, 1972). Their capacity to do so *in vitro*, however, is very variable. For example, *in vitro* seminal vesicle prostaglandin-synthesizing enzymes can convert 75% of substrate to prostaglandins whereas brain tissue converts 1% or less. How this relates to *in vivo* production is unclear but even 1% conversion may represent a level sufficient for the needs of the tissue. A distinct problem when studying *in vitro* synthesis (or *in vivo* synthesis after surgical manipulation) is a transient stimulation of prostaglandin production by trauma unrelated to the normal physiological control mechanisms. Thus unless adequate time is allowed between handling and carrying out measurements, erroneous concentrations may be measured. Notwithstanding these reservations, it is clear that different tissues have varied capacities (qualitatively and quantitatively) to form prostaglandins. Thus platelets can largely (but not exclusively) form TXA_2

when induced to aggregate since they predominantly contain the thromboxane synthesizing enzymes and co-factors to form this compound. On the other hand blood vessels and uteri form predominantly PGI_2, and kidneys PGE_2 and $PGF_{2\alpha}$. The importance of these differences is discussed later but clearly they demonstrate the ways in which selectivity can be present between tissues and indeed between cells. *In vitro* studies of prostaglandin synthesis may be misleading unless careful account is taken of the laboratory conditions used including the addition of co-factors. For example, sheep uterine microsomes and seminal vesicle microsomes form large amounts of PGE_2 and $PGF_{2\alpha}$ in the presence of reduced glutathione but at low substrate concentrations (and without co-factors or with only haemaglobin and tryptophan added) they form largely 6-keto-$PGF_{1\alpha}$ (Dighe *et al.*, 1978; Cottee *et al.*, 1977).

The type of prostaglandin or thromboxane formed in the body can be manipulated by dietary adjustment or by blocking the enzymeq that form a particular prostaglandin. For example, it has been found that an enzyme exists (PGE_2-9-keto reductase) in some tissues that converts PGE_2 to $PGF_{2\alpha}$. The difference in properties of these prostaglandins makes the occurrence of this enzyme of importance. In rats it has been shown that a high salt diet increases the activity of this enzyme 2–3 fold and this can alter renin release and sodium absorption (Weber *et al.*, 1977). The overall prostaglandin formation in the body in man can be increased by feeding a subject arachidonic acid. This increases arachidonate in platelets and significantly increases the aggregation of platelets by adenosine diphosphate (ADP). At the same time the major urinary metabolite of PGE (7α-hydroxy-5,11-di-keto-tetranorprostane-1,16-dioic acid) is also increased. Seyberth *et al.* (1975) administered ethyl arachidonate to man for 2–3 weeks and increased the arachidonate in phospholipids, triglycerides and cholesterol esters. Free arachidonate in plasma was not altered. Dietary factors influencing the prostaglandin forming capacity in lungs have also been established. Meydani, Mathias and Schatte (1978) showed that $PGF_{2\alpha}$, PGE_2 and PGE_1 formation in lungs of rats fed a high (78%) polyunsaturated fatty acid diet (PUFA) was significantly higher than in rats fed a low (5%) PUFA diet. However, no data on thromboxane or PGI_2 formation are available.

Normally in platelets, arachidonic acid is predominant and, with appropriate stimuli, the pro-aggregatory TXA_2 and endoperoxides PGG_2 and PGH_2 are formed and accompany aggregation (Hamberg *et al.*, 1975). The prostaglandins and thromboxanes formed in platelets can be redirected to those of the '1' series by feeding dihomo-γ-linolenic acid, the precursor of prostaglandins and thromboxanes with one unsaturated double bond. Thus, endoperoxides PGG_1 and PGH_1, PGE_1 and possibly TXA_1 are formed with the greater availability of dihomo-γ-linolenic acid and these have less pro-aggregatory action than products formed from arachidonic acid (Falardeau *et al.*, 1976). Kernoff *et al.* (1977) detected reduced plasma heparin-neutralizing activity and reduced platelet aggregation in volunteers fed dihomo-γ-linolenic acid and suggest that this manipulation has potential in treating human thromboembolic disease. However, the discovery by Vane's group (Moncada *et al.*, 1976a) that blood vessel endothelium forms predominantly prostacyclin (PGI_2) from arachidonic acid has necessitated a rethink of the desirability of using dihomo-γ-linolenic acid for treating thromboembolic disease. PGI_2 potently inhibits the adherence of platelets to blood vessel walls. Thus, the increased presence of substrate other than arachidonic acid may inhibit the vascular formation of PGI_2 and, therefore, interfere with the anti-adherent properties of the endothelium. Dihomo-γ-linolenic acid therapy therefore probably does not represent the ideal treatment for thromboembolic disease although further study is clearly warranted.

In the same area, aspirin and sulfinpyrazone have been studied for their ability to prevent myocardial reinfarction. Although pathological studies of the relation between coronary thrombosis and myocardial infarction have yielded conflicting results, much evidence points to occlusive thrombosis being an important factor in myocardial infarction (Chandler *et al.*, 1974). Aspirin in high doses inhibits the cyclo-oxygenase enzymes and, therefore, reduces TXA_2 and PGI_2 formation; the former effect is beneficial in preventing arterial thrombosis but the latter is not. However, although the effect of aspirin on platelet cyclo-oxygenase persists for the duration of the life span of the platelet, the inhibition of vascular enzymes is more transient because of the new protein synthesizing ability of vessels. It is, therefore, likely that modest doses of aspirin will desirably have a greater effect on pro-aggregatory TXA_2 synthesis than on PGI_2 (Vargaftig and Lefort, 1977). Sulfinpyrazone also inhibits prostaglandin formation (Anturane Reinfarction Trial, 1978) and therapy with this drug has had some success in reducing myocardial reinfarction. The ideal therapy in terms of a prostaglandin approach is probably via selective inhibition of TXA_2 synthesis (Moncada and Vane, 1978).

The actions of selective inhibitors of TXA_2 synthesis (such as imidazole and azo analogues of the prostaglandins) make more endoperoxides available for conversion to other prostaglandins (Figure 1.1). Thus, in platelet suspensions in the presence of these selective inhibitors, less thromboxane is formed. Simultaneously, a greater amount of PGE_2 is synthesized (Fitzpatrick and Gorman, 1978). Thus, the effects of induced reduction of a particular prostaglandin may be masked by the presence of greater amounts of others.

Progressive research has identified a number of selective inhibitors of prostaglandin and thromboxane synthesis (see Figure 1.1 for references). These are only relatively specific at moderate dose levels; higher doses reduce selectivity. Phenidone (1-phenyl-3-pyrazolidone) blocks both the lipoxygenase and cyclo-oxygenase pathways in horse platelets and guinea-pig perfused lungs (Blackwell and Flower, 1978) and should be a useful tool for the investigation of the lipoxygenase pathway.

Recent studies involving thromboxanes and platelet aggregation and the effects of commonly used therapeutic agents on this system have helped to explain their unwanted and previously unexplained side-effects. For example, oral contraceptives increase the platelet microsomal content of pro-aggregatory prostaglandins and thromboxane forming enzymes (Schorer *et al.*, 1978). Similar changes occur in smokers (Gerrard *et al.*, 1976) and diabetics (Halushka *et al.*, 1977). Likewise the antithrombotic effects of some therapeutic agents can be explained in terms of prostaglandin drug interaction.

In a recent paper Horrobin *et al.* (1978c) suggest that TXA_2 is a negative feedback regulator of other products formed from arachidonic acid. They confirmed that inhibition of TXA_2 synthesis with imidazole or furosemide or antagonism of TXA_2 action with diazepam leads to greater PGE_2 and $PGF_{2\alpha}$ synthesis. In guinea-pig lung and platelets, the increased prostaglandin synthesis is greater than could be accounted for simply by diversion of endoperoxide to the prostaglandin pathway. Horrobin *et al.* (1978a) evoke the inhibition of TXA_2 as the mechanism of action of dipyridamole in inhibiting platelet aggregation. They suggest that TXA_2 promotes while PGI_2 inhibits calcium release from platelet stores. Dipyridamole inhibits TXA_2 synthesis and prevents calcium mobilization and ensuing aggregation. However, the indirect evidence they present is countered by data of Moncada *et al.* (1978) who showed that dipyridamole does not prevent the conversion of PGH_2 to TXA_2 in rabbit, horse and human platelet preparations. This group suggested that the antithrombotic effect óf dipyridamole (a phosphodiesterase inhibitor) is due to stimulation of cAMP in platelets by PGI_2 (Moncada and Korbut, 1978). PGI_2 released from the pulmonary circulation activates cAMP and this effect is enhanced by dipyridamole. Consistent with this is the greater effect of dipyridamole in arterial than in venous circulation and the antagonism of its action by PGI_2 antiserum and by high doses of aspirin which reduce circulating concentrations of PGI_2. However, Jorgensen and Stoffersen (1978) showed that dipyridamole has an inhibitory effect on platelets which is independent of PGI_2 or TXA_2 but dependent upon albumin concentrations. If prostaglandin and thromboxane synthesis is inhibited by aspirin, dipyridamole in fact enhances thrombin-induced aggregation but increasing albumin concentrations reverse this effect allowing an inhibition of aggregation.

1.3 CENTRAL NERVOUS SYSTEM

The practical implications of the prostaglandins and thromboxanes in CNS function deserve only modest mention at this time although future investigations will certainly alter this as the area is one of continuing research and development. The most widely studied aspect of prostaglandins and brain function is in fever, although they have also been implicated in the mechanisms of action of antidepressant drugs, in analgesia, schizophrenia, cerebral circulation, neuronal transmission and behaviour (see Hillier, 1977 for references).

In recent studies on the role of prostaglandins in controlling body temperature (see Hillier, 1977 for references) it has been shown that intraventricular arachidonic acid causes shivering and dose-related hyperthermia. Additionally, PGE_2 is raised in CSF during certain types of pyrogen fever and can increase temperature in humans in pharmacological doses. Administration of non-steroidal anti-inflammatory drugs to pyrexic animals results in lowered temperature and a parallel decrease in PGE_2 in the CSF. However, evidence that prostaglandins are mandatory mediators of fever is equivocal. Pyrogens can evoke fever in animals that do not respond to prostaglandin administration with hyperthermia (Veale and Cooper, 1975) and elevated levels of prostaglandins are not always seen in pyrogen-induced fever (Cranston *et al.*, 1975). More recently two sub-groups of fever developing after pyrogen administration have been described. The first, seen in animals not previously exposed to pyrogens, had a long latency before hyperthermia, whereas a second sub-group that had on a previous occasion been exposed to pyrogens had a short latency period before hyperthermia on subsequent pyrogen administration. In the latter type, PGE and PGF increased in parallel with the rising body temperature but in the former no significant increase in prostaglandins was noted (Milton *et al.*, 1977). It therefore remains to be decided whether prostaglandins are pathological mediators of pyrogen-induced fever.

Investigations are being carried out in an attempt to link prostaglandins with mental illness. At this time there is little concrete scientific evidence but further investigation is clearly warranted. Horrobin (1977, 1978) has suggested that schizophrenia is a 'prostaglandin-lack disease'. It is hypothesized that schizophrenia is related to excessive functional dopaminergic activity and almost all anti-schizophrenic drugs block dopamine receptors which are involved in stimulating prolactin production and release. Horrobin *et al.* (1978b) have shown that this stimulates prostaglandins. Schizophrenics are said to be resistant to pain and arthritis and prostaglandins have been implicated in these pathological states. Schizophrenia can be transiently relieved by fever (when PGE increases) and platelets from schizophrenics do not produce PGE_1 normally when stimulated by ADP (Abdulla and Hamadah, 1975). High doses of prostaglandin inhibitors cause schizophrenia-like symptoms. More recently, it has been shown that PGE_1 induces a smaller increase in [^{3}H]cyclic AMP in platelet rich plasma from schizophrenics compared with normal individuals (Rotrosen *et al.*, 1978). This suggests that reduced sensitivity as well as inhibition of prostaglandin synthesis is evident in schizophrenics but there is little to explain whether this prostaglandin lack is a cause or an effect of the disease.

However, some anti-schizophrenics such as clozapine do not increase prolactin release and, by inference, prostaglandin synthesis. Tricyclic antidepressants and methyldopa stimulate prolactin release but are not anti-schizophrenic and some studies have shown that rheumatoid arthritis and schizophrenia are not mutually exclusive.

The naturally occurring opiates may also be related to this complex puzzle; β-endorphin and exogenous opiates appear to be able to inhibit prostaglandin synthesis and action (Goldstein *et al.*, 1977; Horrobin, 1978) and endorphins are elevated in schizophrenia (Terenius *et al.*, 1976).

Schizophrenia may, therefore, be related to endorphin excess, prostaglandin deficiency or dopamine supersensitivity, all of which may be interrelated and should be actively studied.

Some clinical data quoted by Horrobin (1978) appear to link prostaglandins to schizophrenia. Penicillin stimulates prostaglandin synthesis without blocking dopamine receptors and this appears to have an anti-psychotic action. 'Evening Primrose Oil' is a rich source of the precursor of PGE_1 (dihomo-γ-linolenic acid) and has been administered with penicillin with initially encouraging results in patients resistant to neuroleptic therapy.

The occurrence of prostaglandins and thromboxanes in the brain is incompletely mapped both in overall formation and in the synthetic capacity of different brain regions. However, Sun *et al.* (1977) and Wolfe *et al.* (1976) showed that rat brain tissue is capable of forming relatively large amounts of PGD_2 and PGE_2, $PGF_{2\alpha}$ and thromboxanes. Sun *et al.* (1977) were unable to identify PGI_2 using radiochemical conversion. However, Chaplin and Hillier (1979) using a sensitive bioassay have shown that rat brain incubates can synthesize a PGI_2-like substance. The identification of new prostaglandins in the brain means that previous studies need to be reconsidered in the light that the newer compounds may have important functions.

If aberrant neurotransmitter behaviour in brain is important in mental illness then prostaglandins may hypothetically be involved. It is now well known that in the peripheral nervous system PGE_2 can inhibit the outflow of noradrenaline from nerve terminals in certain organs (Hedqvist, 1976). The effect of this mechanism may summate with the modulatory influence of presynaptic α-adrenergic receptor stimulation.

In the CNS noradrenaline release has also been shown to be reduced by presynaptic α-receptor stimulation but the action of PGEs is less clear. Recent studies have shown that PGE_2 can reduce [^{3}H]noradrenaline and dopamine overflow from perfused rat cortex slices and may thus contribute to the control of neurotransmitter release in the brain (Bergström *et al.*, 1973; Westfall and Kitay, 1977; Templeton and Hillier, unpublished data). In support of a feedback mechanism, it has also been shown that catecholamines can stimulate prostaglandin synthesis in brain thus completing a feedback loop (Hillier *et al.*, 1976). However, other workers have been unable to show an effect of prostaglandins on spontaneous or evoked ^{3}H overflow in rat brain synaptosomes (Davison, 1977). Thus, the importance of prostaglandins as modulators in the CNS is far from resolved.

1.4 PROSTAGLANDINS AND IMMUNOLOGY

The prostaglandins have consistent effects on immunological systems investigated *in vitro*, but it is as yet generally unclear whether this is of physiological importance *in vivo*. However, the 'spin-off' from these studies has undoubtedly led to a greater understanding of immunological control mechanisms (Pelus and Strausser, 1977).

Prostaglandins appear to regulate the release of humoral antibody or its production, immediate hypersensitivity, cell-mediated immunity and proliferation of lymphoid cells. All of these effects appear to be mediated by an interaction with cyclic AMP and cyclic GMP which are involved in the intracellular control of immune responsiveness.

Classically, the immune system consists of the humoral (B) cells which are bone marrow derived and the cellular or thymus derived (T) cells. Macrophages receive information from, and supply information to, these cells and process antigen. Lymphokines are released from sensitized thymus-dependent lymphocytes following activation with antigen. These exhibit a range of biological actions appropriate to mediators of delayed hypersensitivity reaction, for example mitogenesis and inhibition of macrophage migration, chemotaxis and macrophage activation. The release of lymphokines (the product of antigen-activated thymus-dependent lymphocytes) is potently inhibited by PGE_1 (Gordon *et al.*, 1976; Bray *et al.*, 1978).

Activation of sensitized thymus-dependent lymphocytes also stimulates E-type prostaglandin production from macrophages; thus, lymphokine production activates a dose-related negative feedback inhibition of the cellular immune response. This inhibition by PGE_1 can be extended to other types of hypersensitivity reaction including inhibition of histamine secretion by human basophils and antigen-induced SRS-A production by lung fragments. Consistent with this is the finding that indomethacin will enhance SRS-A release from passively sensitized human lung.

Knowledge of prostaglandins and their role in immune responses may also be of considerable help in understanding excessive immune/inflammatory responses. In rheumatoid arthritis, mediators of inflammation are released into the joint spaces during ingestion of immune complexes by invading PMN or by synovial cells. The potential importance of prostaglandins in this disease has been outlined by Morley (1974). He suggests that lymphokine production may be involved in some of the pathogenic processes observed and postulated that in this disease the lymphocyte response to PGEs is defective, that is PGE does not prevent the release of mediators of inflammation.

In animal models using adjuvant-induced arthritis (which resembles rheumatoid arthritis) treatment with PGE prevents the onset of the disease and attenuates the inflammatory processes (Zurier *et al.*, 1977 for references). PGE may act by reducing lysosomal enzyme and toxic oxygen metabolite release from endocytic cells. In patients with systemic lupus erythematosus

(SLE) there is an excessive B-cell production of antibody while T-cell activity is suppressed. In animals with murine lupus, which is similar to SLE, injection of PGE_1 prolongs survival time. It appears that in part PGE_1 preserves T-lymphocyte function and cellular immune responsiveness (Krakauer *et al.*, 1978).

The prostaglandins may also be involved in the depressed cellular immunity seen in patients with Hodgkin's disease (Goodwin *et al.*, 1977). These patients have depressed cellular immunity manifested by skin-test anergy, or hypo-responsiveness, decreased homograft rejection, increased susceptibility to certain infections and impaired *in vitro* responses to T-cell mitogens. The defect in the cell-mediated immunity is thought to be caused by the presence of circulating suppressor cells and Goodwin *et al.* (1977) identified a glass adherent cell which suppresses T-cell mitogenesis with only minor effects on B cells. This cell produces four times more PGE_2 than normal lymphocytes. Confirmation that the suppressor effect was due to PGE_2 was achieved by adding PGE_2 into phytohaemagglutinin-stimulated cultures which inhibited [^{3}H]thymidine incorporation by 50% at 10^{-8} M. Indomethacin on the other hand caused a marked increase in [^{3}H]thymidine incorporation.

Whether indomethacin has a similar action *in vivo* is as yet unanswered.

1.5 RESPIRATORY SYSTEM

1.5.1 Vasomotor and allergic rhinitis

The subject is discussed in detail by Adaikan, Karim and Kunaratnam in Chapter 2. The two prostaglandins (PGE_2 and $PGF_{2\alpha}$) present in the nasal mucosa produce constriction of the mucosal blood vessels and increase nasal patency. A possible deficiency of these prostaglandins may be involved in nasal congestion associated with rhinitis. Recent observations that intranasal administration of PGI_2 decreases nasal patency, suggest that this prostaglandin may be released in vasomotor and allergic rhinitis (Karim and Adaikan, 1979).

1.5.2 Asthma

The bronchodilator effect of E prostaglandins (particularly PGE_1) has been recognized for many years. Although a definite role for prostaglandins in the lung has yet to be defined, it seems likely that they act as autoregulatory agents. Prostaglandins are released in asthma but their role is thought to be secondary and may be related to physiological attempts to restore the bronchi to a more normal state. Prostaglandins may be involved in the maintenance of normal bronchial tone and thereby adjust local ventilation perfusion ratio in the lungs. However, the use of E series prostaglandins in the treatment of patients with asthma has proved disappointing because of their irritant effect when given by inhalation and their loss of potency when given intravenously (see Smith, 1976 for a detailed review).

Several prostaglandin analogues have been evaluated in laboratory animals and on human respiratory tract muscle *in vitro*. Most of these, however, are potent bronchoconstrictors including those of the E series (Karim and Adaikan, 1976; Strandberg and Hedqvist, 1977). Some of the trinor-inter-*m*-phenylene analogues of PGE_1 are potent in relaxing human respiratory tract smooth muscle *in vitro* and in decreasing histamine-induced lung resistance in anaesthetized guinea-pigs *in vivo* (Table 1.1). These compounds are currently under evaluation for their bronchial effect in asthmatics (Adaikan and Karim, 1979).

Table 1.1 Effects of 4,5,6-trinor-3,7-inter-*m*-phenylene analogues of PGE_1 on respiratory tract smooth muscle

Prostaglandin	*Guinea-pig*		*Human*		
	Trachea in vitro	*Lung resistance* in vivo	*Tracheal strips*	*Bronchial strips*	*Bronchiole strips*
Rac-4,5,6-trinor-3, 7-inter-*m*-phenylene PGE_1 methyl ester	0.28 (3)	0.002 (3)	0.89 (3)	0.66 (3)	0.62 (2)
4,5,6-trinor-3,7-inter-*m*-phenylene-3-oxa-PGE_1 methyl ester	0.38 (3)	0.02 (3)	6.52 (4)	1.28 (3)	0.52 (1)
4,5,6-trinor-3-oxa-3-7-inter-*m*-phenylene PGE_1	0.17 (3)	10.73 (4)	5.86 (3)	0.75 (2)	2.25 (4)

(a) The three analogues produced relaxation in all five systems
(b) Potency compared with PGE_1 (taken as 1) except for guinea-pig trachea *in vitro* where the potency was compared with PGE (taken as 1)
(c) Figures in parenthesis = Number of experiments
Data from Adaikan and Karim (1979)

More recently the effect of PGI_2 on the respiratory tract has been studied. Wasserman and Griffin (personal communication) showed that this prostaglandin induces a step-wise relaxation of guinea-pig tracheal (spiral) strips after sustained contractions are induced with carbachol. In contrast, Omini *et al.* (1977) and Karim and Adaikan (1979) found that PGI_2 contracts guinea-pig tracheal chain preparations. In anaesthetized guinea-pigs intravenously administered PGI_2 was twice as potent as PGE_1 in reducing histamine-induced lung resistance (Karim and Adaikan, 1979). The bronchodilator action of intravenously administered PGI_2 in anaesthetized dogs has also been shown by Wasserman and Griffin (personal communication).

PGI_2 relaxes the human tracheal and bronchial smooth muscles *in vitro*

(Karim and Adaikan, 1979). When given as an aerosol in doses up to 500 μg PGI_2 failed to reverse exercise-induced bronchoconstriction in asthmatics. However, prior administration of this prostaglandin prevented exercise and water mist-induced bronchoconstriction in asthmatics (Bianco *et al.*, 1978). The lack of bronchodilator effect of intravenously and locally administered PGI_2 in healthy volunteers and in asthmatics has also been reported by Szczeklik *et al.*, 1978a).

1.6 CARDIOVASCULAR EFFECTS

Some effects of prostaglandins on the cardiovascular system are reviewed in individual chapters that follow. In this section the effects of PGI_2 and thromboxanes and their practical implications in the cardiovascular system will be discussed.

1.6.1 Prostacyclin (PGI_2) and thromboxanes (TX)

The potent effects of prostaglandin endoperoxides (PGG_2 and PGH_2) and TXA_2 may explain why platelets sometimes stick to the walls of arteries and cause thrombus formation. The search for an answer as to 'why platelets do not stick to the walls of healthy arteries' led to the discovery of PGI_2 (PGX, prostacyclin) with exciting pharmacological properties and potential practical applications. PGI_2 in most respects is the biological opposite of TXA_2, being a potent inhibitor of platelet aggregation and a relaxant of vascular and bronchial smooth muscle (Moncada *et al.*, 1976a, 1976b; Gryglewski *et al.*, 1976; Bunting *et al.*, 1976).

1.6.2 Practical implications of thromboxanes

Although TXA_2 is important in platelet aggregation and thrombus formation, it is difficult to visualize any important practical application of this compound or its analogues. However, selective inhibitors of thromboxane synthesis should prove useful in the prevention of thrombosis by controlling platelet aggregation. Benzydamine, N 0164, imidazole and burimamide have been reported to selectively inhibit thromboxane synthesis (Moncada, Needleman *et al.*, 1976; Eakins and Kulkarni, 1977; Allan and Eakins, 1978) (Figure 1.1). These compounds are only relatively specific at small concentrations; higher doses reduce selectivity. The search for more selective analogues of thromboxane synthesis that could be used in man continues.

It has been known for many years that non-steroidal anti-inflammatory drugs like aspirin inhibit the biosynthesis of prostaglandins. These drugs are now known also to inhibit the synthesis of PGI_2 and thromboxanes. There is some evidence to suggest that at small doses aspirin selectively inhibits the synthesis of thromboxanes. In rabbits low doses of aspirin increase bleeding time and have an antithrombotic effect. At high doses these effects are absent (see O'Grady and Moncada, 1978). The above findings have recently been confirmed in human volunteers (O'Grady and Moncada, 1978; Treacher *et al.*, 1978; Rajah *et al.*, 1978).

1.6.3 Practical implications of prostacyclin

PGI_2 is more potent than other prostaglandins (PGE_1 and PGD_2) in inhibiting platelet aggregation *in vitro* induced by arachidonic acid, ADP or collagen (Moncada *et al.*, 1976a, 1976b). It is also able to disaggregate platelets after ADP or arachidonic acid-induced aggregation (Moncada *et al.*, 1976b). Intravenous infusion of PGI_2 at 10–50 (ng/kg)/min in man also inhibits platelet aggregation induced by ADP and increases bleeding time. Effective rates of infusion of PGI_2, however, consistently lowered diastolic blood pressure while in most subjects the systolic pressure increased. The effect on the blood pressure was preceded by a rise in heart rate. In addition there was erythema of the face and palms, increase in skin temperature and venous blood arterialization (Szczeklik *et al.*, 1978b). The inhibition of platelet aggregation and cardiovascular effects described above have also been observed when PGI_2 is given by inhalation aerosol in doses of 200–400 μg (Szczeklik *et al.*, 1978a). The side-effects of PGI_2 and its chemical instability in solution may limit its clinical usefulness but synthetic analogues with a more selective action on platelets may fulfil the promise.

1.6.3.1 *Thrombosis*

It has been suggested that the property of PGI_2 (or its analogues) in inhibiting platelet aggregation can be utilized to (a) disperse a clot which is building up, e.g. after a heart attack; (b) to prevent recurrence of a second heart attack; and (c) prophylactically in subjects 'at risk' of a heart attack, e.g. in overweight middle-aged man (Moncada and Vane, 1978).

A reversal of blockage of the narrowed lumen of the coronary vessels due to platelet aggregation in an experimental dog model with PGI_2 has been reported by Aiken *et al.* (1979).

1.6.3.2 *Antihypertensive effect*

PGI_2 is a depressor agent with vasodilator activity in the peripheral, coronary and pulmonary vasculature (Armstrong *et al.*, 1977; DuCharme *et al.*, 1979; Dusting *et al.*, 1977). Since it is not inactivated during passage through the lungs, it may be a factor in controlling blood pressure (Armstrong *et al.*, 1977, 1978; Pace-Asciak *et al.*, 1978a, 1978b). Weeks and Sutter (1979) showed that intravenous infusion of PGI_2 inhibits the development of experimental renal hypertension in the rat at doses that did not lower arterial blood pressure. The effect of PGI_2 in established hypertension or other types of hypertension is not known.

1.6.3.3 *Extracorporeal circulation*

Although the use of heparin during haemodialysis prevents gross clotting of blood, interaction of coagulation factors and blood cells with the artificial surfaces of the dialyser lines and membranes results in deposition of fibrin. Such thrombus formation contributes to residual blood loss within the dialyser because erythrocytes are trapped on the membrane. This may aggravate the anaemia of dialysis patient (see Woods *et al.*, 1978). In anaesthetized greyhounds, Woods *et al.* (1978) showed that during haemodialysis, PGI_2 prevented thrombocytopenia, reduced platelet losses within the dialyser and abolished microembolization. With the use of PGI_2, dialysis could be performed without heparin and there was no blood clotting within the dialyser circuit. The authors have suggested that the use of PGI_2 during extracorporeal circulation may permit reduction of the use of heparin for such procedures. A heparin-sparing effect would be desirable in situations where haemorrhage might complicate extracorporeal haemoperfusion such as cardiac surgery, hepatic failure, post-operative dialysis or in patients with pericarditis in danger of haemopericardium. Osteoporosis is another complication of long-term administration of heparin. If the observed effects of PGI_2 in the dog can be confirmed in man, the drug could prove useful during haemodialysis.

1.7 URINARY BLADDER

Results of preliminary studies indicate that prostaglandins may be useful in the treatment of post-surgical and chronic retention of urine.

Naimzada (1967) showed that PGE_1 increases the tone and motility of the guinea-pig and rat bladder *in situ* but not *in vitro*. Ambache and Zar (1970) demonstrated sluggish, long-lasting contractions of the isolated guinea-pig bladder. PGE_1 and PGE_2 relaxed the isolated perfused bladder–urethra junction in the cat (Persson, 1976). Injection of $PGF_{2\alpha}$ into the caudal vesical artery of the dog produced a slow developing sustained increase in bladder tone (Taira, 1974).

The actions of prostaglandins on the human bladder *in vitro* and *in vivo* have been reported by several investigators. Karim *et al.* (1972) showed that both PGE_2 and $PGF_{2\alpha}$ produce sustained contractions of strips of human and baboon bladder *in vitro*. Abrams and Feneley (1976) reported that isolated strips of human urinary bladder are contracted by $PGF_{1\alpha}$, $PGF_{2\alpha}$, PGE_1 and PGE_2. $PGF_{2\alpha}$ was the most potent of all prostaglandins studied. Compared with the contractions of bladder muscle induced by acetylcholine, the response to prostaglandins was slower in onset and longer lasting. These findings have been confirmed by Andersson and Persson (1977) who also confirmed that E prostaglandins relax and F prostaglandins contract human urethral muscle *in vitro*.

There is some speculation on the physiological function of prostaglandins in bladder emptying. Relaxation of the urethra and contraction of the bladder by E prostaglandins seem to be functionally appropriate for such a role (Abrams and Feneley, 1976; Andersson and Persson, 1976). Prostaglandin-like substances have been found in vesical vein blood taken from dogs undergoing bladder distension. This local release of prostaglandins may be designed to accommodate or resist bladder filling (Gilmore and Vane, 1971; Larsson, 1978). The spontaneous activity and tone of isolated strips of bladder muscle from several species including man is reduced by indomethacin, meclofenamic acid and flufenamic acid (all inhibitors of prostaglandin biosynthesis) (Hills, 1976; Johns and Paton, 1976; Bultitude *et al.*, 1976). Indomethacin also abolished PGE_2-like activity in the fluid bathing an isolated strip of rabbit detrusor muscle (Bultitude *et al.*, 1976). It should however be remembered that the use of drugs that inhibit prostaglandin synthesis is not normally associated with retention of urine in the bladder. The effect of PGE_2 and $PGF_{2\alpha}$ on the human bladder has also been investigated. Karim *et al.* (1972) found that inadvertent injection of $PGF_{2\alpha}$ into the bladder in a woman undergoing second trimester pregnancy termination resulted in micturition accompanied by a sustained contraction of the bladder and micturition.

Bultitude *et al.* (1976) studied the effect of PGE_2 in 21 female patients with difficulty in micturition who were found to be in varying degrees of chronic retention. PGE_2 in a dose of 0.5 mg in 40 ml sterile saline was administered into the emptied bladder through a urethral catheter. Fourteen patients responded by a voluntary sustained detrusor contraction with voiding. The bladder was emptied to a far greater degree than before. In most of these patients their ability to contract the detrusor was apparently retained for over 2 years.

Ratnam *et al.* (1979) have also successfully used $PGF_{2\alpha}$ for acute urinary retention after gynaecological surgery. Doses of 1 or 2 mg of this prostaglandin were usually sufficient to cause micturition without producing any side-effects.

1.8 SKIN

1.8.1 Sunburn

Concentrations of prostaglandins and their precursors and metabolites are increased in exudates from human skin irradiated with 'sunburn' (290–320 nm) u.v. *in vivo* (see Greaves, 1978 for references). Inhibition of prostaglandin synthesis by aspirin or indomethacin injected intradermally was first shown to delay and decrease u.v. erythema by Snyder and Eaglstein (1974a). Topical application of 2.5% w/v indomethacin cream to sunburned skin decreased the symptoms which result from exposure to u.v. While indomethacin reduced the dermal components of u.v.-induced inflammation, there was little or no effect on the u.v.-induced epidermal damage in human skin (Snyder and Eaglstein, 1974b). These authors also observed decreased tanning in two volunteers. They concluded that 'as hyperpigmentation is not seen in skin reddened by intradermal injections of prostaglandins, it seems unlikely that indomethacin interferes with melanogenesis by preventing the synthesis of prostaglandins'. Topical indomethacin was found to be superior to one of the most potent steroid creams in decreasing the inflammatory response induced by sunburn and 'might prove useful in separating the direct effects of UVR on melanocytes from possible indirect effects of UVR on melanogenesis'. The optimal concentrations of indomethacin and other prostaglandin synthesis inhibitors and their systemic toxicity remain to be evaluated before these substances can be recommended for widespread use.

The role of prostaglandins in sunburn also needs to be explored further. Studies on the appearance and disappearance of prostaglandins and their precursors and metabolites in the presence and absence of indomethacin suggest that inflammatory changes in irradiated skin cannot be satisfactorily explained by the actions of these agents alone. Exudate from human skin irradiated with three times the minimum erythema dose of long-wavelength u.v. following systemic photosensitizing psoralen pretreatment shows no increase in prostaglandin activity (see Greaves, 1978).

Greaves (1978) has hypothesized that evoked prostaglandin formation has a protective effect on the epidermis of sun-exposed skin. 'The presence of raised levels of PGE_2 in u.v. irradiated human skin would be expected to protect epidermal cells from the mutagenic effect of u.v. by increasing cyclic-AMP formation and thus reducing the vulnerable pool of actively dividing cells.' It is therefore conceivable that long-term treatment of sunburn with inhibitors of prostaglandin synthesis might result in increased incidence of skin carcinoma, especially in fair-skinned people in sunny climates (Greaves, 1978).

1.8.2 Psoriasis

It has been reported that levels of PGE_2 and $PGF_{2\alpha}$ are several times lower in psoriatic skin compared to normal skin (Aso *et al.*, 1973). Based on these data Jacobs and Jacobs (1974) have tested a hypothesis that 'topical application of either PGE_1, PGE_2 or $PGF_{2\alpha}$ might penetrate the scaling epidermal layer and perhaps replenish the lowered prostaglandin level and hence cause improvement of involved psoriatic skin'. Topical applications of $PGF_{1\alpha}$ or PGE_2 for 53 and 27 days respectively produced no significant change in the involved skin. 'In contrast, PGE_1 treatment elicited dramatic and distinct alterations in the treated psoriatic skin and there was decreased scaling and thinning of the plaque following treatment for 28 days.

Further studies are required to establish a role for endogenous prostaglandin in psoriasis and the use of exogenous prostaglandins in the treatment of this condition.

1.9 POST-PARTUM HAEMORRHAGE

In spite of considerable interest in evaluating the role of prostaglandins in human reproduction and in developing practical applications of prostaglandins in obstetrics and gynaecology, the use of these substances in the control or prevention of post-partum haemorrhage remains almost unexplored.

Roth-Brandel *et al.* (1970) compared the effectiveness of PGE_1 (100 μg) ergometrine (200 μg), oxytocin (3 IU) and a combination of ergometrine (200 μg) and PGE_1 (100 μg) on blood loss and placental separation in the third stage of labour in a total of 188 women after delivery of the foetus. All drugs were injected intravenously. The authors found that although PGE_1 produced sustained contraction of the post-partum uterus, it did not reduce blood loss or shorten the time for placental separation.

After successfully inducing labour with $PGF_{2\alpha}$ in 21 women at term, Persianinov *et al.* (1973) continued infusing $PGF_{2\alpha}$ during the third stage and found that the amount of blood loss was less than when oxytocin was used.

Takagi *et al.* (1976) injected $PGF_{2\alpha}$ directly into the uterine muscle in 38 patients with severe post-partum haemorrhage. The authors claimed that the treatment was 'very highly effective in affecting post-partum haemostasis'. The same prostaglandin given intravenously or intramuscularly into the gluteal muscle did not have any effect on post-partum haemorrhage.

Intravenous and intrauterine administration of $PGF_{2\alpha}$ or 15(S)15-methyl-$PGF_{2\alpha}$ has also been successfully used in the treatment of severe uterine bleeding by Zahradnik *et al.* (1977).

The amount of blood loss after delivery in two groups of patients given syntometrine (5 IU oxytocin and 0.5 mg ergometrine) or sulprostone (16-phenoxy-ω-17,18,19,20-tetranor-PGE_2 methyl sulphonylamide) intramuscularly at crowning was compared in a preliminary study by Ruoff *et al.* (see Karim, 1979). The total amount of blood loss after delivery of the foetus and during the subsequent 24 h was measured. The mean amount of blood loss at delivery in the 10 patients treated with syntometrine was 225.5 ml (range 64–540 ml) and the mean amount during the subsequent 24 h was 101.1 ml (range 52–533 ml). In the sulprostone group the amount of blood loss after delivery averaged 144.6 ml (range 87.3–182.5 ml). Blood loss in this group during the subsequent 24 h was 94.0 ml (range 58.9–119.5 ml). One patient in the syntometrine group required a transfusion. There were no side-effects in any patients in both groups.

References

Abdulla, Y. H. and Hamadah, K. (1975). Effect of ADP on PGE_1 formation in blood platelets from patients with depression, mania and schizophrenia. *Br. J. Psychiatry*, **127**, 591

Abrams, P. H. and Feneley, R. C. L. (1976). The actions of prostaglandins on the smooth muscle of the human urinary tract *in vitro*. *Br. J. Urol.*, **47**, 909

Adaikan, P. G. and Karim, S. M. M. (1979). Effects of some trinor inter-*m*-phenylene analogues of PGE_1 on the respiratory tract smooth muscle of guinea-pig and man. (In press)

Aiken, J. W., Gorman, R. R., and Shebuski, R. J. (1979). Prostacyclin prevents blockage of partially obstructed coronary arteries. In: J. R. Vane and S. Bergström (eds.). *Advances in Prostaglandin and Thromboxane Research* (New York: Raven Press)

Allan, G. and Eakins, K. E. (1978). Burimamide is a selective inhibitor of thromboxane-A biosynthesis in human platelet microsomes. *Prostaglandins*, **15**, 659

Ambache, N. and Zar, M. A. (1970). Non-cholinergic transmission by post-ganglionic motor neurones in the mammalian bladder. *J. Physiol. (Lond.)*, **210**, 761

Andersson, K. E., Ek, A. and Persson, C. G. A. (1977). Effects of prostaglandins on the isolated human bladder and urethra. *Acta Physiol. Scand.*, **100**, 165

Anturane Reinfarction Trial (1978). Sulfinpyrazone in the prevention of cardiac death after myocardial infarction. *N. Engl. J. Med.*, **298**, 289

Armstrong, J. M., Chapple, D., Dusting, G. J., Hughes, R., Moncada, S. and Vane, J. R. (1977). Cardiovascular actions of prostacyclin (PGI_2) in chloralose anaesthetized dogs. *Br. J. Pharmacol.*, **61**, 136P

Armstrong, J. M., Lattimer, N., Moncada, S. and Vane, J. R. (1978). Comparison of the vasodepressor effects of prostacyclin and 6-oxo-prostaglandin $F_{1\alpha}$ with those of prostaglandin E_2 in rats and rabbits. *Br. J. Pharmacol.*, **62**, 125

Aso, K., Sakamoto, N., Farber, E., Deneau, D., Krulig, D. and Wilkinson, D. (1973). The synthesis of prostaglandins E_2 and $F_{2\alpha}$ in psoriatic skin. *Abst. Soc. for Invest. Dermatol.*, Atlantic City, Maryland, April 1973

Bergström, S., Farnebo, L. O. and Fuxe, K. (1973). Effect of PGE_2 on central and peripheral catecholamine neurones. *Eur. J. Pharmacol.*, **21**, 362

Bianco, S., Robuschi, M., Ceserani, R. and Gandolfi, C. (1978). Prevention of a specifically induced bronchoconstriction by prostaglandin (PGI_2) in asthmatic subjects. *IRCS Med. Sci.*, **6**, 256

Blackwell, G. J. and Flower, R. J. (1978). 1-phenyl-3-pyrazolidone: an inhibitor of arachidonate oxidation in lung and platelets. *Br. J. Pharmacol.*, **63**, 360P

Bray, M. A., Gordon, D. and Morley, J. (1978). Prostaglandins as regulators in cellular immunity. *Prostagl. Med.*, **1**, 183

Bultitude, M. I., Hills, N. H. and Shuttleworth, K. E. D. (1976). Clinical and experimental studies on the action of prostaglandins and their synthesis inhibitors on detrusor muscle *in vitro* and *in vivo*. *Br. J. Urol.*, **48**, 631

Bunting, S., Gryglewski, R. J., Moncada, S. and Vane, J. R. (1976). Arterial walls generate from prostaglandin endoperoxide a substance (prostaglandin X) which relaxes strips of mesenteric and coeliac arteries and inhibits platelet aggregation. *Prostaglandins*, **12**, 897

Chandler, A. B., Chapman, I., Erhardt, L. R., Roberts, W. C., Schwartz, C. J., Sinapius, D., Spain, D. M., Sherry, S., Ness, P. M. and Simon, T. L. (1974). Coronary thrombosis in myocardial infarction. Report of a workshop on the role of coronary thrombosis in the pathogenesis of acute myocardial infarction. *Am. J. Cardiol.*, **34**, 823

Chaplin, D. and Hillier, K. (1979). A prostacyclin-like substance in rat brain. *Br. J. Pharmacol.* (In press)

Christ, E. J. and van Dorp, D. A. (1972). Comparative aspects of prostaglandin biosynthesis in animal tissues. *Biochim. Biophys. Acta*, **270**, 537

Cottee, F., Flower, R. J., Moncada, S., Salmon, J. A. and Vane, J. R. (1977). Synthesis of 6-keto $PGF_{1\alpha}$ by ram seminal vesicle microsomes. *Prostaglandins*, **14**, 413

Cranston, W. I., Hellon, R. F. and Mitchell, D. J. (1975). Fever and brain prostaglandin release. *J. Physiol.*, **248**, 28P

Davison, D. V. (1977). Possible roles of prostaglandins in neurotransmission in the CNS. Ph.D. Thesis, University of Aberdeen.

Dighe, K. K., Jones, R. L. and Poyser, N. L. (1978). Development of a radioimmunoassay for measurement of 6-oxo-prostaglandin $F_{1\alpha}$. *Br. J. Pharmacol.*, **63**, 406P

DuCharme, D. W., DeGraaf, G. L., Humphrey, S. J. and Wending, M. G. (1979). Hemodynamic activity of prostacyclin (PGI_2) as compared to other products of the arachidonic acid cascade. In: A. Scriabine, A. N. Lefer and S. A. Kuehl (eds.), *Prostaglandins in Cardiovascular and Renal Function* (New York: Spectrum Press) (In press)

Dusting, G. J., Moncada, S. and Vane, J. R. (1977). Prostacyclin (PGX) is the endogenous metabolite responsible for relaxation of coronary arteries induced by arachidonic acid. *Prostaglandins*, **13**, 3

Eakins, K. E. and Kulkarni, P. S. (1977). Selective inhibitory actions of sodium-*p*-benzyl-4 [1-oxo-2-(4-chlorobenzyl)-3-phenyl propyl] phenyl phosphonate (N-0164) and indomethacin on the biosynthesis of prostaglandins and thromboxanes from arachidonic acid. *Br. J. Pharmacol.*, **60**, 135

Falardeau, P., Hamberg, M. and Samuelsson, B. (1976). Metabolism of 8,11,14-eicosatrienoic acid in human platelets. *Biochim. Biophys. Acta*, **441**, 193

Fitzpatrick, F. A. and Gorman, R. R. (1978). A comparison of imidazole and 9,11-azo-prosta-5,13-dienoic acid. Two selective thromboxane synthetase inhibitors. *Biochim. Biophys. Acta*, **539**, 162

Flower, R. J. (1974). Drugs which inhibit prostaglandin biosynthesis. *Pharmacol. Rev.*, **26**, 36

Gerrard, J. M., White, J. G. and Krivit, W. (1976). Labile aggregation stimulating substance, free fatty acids and platelet aggregation. *J. Lab. Clin. Med.*, **87**, 73

Gilmore, N. J. and Vane, J. R. (1971). Hormones released into the circulation when the urinary bladder of the anaesthetized dog is distended. *Clin. Sci.*, **41**, 69

Goldstein, A., Cox., B. M., Klee, W. A. and Nirenberg, M. (1977). Endorphin from pituitary inhibits cyclic AMP formation in homogenates of neuroblastoma × glioma hybrid cells. *Nature*, **265**, 362

Goodwin, J. S., Messner, R. P., Bankhurst, A. D., Peake, G. T., Saiki, J. H. and Williams, R. C. (1977). Prostaglandin-producing suppressor cells in Hodgkin's disease. *N. Engl. J. Med.*, **297**, 963

Gordon, D., Bray, M. A. and Morley, J. (1976). Control of lymphokine secretion by prostaglandins. *Nature*, **262**, 401

Greaves, M. W. (1978). Does ultraviolet-evoked prostaglandin formation protect skin from actinic cancer? *Lancet*, **i**, 189

Gryglewski, R. J., Bunting, S., Moncada, S., Flower, R. J. and Vane, J. R. (1976). Arterial walls are protected against deposition of platelet thrombi by a substance (prostaglandin X) which they make from prostaglandin endoperoxides. *Prostaglandins*, **12**, 685

Halushka, P. V., Lurie, D. and Colwell, J. A. (1977). Increased synthesis of prostaglandin-E-like material by platelets from patients with diabetes mellitus. *N. Engl. J. Med.*, **297**, 1306

Hamberg, M., Svensson, J. and Samuelsson, B. (1975). Thromboxanes: a new group of biologically active compounds derived from prostaglandin endoperoxides. *Proc. Natl. Acad. Sci.*, **72**, 2994

Hedqvist, P. (1976). Prostaglandin action on transmitter release at adrenergic neuroeffector junctions. *Advances in Prostaglandin and Thromboxane Research*, Vol. I, p. 357 (New York: Raven Press)

Hillier, K. (1977). Current status of prostaglandin and thromboxane research. *Drugs of Today*, **13**, 418

Hillier, K. (1978). Prostaglandins and thromboxanes. Pharmacologic and biosynthetic aspects. *Semin. Perinatol.*, **2**, 197

Hillier, K., Roberts, P. J. and Woollard, P. (1976). Catecholamine-stimulated prostaglandin synthesis in rat brain synaptosomes. *Br. J. Pharmacol.*, **58**, 426P

Hills, N. H. (1976). Prostaglandins and tone in isolated strips of mammalian bladder. *Br. J. Pharmacol.*, **57**, 464P

Horrobin, D. F. (1977). Schizophrenia as a prostaglandin deficiency disease. *Lancet*, **i**, 936

Horrobin, D. F. (1978). Schizophrenia: a prostaglandin deficiency disease? *Prostagl. Ther.*, **4**, 1

Horrobin, D. F., Ally, A. I. and Manku, M. S. (1978a). Dipyridamole and platelet aggregation. *Lancet*, **ii**, 270

Horrobin, D. F., Manku, M. S. and Karmali, R. (1978b). Prostaglandins as second messengers of prolactin action. In: *Progress in Prolactin Physiology and Pathology*, pp. 189–200 (Amsterdam: Elsevier).

Horrobin, D. F., Manku, M. S., Karmali, R. A., Oka, M., Ally, A. I., Morgan, R. O., Karmazyn, M. and Cunnane, S. C. (1978c). Thromboxane A_2: a key regulator of prostaglandin biosynthesis and of interactions between prostaglandins, calcium and cyclic nucleotides. *Med. Hypotheses*, **4**, 178

Jacobs, K. F. and Jacobs, M. M. (1974). Prostaglandin treatment of psoriatic skin. *Rocky Mountain Med. J.*, **71**, 507

Johns, A. and Paton, D. M. (1976). Evidence for a role of prostaglandins in atropine-resistant transmission in the mammalian urinary bladder. *Prostaglandins*, **11**, 595

Jorgensen, K. A. and Stoffersen, E. (1978). Dipyridamole and platelet function. *Lancet*, **ii**, 1258

Karim, S. M. M. (1979). Prostaglandins in obstetrics and gynaecology. *Proceedings of International Sulprostone Symposium*, Vienna, Oct., 1978. (Pfizer-Schering)

Karim, S. M. M. and Adaikan, P. G. (1979). Some pharmacological studies with prostacyclins in baboon and man. In: J. R. Vane and S. Bergström (eds.), *Advances in Prostaglandin and Thromboxane Research* (New York: Raven Press) (In press)

Karim, S. M. M., Sharma, S. D. and Filshie, G. M. (1972). Termination of second trimester pregnancy with intra-amniotic administration of prostaglandins E_2 and $F_{2\alpha}$. In: E. M. Southern (ed.), *Prostaglandins: Clinical Applications and Human Reproduction*, p. 403 (Mount Sisco, N.Y.: Futura)

Kernoff, P. B. S., Willis, A. L., Stone, K. J., Davies, J. A. and McNicol, G. P. (1977). Antithrombotic potential of dihomo-gamma-linolenic acid in man. *Br. Med. J.*, **2**, 1441

Krakauer, K., Torrey, S. B. and Zurier, R. B. (1978). Prostaglandin E_1 treatment of NZB/W mice. III. Preservation of spleen cell concentrations and mitogen-induced proliferative responses. *Clin. Immunol. Immunopathol.* (In press) Quoted by Zurier (1978)

Lands, W. E. M. and Rome, L. H. (1976). Inhibition of prostaglandin biosynthesis. In: S. M. M. Karim (ed.), *Prostaglandins: Chemical and Biochemical Aspects*, p. 87 (Lancaster: MTP Press)

Larsson, C. (1978). Effects of prostaglandins on the field stimulated rat isolated urinary bladder. *Prostaglandins*, **15**, 701

Meydani, S. N., Mathias, M. M. and Schatte, C. L. (1978). Dietary fat type and ambient oxygen tension influence pulmonary prostaglandin synthetic potential. *Prostagl. Med.*, **1**, 241

Milton, A. S., Smith, S. and Tomkins, K. B. (1977). Levels of prostaglandin F and E in cerebrospinal fluid of cats during pyrogen-induced fever. *Br. J. Pharmacol.*, **59**, 447P

Mitchell, S., Poyser, N. L. and Wilson, N. H. (1977). Effect of *p*-bromophenacyl bromide, an inhibitor of phospholipase A_2 on arachidonic acid release and prostaglandin synthesis by the guinea-pig uterus *in vitro*. *Br. J. Pharmacol.*, **59**, 107

Moncada, S., Flower, R. J. and Russell-Smith, N. (1978). Dipyridamole and platelet function. *Lancet*, **ii**, 1257

Moncada, S., Gryglewski, R., Bunting, S. and Vane, J. R. (1976a). An enzyme isolated from arteries transforms prostaglandin endoperoxides to an unstable substance that inhibits platelet aggregation. *Nature*, **263**, 663

Moncada, S., Gryglewski, R., Bunting, S. and Vane, J. R. (1976b). A lipid peroxide inhibits the enzyme blood vessels microsomes that generate the substance (prostaglandin X) which prevents platelet aggregation. *Prostaglandins*, **12**, 715

Moncada, A. S. and Korbut, R. (1978). Dipyridamole and other phosphodiesterase inhibitors act as antithrombotic agents by potentiating endogenous prostacyclin. *Lancet*, **i**, 1286

Moncada, S., Needleman, P., Bunting, S. and Vane, J. R. (1976). Prostaglandin endoperoxide and thromboxane generating systems and their selective inhibition. *Prostaglandins*, **12**, 323

Moncada, S. and Vane, J. R. (1978). Unstable metabolites of arachidonic acid and their role in haemostasis and thrombosis. *Br. Med. Bull.*, **34**, 129

Morley, J. (1974). Prostaglandin and lymphokines in arthritis. *Prostaglandins*, **8**, 315

Myatt, L. and Elder, M. G. (1977). Inhibition of platelet aggregation by a placental substance with prostaglandin-like activity. *Nature*, **268**, 159

Naimzada, K. (1967). Azione della prostaglandin E_1 sulla vesica (esperienza nella caviae nel ratto). *Boll. Soc. Ital. Biol. Sperim.*, **43**, 518

Nijkamp, F. P., Flower, R. J., Moncada, S. and Vane, J. R. (1976). Partial purification of rabbit aorta contracting substance releasing factor and inhibition of its activity by anti-inflammatory steroids. *Nature*, **263**, 479

Nijkamp, F. P., Moncada, S., White, H. L. and Vane, J. R. (1977). Diversion of prostaglandin endoperoxide metabolism by selective inhibition of thromboxane A_2 biosynthesis in lung, spleen or platelets. *Eur. J. Pharmacol.*, **44**, 179

O'Grady, J. and Moncada, S. (1978). Aspirin: A paradoxical effect on bleeding time. *Lancet*, **ii**, 780

Omini, C., Moncada, S. and Vane, J. R. (1977). The effects of prostacyclin (PGI_2) on tissues which detect prostaglandins (PGs). *Prostaglandins*, **14**, 625

Pace-Asciak, C. R., Carrara, M. C. and Nicolaou, K. C. (1978a). Prostaglandin I_2 has more potent hypotensive properties than prostaglandin E_2 in the normal and spontaneously hypertensive rat. *Prostaglandins*, **15**, 999

Pace-Asciak, C. R., Carrara, M. C., Rangaraj, G. and Nicolaou, K. C. (1978b). Enhanced formation of PGI_2, a potent hypotensive substance, by aortic rings and homogenates of the spontaneously hypertensive rat. *Prostaglandins*, **15**, 1005

Pelus, L. M. and Strausser, H. R. (1977). Prostaglandins and the immune response. *Life Sci.*, **20**, 903

Persianinov, L. S., Manuilova, I. A. and Chernukha, E. A. (1973). The result of using prostaglandin $F_{2\alpha}$ for induction and stimulation of labor. In: S. M. Bergström and S. Bernhard (eds.), *Advances in Biosciences*, **9**, 585 (New York: Vieweg, Pergamon Press)

Persson, C. G. A. (1976). Inhibitory effect at the bladder-urethral junction. *Acta Physiol. Scand.*, **97**, 139

Rajah, S. M., Penny, A. and Kester, R. (1978). Aspirin and bleeding time. *Lancet*, **ii**, 1104

Ratnam, S. S., Prasad, R. N. V. and Karim, S. M. M. (1979). Management of post-surgical urinary retention with prostaglandin $F_{2\alpha}$. *Singapore J. Obstet. Gynaecol.*, **10**, 23

Roth-Brandel, U., Bygdeman, M. and Wiqvist, N. (1970). A comparative study on the influence of prostaglandin E_1 oxytocin and ergometrine on the pregnant human uterus. *Acta Obstet. Gynecol. Scand.*, **49** (Suppl. 5), 1

Rotrosen, J., Miller, A. D., Mandio, D., Traficante, L. J. and Gershon, S. (1978). Reduced PGE_1 stimulated ^3H-cAMP accumulation in platelets from schizophrenics. *Life Sci.*, **23**, 1989

Schorer, A. E., Gerrard, J. M., White, J. G. and Krivit, W. (1978). Oral contraceptive use alters the balance of platelet prostaglandin and thromboxane synthesis. *Prostagl. Med.*, **1**, 5

Seyberth, H. W., Oelz, O., Kennedy, T., Sweetman, B. J., Danon, A., Frolich, J. C., Heimberg, M. and Oates, J. A. (1975). Increased arachidonate in lipids after administration to man. Effects on prostaglandin biosynthesis. *Clin. Pharmacol. Ther.*, **18**, 521

Smith, A. P. (1976). Prostaglandins and the respiratory system. In: S. M. M. Karim (ed.), *Advances in Prostaglandin Research: Prostaglandins: Physiological, Pharmacological and Pathological Aspects*, pp. 83–102 (Lancaster: MTP Press)

Snyder, D. S. and Eaglstein, W. H. (1974a). Intradermal anti-prostaglandin agents and sunburn. *J. Invest. Dermatol.*, **62**, 47

Snyder, D. S. and Eaglstein, W. H. (1974b). Topical indomethacin and sunburn. *Br. J. Dermatol.*, **90**, 91

Strandberg, K. and Hedqvist, P. (1977). Bronchial effects of some prostaglandin E and F analogues. *Acta Physiol. Scand.*, **100**, 172

Sun, F. F., Chapman, J. P. and McGuire, J. G. (1977). Metabolism of prostaglandin endoperoxides in animal tissues. *Prostaglandins*, **14**, 1055

Szczeklik, A., Gryglewski, R. J., Nizankowska, E., Nizankowski, R. and Musial, J. (1978a). Pulmonary and anti-platelet effects of intravenous and inhaled prostacyclin in man. *Prostaglandins*, **16**, 651

Szczeklik, A., Gryglewski, R. J., Nizankowski, R., Musial, J., Picton, R. and Mruk, J. (1978b). Circulatory and anti-platelet effects of intravenous prostacyclin in healthy men. *Pharmacol. Res. Commun.*, **10**, 545

Taira, N. (1974). Mode of actions of prostaglandin $F_{2\alpha}$ on the urinary bladder and its arterial bed in the dog. *Eur. J. Pharmacol.*, **29**, 30

Takagi, S., Yoshida, T., Yogo, T., Abe, M., Tochigi, H., Sakata, H. and Takahashi, H. (1976). The effects of uterine intramuscular injection of $PGF_{2\alpha}$ on severe post-partum haemorrhage. In: B. Samuelsson and R. Paoletti (eds.), *Advances in Prostaglandin and Thromboxane Research*, Vol. II, p. 1003 (New York: Raven Press)

Terenius, L., Wahlstrom, A., Linstrom, L. and Widerlow, E. (1976). Quoted by Rotrosen *et al.* (1978)

Treacher, D., Warlow, C. and McPherson, K. (1978). Aspirin and bleeding time. *Lancet*, **ii**, 1378

Vane, J. R. (1978). Inhibitors of prostaglandin, prostacyclin and thromboxane synthesis. In: F. Coceani and P. M. Olley (eds.), *Advances in Prostaglandin and Thromboxane Research*, Vol. IV, pp. 27–44 (New York: Raven Press)

Vargaftig, B. B. and Dao Hai, N. (1972). Selective inhibition by mepacrine of the release of rabbit aorta contracting substance evoked by administration of bradykinin. *J. Pharm. Pharmacol.*, **24**, 159

Vargaftig, B. B. and Lefort, J. (1977). Acute hypotension due to carrageenan: arachidonic acid and slow reacting substance C in the rabbit: role of the platelets and nature of pharmacological antagonism. *Eur. J. Pharmacol.*, **43**, 125

Veale, W. L. and Cooper, K. E. (1975). In: *Temperature Regulation and Drug Action* (P. Lomax *et al.*, eds.), p. 218 (Basel: Karger)

Wasserman, M. A. (1976). Bronchopulmonary pharmacology of some prostaglandin endoperoxide analogs in the dog. *Eur. J. Pharmacol.*, **36**, 103

Weber, P. C., Larsson, C., Anggard, E., Hamberg, M., Corey, E. J., Nicolaou, K. C. and Samuelsson, B. (1976). Stimulation of renin release from rabbit renal cortex by arachidonic acid and prostaglandin endoperoxides. *Circ. Res.*, **39**, 868

Weber, P. C., Larsson, C. and Scherer, B. (1977). Prostaglandin E_2-9-keto reductase as a mediator of salt intake-related prostaglandin renin interaction. *Nature*, **266**, 65

Weeks, J. R. and Sutter, D. M. (1979). An antihypertensive effect of prostacyclin. In: J. R. Vane and S. Bergström (eds.), *Advances in Prostaglandin and Thromboxane Research*, (New York: Raven Press) (In press)

Westfall, T. C. and Kitay, D. (1977). Effect of prostaglandins on release of (^{3}H) dopamine from superfused slices of rat striatum following electrical stimulation. *Proc. Soc. Exp. Biol. Med.*, **155**, 305

Wolfe, L. S., Rostorowski, K. and Marion, J. (1976). Endogenous formation of the prostaglandin endoperoxide metabolite thromboxane B_2 by brain tissue. *Biochem. Biophys. Res. Commun.*, **70**, 907

Woods, H. F., Ash, G., Weston, M. J., Bunting, S., Moncada, S. and Vane, J. R. (1978). Prostacyclin can replace heparin in haemodialysis in dogs. *Lancet*, **ii**, 1075

Zahradnik, H. P., Steiner, H., Hillemanns, H. G., Breckwoldt, M. and Ardelt, W. (1977). Prostaglandin $F_{2\alpha}$ und 15-methyl prostaglandin $F_{2\alpha}$ Anwendung bei massiven uterinen Blatungen. *Geburtshu. Frauenheilk*, **37**, 493

Zurier, R. B. (1978): PGs, inflammation and immune responses. *Prostagl. Ther.*, **5**, 1–4

Zurier, R. B., Sayadoff, D. M., Torrey, S. B. and Rothfield, N. F. (1977). Prostaglandin E_1 treatment of NZB/W mice. 1: Prolonged survival of female mice. *Arthritis Rheum.*, **20**, 723

2
Prostaglandins and Nasal Patency

P. G. ADAIKAN, S. M. M. KARIM and N. KUNARATNAM

2.1 INTRODUCTION

Allergic diseases of the nose and paranasal sinuses are among the most common problems encountered in otorhinolaryngology and respiratory medicine. However, allergy is not the only cause of non-infectious sneezing, rhinorrhoea and nasal blockage. Such symptoms may also arise from autonomic imbalance associated with relative hyper-reactivity of the parasympathetic nervous system. Thus patients with vasomotor rhinitis can be sub-divided into those with or without an allergic cause.

The management of vasomotor rhinitis and hay fever includes:

(1) Elimination or reduction in exposure of the patients to predisposing factors,
(2) Hyposensitization,
(3) Symptomatic treatment, and
(4) Corrective surgery.

The presence of a large number of blood vessels in the nasal mucous membrane lends the mucosa readily to engorgement and oedema as in allergic vasomotor rhinitis. Excessive congestion of the blood vessels of the nasal mucosa produces nasal obstruction. Topical application of decongestants to nasal mucosa in the form of drops or sprays produces symptomatic relief. There are at present a large number of proprietary preparations of decongestants on the market (Shaw, 1964). Prolonged use of some of these decongestants may lead to rhinitis medicamentosa or allergic hypersensitivity and swelling of the nasal mucosa. Frequent use of decongestants by patients may result in rebound vasodilatation with a more distressing manifestation of nasal symptoms than was originally present.

The three types of compounds which are frequently used in nasal solutions either as a combination or individually include: (1) the antihistamines, (2) the sympathomimetics, and (3) the corticosteroids.

Antihistamines readily prevent sneezing and rhinorrhoea but are relatively ineffective in relieving nasal obstruction. Antihistamines block histamine receptors at cellular level and act as pharmacological histamine antagonists (Mygind, 1978) in addition to causing a shrinkage of the mucosa (Shaw, 1964). In therapeutic doses antihistamines cause sedation and dryness of mouth and mucous membrane (Mygind, 1978).

Sympathomimetic drugs act directly on the adrenergic α-receptors of smooth muscle of the arterioles producing vasoconstriction leading to a reduction in blood flow and decrease in the thickness of the oedematous nasal mucosa. These changes produce a concomitant increase in nasal patency (Harrison, 1976). Prolonged usage of all such drugs results in secondary vasodilatation (Shaw, 1964).

Topical corticosteroids may produce relief in patients with allergic rhinitis, particularly during the hay fever season (Harrison, 1976). The value of topical steroid solutions in the treatment of rhinitis is doubtful although greater benefit may be derived from their systemic use (Shaw, 1964).

It is 12 years since the effect of prostaglandins (PG) on the nasal blood flow in the dog was first reported (Stovall and Jackson, 1967). Subsequent studies with natural prostaglandins in human volunteers have been discouraging due to unpredictable results and side-effects (Anggård, 1969; Jackson, 1970; Karim *et al.*, 1976, 1978). Results of studies in healthy human volunteers and in patients with vasomotor rhinitis with some prostaglandin analogues are promising (Karim *et al.*, 1978; Adaikan *et al.*, 1978; Karim *et al.*, 1979) (Figure 2.1).

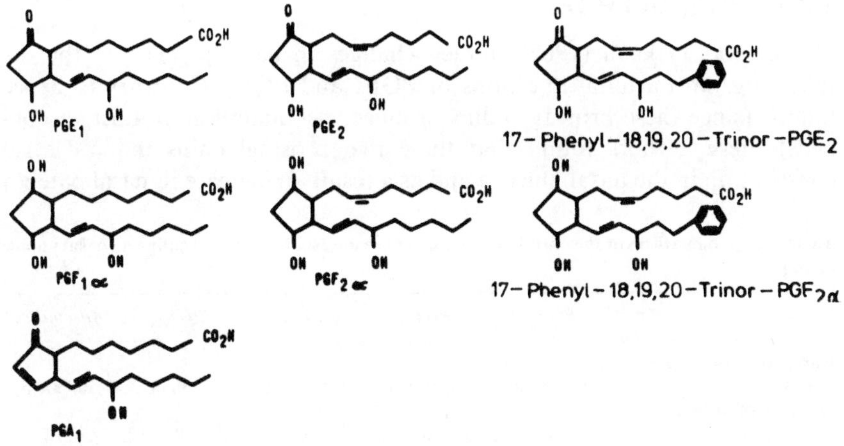

Figure 2.1 Chemical structures of prostaglandins referred to in this review

2.2 PRESENCE OF PROSTAGLANDINS IN NASAL TISSUE AND SECRETIONS

Toh and Mohiuddin (1958) found two pharmacologically active substances in the nasal mucosa of dog and sheep. One of these was shown to be histamine and the other was thought to be an unsaturated acid. The authors wrote 'The presence of another smooth muscle stimulating substance besides histamine in the nasal mucosa lends interest to the problem of allergic rhinitis. It may be that these substances are released in this condition to produce vascular engorgement and subsequent oedema'. Further studies have led to the identification of PGE compounds in the nasal mucosa of the sheep and a mixture of PGE and PGF compounds in extracts of human nasal mucosa (Chow *et al.*, 1976).

More recently, Okazaki *et al.* (1977) found PGE in the nasal secretions of six out of 12 patients with hay fever and in pooled nasal washings from normal subjects.

Since PGE and PGF are present in the nasal mucosa, and topical applications of these prostaglandins decrease resistance to nasal breathing, it is likely that these substances are involved in maintaining nasal patency in the normal situation. It is as yet not known whether there is a deficiency of prostaglandins in the nasal mucosa in subjects with nasal congestion.

2.3 EFFECT OF PROSTAGLANDINS ON NASAL AIRWAY RESISTANCE IN THE DOG

2.3.1 PGE_1 and PGE_2

Stovall and Jackson (1967) studied changes in nasal patency in the dog following intra-arterial injections of PGE_1 and PGE_2. Contrary to expectations (since these prostaglandins produce vasodilatation in most vascular beds) these authors found that these two prostaglandins induced vasoconstriction in the nasal mucosa and as a result an increase in nasal patency.

Table 2.1 Comparison of the duration of action of prostaglandins and adrenaline on nasal patency in dog

	PGE_1	PGE_2	*PGA*	$PGF_{2\alpha}$	*Adrenaline**
Range of doses (per 10 kg)	50–500 ng	50–500 ng	0.5–10 μg	1–50 μg	50–500 ng
Number of animals tested	9	6	6	8	16
Mean ± s.d. of duration of responses	7.4 ± 4.5	7.2 ± 4.1	1.9 ± 1.4	3.0 ± 1.5	1.0

* Duration of equipotent adrenaline response set at 1.0
Data from Stovall and Jackson (1967)

Absolute changes in nasal resistance and the duration of response to prostaglandins varied considerably from animal to animal. The authors found that adrenaline and PGE_1 or PGE_2 were equipotent in producing an increase in nasal patency when administered in identical quantities. However, the duration of effect was more than seven times longer with PGE_1 and PGE_2 compared to adrenaline (Table 2.1, Figure 2.2).

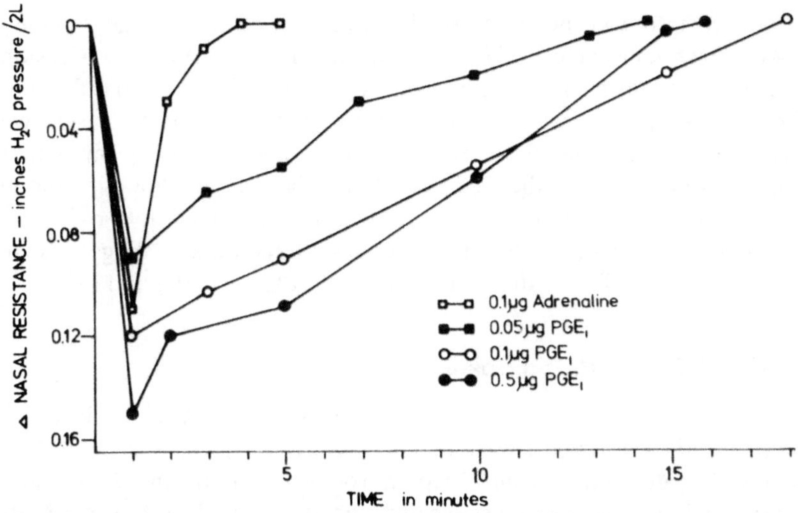

Figure 2.2 Decrease in nasal resistance in dogs induced by three doses of PGE_1 and adrenaline. Figure is from Stovall and Jackson (1967) by courtesy of *Ann. Otol.*

2.3.2 PGA_1 and $PGF_{1\alpha}$

PGA_1 and $PGF_{1\alpha}$ were equipotent in increasing nasal patency in the dog. They were about 100 times less potent than PGE compounds (Stovall and Jackson, 1967).

2.3.3 Mode of action

The lower doses of PGE_1 and PGE_2 produced a decrease in nasal resistance. Depending upon the dose used there was either a fall in blood pressure or no change in this parameter. Simultaneous recording of nasal resistance and blood pressure in dogs showed that the former effect was not dependent on the latter (Stovall and Jackson, 1967). Papaverine increased nasal resistance in dogs while PGE decreased it. Both papaverine and PGE, however, produced a fall in blood pressure. Furthermore, the increase in nasal patency paralleled a decrease in nasal temperature. These results suggest that PGEs have a direct vasoconstrictor action in the nose in contrast to their dilatory action in other vascular beds (Stovall and Jackson, 1967).

2.4 EFFECT OF PROSTAGLANDINS ON NASAL AIRWAY RESISTANCE IN HEALTHY HUMAN VOLUNTEERS

2.4.1 PGE_1, PGE_2 and $PGF_{1\alpha}$ (10–15 μg doses)

Anggård (1969) studied the effects of PGE_1 and $PGF_{1\alpha}$ on nasal airway resistance in seven normal subjects. The test solution (50 μg/ml) was introduced into each nostril through a nebulizer in an average volume of 0.24 ml. Each subject received PGE_1, PGE_2 and $PGF_{1\alpha}$ on different occasions. In four of the subjects PGE_1 and PGE_2 decreased resistance to nasal airflow. The onset of this effect was slow. It was maximal at 10 minutes and lasted, with a gradual decline, for 30–60 minutes. PGE_1 and PGE_2 appeared to be equipotent in producing these effects. Three other subjects however, did not respond to PGE_1 and PGE_2. $PGF_{1\alpha}$ at the doses tested did not produce any changes in nasal resistance in all of the seven subjects studied. Anggård did not observe any side-effects with 10–15 μg doses of PGE_1, PGE_2 and $PGF_{1\alpha}$.

2.4.2 PGE_1 (37–100 μg doses)

In order to find the clinically useful dose of PGE_1 that would reduce nasal congestion, Jackson (1970) tested higher doses of PGE_1 (37, 50, 75 and 100 μg) in 15 adult male volunteers on 39 separate occasions. PGE_1 in 0.2 ml solution was sprayed into one nostril using calibrated atomizer while the other nostril received 0.2 ml of the vehicle.

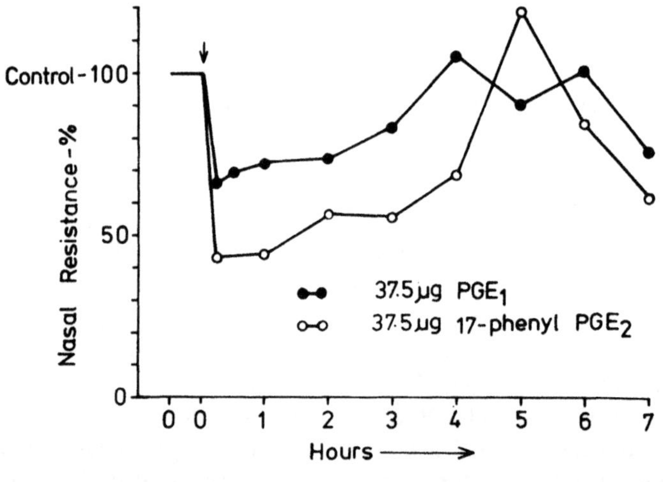

Figure 2.3 Comparative effects of PGE_1 and 17-phenyl-trinor-PGE_2 on nasal resistance in a male volunteer. Figure is from Karim *et al.* (1978) by courtesy of *Prostaglandins*

There was a variable increase in nasal patency with PGE_1. Out of the 39 tests, the results of 25 were considered good to excellent while 14 tests were found to be poor. Three of the subjects failed to respond to PGE_1 on two occasions. Seven out of the 15 subjects responded to one drug application but did not respond on the second occasion. Five subjects gave good response on repeated testing. Side-effects occurred only with doses of 100 μg. This dose produced some degree of nasal irritation in all subjects. In some, this was in the form of mild burning sensation while in others it was a burning sensation followed by lacrimation and nasal throbbing. There were no drug related changes in blood pressure or pulse rate.

Karim *et al.* (1976, 1978) have confirmed and extended the above findings with PGE_1 in man. The effect of a single topical dose of PGE_1 (37.5 μg) on nasal patency was studied in six adult healthy male volunteers. PGE_1 increased nasal patency in four out of six healthy volunteers. This effect lasted for 3–7 hours. In two other subjects there was little increase in nasal patency which lasted for less than 30 minutes (Figure 2.3). Four out of the six subjects experienced side-effects which included strong burning sensation inside the nose, nasal throbbing, lacrimation, headache and sore throat. The symptoms lasted for 15–60 minutes.

2.4.3 17-phenyl-trinor-PGE_2

As an extension of the above study, Karim *et al.* (1976, 1978) studied the effect of 17-phenyl-trinor-PGE_2 (a synthetic analogue of natural PGE_2) applied topically in the same six volunteers on different occasions. Intranasal administration of 37.5 μg of 17-phenyl-trinor-PGE_2 increased nasal patency in all the six volunteers. The effect lasted for 2 hours in two subjects, 4–5 hours in two and for more than 7 hours in the remaining two subjects (Figure 2.3). No side-effects were encountered with this prostaglandin.

2.5 EFFECT OF PROSTAGLANDINS ON NASAL AIRWAY RESISTANCE IN PATIENTS WITH VASOMOTOR AND ALLERGIC RHINITIS

2.5.1 17-phenyl-trinor-PGE_2

Twenty patients with vasomotor and allergic rhinitis (6 male and 14 female) received a single dose of 50 μg 17-phenyl-trinor-PGE_2 instilled into one nostril (Karim *et al.*, 1978). Nasal patency was measured over a period of 7 hours. 17-phenyl-trinor-PGE_2 increased the nasal patency in all of these patients. The effect lasted for over 7 hours in 18 patients and for 4–5 hours in the remaining two. All patients experienced symptomatic relief which lasted for more than 7 hours (Figure 2.4). In contrast there was some increase in resistance in the untreated nostril. In another group of six patients who received 17-phenyl-trinor-PGE_2 (50 μg) in both nostrils, the increase in nasal patency was similar in both nostrils and the effect lasted for more than 7 hours (Figure 2.5).

Out of the 26 subjects treated with 17-phenyl-trinor-PGE_2, only four complained of local nasal irritation which lasted for 5–10 minutes. There were no other side-effects.

2.5.2 $PGF_{2\alpha}$

In a subsequent study (Adaikan *et al.*, 1978) the effect of 17-phenyl-trinor-PGE_2 on nasal patency was compared with $PGF_{2\alpha}$ in eight patients with vasomotor rhinitis. $PGF_{2\alpha}$ (50, 100 and 200 μg) or 17-phenyl-trinor-PGE_2 (50 μg) were used on four separate occasions separated by 7 days. Both 17-phenyl-trinor-PGE_2 (50 μg) and $PGF_{2\alpha}$ (50, 100 and 200 μg), increased nasal patency in all eight subjects. The only side-effect encountered with 17-phenyl-trinor-PGE_2 was transient nasal irritation in two subjects.

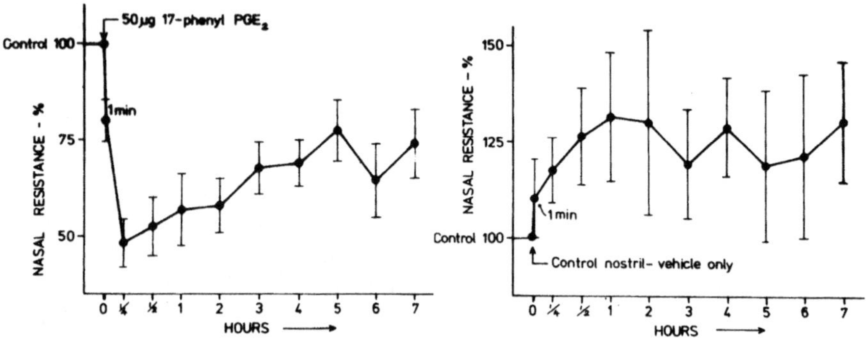

Figure 2.4 Effect of a single dose of 17-phenyl-trinor-PGE_2 (50 μg) instilled in one nostril in 20 patients with vasomotor and allergic rhinitis. Standard error of the mean is indicated by vertical bars. Figure is from Karim *et al.* (1978) by courtesy of *Prostaglandins*

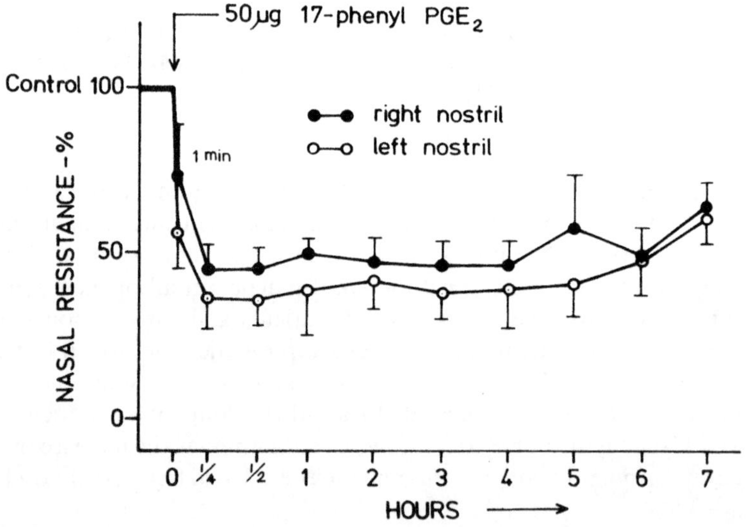

Figure 2.5 Effect of 17-phenyl-trinor-PGE_2 instilled into both nostrils in six patients with vasomotor rhinitis. Standard error of the mean is indicated by vertical bars. Figure is from Karim *et al.* (1978) by courtesy of *Prostaglandins*

The increase in nasal patency and the duration of effect of $PGF_{2\alpha}$ was dose dependent (Table 2.2, Figure 2.6). The effect of the highest dose of $PGF_{2\alpha}$ (200 μg) was comparable to that produced by 50 μg of 17-phenyl-trinor-PGE_2 both in terms of magnitude and duration of action. The effect lasted for more than 7 hours in most subjects. However, $PGF_{2\alpha}$ at a 200 μg dosage produced

Table 2.2 Duration of increase in nasal patency after local administration of prostaglandins

Dose	*No. of patients*				
	0–30 min	*1–2 h*	*3–6 h*	*Over 7 h*	*Total no. of patients*
$PGF_{2\alpha}$ 50 μg	1	4	2	1	8
$PGF_{2\alpha}$ 100 μg	1	—	6	1	8
$PGF_{2\alpha}$ 200 μg	1	—	2	5	8
17-PhE_2 50 μg	—	—	2	6	8

Data from Adaikan *et al.* (1978)

headache and lacrimation (one patient each), sore throat (two patients) and nasal irritation (three patients). These side-effects would tend to limit the usefulness of this prostaglandin as a nasal decongestant. The lower doses of $PGF_{2\alpha}$ (50 μg and 100 μg) which are free from side-effects may be of some value although the duration of action is short.

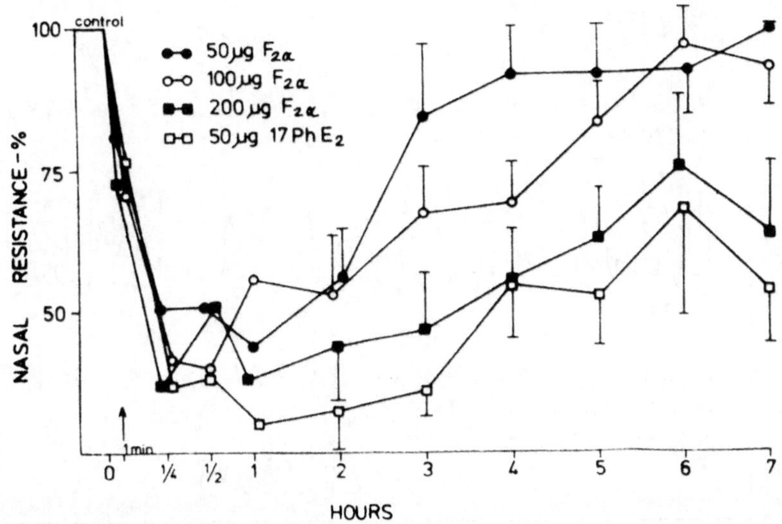

Figure 2.6 Effect of $PGF_{2\alpha}$ and 17-phenyl-trinor-PGE_2 on nasal patency in eight subjects with vasomotor rhinitis. Vertical bar indicates standard error of the mean. (Omitted for clarity for observations $t < 2$ h). Figure is from Adaikan *et al.* (1978) by courtesy of *IRCS Medical Science*

2.5.3 17-phenyl-trinor-PGF$_{2\alpha}$

Recently the effect of a single dose of 17-phenyl-trinor-PGF$_{2\alpha}$ (a synthetic analogue of natural PGF$_{2\alpha}$) at 12.5 μg, 25 μg and 50 μg was studied in 14 patients with vasomotor rhinitis on separate occasions. 17-phenyl-trinor-PGF$_{2\alpha}$ increased nasal patency in all patients. The magnitude and duration of action were dose-dependent (Figures 2.7, 2.8, Table 2.3). Out of 37 tests in 14 subjects with 17-phenyl-trinor-PGF$_{2\alpha}$ (12.5 μg, 25 μg and 50 μg) local irritation was encountered in four tests and lacrimation in two tests.

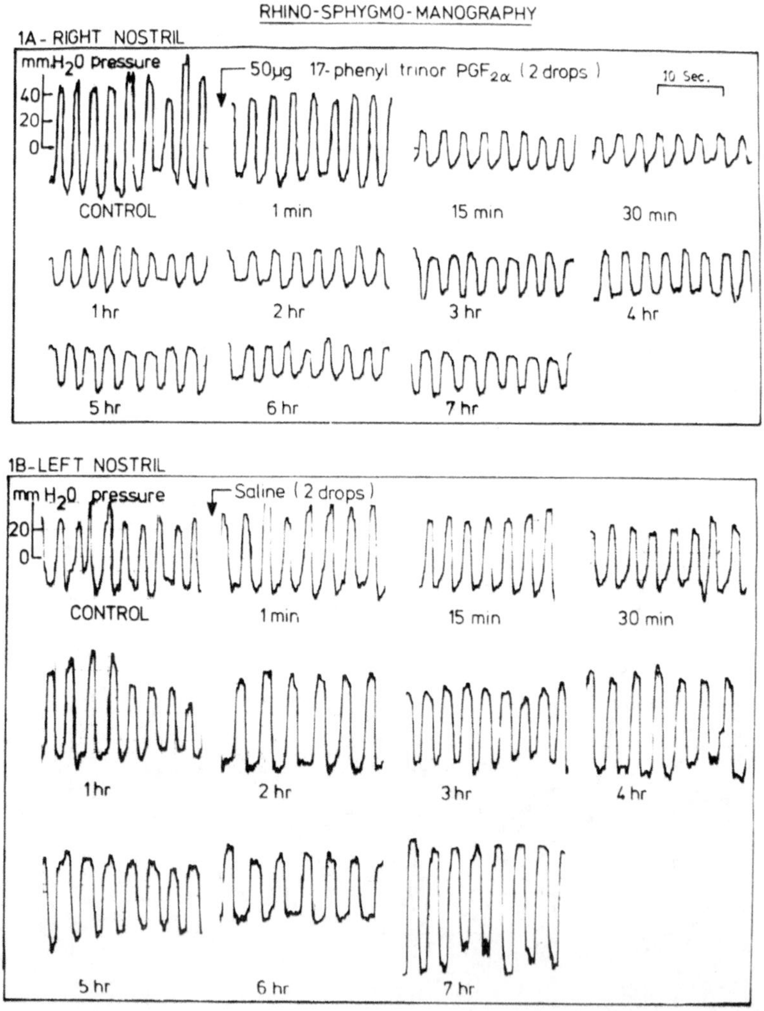

Figure 2.7 A typical record of sphygmomanography. 1A: Effect of a single dose of 17-phenyl-trinor-PGF$_{2\alpha}$ instilled into the congested nostril of a patient with vasomotor rhinitis. 1B: Control nostril, saline only. (Karim *et al.*, 1979)

The magnitude and duration of action of 17-phenyl-trinor-$PGF_{2\alpha}$ and of 17-phenyl-trinor-PGE_2 were similar. These compounds are 4–8 times more potent than $PGF_{2\alpha}$ (Karim *et al.*, 1979).

17-phenyl-trinor-$PGF_{2\alpha}$ is chemically more stable in aqueous solution than 17-phenyl-trinor-PGE_2. The former compound therefore is a preferred candidate for further development.

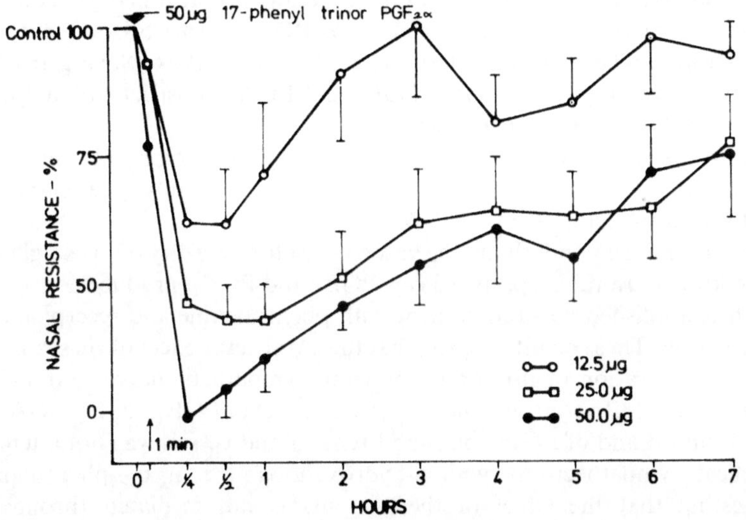

Figure 2.8 Effect of 17-phenyl-trinor-$PGF_{2\alpha}$ on nasal patency in 14 subjects with vasomotor rhinitis. Vertical bar indicates standard error of the mean. (Karim *et al.*, 1979)

Table 2.3 Duration of increase in nasal patency after local administration of 17-phenyl-trinor-$PGF_{2\alpha}$

Dose	*No. of patients*				
	0–30 min	*1–2 h*	*3–6 h*	*Over 7 h*	*Total no. of patients*
12.5 µg	2	6	3	3	14
25.0 µg	—	4	5	8	14
50.0 µg	—	—	6	8	14

Data from Karim *et al.*, 1979

2.6 MECHANISM OF ACTION

Generally prostaglandins of the E series are vasodilators and those of the F series vasoconstrictors. PGE_1 is a potent vasodilator in guinea-pig and human skin. Single intradermal injections of PGE_1 in man produced vasodilatation and a long-lasting erethema persisting for up to 10 hours (Solomon *et al.*, 1968).

PGE_1 and PGE_2 increased blood flow and decreased vascular resistance in human forearm (Robinson *et al.*, 1973). Intra-arterial administration of $PGF_{2\alpha}$ in small doses caused a fall in forearm blood flow. $PGF_{2\alpha}$ also caused constriction of the superficial hand veins in man (Robinson *et al.*, 1973).

On the other hand, PGE_1 and PGE_2 generally produce a constrictor effect in isolated vascular smooth muscles *in vitro*. PGE_1 constricts isolated strips of rabbit aorta and cat carotid artery (Khairallah *et al.*, 1967). Strong and Bohr (1967) also reported that PGE_1, PGE_2 and PGA_1 constrict isolated rabbit aorta and dog coronary artery strips.

From the study of Stovall and Jackson (1967) on dog nasal mucosa (see 2.3.3) it is apparent that prostaglandins decrease nasal airway resistance by a local vasoconstrictor effect.

The mechanism underlying the vasoconstrictor property of prostaglandins is not known. In rabbit perfused ear, PGE_1 and $PGF_{2\alpha}$ produce constriction which is abolished by pretreatment with phentolamine and reserpine or by denervation. These results suggest that the constrictor effect of these agents is due to a liberation of noradrenaline from sympathetic nerves (Al Tai and Graham, 1972). In contrast, the constrictor effect of PGE_1, PGE_2, PGA_2 and $PGF_{2\alpha}$ on rat and of $PGF_{2\alpha}$ on rabbit renal blood vessels was not altered by chemical sympathectomy with 6-hydroxydopamine or by phentolamine, suggesting that the effect of these agents is not mediated through the adrenergic mechanism (Malik and McGiff, 1975).

It is not known whether the increase in nasal patency caused by prostaglandin in human nasal mucosa is dependent on the adrenergic system. It is unlikely to be mediated through histamine release, since histamine decreases nasal patency (unpublished observations).

It is likely that the constriction produced by prostaglandins on nasal mucosa is due to a direct effect on the vascular smooth muscle. The precise mode of action of prostaglandins on nasal vascular smooth muscle is under investigation.

2.7 OTHER RELATED AREAS OF APPLICATION

The efficacy of prostaglandins in increasing nasal patency may be beneficial in the following related areas:

(1) *Sinus headache*

Acute sinus infection also causes blocking of fronto-nasal duct and other ostia. A single dose of a decongestant solution applied at the middle meatus could be beneficial.

(2) *Acute otitis media and Eustachian obstruction*
In conditions of acute otitis media and obstruction of Eustachian tube (especially in children) application of prostaglandin at nasopharyngeal level may help to restore or maintain its patency.

(3) *Intra-nasal surgery*
During the period following intra-nasal surgery the decongestant prostaglandin may prove useful in clearing crusts and debris from the nose.

(4) *During flight*
Nasal decongestants could be utilized before, during and after flight for patients who are prone to barotrauma affecting the sinuses or the middle ear.

2.8 CONCLUSIONS AND COMMENTS

Available data suggest that prostaglandins are involved in the physiology of nasal patency. This evidence is based on the fact that human nasal mucosa and nasal secretions contain prostaglandins and that prostaglandins readily relieve nasal congestion in human volunteers and patients suffering from vasomotor and allergic rhinitis.

The promising results with prostaglandin analogues, 17-phenyl-trinor-PGE_2 and 17-phenyl-trinor-$PGF_{2\alpha}$, and the general lack of side-effects warrant an extension of these studies to a larger population.

References

Adaikan, P. G., Kunaratnam, N. and Karim, S. M. M. (1978). Effect of prostaglandin $F_{2\alpha}$ on nasal patency in man: comparison with 17-phenyl-trinor-PGE_2. *IRCS Med. Sci.*, **2**, 206

Al Tai, S. A. and Graham, J. D. P. (1972). The actions of prostaglandins E_1 and $F_{2\alpha}$ on the perfused vessels of the isolated rabbit ear. *Br. J. Pharmacol.*, **44**, 699

Anggård, A. (1969). The effect of prostaglandins on nasal airway resistance in man. *Ann. Otol.*, **78**, 657

Chow, M. T., Salmon, J. A., Karim, S. M. M. and Kunaratnam, N. (1976). Identification of prostaglandins in human nasal mucosa. *South East Asian/Western Pacific Regional Meeting of Pharmacologists*. Abstract 103. 11–14 May, 1976, Singapore

Harrison, D. F. N. (1976). Nasal drops, spray and inhalations. *Prescribers' J.*, **16**, 69

Jackson, R. T. (1970). Prostaglandin E_1 as a nasal constrictor in normal human volunteers. *Curr. Ther. Res.*, **12**, 711

Karim, S. M. M., Adaikan, P. G. and Kunaratnam, N. (1976). Effect of prostaglandins on nasal patency in man. *South East Asian/Western Pacific Regional Meeting of Pharmacologists*. Abstract 104. 11–14 May, 1976, Singapore

Karim, S. M. M., Adaikan, P. G. and Kunaratnam, N. (1978). Effect of topical prostaglandins on nasal patency in man. *Prostaglandins*, **15**, 457

Karim, S. M. M., Adaikan, P. G. and Kunaratnam, N. (1979). Effect of 17-phenyl-trinor-$PGF_{2\alpha}$ on nasal patency in man. *Prostagl. Med.* (In press)

Khairallah, P. A., Page, I. H. and Turker, R. K. (1967). Some properties of prostaglandin E_1 action on muscle. *Arch. Int. Pharmacodyn. Ther.*, **169**, 328

Malik, K. U. and McGiff, J. C. (1975). Modulation by prostaglandins of adrenergic transmission in the isolated perfused rabbit and rat kidneys. *Circ. Res.*, **36**, 599

Mygind, N. (1978). Conventional medical treatment. In: N. Mygind, *Nasal Allergy* (Oxford: Blackwell Scientific Publications)

Okazaki, T., Reisman, R. E. and Arbesman, C. E. (1977). Prostaglandin E in the secretions of allergic rhinitis. *Prostaglandins*, **13**, 681

Robinson, B. F., Collier, J. G., Karim, S. M. M. and Somers, K. (1973). Effect of prostaglandins A_1, A_2, B_1, B_2, E_2 and $F_{2\alpha}$ on forearm arterial bed and superficial hand veins in man. *Clin. Sci.*, **44**, 367

Shaw, H. (1964). Nasal drops and sprays. *Prescribers' J.*, **4**, 6

Solomon, L. M., Juhlin, L. and Kirschenbaum, B. (1968). Prostaglandin on cutaneous vasculature. *J. Invest. Dermatol.*, **51**, 280

Strong, C. G. and Bohr, D. F. (1967). Effects of prostaglandins E_1, E_2, A_1 and $F_{1\alpha}$ on isolated vascular smooth muscle. *Am. J. Physiol.*, **213**, 725

Stovall, R. and Jackson, R. T. (1967). Prostaglandins and nasal blood flow. *Ann. Otol.*, **76**, 1051

Toh, C. C. and Mohiuddin, A. (1958). Vasoactive substances in the nasal mucosa. *Br. J. Pharmacol.*, **13**, 113

3
PGE_1 in Ischaemic Peripheral Vascular Disease

L. A. CARLSON and A. G. OLSSON

3.1 INTRODUCTION

Some of the many biological effects of prostaglandin E_1 (PGE_1) may be beneficial when given to ischaemic tissues or organs. This prostaglandin is a potent vasodilator and an efficient inhibitor of platelet aggregation *in vitro* (Bergström *et al.*, 1968). It also stabilizes lysosomal membranes (Raflo, *et al.*, 1973). This prevents the release of lysosomal proteases and phospholipases which, when liberated, damage other tissue membranes and degrade or denature important cellular proteins. PGE_1 may also protect other membranes such as those of red blood cells resulting in better oxygen delivery and more efficient utilization of delivered oxygen by cells in ischaemic states. Another possible mechanism of the beneficial effect of PGE_1 may involve an antagonism of some of the anti-inflammatory effects of kinins such as bradykinin. PGE_1 may influence the oxidative metabolism of the tissue and save oxygen since it is a potent inhibitor of lipolysis (Carlson, 1967). Furthermore there is evidence that PGE_1 stimulates epidermal growth (Bentley-Phillips *et al.*, 1977).

However, when PGE_1 is injected intravenously into healthy human subjects in doses of 0.1 (μg/kg)/min, it invariably causes distressing subjective effects such as headache, flush, abdominal cramps and nausea (Carlson *et al.*, 1968). These effects limit the use of PGE_1 by the *intravenous* route in clinical situations such as ischaemia of the lower limbs.

In order to overcome this problem, the *local* effects of PGE_1 when given *intra-arterially* in smaller doses were studied. PGE_1 infused into the brachial artery in dose of 0.001 (μg/kg)/min in healthy volunteers (Bevegård and Orö, 1969) produced a dramatic increase in forearm blood flow without any disturbing subjective side-effects. Intra-arterial administration of PGE_1 in small doses to an ischaemic area is therefore a possible way of overcoming the unpleasant side-effects associated with intravenous infusion. The ischaemic limb was chosen because the artery to this tissue is easily accessible and the effect of PGE_1 easily measured.

3.2 EXPERIENCE WITH PROSTAGLANDINS IN PERIPHERAL ARTERY DISEASE

3.2.1 Intra-arterial infusion

The first clinical study with PGE_1 in pronounced ischaemia of the lower limbs was carried out by local intra-arterial infusion of PGE_1 in the diseased leg. The drug was given to six patients with severe symptoms of peripheral artery disease (Table 3.1). All patients except one had intense resting pains, three had ischaemic ulcers and two had dry apical gangrene with mummification of one or several toes. Three of the patients had diabetes; the others obliterative arteriosclerosis.

PGE_1 was given via a catheter in the femoral artery of the affected limb with an infusion pump in a dose of 0.0015 (μg/kg)/min for 10 min every hour for 72 h. This treatment was often repeated after an interval of approximately 1 month.

The effect on the severe resting pain (Table 3.1) was very dramatic in all patients with or without ulcers with complete or almost complete abolition of the pain within the first 24 hours of treatment. Rapid changes in the ulcers also occurred. Oedema disappeared and the ulcer surfaces dried. Healing started and was complete after 3 months in two of the subjects. The patients with distal mummified gangrene also responded with a transient pain relief but

Table 3.1 Clinical findings and effect of intra-arterial infusion of PGE$_1$ in peripheral artery disease

Case	*Diagnosis*	*Sex*	*Age (years)*	*Resting pains*	*Ulcer*	*Gangrene*	*Effect*	
							Resting pains	*Healing*
1	D.m.	M	74	++	++	—	↓↓	+++
2	Art. obl.	F	69	·	+	—	—	++
3	D.m.	M	74	+++	+++		↓↓↓	+++
4	Art. obl.	F	81	+++	—	—	↓↓↓	—
5	Art. obl.	M	61	+++	—	+	—	—
6	D.m.	F	69	+++		+	·	·

Art. obl. = arteriosclerosis obliterans
D.m. = diabetes mellitus

there was no healing. One example of ulcer healing (Case 1) is shown (Figures 3.1–3.3).

Side-effects noted with intra-arterial infusions included slight flush and increased venous filling of the treated leg. A slight oedema could be seen in the

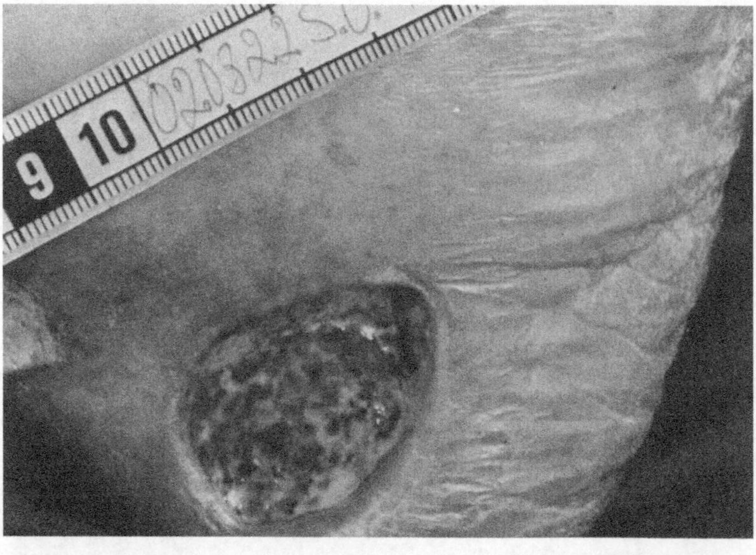

Figure 3.1 Medical aspect of left heel of patient No. 1 (Table 3.1) before intra-arterial infusion of PGE$_1$

foot. These disappeared on decreasing the dose. Body temperature increased by 0.2–1.0 °C and loose stools were occasionally noted. Heart rate and blood pressure, measured hourly during the infusion, were not affected with the doses used.

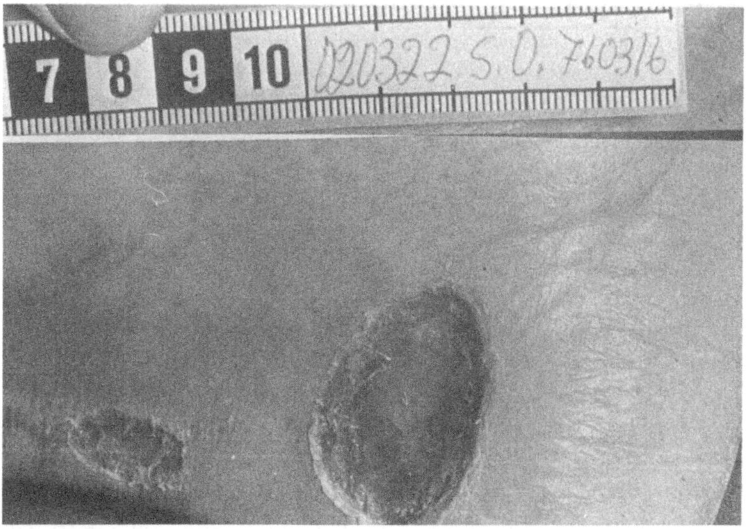

Figure 3.2 The same ulcer as in Figure 3.1 during the 72 hours of intra-arterial infusion of PGE_1

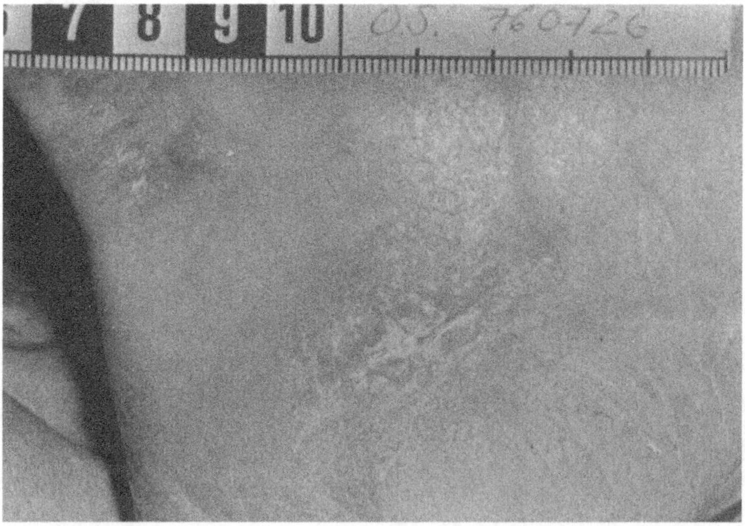

Figure 3.3 Healed ulcers 4 months after intra-arterial infusion of PGE_1

3.2.2 Intravenous infusion

During continued intra-arterial treatment of additional patients with severe ischaemia of the legs (where no further medical or surgical treatment was available) we observed in two cases with bilateral ulcers of the feet, a pain-relieving and healing effect in the leg not given intra-arterial infusion. If this effect was due to PGE$_1$ then the drug may also be given *intravenously* in doses low enough not to produce side-effects.

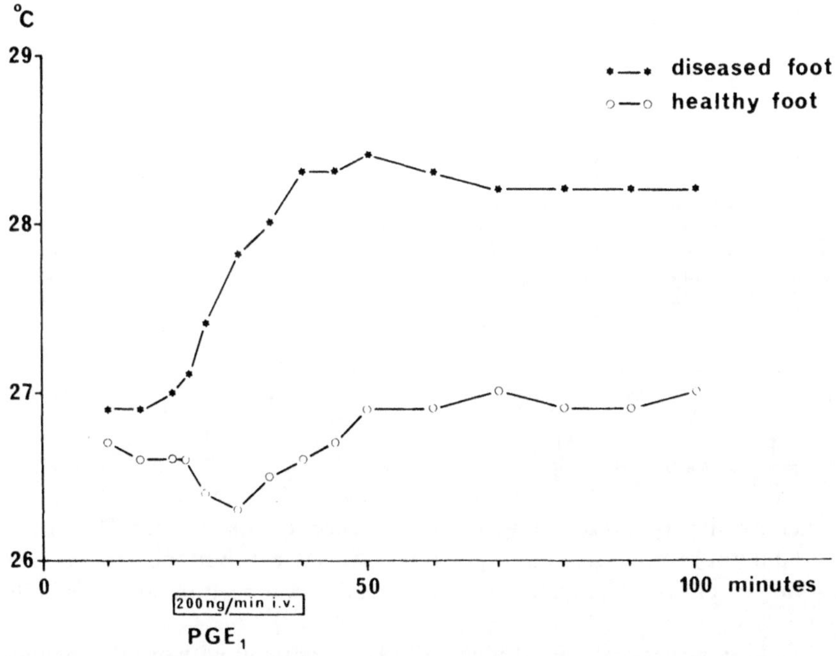

Figure 3.4 Skin temperature of the big toe of *diseased* and *healthy* foot before, during and after intravenous infusion with PGE$_1$

Although PGE$_1$ to a large extent is inactivated during passage through the pulmonary circulation (Mathé *et al.*, 1977) we could demonstrate a therapeutic effect in the periphery after intravenous infusion of low doses of this compound without any side-effects. This is illustrated in Figure 3.4 which shows the skin temperature of the feet in a 68-year-old diabetic woman (Case 2, Table 3.2) with multiple ischaemic ulcers of the left foot (diseased foot). The right foot was unaffected by pain and ulcers (healthy foot). Intravenous infusion of PGE$_1$ in the dose 0.003 (μg/kg)/min caused an immediate rise of 1.5 °C in skin temperature in the diseased foot. This increase in temperature persisted for 60 minutes after the infusion was stopped. There was no rise in skin temperature in the *healthy* foot. Further, during the first 24 hours of treatment oedema of the foot subsided, the wet ulcer surface dried up and the severe pain vanished. The ulcers started to heal and healing was subsequently complete.

In a series of nine patients with peripheral artery disease (with symptoms similar to those described in Section 3.2.1), intravenous infusions of PGE_1 in doses of 0.001 (μg/kg)/min for 72 h were given. This represented approximately six times the intra-arterial dose (Table 3.2). Four out of the five

Table 3.2 Clinical findings and effect of intravenous infusions of PGE_1 in peripheral artery disease

Case	*Diagnosis*	*Sex*	*Age (years)*	*Resting pains*	*Ulcer*	*Effect*	
						Resting pains	*Healing*
1	Art. obl.	F	81	++	++	↓	+[2]
2	D.m.	F	68	+++	++	↓↓↓	+++
3	Art. obl.	F	85	+	++	↓	+[2]
4	Art. obl.	F	65	+++	+++	—	—
5	Art. obl.	F	77	—	+++		+[2]
6	Art. obl.	M	71	—	+		+
7	Art. obl.	F	71	+++	++	↓↓↓	+
8	D.m.	F	61	+++	—	↓↓↓	
9	D.m.	M	60	+++	+[1]	↓↓↓	—

Art. obl. = arteriosclerosis obliterans
D.m. = diabetes mellitus

[1] apical gangrene
[2] after partial skin transplantation

patients with very severe resting pains experienced complete relief. The patient who did not respond had distal gangrene. All subjects but one had ulcers of varying extension. Complete or partial healing was seen in six out of nine patients.

In addition to the beneficial effect of PGE_1 in patients with distal ischaemia caused by arteriosclerosis or diabetes, we have also successfully used PGE_1 in patients with thromboangiitis obliterans. The following case is illustrative[1]:

A 47-year-old unmarried female clerk (born 1930). Normal menstruations. Her father had rheumatoid arthritis – otherwise no known chronic illness in the family. She was a rather heavy smoker through the years 1947–9 and 1969–76 (about 20 cigarettes per day). During most of the 1960s she smoked only occasionally. At the age of 23 infiltrates and nodules were found on the dorsal of her left foot and on her lower left leg. Recurrent infiltrates and nodules occurred during the following years. At the age of 26, symptoms of Raynaud's phenomenon appeared on her hands and claudication on walking. She also had slow healing paronychiae on the left foot. Arteriography failed to

[1] In collaboration with Professor Nils Thyresson, Department of Dermatology, Karolinska Hospital, Stockholm (Olsson and Thyresson, 1978).

show any pathological changes but oscillometry demonstrated low amplitudes over the calves. The patient was treated with vasodilator drugs and was encouraged to stop smoking. During the sixties she did not suffer from ischaemic problems. However, she occasionally had fissures between the toes and eczematous lesions on the feet and hands. She was also found to have contracted an allergic contact dermatitis and to have been sensitized to formalin and certain rubber chemicals.

After taking up smoking in the early 1970s, her feet became acrocyanotic and cold sensitive. Ulcerating nodules of the dorsum of the left foot occurred in 1974. Oscillometrical and plethysmographical signs of obliterating lesions were found in the arteries of both lower legs. Pathological plethysmography was also found over her left hand. The ulcer on the foot caused intense pain and healed only slowly during the course of 1 year. She was given topical dermatological treatment and for some months oral prednisolone was also prescribed.

In February 1976 the patient got ulcers in the first and second toes of the left foot after a minor trauma. The ulcers increased gradually and became extremely tender and painful. Continuous pain occurred both day and night and she had to hang the left leg outside the bed during the night. The patient was admitted to hospital in July 1976. Arteriography showed advanced

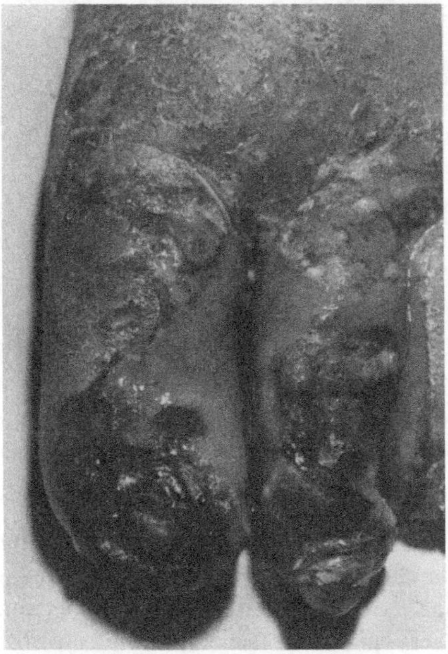

Figure 3.5 Ulcers in a 47-year-old female with thromboangiitis obliterans before treatment with PGE_1

arterial obstructions and occlusions from below the knee of the left leg and also of the right leg. She was treated with infusions including penicillin because of septic infections and with the thrombolytic drug Brinastrase(R) (Astra Läkemedel AB, Sweden) containing the proteolytic enzyme brinase from *Aspergillus oryzae*. The treatment had no effect on either resting pains or ulcers. The situation was desperate, with incipient gangrene of the toes. Amputation of the lower leg was seriously considered by a consulting orthopaedist. Because of the promising results achieved with PGE_1, it was decided to give this treatment a trial. At the start of the treatment the patient had dark-coloured infected ulcers with β-haemolysing streptococci group A and some klebsiella on her first and second toes (Figure 3.5). X-ray revealed signs of osteitis in both digit I and II of the phalanges.

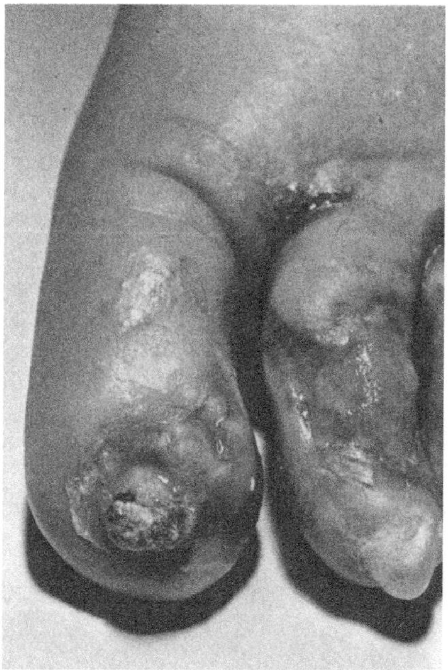

Figure 3.6 The same toes as in Figure 3.5 after 4 months. The patient was given intravenous infusions of PGE_1 in the dose of 0.001 (μg/kg)/h for 72 hours at monthly intervals. Picture after three treatments

The subjective effect of the treatment was noticeable during the first 24-hour infusion. The main effect was an almost immediate pain relief. Even on the first night the patient no longer needed to keep the leg outside the bed, as had been necessary every night for several months prior to treatment. The tenderness also disappeared and the patient could support herself on the foot without pain during the second day of infusion.

The objective effects were also evident during the first 24 hours of treatment.

The oedema subsided and drying of the ulcers was noted during the first days of treatment. Healing started with pink dry granulations and the ulcers were continuously epithelialized (Figure 3.6). Non-vital parts of the distal phalanx of the left big toe were slowly delimited and finally amputated spontaneously 8 months after the first treatment. The ulcers healed completely. The pain disappeared and has not recurred. The patient is still free from pain and ulcers in December 1978 (Figure 3.7).

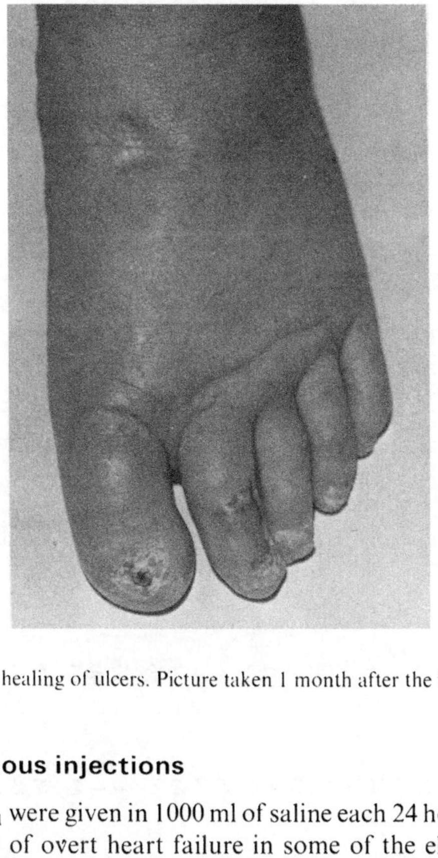

Figure 3.7 Complete healing of ulcers. Picture taken 1 month after the fifth and last treatment

3.2.3 Intravenous injections

Infusions of PGE_1 were given in 1000 ml of saline each 24 hours. This not only increased the risk of overt heart failure in some of the elderly patients but could also theoretically influence flow properties of the blood. The beneficial effect of the treatment therefore cannot be attributed only to the effect of PGE_1 but also to decreased blood viscosity resulting in better microcirculation in affected areas.

To overcome this problem, we gave PGE_1 in repeated bolus intravenous injections. The results of this treatment are summarized in Table 3.3.

Twenty-two subjects – all with ischaemic ulcers of the lower limbs and with varying degree of resting pain – were treated with 20 μg PGE_1 given intravenously for 5 minutes every second hour, seven times a day for 3 days. They

Table 3.3 Clinical findings and effect of intravenous injections of PGE_1 in peripheral artery disease

Case	*Diagnosis*	*Sex*	*Age (years)*	*Resting pain*	*Ulcer area*	*No. of treatments*	*Follow up time (months)*	*Effect*	
								Resting pain	*Ulcer healing*
1	Art. obl.	M	60	+++	++	2	3	+++	+++
2	Art. obl.	M	67	+++	+++	3	13	+++	+++
3	Art. obl.	M	69	+++	+++	1	1	+++	+
4	Art. obl.	M	76	+++	++	2	6	+++	+++
5	Art. obl.	M	81	+++	+++	2	5	++	+
6	Art. obl.	M	55	+++	++	1	2	++	0
7	Art. obl.	M	52	++	++	1	1	+++	+++
8	Art. obl.	M	52	++	+++	1	1	++	+
9	D.m.	F	71	++	+++	1	1	+++	++
10	D.m.	M	67	++	+++	1	1	+++	++
11	Art. obl.	M	69	++	+++	1	1	++	++
12	Art. obl.	M	65	++	+++	1	6	+	0
13	Art. obl.	M	64	++	++	3	6	+[1]	0
14	Art. obl.	M	66	++	+++	3	3	++[1]	+
15	Art. obl.	F	75	+	+++	3	10	+++	+++
16	D.m.	F	40	+	++	3	6	+++	+++
17	Art. obl.	M	65	+	+++	1	2	+++	+++
18	Bürger	M	51	+	+++	2	3	++	+
19	D.m.	M	75	+	+++	4	9	++	++
20	Art. obl.	M	72	+	+	1	1	+++	+++
21	D.m.	M	54	0	++	3	8		+++
22	D.m.	M	40	0	+++	2	9		+++

Resting pain: +++ very intense, ++ intense, + moderate, 0 no pain
Ulcer area: +++ multiple ulcers or one $>2 cm^2$, ++ 1–$2 cm^2$, + $<1 cm^2$
Effects on resting pain: +++ complete abolition, ++ almost complete abolition, + moderate
Ulcer healing: +++ complete healing, ++ almost complete healing, + partial healing, 0 no healing
[1] initially good effect but worse later

all had very extensive and pronounced peripheral atherosclerotic vascular disease. Any further vascular surgical or medical treatment was not possible. This treatment was often repeated one or more times (Table 3.3) upon request of the patients.

3.2.3.1 *Effect on resting pains* (Table 3.3)

Six subjects had very severe disabling resting pain which necessitated taking strong analgesics and sedatives and hanging the afflicted leg outside and below the bed every night. Four of these subjects experienced a complete pain relief after one to three treatments with PGE_1. Two additional patients with severe resting pain also experienced almost complete pain relief with one and two treatments respectively.

An additional eight out of the 22 patients had intense ischaemic pain before treatment. Three of these experienced complete pain relief during the first treatment, three had moderate relief and two had slight relief.

There was complete disappearance of pain in four out of six patients with moderate initial ulcer pain.

3.2.3.2 *Effect on ulcer healing*

Of the six patients with ischaemic ulcers and very intense pains three had complete ulcer healing within the period of observation. Complete healing might be expected in an additional two subjects with so far short observation time. No effect was seen in one subject (Table 3.3).

Most of the eight patients with intense resting pains have so far not been observed for sufficiently long times but nevertheless the ulcer has healed completely in one patient and almost completely in four others. There was no healing in two subjects and only a transient healing in one.

Of the six patients with ulcers and slight pains, the ulcers in four healed completely. The ulcers in the two diabetic patients without associated pain also healed.

3.3 COMMENTS

In patients with advanced ischaemic symptoms of peripheral artery disease, we have observed striking effects of the infusion of PGE_1 both on relief of resting pains and on ulcer healing. The effect was similar irrespective of the route of drug administration.

In spite of the dramatic therapeutic effects, it should be emphasised that our experience so far is derived from uncontrolled trials. Therefore we are starting a controlled study on the effect of ulcer healing following PGE_1 injection.

The following facts make us believe that the beneficial effect is due to the action of PGE_1: (1) All subjects had severe and pronounced disease and had been treated optimally before PGE_1 was given. They were referred to us from specialist clinics such as the Department of Dermatology or Endocrinology or the Department of Vascular Surgery and had been treated for a long time with antibiotic infusions, local medication, surgery, etc. without any effect. (2) The effect of PGE_1 was immediate and both subjective (pain relief) and objective (ulcer healing) effects were often noted already during the first 24 hours of treatment.

We feel that the use of PGE_1 in severe peripheral vascular disease where no further treatment except amputation was possible is an example of what can be achieved when basic and clinical research are co-ordinated. We were given the opportunity in the early 1960s to collaborate with Professor S. Bergström and work with the then recently isolated prostaglandins and test them for their pharmacological and metabolic properties in healthy subjects. Based on the results of these studies we started to use PGE_1 in patients with peripheral vascular disease. We are presently not able to ascribe the often striking clinical results we have obtained to any specific effect of PGE_1 (on, e.g., platelet aggregation, microcirculation or other processes), but we feel that this is an area well worth further clinical and biochemical studies. A better understanding of the mechanism behind the observed clinical effects may lead to even better treatment of ischaemic tissues with other prostaglandins.

3.4 SUMMARY

The effect of PGE_1 was studied in patients suffering from advanced arteriosclerosis of the legs with chronic ischaemic ulcers and resting pains. When PGE_1 was given as intra-arterial (six patients) or intravenous infusions (nine patients) or as intravenous injections (22 patients), in a 24-hour dose of 0.25–2.00 μg/kg for 72 h, almost all patients experienced an immediate and complete relief from pain. Chronic ulcers started to heal immediately and continued to do so until complete healing was achieved in many cases. Our good clinical experience with PGE_1 in chronic ischaemia of the lower limbs is encouraging and calls for further controlled studies.

Acknowledgements

Supported by grants from Petrus och Augusta Hedlunds Stiftelse, Tore Nilsons Fond för Medicinsk Forskning, Hans och Loo Ostermans fond and by the Swedish Medical Research Council (19X-204).

References

Bentley-Phillips, C. G., Paulli-Jorgensen, H. and Marks, R. (1977). The effects of prostaglandins E_1 and $F_{2\alpha}$ on epidermal growth. *Arch. Derm. Res.*, **257**, 233

Bergström, S., Carlson, L. A. and Weeks, J. R. (1968). The prostaglandins: A family of biologically active lipids. *Pharmacol. Rev.*, **20**, 1

Bevegård, S. and Orö, L. (1969). Effect of prostaglandin E_1 on forearm blood flow. *Scand. J. Clin. Lab. Invest.*, **23**, 347

Carlson, L. A. (1967). Cardiovascular and metabolic effects of prostaglandins. *Progr. Biochem. Pharmacol.*, **3**, 94

Carlson, L. A., Ekelund, L. G. and Orö, L. (1968). Clinical and metabolic effects of different doses of prostaglandin E_1 in man. *Acta Med. Scand.*, **183**, 423

Mathé, A. A., Hedqvist, P., Strandberg, K. and Leslie, C. A. (1977). Aspects of prostaglandin function in the lung (First of two parts). *N. Engl. J. Med.*, **296**, 850

Olsson, A. G. and Thyresson, N. (1978). Healing of ischaemic ulcers by intravenous prostaglandin E_1 in a woman with thromboangitis obliterans. *Acta Dermatovener.*, **58**, 467

Raflo, G. T., Wangensteen, S. L., Glenn, T. M. and Lefer, A. M. (1973). *Eur. J. Pharmacol.*, **24**, 86

4
Prostaglandins, their Synthesis Inhibitors and Ductus Arteriosus

F. COCEANI and P. M. OLLEY

4.1 INTRODUCTION

The ductus arteriosus is a major foetal blood vessel connecting the pulmonary artery to the descending portion of the aortic arch and carries 90% of the right ventricular output thus bypassing the foetal lungs. At birth, the ductus ceases its function and undergoes constriction followed by permanent closure. Of the two states of this vessel (prenatal patency and postnatal closure) the latter has generally attracted greater attention because of its abrupt occurrence and its association with other postnatal circulatory changes. Ductal patency, on the other hand, has been considered a passive process subject to extraductal factors such as right ventricular output and the pressure gradient between pulmonary and systemic circulations (Heymann and Rudolph, 1975).

Recent findings suggesting that a prostaglandin (PG) keeps the ductus patent in the foetus have added a new perspective to work in this field. This concept not only has stimulated much research on the ductus but has also provided fresh impetus to investigations of the role of prostaglandins in the foetal circulation and in the circulatory adjustments to postnatal life. Furthermore, knowledge of the involvement of prostaglandins in the ductus has afforded a new approach in the management of pathological conditions of the infant requiring ductus patency or closure.

Most of the evidence implicating a prostaglandin mechanism in the control of ductal tone has been gathered from studies in the lamb. Other species, including man, appear to respond to prostaglandins in a manner similar to the lamb. Nevertheless, some differences between species have been described and they will be discussed separately.

4.2 DUCTUS PATENCY

In 1973, we reported (Coceani and Olley, 1973) that PGE_1 and PGE_2 relax the lamb ductus arteriosus *in vitro* and that this effect was more pronounced in a low oxygen environment. On the basis of that observation and the concomitant demonstration of PGE-like material in ductal tissue, we postulated that a prostaglandin might maintain prenatal patency of the vessel. This suggestion is now well supported by a variety of findings in several animal species.

Inhibitors of prostaglandin synthesis, such as the non-steroidal anti-inflammatory drugs and 5,8,11,14-eicosatetraynoic acid (ETA), constrict ductus arteriosus of foetal lambs (Coceani *et al.*, 1975; Olley *et al.*, 1975; Heymann and Rudolph, 1976; Clyman *et al.*, 1978a; Friedman, W. F. *et al.*, 1978), rats (Sharpe *et al.*, 1974, 1975), and rabbits (Sharpe *et al.*, 1975). Non-steroidal anti-inflammatory drugs have been used more often and their relative activity on the ductus, both *in vitro* (Coceani *et al.*, 1978c) and *in vivo* (Sharpe *et al.*, 1974, 1975; Heymann and Rudolph, 1976; Coceani *et al.*,

1978c; Friedman, W. F. *et al.*, 1978), correlates with their potencies in blocking the prostaglandin synthetase enzyme system (cf. Flower, 1974). However, these drugs are effective in constricting the ductus arteriosus at lower doses than those used therapeutically. Friedman, W. F. *et al.* (1978) have shown that indomethacin given intravenously to mature foetal lambs constricts the ductus at a dose of 10 μg per kilogram body weight. Constriction of the ductus *in vitro* and *in vivo* following blockade of prostaglandin synthesis is fully reversed by treatment with PGE_1 or PGE_2 (Coceani *et al.*, 1975; Friedman, W. F. *et al.*, 1978). These data indicate that the foetal ductus is kept patent by a relaxant prostaglandin. Moreover, *in vitro* findings imply that most, if not all, of the active compound is formed intramurally in the ductus.

While this concept is now well established, the identity of the active prostaglandin remains controversial. Theoretically, several different compounds could play this role because arachidonic acid, the predominant polyunsaturated fatty acid in mammalian cells, is converted via the cyclo-oxygenase pathway to a variety of vasoactive products (prostaglandin endoperoxides, thromboxane A_2, PGI_2, primary prostaglandins). However, results of biochemical and pharmacological studies limit the choice to two compounds, PGE_2 and PGI_2.

Work from different laboratories (Pace-Asciak and Rangaraj, 1977, 1978b; Powell and Solomon, 1977; Friedman, 1978; Terragno *et al.*, 1978) has established that 6-keto-$PGF_{1\alpha}$ (a metabolite of PGI_2) is the major product of arachidonic acid metabolism in the ductus arteriosus from mature foetal lambs and calves. PGE_2 and $PGF_{2\alpha}$ are formed in small amounts while PGD_2 and TXB_2 are not formed at all. These findings imply the occurrence of PGI_2 in the vessel. Indeed, a compound with the anti-aggregatory action of PGI_2 on platelets has been detected in the fluid bathing an isolated preparation of lamb ductus (Clyman *et al.*, 1978b). The relative amounts of PGI_2 (in 6-keto-$PGF_{1\alpha}$ equivalents) and PGE_2 generated in specimens of whole ductus vary with species. Thus, in the lamb PGE_2 synthesis ranges between 10% and 20% of PGI_2 synthesis (Pace-Asciak and Rangaraj, 1977, 1978b), whereas in the calf PGE_2 synthesis never exceeds 10% of the PGI_2 value (Terragno *et al.*, 1978). In either species, the location of the prostaglandin synthetase enzymes is not known, nor is it known whether the proportions of PGE_2 and PGI_2 formed, remain constant across the vessel wall. It is likely that in the ductus, as in other vessels, PGI_2 synthesis occurs primarily in the endothelium (Moncada *et al.*, 1977).

The effects of arachidonic acid and its metabolites on the isolated preparation of lamb ductus at PO_2 levels mimicking the foetal condition have been studied. Table 4.1 gives the results of this screening. As shown, PGE_2 is the most potent among the relaxant prostaglandins formed in the tissue, its threshold concentration being lower than that of PGI_2 by several orders of magnitude. The relatively low activity of PGI_2 is unlikely to be due to its breakdown to 6-keto-$PGF_{1\alpha}$ in the bath/extracellular fluid compartment because identical results are obtained in the guinea-pig ductus (Coceani *et al.*, 1979) which, by virtue of its smaller size, must have more accessible target sites. Prostaglandin endoperoxides are second in order of potency to PGE_2 in relaxing the ductus. However, their action on the muscle results from transformation to another compound (Coceani *et al.*, 1978a). Likewise, arachidonic acid has little or no activity *per se* on the ductus since its action is inhibited by pre-treatment with blockers of prostaglandin synthesis (Coceani *et al.*, 1978c). Judging from the relative potencies of endoperoxide derivatives, PGE_2 is the most likely candidate for mediating the response to PGG_2/PGH_2. Consistent with this possibility is the finding that PGH_1, which is not a substrate for the PGI_2 synthetic reaction, is as potent as PGH_2 in relaxing the ductal tissue (Coceani *et al.*, 1979).

Table 4.1 Effects of arachidonic acid and its metabolites on the ductus arteriosus from near-term foetal lambs

Compound	*Relaxation*	*Contraction*	*No effect*
Arachidonic acid	10^{-6} to 10^{-4}		
PGG_2	10^{-9} to 10^{-7}		
PGH_2	10^{-9} to 10^{-7}		
TXA_2			10^{-6}
TXB_2			10^{-7}
PGI_2	10^{-6}		
6-keto-$PGF_{1\alpha}$			10^{-6}
PGE_2	10^{-12} to 10^{-10}		
PGD_2	10^{-5}		
$PGF_{2\alpha}$		10^{-7} to 10^{-5}	

Compounds were tested on an isolated circular strip of ductus arteriosus (PO_2, 8–16 mmHg). Figures are molar concentrations in the bath fluid and apply to threshold concentrations for a given effect or to maximal concentration tested when compounds were inactive. Thromboxane A_2 (TXA_2) was generated enzymatically and its concentration is expressed in endoperoxide equivalents. PGE_1 was as potent as PGE_2 in relaxing the ductus, whereas PGE_1 (and presumably PGE_2) metabolites (15-keto and 15-keto-13,14-dihydro) had little relaxant activity (threshold, 10^{-7} to 10^{-6} M). (From Coceani and Olley, 1973; Coceani *et al.*, 1975, 1978a, b and c).

In brief, the pertinent question is whether prenatal patency of the ductus is determined by the more *active* PGE_2 or the more *abundant* PGI_2.

The idea that PGE_2 is implicated in ductus patency has been challenged on two grounds (cf. Coceani *et al.*, 1979). It has been suggested that PGE_2 is formed non-enzymatically (Friedman, 1978)–a possibility supported by findings in the porcine aorta (Salmon *et al.*, 1978)–and, secondly, that different responsiveness of the ductus to PGE_2 and PGI_2 *in vitro* may not necessarily occur *in vivo*. While the latter issue cannot be resolved without further work, one may also argue that studies showing little formation of PGE_2 in the foetal ductus *in vitro* (Pace-Asciak and Rangaraj, 1977, 1978b; Powell and Solomon, 1977; Friedman, 1978; Terragno *et al.*, 1978) would also require verification *in vivo*. The demonstrated relaxant effect of reduced glutathione (Coceani *et al.*, 1976) implies that a functional endoperoxide isomerase exists in ductal tissue. In this context, it should be noted that 15-hydroperoxy arachidonic acid, an inhibitor of PGI_2 synthesis, enhances the response to PGH_2 (Coceani *et al.*, 1979); presumably, interference with the PGI_2 synthetic reaction results in a greater conversion of PGH_2 to PGE_2.

In our view, the sum of data strongly suggest that the foetal ductus is maintained in a relaxed state by intramural generation of PGE_2. PGI_2, however, may complement PGE_2 action on muscle cells and prevent mechanical obstruction of the vessel by platelet aggregates. Other factors may also contribute to ductus patency. We reported the formation of ductus-relaxing activity during PGI_2 biosynthesis which could not be ascribed to PGI_2 or PGE_2 (Coceani *et al.*, 1978a). The identity of this agent (or agents) remains to be elucidated. Furthermore, ductal tone may be influenced by blood-borne prostaglandins. Indeed, several authors (Challis *et al.*, 1976, 1978; Friedman, W. F. *et al.*, 1978; Lewis *et al.*, 1978) have shown that PGE and PGF compounds (possibly PGE_2 and $PGF_{2\alpha}$) are more abundant in the foetal than in the maternal plasma of sheep and that prostaglandin levels fall abruptly after birth. The ratio of PGE to PGF in foetal plasma varies between investigators. However, all reports are consistent in showing that the amount of circulating PGE is sufficient to exert an effect on the ductus.

The scheme involving a prostaglandin, specifically PGE_2, in ductus patency is based on work in the lamb and, possibly, it also applies to the rat (Sharpe *et al.*, 1974; Sharpe and Larsson, 1975; Sharpe *et al.*, 1975), rabbit (Sharpe and Larsson, 1975; Sharpe *et al.*, 1975), and man (see Section 4.4). Some species, however, may lack this prostaglandin mechanism. Starling and Elliott (1974) reported that inhibitors of prostaglandin synthesis (indomethacin, naproxen) relax rather than contract an isolated preparation of calf ductus arteriosus. On the basis of this and other findings (see Section 4.3) the authors have suggested that prostaglandins may play a role in ductus closure. While their hypothesis will require verification *in vivo*, it may not be a coincidence that the calf ductus generates only minute amounts of PGE_2 (Terragno *et al.*, 1978). Furthermore, according to Starling and Elliott (1974) the action of PGE_2 in the calf at low PO_2 (15–20 mmHg) is biphasic and consists of an initial contraction followed by a relaxation, the latter being abolished by raising the PO_2 to 80–100 mmHg. Another exception, documented by work in our laboratory (unpublished) is that in the guinea-pig inhibitors of prostaglandin synthesis of diverse structure and mechanism of action (i.e. indomethacin, meclofenamate, aspirin, ETA) produce only a marginal ductal contraction *in vitro* or have no effect at all, even at exceedingly high doses (e.g. indomethacin 2.8×10^{-4}/M).

4.2.1 Ontogeny of the prostaglandin mechanism

It is now known that foetal organs acquire an active enzyme system for the synthesis of prostaglandins at an early age (Pace-Asciak, 1978; Pace-Asciak and Rangaraj, 1978a). The same enzymes occur in developing blood vessels, including the ductus arteriosus. Biochemical studies (Powell and Solomon, 1977; Pace-Asciak and Rangaraj, 1978b) have shown that prostaglandin synthetic activity is fully developed in the ductus of foetal lambs and calves at respectively 0.7 and 0.4 gestation. In fact, according to Clyman *et al.* (1978b) PGI_2 synthesis is greater in immature (0.6 gestation) than in mature ductal preparations *in vitro*. Whether this difference is a true feature or rather a reflection of the relatively greater thickness of the intimal layer in the immature vessel (cf. Cassels, 1973) remains to be established. Consistent with an early development of the prostaglandin system is the demonstration of PGE and PGF in the circulation of foetal lambs from 0.7 gestation onwards (Challis *et al.*, 1976).

In vitro experiments with blockers of prostaglandin synthesis indicate that prostaglandins formed in the wall of the immature ductus exert a relaxant action on the muscle (Olley *et al.*, 1976b; Clyman *et al.*, 1978a; Coceani *et al.*, 1978c). Indeed, this prostaglandin relaxing mechanism is more effective in the preterm (0.7 gestation) than in the term ductus and is strong enough to curtail the response of muscle cells to oxygen. It is an outstanding question whether the greater sensitivity of the immature ductus to the blockers reflects a more active synthesis of prostaglandins, as suggested by the findings of Clyman *et al.* (1978b) with PGI_2, or an increased responsiveness to prostaglandins. While active *in vitro*, aspirin is inactive on the ductus of premature lambs (0.6–0.7 gestation) *in vivo* (Rudolph and Heymann, 1978), possibly because the drug does not reach adequate levels in the circulation (cf. Rudolph, 1978a). The same explanation may apply to negative findings in the immature rat (Sharpe *et al.*, 1975).

4.3 DUCTUS CLOSURE

Although it has been known for some time that the rise in blood oxygen tension at birth is the prime stimulus to ductus closure, the mechanism of action of oxygen remains unclear. Several investigators (Kovalčík, 1963; cf. Heymann and Rudolph, 1975) have considered the possibility that oxygen induces ductus closure by eliciting the intramural release of a humoral, or neurohumoral, agent but none of the several substances examined (i.e. acetylcholine, norepinephrine, histamine) fits the role. It is possible, however, that local or blood-borne vasoconstrictors (e.g. bradykinin) contribute to ductus closure by facilitating the action of oxygen (McMurphy *et al.*, 1972; Ikeda *et al.*, 1973; Noel and Cassin, 1976). Alternatively, it has been proposed (Kovalčík, 1963; Fay, 1971) that oxygen acts directly on muscle cells by affecting enzymatic reactions which are essential for the contraction. Regardless of whether the action of oxygen is direct or mediated indirectly, factors other than oxygen, which may or may not be humoral (cf. Ikeda *et al.*, 1973;

Smieško *et al.*, 1978), are likely to be involved in this event and their importance becomes manifest under certain conditions. For example, in obstructive right heart malformations, such as atresia of the pulmonary artery, the ductus often closes despite the severe hypoxaemia. Conversely, the ductus may remain patent in premature infants with normal or near-normal blood oxygen tension.

Prostaglandins and thromboxanes have also been implicated in ductus closure. However, there is no agreement among investigators on the identity of the active substance and its mode of action. Following studies in an isolated preparation of calf ductus, Starling and Elliott (1972, 1974) proposed that prostaglandins play an intermediary role in the sequence of events leading to ductus closure. Their hypothesis, which envisages $PGF_{2\alpha}$ as the *messenger* of the oxygen response, receives support from the demonstration that this compound constricts the ductus (see Table 4.1) and that this effect is oxygen-dependent. Inhibitors of prostaglandin synthesis and action reverse the effect of oxygen on the ductus. Additional support comes from the notion that prostaglandin biosynthesis requires molecular oxygen (Nugteren and Van Dorp, 1965; Samuelsson, 1965) and the finding that $PGF_{2\alpha}$, unlike PGE_2, is not degraded by ductal enzymes (Pace-Asciak and Rangaraj, 1978b). $PGF_{2\alpha}$ may therefore accumulate in ductal tissue following postnatal elevation of blood oxygen tension. Although attractive, the proposal of Starling and Elliott has not been confirmed by findings in other species. Different investigators (Coceani *et al.*, 1975, 1978c; Clyman *et al.*, 1978a) have shown that the constrictor response of the isolated lamb ductus to oxygen remains unchanged or is enhanced by treatment with inhibitors of prostaglandin synthesis. Moreover, $PGF_{2\alpha}$ does not constrict the patent ductus *in vivo*, both prenatally (lamb) (Friedman, W. F. *et al.*, 1978) and postnatally (infant) (Starling *et al.*, 1978a), and may even re-open the closing ductus (rat) (Sharpe and Larsson, 1975). Whether *in vitro* or *in vivo*, effective doses of $PGF_{2\alpha}$ are far greater than those of PGE_1 or PGE_2 (Coceani *et al.*, 1975; Sharpe and Larsson, 1975; Clyman *et al.*, 1978c), which may indicate a pharmacological action rather than a physiological function. In summary, the evidence is overwhelmingly against a direct role of $PGF_{2\alpha}$ in ductus closure and findings in the calf, if verified *in vivo*, would signify a peculiar evolutionary departure.

An alternative scheme implicating a member of the prostaglandin system in ductus closure has been proposed by Friedman (1978). In his view, TXA_2, which is the most potent vasoconstrictor derived from arachidonic acid, is responsible (presumably in concert with oxygen although this is not discussed) for the contraction of ductal muscle at birth. Since ductal tissue lacks the TXA_2 synthetic enzyme (Pace-Asciak and Rangaraj, 1977, 1978b; Powell and Solomon, 1977; Friedman, 1978; Terragno *et al.*, 1978), Friedman assumes that TXA_2 acting on the ductus originates from the lungs and that a greater amount of TXA_2 is released during the immediate postnatal period. Indeed, TXA_2 synthetic activity is lower in foetal than in neonatal or adult lungs of sheep (Friedman, 1978), ox (Powell and Solomon, 1978) and rabbit (Sun and McGuire, 1978). However, there are several facts which argue against Friedman's proposal. TXA_2 is inactive on ductal muscle, at least *in vitro* (Coceani *et al.*, 1978a). Secondly, TXA_2 is an exceedingly labile compound (Dusting *et al.*, 1978) and would appear unsuitable as a circulating hormone and the cause of a sustained contraction of the ductus. Moreover, TXA_2 is released from lungs only under extreme, and quite unphysiological, conditions (e.g. anaphylactic shock) (Palmer *et al.*, 1973; cf. Gryglewski *et al.*, 1978). Finally, the TXA_2 synthesis enzymes are apparently absent in the lungs of certain species, including man (Sun *et al.*, 1977).

Although $PGF_{2\alpha}$ and TXA_2 are probably not important as ductal constrictors, some prostaglandins may contribute to ductus closure by other means.

One possibility, suggested by our work *in vitro* (Coceani and Olley, 1973; Coceani *et al.*, 1975, 1978a), is that PGE_2 becomes less effective postnatally, thus removing its relaxant effect on the ductus. Our results, however, are at variance with those of Clyman *et al.* (1977, 1978c) who found that the threshold of action of PGE_1 and PGE_2 at low and high PO_2 is identical. The reason for this discrepancy is not clear, though technical factors may be important (Coceani and Olley, 1977). Experiments *in vivo* cannot provide a precise measurement of effectiveness of PGE_2 under different levels of blood oxygenation because, prenatally, the ductus is maximally or near maximally dilated and, postnatally, the magnitude of response depends not only on the intrinsic sensitivity of muscle cells to the compound but also on the amount of compound reaching the vessel after pulmonary and systemic inactivation, and on the occurrence of biochemical (Frazer and Brady, 1978) and structural (Hörnblad, 1967; Hörnblad *et al.*, 1969; Fay and Cooke, 1972) changes in ductal tissue which may affect the viability of the muscle. Nevertheless, intravenous doses of PGE_1 and PGE_2 required for re-opening a closing ductus in newborn pigs with normal blood oxygenation (Starling *et al.*, 1976) are 10–20 times higher than those effective in hypoxaemic infants (see Section 4.4.1.1).

Alternatively, it has been speculated that the postnatal rise in blood oxygen tension may induce ductus closure by reducing the endogenous synthesis of PGE_2 in favour of the less active PGI_2. This possibility, raised by Vane (cf. Coceani *et al.*, 1979), is not supported by studies of prostaglandin biosynthesis in homogenates of foetal and neonatal lamb ductus (Pace-Asciak and Rangaraj, 1978b). However, further work employing the intact ductus will be required to settle this question.

4.4 CLINICAL EXPERIENCE

The evidence that patency of the foetal ductus arteriosus is an active process mediated by a prostaglandin and the demonstration that the ductus could be closed *in utero* by inhibition of prostaglandin synthesis led to pharmacological manipulation of this vessel in the clinical situations. This provides an example of basic research leading directly to an advance in patient care.

4.4.1 Treatment with prostaglandins

During intrauterine life the arrangement of the circulation often minimizes the effect of many congenital heart malformations. At birth as the circulation adapts to an independent existence, the full effects of such malformations become manifest. Prolongation of ductus patency by an infusion of PGE_1 or PGE_2 has proved valuable in many such patients (Elliott *et al.*, 1975; Christensen and Fabricus, 1975; Olley *et al.*, 1976a; Heymann and Rudolph, 1977; Neutze *et al.*, 1977).

4.4.1.1 *Ductus-dependent pulmonary blood flow*

Pulmonary atresia and tricuspid atresia typify a group of malformations in which pulmonary blood flow through the normal channels is impossible or markedly reduced. In these lesions the ductus arteriosus may be the only major channel by which desaturated blood can reach the lungs and undergo gas exchange. Fortunately for such patients normal ductus closure is often delayed for several hours or even days permitting recognition of the heart defect and time for intervention. However, despite the fact that the major stimulus to ductus closure (i.e. the rise in arterial oxygen saturation) is lacking, the ductus does begin to close, producing progressive reduction in pulmonary blood flow and consequently in the volume of oxygenated blood returning to the left atrium. This results in a progressive fall in systemic arterial oxygen saturation and eventually metabolic acidosis which both tend to increase pulmonary vasoconstriction and further compromise pulmonary blood flow. Without intervention, these patients usually die within a few days of birth. The expression 'ductus-dependent pulmonary blood flow' embraces all such lesions.

An infusion of PGE_1, or PGE_2, is an alternative to emergency surgery in such patients. By reversing systemic hypoxia it provides time to correct metabolic acidosis and to schedule surgery on a semi-elective basis.

PGE_1, 0.03–0.10 (μg/kg)/min can be given either intra-arterially via an umbilical artery catheter positioned with its tip just proximal to the aortic end of the ductus arteriosus or intravenously. Most patients so treated have been less than 24 hours of age. However, the oldest patient to respond successfully was 29 days old. The effectiveness of PGE_1 is demonstrated by a rise in arterial PO_2 in excess of 10 mmHg which usually occurs within a few minutes of starting the infusion. Enlargement of the ductus arteriosus can be confirmed angiographically. Because these patients have initial PaO_2s which fall on the steepest portion of the oxygen dissociation curve, PGE_1 action leads to a marked increase in arterial oxygen saturation and hence in the amount of oxygen available to tissues. Occasionally, the response may be more delayed, or an initial rise in PaO_2 may be followed by a further increase over the next few hours. While the major benefit is due to dilatation of the ductus arteriosus, PGE_1 also produces pulmonary vasodilatation (Carlson *et al.*, 1969; Kadowitz *et al.*, 1974) which should help to increase pulmonary blood flow.

PGE_1 has been used mainly as a short-term emergency measure, followed by semi-elective palliative surgery once the patient's condition has stabilized. Lewis and Lurie (1978), however, reported successful prolonged use of PGE_1, 0.1 (μg/kg)/min without significant side-effects in a premature infant with severe tetralogy of Fallot. PGE_1 was initially given intra-arterially followed by intravenously for a total of 29 days during which the ductus remained fully responsive. Within 3 hours of stopping the infusion the ductus constricted, but dilated again when PGE_1 infusion was restarted.

Whatever the underlying cardiac defect, the response to PGE_1 is remarkably consistent and tolerance does not appear to develop. In practice, it is often possible to reduce the dosage while maintaining an adequate response. PGE_2, used in a few patients, is as effective as PGE_1 in dilating the ductus and elevating the PaO_2 (Olley *et al.*, 1978b).

Failure to respond to intra-arterial infusions of prostaglandins may result from an incorrect catheter position or be due to an abnormally situated ductus. With intravenous infusions, the large right-to-left atrial shunt invariably present in these cardiac malformations ensures that an adequate dose of PGE_1 reaches the ductus before significant inactivation occurs. A totally closed ductus is unlikely to respond to PGE_1. Indeed, we have been unable to re-open the ductus arteriosus in newborn lambs varying from a few days to 3–4 weeks of age even with doses 10–100 times higher than those used clinically (Olley *et al.*, 1978a). Occasional failures may also be ascribed to congenital absence or intra-uterine closure of the ductus.

4.4.1.2 *Ductus-dependent systemic circulation*

Aortic atresia is not an uncommon congenital heart malformation and is usually associated with severe hypoplasia of the left ventricle and mitral atresia. This particular malformation is surgically not correctable, but illustrates a situation in which the entire systemic blood flow, including the coronary circulation, is supported by the right ventricle and depends on right-to-left flow through the ductus arteriosus. When the ductus begins to close, systemic perfusion falls, resulting in myocardial failure and severe tissue hypoxia with secondary metabolic acidosis. Such patients succumb within the first days of life and few cardiologists would consider intervention. However, there are other malformations which carry a better overall prognosis in which the systemic circulation is partially ductus-dependent.

In most examples of interruption of the aortic arch, blood flow to the descending aorta is also derived from the right ventricle via the ductus arteriosus. Furthermore, Rudolph (1978b) has shown how the ductus, when patent, can act as a bypass for severe juxtaductal aortic coarctations. In both conditions, the onset of ductal closure compromises blood flow in the descending aorta causing progressive metabolic acidosis, decreased responsiveness to diuretics and difficulty in adjusting digoxin dosage. Medical treatment for such patients is notoriously unsuccessful and surgery carries an extremely high risk largely due to their poor pre-operative condition.

PGE_1, infused into the pulmonary artery end of the ductus arteriosus, can restore systemic perfusion and provide time to correct the metabolic consequences of the heart defect. Although these patients are usually much less hypoxic than patients with ductus-dependent pulmonary blood flow, the ductus still appears to respond to PGE_1 as judged by abolition of pressure gradients between the pulmonary artery and the descending aorta, by clinical reappearance of palpable femoral pulses, and by restored responsiveness to diuretics. We have reported the successful use of PGE_2 in a patient with aortic interruption (Radford *et al.*, 1976) while Lang *et al.* (1977) used PGE_1. Berman *et al.* (1978) recently described the use of PGE_1 in 13 non-hypoxic infants with aortic arch lesions. Each of the four patients with interruption and a patent ductus showed an increase in descending aorta pressure and a reduced pressure gradient between the pulmonary artery and the descending aorta in response to PGE_1, 0.025–0.100 (μg/kg)/min. Six out of seven patients with coarctation and a patent ductus also benefited from PGE_1 treatment. Two infants in whom the ductus was completely closed and a third with a patent ductus who was 5 months old failed to respond.

Thus, it appears that patients with ductus-dependent systemic blood flow can benefit from pre-operative infusion of PGE_1. The effect on the ductus outweighs any potentially adverse effect which might result from pulmonary vasodilatation.

4.4.1.3 *Transposition of the great arteries*

Patients with complete transposition of the great arteries (TGA) depend for survival on mixing between the systemic and pulmonary circulations. While this mixing may occur at atrial, ventricular or ductal level, the ventricular septum is often intact. Atrial septostomy using a balloon-tipped catheter improves arterial oxygen saturation in these severely hypoxic infants but occasionally little improvement occurs despite an apparently adequate atrial tear. This poor response may be due to a relatively low pulmonary blood flow in this haemodynamic situation. By dilating the ductus arteriosus with an infusion of PGE_1 it is possible to increase systemic-to-pulmonary artery shunting and consequently pulmonary blood flow. Increased pulmonary venous return to the left atrium tends to stretch that chamber and increase left-to-right (i.e. pulmonary-to-systemic) shunting. The overall effect is an improved mixing between the two circuits.

Ten newborns with complete TGA and a patent ductus arteriosus, who were hypoxaemic despite an apparently successful septostomy, have been treated with PGE_1 (Olley *et al.*, 1979). Six of these patients had an intact ventricular septum. PGE_1 at a dose of 0.1 (μg/kg)/min had a beneficial effect in eight out of the 10 infants. Systemic oxygen saturation rose from an average value of 26% to 53%. In the remaining two patients, PGE_1 had no effect; however, treatment lasted only 10 minutes. Unfortunately all patients experienced a fall in blood oxygen levels as soon as the infusion was discontinued and all eventually had to have a surgical septostomy. Two patients were also given PGE_1 after surgery and were successfully weaned a few days later. Neutze *et al.* (1977) have also reported similar results in three patients with transposition and speculate that at least part of the beneficial effect depends on pulmonary vasodilatation rather than increased ductal shunting.

Dilatation of the ductus arteriosus and increased pulmonary blood flow are not entirely beneficial in TGA and may indeed precipitate congestive heart failure especially if the atrial communication is inadequate. PGE_1 is, therefore, most useful as a temporary therapy until a more definitive treatment can be arranged.

4.4.1.4 *Other lesions*

PGE_1 can be used as a therapeutic challenge in patients with pulmonary atresia or severe pulmonary stenosis combined with an anomalous and possibly obstructed pulmonary venous drainage (Freedom *et al.*, 1978). This combination may occur in the asplenia syndrome. If PGE_1 produces radiographic pulmonary oedema, it suggests that the pulmonary veins are indeed obstructed and that a surgical anastomosis to increase pulmonary blood flow is unlikely to benefit the patient.

Ebstein's anomaly (in which the septal leaflet of the tricuspid valve is displaced into the right ventricle), and congenital tricupsid incompetence often result in inadequate forward flow from the right ventricle especially when pulmonary vascular resistance remains high. Right-to-left atrial shunting, secondary to the tricuspid valve problem, causes severe systemic hypoxia. PGE_1 might help such patients by opening the ductus and perhaps by reducing pulmonary vascular resistance thus allowing the right ventricle to eject against a lower resistance. We have observed a rise in arterial oxygen saturation following PGE_1 in three newborns with Ebstein's anomaly. Unfortunately, however, the effect of PGE_1 was not sustained and all three patients eventually succumbed.

4.4.1.5 *Side-effects*

Side-effects associated with PGE_1 treatment are not infrequent and are more common with intravenous than with intra-arterial administration because a significant proportion of the compound reaches the central nervous system (Heymann and Rudolph, 1977; Olley *et al.*, 1978b). Regardless of the route of PGE_1 administration, however, side-effects rapidly subside upon stopping the treatment.

Pyrexia occurs in approximately one-third of the patients given intravenous PGE_1 but is never severe enough to justify discontinuation of the infusion. This complication probably results from a direct action of the compound on anterior hypothalamic neurons (cf. Coceani and Pace-Asciak, 1976).

Apnoea has also been encountered in several patients receiving intravenous PGE_1. The mechanism of this effect is unclear, though it is known that prostaglandins act upon respiratory centres (cf. Coceani and Pace-Asciak, 1976). The risk of apnoea necessitates constant monitoring of all patients during prostaglandin administration.

Mild hypotension due to systemic vasodilatation is also common but in our experience has never been severe nor has it created problems during subsequent surgery.

Patients may also manifest a rather curious muscular hyperactivity often referred to by the attending nurse as the baby being 'jittery'. We have observed the same phenomenon in unsedated newborn lambs during PGE_1 infusion in a dose range between 1 and 10 (μg/kg)/min. Its mechanism remains unexplained. Fariello *et al.* (1977), while monitoring the EEG in eight patients during PGE_1 or PGE_2 infusion, did not observe any seizure activity and, in fact, reported a trend for the tracing to become better organized.

Intra-arterial infusion of PGE_1 may be associated with regional cutaneous flushing due to the dilatory action of the compound on a territorial artery. The flush often fades within 20–30 minutes even without a reduction in dosage and does not limit therapy, although it may produce a dramatic Harlequin effect.

Because the most troublesome complications of PGE_1 therapy result from a disturbance of CNS function, PGI_2, which is seemingly free of central effects (O'Grady, 1979), would be an attractive alternative agent even though it is a weak ductal relaxant. However, PGI_2 is not easily administered due to its lability in aqueous medium at physiological pH. Possibly, stable analogues of PGI_2 may become available for trial in the future.

Recently we have observed two serious complications of prolonged umbilical artery catheterization which has led us to limit the use of this route of administration to 48 hours. One patient experienced a non-fatal caecal perforation while a second had a massive and fatal hepatic infarction.

Gittenberger-De Groot *et al.* (1978) have described histological changes consisting of medial oedema, separation of medial components, pathological interruptions of the internal elastic lamina and intimal lacerations extending into the media, in the ductus of four patients who had received PGE_1 (0.10 (μg/kg)/min from 10 hours to 3 days). They suggested that PGE_1 might have a specific weakening effect on the ductal wall rendering it liable to laceration. Subsequent studies by Dr Gittenberger-De Groot on material from patients given much lower doses of PGE_1, 0.01 (μg/kg)/min failed to show the same changes (personal communication). Clearly, further studies are required. However, no reports of haemorrhage or ductus rupture in patients given PGE_1 have so far appeared, nor have we encountered a ductus aneurysm or any abnormal dilatation of the aortic wall in our follow-up studies which include repeat cardiac catheterization in 11 patients.

4.4.1.6 *Benefits*

As a short-term procedure the beneficial effect of PGE_1 is often dramatic and can probably be maintained for as long as one wishes to continue an intravenous infusion. This is impractical for more than a few weeks, and an alternative agent effective by the oral or subcutaneous route would be desirable.

Starling *et al.* (1978b) have studied the effects of three methylated analogues of PGE_1 and PGE_2 on the ductus arteriosus of swine *in vivo*. All three compounds re-opened the ductus when given intravenously, intramuscularly or orally and the effect of each dose persisted for 4 hours, or more, in many instances. Side-effects included sedation, apnoea, and a transient drop in heart rate and blood pressure. More animal studies are probably needed before human trials of long-term oral treatment are initiated. However, the possibility of maintaining ductus patency beyond the immediate postnatal period would eliminate the necessity of palliative surgery in many ductus-dependent lesions or, at least, would defer it for several months.

While the use of PGE_1 reduces the peri-operative mortality of palliative surgery performed soon after birth, it remains to be demonstrated whether it will have a significant impact on long-term survival of patients with complex cardiac malformations. Perhaps, the most significant effect will be on the group of infants with aortic arch lesions in whom the long-term prognosis is good provided they can survive corrective surgery in the neonatal period.

4.4.2 Treatment with inhibitors of prostaglandin synthesis

Persistent ductus arteriosus (PDA) in premature infants, with or without the respiratory distress syndrome, is a common problem in newborn nurseries and is almost always due to failure of the oxygen-triggered mechanism(s) normally responsible for its closure. In contrast, PDA beyond the neonatal period is probably due to inadequate development of the ductal muscle or some other structural anomaly of the vessel wall and attempts to induce closure with indomethacin have been unsuccessful (Kostis, 1977; McCarthy *et al.*, 1977; McGrath *et al.*, 1977).

The incidence of PDA increases with prematurity and may be greater than 80% with infants under 1000 g birth weight. When the patent ductus causes a significant left-to-right shunting, it may compromise recovery from the respiratory distress syndrome and result in a progressive deterioration in pulmonary function with the possible development of bronchopulmonary dysplasia. This high incidence of ductus patency may reflect decreased sensitivity of the immature ductus to oxygen (McMurphy *et al.*, 1972; Noel and Cassin, 1976), increased activity of the intramural prostaglandin mechanism (Olley *et al.*, 1976b; Clyman *et al.*, 1978a; Coceani *et al.*, 1978c), or a combination of both. Blood-borne prostaglandins may also contribute to ductus patency. Indeed, there is evidence that PGE levels may be increased in infants with both respiratory distress syndrome and PDA (Friedman and Demers, 1978; Lucas and Mitchell, 1978), but this needs confirmation (Mitchell *et al.*, 1978).

In 1976, two groups of investigators (Friedman *et al.*, 1976; Heymann *et al.*, 1976) simultaneously reported the result of their initial trials of pharmacologic closure of the ductus. Large doses of indomethacin (2.5–5.0 mg/kg) given orally or rectally caused the ductus to close but the treatment was associated with significant renal dysfunction (Friedman *et al.*, 1976). Salicylates although successful in one patient were not generally effective but indomethacin in doses of 0.1–0.2 mg/kg produced ductus closure without evidence of renal dysfunction (Heymann *et al.*, 1976). Both groups have recently published follow-up studies on a larger number of patients (Heymann, 1978; Merritt *et al.*, 1978). Using an indomethacin dose schedule of 0.2 mg/kg (orally or intravenously) every 24 hours to a maximum of 0.6 mg/kg per treatment course, Merritt *et al.* (1978) obtained prompt constriction of the ductus arteriosus in 31 out of 35 patients with consequent alleviation of left-to-right shunting. The remaining four patients underwent PDA ligation because of worsening cardiopulmonary function. In 19 of the successfully treated infants, the ductus re-opened and in 10 out of 11 given a second course of indomethacin, the ductus closed again. In the remaining eight patients spontaneous closure of the ductus ultimately occurred. The mean gestational age of their patients was around 30 weeks with an average birth weight of 1361 g. Thirty-nine out of 60 infants (65%) treated with indomethacin by Heymann (1978) showed a significant reduction of shunting with eventual disappearance of the murmur, alleviation of symptoms, presumably as a result of ductus closure. A further 14 out of the 60 infants (23%) showed a marked improvement and six a moderate improvement. Thus only one patient failed to respond to indomethacin. Eight out of the 60 patients eventually underwent surgical ligation after responding only partially or relapsing after a good initial response. In both these studies indomethacin was first given to most patients within 2–5 days of the onset of heart failure.

In contrast to these successful results, Neal *et al.* (1977) succeeded in closing the ductus in only two out of 11 patients. However, their patients received indomethacin at an older age and had more severe lung disease. McCarthy *et al.* (1978) attempted to relate indomethacin responsiveness to *actual age* at time of therapy. Of their 18 patients, eight responded to indomethacin with closure of the ductus. All these eight infants were 33 weeks actual age or younger, while patients 34–36 weeks of age improved without complete closure and those over 36 weeks failed to respond. This experience would accord with experimental data reviewed above (see Section 4.2.1).

Indomethacin is sparingly soluble in an aqueous medium (Krasowska *et al.*, 1972) and is often administered as a suspension either rectally or via a nasogastric tube. This raises the possibility that variable dosage or inadequate absorption may be responsible for some or all infants who failed to respond to indomethacin. We have measured plasma concentrations of indomethacin in 50 patients given 65 courses of the drug. In our series, the drug was completely dissolved in phosphate buffer. Eighteen out of the 50 patients underwent complete ductal closure while a further 15 had echocardiographic or clinical evidence of reduced left-to-right shunting. Plasma concentrations in those treated successfully were not significantly different from those who failed to respond to indomethacin. There was no difference in gestational age, birth weight, time of appearance of the ductal shunt, time of onset of heart failure, or duration of medical therapy prior to indomethacin in the two groups. Friedman, Whitman *et al.* (1978) measured plasma levels in two premature infants given indomethacin and found a considerably prolonged half-life (21–24 h) compared with full-term healthy newborns (14.7 h) or with healthy adults (2–3 h). Thus, in our experience there appears to be no distinguishing feature to identify patients unlikely to respond to prostaglandin synthetase blockade. A possible factor, as yet uninvestigated, might be the concentration of circulating PGE and, indeed, the level of endogenous prostaglandin production in all tissues. Conceivably, patients with high blood levels of prostaglandins might more easily escape from prostaglandin synthetase blockade or may require higher doses of indomethacin over a longer period of time to achieve ductus closure (cf. Lucas and Mitchell, 1978). If such escape from blockade does occur then the ductus is likely to respond to circulating PGE with a greater relaxation (Coceani *et al.*, (1978a).

We have also used ibuprofen (Motrin) as an alternative to indomethacin in three patients. Results were negative; however, blood levels of the drug were below the usual therapeutic range in adults.

The use of indomethacin is associated with potential complications. With large doses, renal function is temporarily impaired. Heymann (1978) has described one patient who developed nephrotic syndrome at the age of 4 months and subsequently recovered. It is not clear whether this episode was related to the use of indomethacin. Necrotizing enterocolitis, increased incidence of intracranial haemorrhage and gastro-intestinal haemorrhage are additional potential complications which have occurred in patients given indomethacin. However, these are common problems in the newborn nursery and to date there is no evidence that their incidence is increased in patients receiving indomethacin. Nevertheless, Friedman, Whitman *et al.* (1978) have confirmed that platelet aggregation may be suppressed for up to 4 days after indomethacin. Indomethacin (1.9–2.5 mg/kg) has been shown to increase the constrictor response of the pulmonary circulation to hypoxia in neonatal goats (Tyler *et al.*, 1975) but there is no evidence as yet that this causes any problems in clinical usage.

Chloroquine (possibly acting as a prostaglandin antagonist, Manku and Horrobin, 1976), has also been used to close the ductus arteriosus in one full term and two premature infants (Collins *et al.*, 1976). All three patients were given intravenous or intramuscular doses of 3–4 mg/kg of the drug and all showed a rapid clinical response. No side-effects were observed but no long-term follow-up especially relating to the possible occurrence of retinopathy has been reported.

In summary, the ductus can be completely closed with indomethacin in about 50% of premature infants especially those under 35 weeks of age. Most of the remainder show evidence of reduced left-to-right shunt and may subsequently undergo spontaneous closure. However, some patients do not respond or relapse after apparently successful closure and eventually require surgical ligation. The factors which determine responsiveness of the ductus to drugs remain unknown, but may be related to the age and the activity of the prostaglandin synthesis enzyme in the ductus and other organs. The final role for 'medical closure' of the ductus needs to be defined by carefully conducted randomized trials in which both the time and type of intervention are compared. Surgical ligation remains a safe, rapid and certain alternative to indomethacin.

4.5 CONCLUSION

Research in the past few years has established that prenatal patency of the ductus arteriosus is determined by an endogenous prostaglandin. There is debate on whether the active compound is PGE_2 or PGI_2. In our view the evidence favours PGE_2 for this role. PGI_2, though a weaker ductal relaxant than PGE_2, may complement PGE_2 action on muscle cells and may also contribute to ductus patency through its antithrombotic action. This prostaglandin-mediated relaxing mechanism develops at an early age, reaches maximal activity at 0.7 gestation and abates thereafter. It is conceivable that the loss in prostaglandin activity from 0.7 gestation onwards represents a priming mechanism for postnatal closure of the vessel. Knowledge of prostaglandin function in ductal muscle has afforded a new approach to the management of children in whom ductus patency or closure may be beneficial.

Several outstanding issues, both conceptual and practical, remain to be settled and they are listed below.

(1) The presence and activity in ductal tissue of the enzyme catalyzing the formation of PGE_2 (the putative effector of ductus patency) needs to be established by unequivocal means.

(2) The relative importance of local vs. blood-borne PGE_2 in determining prenatal patency of the ductus.
(3) The role of prostaglandins in ductus closure.
(4) The involvement of prostaglandins in extraductal events contributing to foetal vascular homeostasis and postnatal adjustments of the circulation.

Questions relating to the clinical use of prostaglandins and blockers of prostaglandin synthesis are:

(1) Safety of prolonged administration of prostaglandins to the newborn.
(2) Safety and effectiveness of presently available prostaglandin synthetase inhibitors in closing the ductus of the premature infant when compared with other possible methods such as surgery or controlled high FIO_2 (Yamanouchi, 1978). The concurrent use of indomethacin with a high FIO_2 may be more effective than either method used separately.
(3) Safety of treating the pregnant mother with inhibitors of prostaglandin synthesis.

In the future, the development of long-acting analogues of PGE_2 and PGI_2 and of more specific inhibitors of prostaglandin synthesis and action, along with readily available methods of monitoring blood levels of prostaglandins should result in further exciting clinical applications.

Acknowledgements

The authors acknowledge the contribution of the staff and fellows in the Divisions of Cardiology and Neonatology to the clinical studies, and in particular the support of Drs R. D. Rowe and P. R. Swyer. The contribution of Dr I. Bishai and Mrs E. Bodach, Mr F. Hamilton, and Mrs E. White to the animal studies is also gratefully recognized. Mrs D. Campbell provided expert secretarial assistance during the preparation of this manuscript. Financial support was received from the Ontario Heart Foundation and the Upjohn Company.

References

Berman, W., Heymann, M. A., Whitman, V. and Rudolph, A. M. (1978). Dilatation of the ductus arteriosus by prostaglandin E_1 in aortic arch abnormalities. *Circulation*, **58 (Suppl. 2)**, 44

Carlson, L. A., Ekelund, L. G. and Orö, L. (1969). Circulatory and respiratory effects of different doses of prostaglandin E_1 in man. *Acta Physiol. Scand.*, **75**, 161

Cassels, D. E. (1973). *The Ductus Arteriosus*, pp. 37–50 (Springfield: Charles C. Thomas)

Challis, J. R. G., Dilley, S. R., Robinson, J. S. and Thorburn, G. D. (1976). Prostaglandins in the circulation of the foetal lamb. *Prostaglandins*, **11**, 1041

Challis, J. R. G., Hart, I., Louis, T. M., Mitchell, M. D., Jenkin, G., Robinson, J. S. and Thorburn, G. D. (1978). Prostaglandins in the sheep fetus: implications for fetal function. In:

F. Coceani and P. M. Olley (eds.). *Prostaglandins and Perinatal Medicine, Advances in Prostaglandin and Thromboxane Research*, Vol. IV, pp. 115–132 (New York: Raven Press)

Christensen, N. C. and Fabricus, J. (1975). Medical manipulation of the ductus arteriosus. *Lancet*, **ii**, 406

Clyman, R. I., Heymann, M. A. and Rudolph, A. M. (1977). Ductus arteriosus: responses to prostaglandin E_1 at high and low oxygen concentrations. *Prostaglandins*, **13**, 219

Clyman, R. I., Mauray, F., Heymann, M. A. and Rudolph, A. M. (1978a). Ductus arteriosus: developmental response to oxygen and indomethacin. *Prostaglandins*, **15**, 993

Clyman, R. I., Mauray, F., Koerper, M. A., Wiemer, F., Heymann, M. A. and Rudolph, A. M. (1978b). Formation of prostacyclin (PGI_2) by the ductus arteriosus of foetal lambs at different stages of gestation. *Prostaglandins*, **16**, 633

Clyman, R. I., Wong, L., Heymann, M. A. and Rudolph, A. M. (1978c). Responsiveness of the lamb ductus arteriosus to prostaglandins and their metabolites. *Prostaglandins*, **15**, 325

Coceani, F., Bishai, I., Bodach, E. P., White, E. P. and Olley, P. M. (1979). On the evidence implicating PGE_2 rather than PGI_2 in the patency of the foetal ductus arteriosus. In: *Workshop on Prostacyclin and its Analogues* (S. Bergström and J. R. Vane, eds.) (New York: Raven Press) (In press)

Coceani, F., Bishai, I., White, E., Bodach, E. and Olley, P. M. (1978a). Action of prostaglandins, endoperoxides, and thromboxanes on the lamb ductus arteriosus. *Am. J. Physiol.*, **234**, H117

Coceani, F., Bodach, E., White, E., Bishai, I. and Olley, P. M. (1978b). Prostaglandin I_2 is less relaxant than prostaglandin E_2 on the lamb ductus arteriosus. *Prostaglandins*, **15**, 551

Coceani, F. and Olley, P. M. (1973). The response of the ductus arteriosus to prostaglandins. *Can. J. Physiol. Pharmacol.*, **51**, 220

Coceani, F. and Olley, P. M. (1977). Letter to the Editor. Oxygen tension and the response of the ductus arteriosus to prostaglandins E_1 and E_2. *Prostaglandins*, **14**, 595

Coceani, F., Olley, P. M., Bishai, I., Bodach, E. and White, E. P. (1978c). Significance of the prostaglandin system to the control of muscle tone of the ductus arteriosus. In: F. Coceani and P. M. Olley (eds.), *Prostaglandins and Perinatal Medicine, Advances in Prostaglandin and Thromboxane Research*, Vol. IV, pp. 325–333 (New York: Raven Press)

Coceani, F., Olley, P. M. and Bodach, E. (1975). Lamb ductus arteriosus: effect of prostaglandin synthesis inhibitors on the muscle tone and the response to prostaglandin E_2. *Prostaglandins*, **9**, 299

Coceani, F., Olley, P. M. and Bodach, E. (1976). Prostaglandins: a possible regulator of muscle tone in the ductus arteriosus. In: B. Samuelsson and R. Paoletti (eds.), *Advances in Prostaglandin and Thromboxane Research*, Vol. I, pp. 417–424 (New York: Raven Press)

Coceani, F. and Pace-Asciak, C. R. (1976). Prostaglandins and the central nervous system. In: S. M. M. Karim (ed.), *Prostaglandins: Physiological, Pharmacological and Pathological Aspects*, pp. 1–36 (Lancaster: MTP Press)

Collins, G., Outerbridge, E., Manku, M. S. and Horrobin, D. F. (1976). Chloroquine as prostaglandin antagonist in treatment of patent ductus arteriosus. *Lancet*, **ii**, 810

Dusting, G. J., Moncada, S., Mullane, K. M. and Vane, J. R. (1978). Biotransformation of arachidonic acid in the circulation of the dog. *Br. J. Pharmacol.*, **63**, 359P

Elliott, R. B. and Starling, M. B. (1972). The effect of prostaglandin $F_{2\alpha}$ in the closure of the ductus arteriosus. *Prostaglandins*, **2**, 399

Elliott, R. B., Starling, M. B. and Neutze, J. M. (1975). Medical manipulation of the ductus arteriosus. *Lancet*, **i**, 140

Fariello, R., Olley, P. M. and Coceani, F. (1977). Neurological and electroencephalographic changes in newborns treated with prostaglandins E_1 and E_2. *Prostaglandins*, **13**, 901

Fay, F. S. (1971). Guinea-pig ductus arteriosus. I. Cellular and metabolic basis for oxygen sensitivity. *Am. J. Physiol.*, **221**, 470

Fay, F. S. and Cooke, P. H. (1972). Guinea-pig ductus arteriosus. II. Irreversible closure after birth. *Am. J. Physiol.*, **222**, 841

Flower, R. J. (1974). Drugs which inhibit prostaglandin biosynthesis. *Pharmacol. Rev.*, **26**, 33

Frazer, P. D. and Brady, F. O. (1978). Superoxide dismutase in bovine fetal ductus arteriosus, thoracic aorta, and pulmonary and umbilical arteries. *Proc. Soc. Exp. Biol. Med.*, **159**, 30

Freedom, R. M., Olley, P. M., Coceani, F. and Rowe, R. D. (1978). The prostaglandin challenge: a test to unmask obstructed total anomalous pulmonary venous connections in the asplenia syndrome. *Br. Heart J.*, **40**, 91

Friedman, W. F. (1978). Studies of the response of the ductus arteriosus. In: *The Ductus Arteriosus, Proceedings of the Seventy-fifth Ross Conference on Pediatric Research*, p. 93 (Columbus: Ross Laboratories)

Friedman, W. F., Hirschklau, M. J., Printz, M. P., Pitlick, P. T. and Kirkpatrick, S. E. (1976). Pharmacologic closure of patent ductus arteriosus in the premature infant. *N. Engl. J. Med.*, **295**, 526

Friedman, W. F., Printz, M. P. and Kirkpatrick, S. E. (1978). Blockers of prostaglandin synthesis: a novel therapy in the management of the premature human infant with patent ductus arteriosus. In: F. Coceani and P. M. Olley (eds.), *Prostaglandins and Perinatal Medicine, Advances in Prostaglandin and Thromboxane Research*, Vol. IV, pp. 373–381 (New York: Raven Press)

Friedman, Z. and Demers, L. M. (1978). Essential fatty acids, prostaglandins, and respiratory distress syndrome of the newborn. *Pediatrics*, **61**, 341

Friedman, Z., Whitman, V., Maisels, M. J., Berman, W. Jr., Marks, K. H. and Vesell, E. S. (1978). Indomethacin disposition and indomethacin-induced platelet dysfunction in premature infants. *J. Clin. Pharmacol.*, **18**, 272

Gittenberger-De Groot, A. C., Moulaert, A. J., Harinck, E. and Becker, A. E. (1978). Histopathology of the ductus arteriosus after prostaglandin E_1 administration in ductus-dependent cardiac anomalies. *Br. Heart J.*, **40**, 215

Gryglewski, R. J., Korbut, R., Ocetkiewicz, A., Splawinski, J., Wojtaszek, B. and Sweis, J. (1978). Lungs as a generator of prostacyclin-hypothesis on physiological significance. *Naunyn-Schmiedeberg's Arch. Pharmacol.*, **304**, 45

Heymann, M. A. (1978). Management of patent ductus arteriosus with prostaglandin synthetase inhibitors. In: *The Ductus Arteriosus, Proceedings of the Seventy-fifth Ross Conference on Pediatric Research*, p. 166 (Columbus: Ross Laboratories)

Heymann, M. A. and Rudolph, A. M. (1975). Control of the ductus arteriosus. *Physiol. Rev.*, **55**, 62

Heymann, M. A. and Rudolph, A. M. (1976). Effects of acetylsalicyclic acid on the ductus arteriosus in foetal lambs *in utero*. *Circ. Res.*, **38**, 418

Heymann, M. A. and Rudolph, A. M. (1977). Ductus arteriosus dilatation by prostaglandin E_1 in infants with pulmonary atresia. *Pediatrics*, **59**, 325

Heymann, M. A., Rudolph, A. M. and Silverman, N. H. (1976). Closure of the ductus arteriosus in premature infants by inhibition of prostaglandin synthesis. *N. Engl. J. Med.*, **295**, 530

Hörnblad, P. Y. (1967). Studies on closure of the ductus arteriosus. III. Species differences in closure rate and morphology. *Cardiologia*, **51**, 262

Hörnblad, P. Y., Larsson, K. S. and Marsk, L. (1969). Studies on closure of the ductus arteriosus. VII. Closure rate and morphology of the ductus arteriosus in the lamb. *Cardiologia*, **54**, 336

Ikeda, M., Rubinstein, E. H. and Sonnenschein, R. R. (1973). Interaction of three factors in the closure of the ductus arteriosus. *Proc. Soc. Exp. Biol. Med.*, **143**, 354

Kadowitz, P. J., Joiner, P. D. and Hyman, A. L. (1974). Influence of prostaglandins E_1 and $F_{2\alpha}$ on pulmonary vascular resistance in the sheep. *Proc. Soc. Exp. Biol. Med.*, **145**, 1258

Kostis, J. B. (1977). Patent ductus arteriosus. *N. Engl. J. Med.*, **296**, 106

Kovalčík, V. (1963). The response of the isolated ductus arteriosus to oxygen and anoxia. *J. Physiol. (Lond.)*, **169**, 185

Krasowska, H., Krówczynski, L. and Glab, E. (1972). Solubility of indomethacin in organic solvent and solvent-water systems. *Dissert. Pharm. Pharmacol.*, **24**, 623

Lang, P., Freed, M. D., Rosenthal, A., Castaneda, A. R. and Nadas, A. S. (1977). The use of prostaglandin E_1 in an infant with interruption of the aortic arch. *J. Pediatr.*, **91**, 805

Lewis, A. B. and Lurie, P. R. (1978). Prolonged prostaglandin E_1 infusion in an infant with cyanotic congenital heart disease. *Pediatrics*, **61**, 534

Lewis, P. E., Cefalo, R. C., Naulty, J. S., Fletcher, J. R. and Ramwell, P. W. (1978). Maternal and foetal prostaglandin levels during acute maternal hypoxia in the pregnant ewe. In: F. Coceani and P. M. Olley (eds.), *Prostaglandins and Perinatal Medicine, Advances in Prostaglandin and Thromboxane Research*, Vol. IV, pp. 133–135 (New York: Raven Press)

Lucas, A. and Mitchell, M. D. (1978). Plasma prostaglandins in pre-term neonates before and after treatment for patent ductus arteriosus. *Lancet*, **ii**, 130

Manku, M. S. and Horrobin, D. F. (1976). Chloroquine, quinine, procaine, quinidine and clomipramine are prostaglandin agonists and antagonists. *Prostaglandins*, **12**, 789

McCarthy, J., Juris, A., Zies, L., Ferrero, F., Kaiser, G., Garcia, O. and Tamer, D. (1977). Failure of indomethacin to close the ductus arteriosus. *Pediatr. Res.*, **11**, 395

McCarthy, J. S., Zies, L. G. and Gelband, H. (1978). Age-dependent closure of the patent ductus arteriosus by indomethacin. *Pediatrics*, **62**, 706

McGrath, R. L., Wolfe, R. R., Simmons, M. A. and Nora, J. J. (1977). Patent ductus arteriosus. *N. Engl. J. Med.*, **296**, 106

McMurphy, D. M., Heymann, M. A., Rudolph, A. M. and Melmon, K. L. (1972). Developmental changes in constriction of the ductus arteriosus: responses to oxygen and vasoactive agents in the isolated ductus arteriosus of the foetal lamb. *Pediatr. Res.*, **6**, 231

Merritt, T. A., DiSessa, T. G., Feldman, B. H., Kirkpatrick, S. E., Gluck, L. and Friedman, W. F. (1978). Closure of the ductus arteriosus with ligation and indomethacin. A consecutive experience. *J. Pediatr.*, **93**, 639

Mitchell, M. D., Lucas, A., Whitfield, M., Etches, P., Brunt, J. D. and Turnbull, A. C. (1978). Selective elevation of circulating prostaglandin concentrations in hyaline membrane disease in pre-term infants. *Prostagland. Med.*, **1**, 207

Moncada, S., Herman, A. G., Higgs, E. A. and Vane, J. R. (1977). Differential formation of prostacyclin (PGX or PGI_2) by layers of the arterial wall. An explanation for the anti-thrombotic properties of vascular endothelium. *Thromb. Res.*, **11**, 323

Neal, W. A., Kyle, J. M. and Mullett, M. D. (1977). Failure of indomethacin therapy to induce closure of the ductus arteriosus in premature infants with respiratory distress syndrome. *J. Pediatr.*, **91**, 621

Neutze, J. M., Starling, M. B., Elliott, R. B. and Barratt-Boyes, B. G. (1977). Palliation of cyanotic congenital heart disease in infancy with E type prostaglandins. *Circulation*, **55**, 238

Noel, S. and Cassin, S. (1976). Maturation of contractile response of ductus arteriosus to oxygen and drugs. *Am. J. Physiol.*, **231**, 240

Nugteren, D. H. and Van Dorp, D. A. (1965). The participation of molecular oxygen in the biosynthesis of prostaglandins. *Biochim. Biophys. Acta*, **98**, 654

O'Grady, J. (1979). Effects of intravenous prostacyclin infusion in healthy volunteers. Some preliminary observations. In: S. Bergström and J. R. Vane (eds.), *Workshop on Prostacyclin and its Analogues*, (New York: Raven Press) (In press)

Olley, P. M., Bodach, E., Heaton, J. and Coceani, F. (1975). Further evidence implicating E type prostaglandins in the patency of the lamb ductus arteriosus. *Eur. J. Pharmacol.*, **34**, 247

Olley, P. M., Coceani, F. and Bodach, E. (1976a). E type prostaglandins. A new emergency therapy for certain cyanotic congenital heart malformations. *Circulation*, **53**, 728

Olley, P. M., Coceani, F. and Rowe, R. D. (1978b). The role of prostaglandin E_1 and E_2 in the management of neonatal heart disease. In: F. Coceani and P. M. Olley (eds.), *Prostaglandins and Perinatal Medicine, Advances in Prostaglandin and Thromboxane Research*, Vol. IV, pp. 345–353 (New York: Raven Press)

Olley, P. M., Heaton, J. and Coceani, F. (1978a). Circulatory effects of a continuous infusion of E type prostaglandins in the newborn lamb. In: F. Coceani and P. M. Olley (eds.), *Prostaglandins and Perinatal Medicine, Advances in Prostaglandin and Thromboxane Research*, Vol. IV, pp. 239–247 (New York: Raven Press)

Olley, P. M., Rowe, R. D., Freedom, R. M., Swyer, P. R. and Coceani, F. (1979). Pharmacological manipulation of the ductus arteriosus. In: M. Godman and R. M. Marquis (eds.), *Pediatric Cardiology 1978: Heart Disease in the Neonate*, (Edinburgh: Churchill Livingstone) (In press)

Olley, P. M., White, E. P., Bodach, E., Heaton, J. and Coceani, F. (1976b). The contractile response of the developing lamb ductus arteriosus to ibuprofen. *Circulation*, **54 (Suppl. 2)**, 168

Pace-Asciak, C. R. (1978). Prostaglandin biosynthesis and catabolism in several organs of developing fetal and neonatal animals. In: F. Coceani and P. M. Olley (eds.), *Prostaglandins and Perinatal Medicine, Advances in Prostaglandin and Thromboxane Research*, Vol. IV, pp. 45–49 (New York: Raven Press)

Pace-Asciak, C. R. and Rangaraj, G. (1977). The 6-keto prostaglandin $F_{1\alpha}$ pathway in the lamb ductus arteriosus. *Biochim. Biophys. Acta*, **486**, 583

Pace-Asciak, C. R. and Rangaraj, G. (1978a). Distribution of prostaglandin biosynthetic pathways in organs and tissues of the foetal lamb. *Biochim. Biophys. Acta*, **528**, 512

Pace-Asciak, C. R. and Rangaraj, G. (1978b). Prostaglandin biosynthesis and catabolism in the lamb ductus arteriosus, aorta and pulmonary artery. *Biochim. Biophys. Acta*, **529**, 13

Palmer, M. A., Piper, P. J. and Vane, J. R. (1973). Release of rabbit aorta contracting substance (RCS) and prostaglandins induced by chemical or mechanical stimulation of guinea-pig lungs. *Br. J. Pharmacol.*, **49**, 226

Powell, W. S. and Solomon, S. (1977). Formation of 6-oxoprostaglandin $F_{1\alpha}$ by arteries of the foetal calf. *Biochim. Biophys. Res. Commun.*, **75**, 815

Powell, W. S. and Solomon, S. (1978). Biosynthesis of prostaglandins and thromboxane B_2 by foetal lung homogenates. *Prostaglandins*, **15**, 351

Radford, D. R., Bloom, K. R., Coceani, F., Fariello, R. and Olley, P. M. (1976). Prostaglandin E_1 for interrupted aortic arch in the neonate. *Lancet*, **ii**, 95

Rudolph, A. M. (1978a). The role of the ductus arteriosus in the foetus and postnatal circulatory changes. In: *The Ductus Arteriosus, Proceedings of the Seventy-fifth Ross Conference on Pediatric Research*, p. 116 (Columbus: Ross Laboratories)

Rudolph, A. M. (1978b). Role of the ductus arteriosus in congenital heart disease. In: *The Ductus Arteriosus, Proceedings of the Seventy-fifth Ross Conference on Pediatric Research*, p. 194 (Columbus: Ross Laboratories)

Rudolph, A. M. and Heymann, M. A. (1978). Hemodynamic changes induced by blockers of prostaglandin synthesis in the foetal lamb *in utero*. In: F. Coceani and P. M. Olley (eds.), *Prostaglandins and Perinatal Medicine, Advances in Prostaglandin and Thromboxane Research*, Vol. IV, pp. 231–237 (New York: Raven Press)

Salmon, J. A., Smith, D. R., Flower, R. J., Moncada, S. and Vane, J. R. (1978). Further studies on the enzymatic conversion of prostaglandin endoperoxide into prostacyclin by porcine aorta microsomes. *Biochim. Biophys. Acta*, **523**, 250

Samuelsson, B. (1965). On the incorporation of oxygen in the conversion of 8,11,14-eicosatrienoic acid to prostaglandin E_1. *J. Am. Chem. Soc.*, **87**, 3011

Sharpe, G. L. and Larsson, K. S. (1975). Studies on closure of the ductus arteriosus. X. *In vivo* effect of prostaglandin. *Prostaglandins*, **9**, 703

Sharpe, G. L., Larsson, K. S. and Thalme, B. (1975). Studies on closure of the ductus arteriosus. XII. *In utero* effect of indomethacin and sodium salicylate in rats and rabbits. *Prostaglandins*, **9**, 585

Sharpe, G. L., Thalme, B. and Larsson, K. S. (1974). Studies on closure of the ductus arteriosus. XI. Ductal closure *in utero* by a prostaglandin synthetase inhibitor. *Prostaglandins*, **8**, 363

Smieško, V., Kriška, M. and Kovalčík, V. (1978). Bayliss myogenic response in the isolated ductus arteriosus of guinea-pig and rabbit foetuses. *Experientia*, **34**, 745

Starling, M. B. and Elliott, R. B. (1974). The effects of prostaglandins, prostaglandin inhibitors, and oxygen on the closure of the ductus arteriosus, pulmonary arteries and umbilical vessels *in vitro*. *Prostaglandins*, **8**, 187

Starling, M. B., Neutze, J. M. and Elliott, R. B. (1978a). Effect of prostaglandins and some methyl derivatives on the ductus arteriosus. In: F. Coceani and P. M. Olley (eds.), *Prostaglandins and Perinatal Medicine, Advances in Prostaglandin and Thromboxane Research*, Vol. IV, pp. 335–343 (New York: Raven Press)

Starling, M. B., Neutze, J. M., Elliott, R. L. and Elliott, R. B. (1976). Studies on the effects of prostaglandins E_1, E_2, A_1, and A_2 on the ductus arteriosus of swine *in vivo* using cineangiography. *Prostaglandins*, **12**, 355

Starling, M. B., Neutze, J. M., Elliott, R. L., Taylor, I. M. M. and Elliott, R. B. (1978b). The effects of some methyl prostaglandin derivatives on the ductus arteriosus of swine *in vivo*. *Prostaglandins and Medicine*, **1**, 267

Sun, F. F., Chapman, J. P. and Mcguire, J. C. (1977). Metabolism of prostaglandin endoperoxide in animal tissues. *Prostaglandins*, **14**, 1055

Sun, F. F. and McGuire, J. C. (1978). Metabolism of prostaglandins and prostaglandin endoperoxides in rabbit tissues during pregnancy: differences in enzyme activities between mother and foetus. In: F. Coceani and P. M. Olley (eds.), *Prostaglandins and Perinatal Medicine, Advances in Prostaglandin and Thromboxane Research*, Vol. IV, pp 75–85 (New York: Raven Press)

Terragno, N. A., McGiff, J. C., Smigel, M. and Terragno, A. (1978). Patterns of prostaglandin production in the bovine fetal and maternal vasculature. *Prostaglandins*, **16**, 847

Tyler, T., Wallis, R., Leffler, C. and Cassin, S. (1975). The effects of indomethacin on the pulmonary vascular response to hypoxia in the premature and mature newborn goat. *Proc. Soc. Exp. Biol. Med.*, **150**, 695

Yamanouchi, P. (1978). Ductal shunt in premature infants observed by tcPO_2 measurements. *Proceedings of the 1st International Symposium on Continuous Transcutaneous Blood Gas Monitoring*. Marburg (In press)

5
Prostaglandins and Angiography

D. LEGGE

5.1 INTRODUCTION

Angiography has developed from the simple demonstration of lesions involving vascular structures to the detailed anatomic study of various organs and systems. Opacification of an organ is made by the injection of contrast medium into its arterial supply. Provided a sufficient bolus of contrast medium is maintained, the organ and its venous drainage will be well shown. Opacification of the venous anatomy is enhanced by administration of a

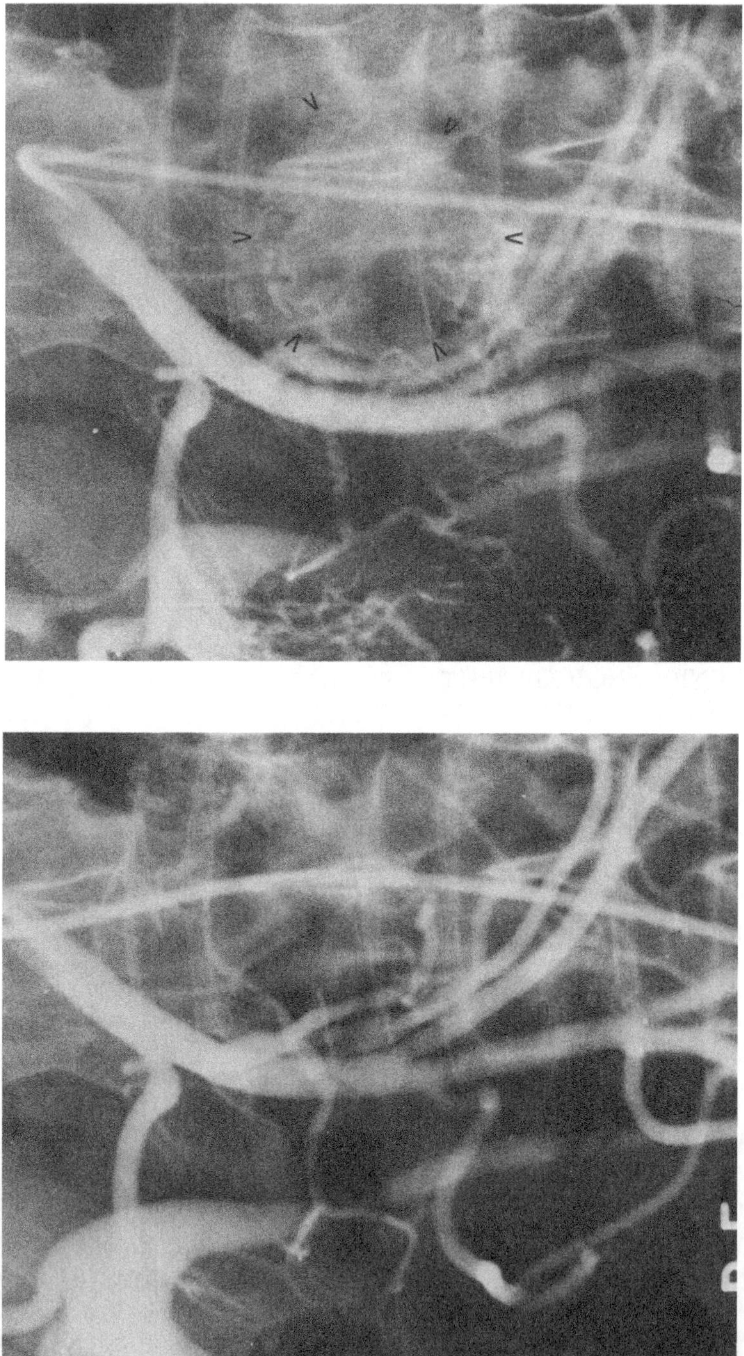

(a) (b)

Figure 5.1 Superior mesenteric angiogram performed on a 42-year-old male who had recurrent episodes of melena for previous 9 months. (a) Control study: normal appearance. (b) After prostaglandin: smaller arteries are opacified showing a vascular tumour in the jejunum, representing a leomyoma (see arrows) vasodilating drug prior to the injection of contrast medium. Several drugs have been used for this purpose including tolazoline and bradykinnin, but these may produce unwanted systemic haemodynamic side-effects and impair the quality of the arterial phase of the study. The prostaglandins have vasodilating properties and prostaglandin $F_{2\alpha}$ ($PGF_{2\alpha}$) has been used for more than 200 visceral angiographic studies performed at the Mater Hospital since April 1975. In this chapter advantages of the use of this drug in selective angiography are described.

5.2 SUPERIOR MESENTERIC STUDIES

In 33 patients angiographic studies of the superior mesenteric artery were obtained before and after the injection of 80 μg of $PGF_{2\alpha}$ (Figure 5.1) (Legge, 1977a). All the studies were improved by the use of this drug, which we now inject routinely for superior mesenteric angiography. The result is a

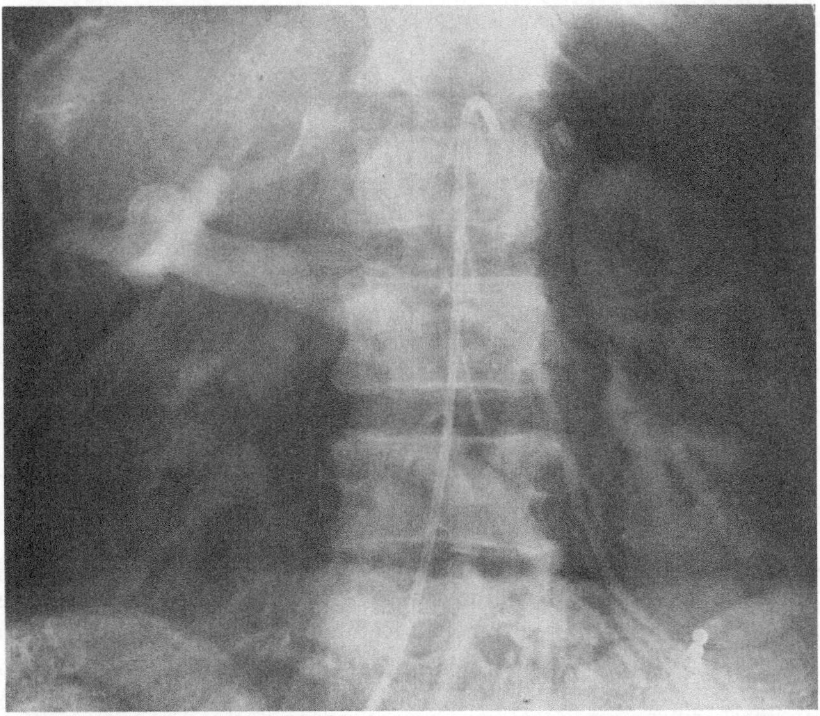

Figure 5.2 Normal venous phase of superior mesenteric angiogram after intra-arterial injection of 80 μg of $PGF_{2\alpha}$. Small vessels draining the wall of the small bowel are well opacified, as is the superior mesenteric and portal vein

measurable increase in the size of the superior mesenteric artery and its branches, and the smaller arterial branches supplying the wall of the bowel are shown in detail. This better demonstrates tumours arising from the bowel such as leomyoma (Figure 5.1), or tumours of the pancreas supplied by the superior mesenteric artery. Demonstration of the superior mesenteric and portal veins are improved by the use of prostaglandin (Figure 5.2), which is of importance in the management of portal hypertension.

5.3 SPLENIC ANGIOGRAPHY

Selective catheterization of the splenic artery is usually easily achieved and the injection of 60 μg of $PGF_{2\alpha}$ enhances demonstration of the splenic circulation. The small vessels in the body of the pancreas which are supplied by the splenic artery are well demonstrated (Figure 5.3). This is of importance when seeking carcinoma in the body of the pancreas, which is usually a poorly vascularized lesion. Opacification of the splenic vein is improved, which is necessary in the study of portal hypertension, both for the demonstration of abnormal collateral branches and normal anatomy.

5.4 PANCREATIC ANGIOGRAPHY

The pancreas is a highly vascular structure and requires injection of contrast medium into one of its smaller vessels (either the gastro-duodenal or the dorsal pancreatic artery) for adequate examination. Even then it is not possible to opacify the smaller vessels within the pancreas without the use of a vasodilator drug (Figure 5.4). Diagnosis of carcinoma of the pancreas depends upon demonstrating fixed irregularities of the small vessels encased by carcinoma and these are well shown after the injection of 60 μg of $PGF_{2\alpha}$ (Figure 5.5) (Legge, 1978).

5.5 HEPATIC ANGIOGRAPHY

Hepatic angiographic studies often give rise to difficulty in diagnosis as many metastatic tumours involving the liver are poorly vascularized. $PGF_{2\alpha}$ has been used extensively to improve opacification of the parenchyma of the liver so that the demonstration of negative defects which represent poorly vascularized metastatic tumour is enhanced (Figure 5.6). Any vascularity present in the rim of metastatic tumour is also better shown using prostaglandin (Figure 5.7). The wall of the gall bladder is better demonstrated after prostaglandin injection and primary carcinoma of the gall bladder is then amenable to diagnosis (Legge, 1977b).

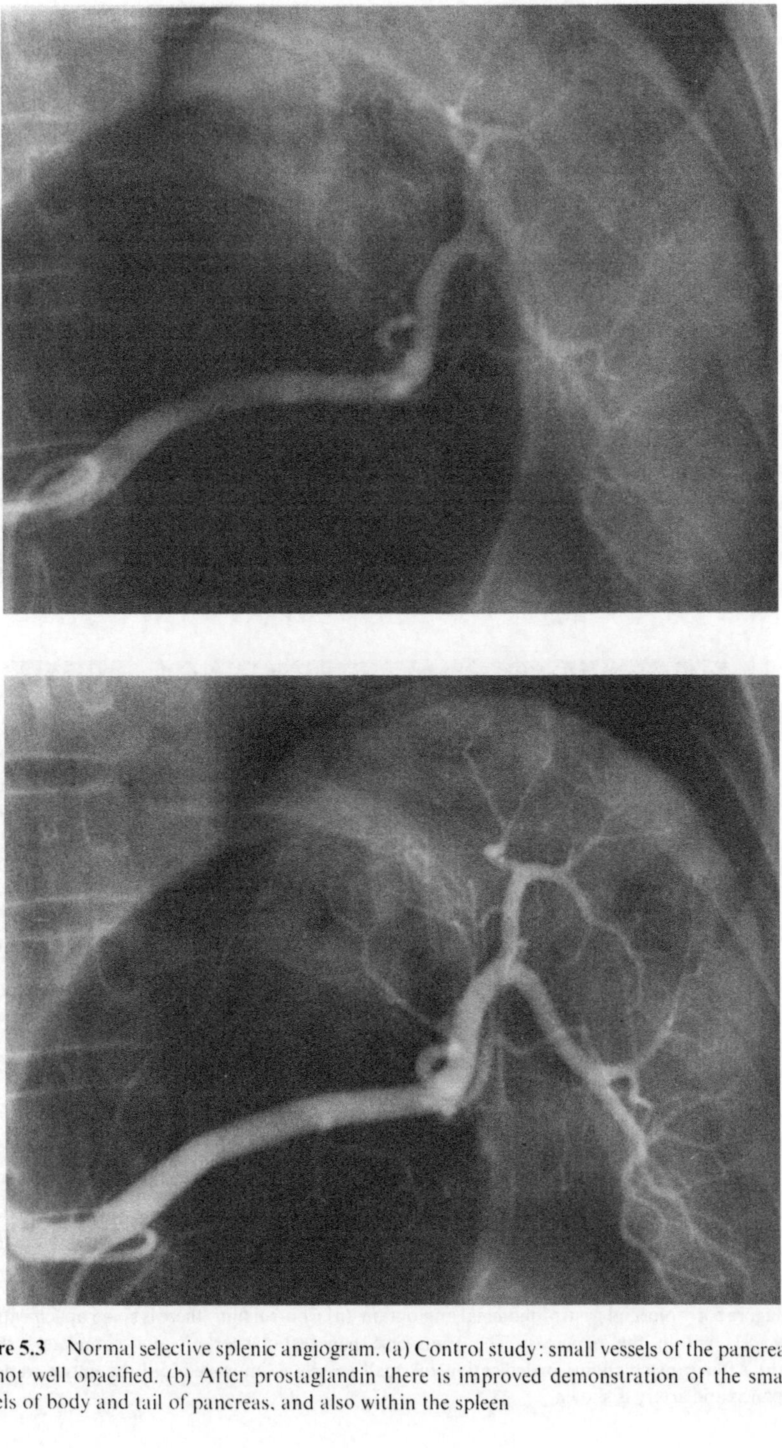

(a)

(b)

Figure 5.3 Normal selective splenic angiogram. (a) Control study: small vessels of the pancreas are not well opacified. (b) After prostaglandin there is improved demonstration of the small vessels of body and tail of pancreas, and also within the spleen

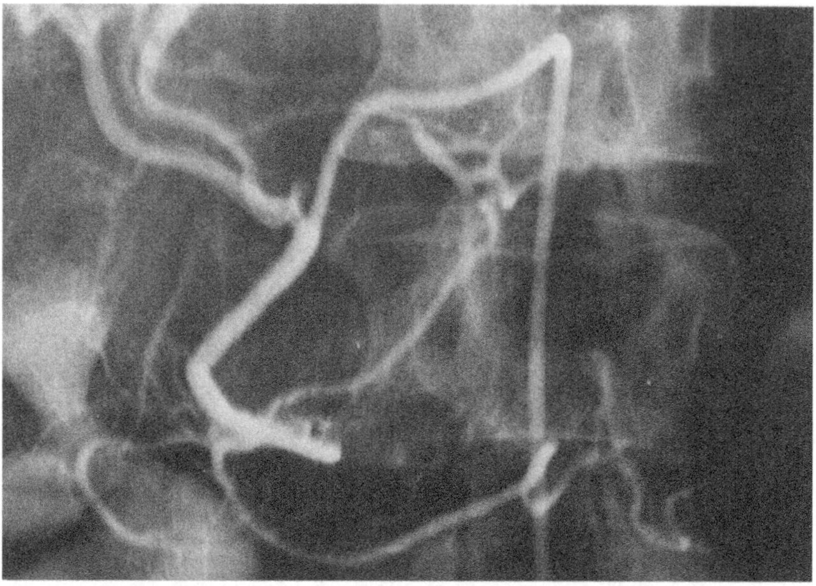

(a)

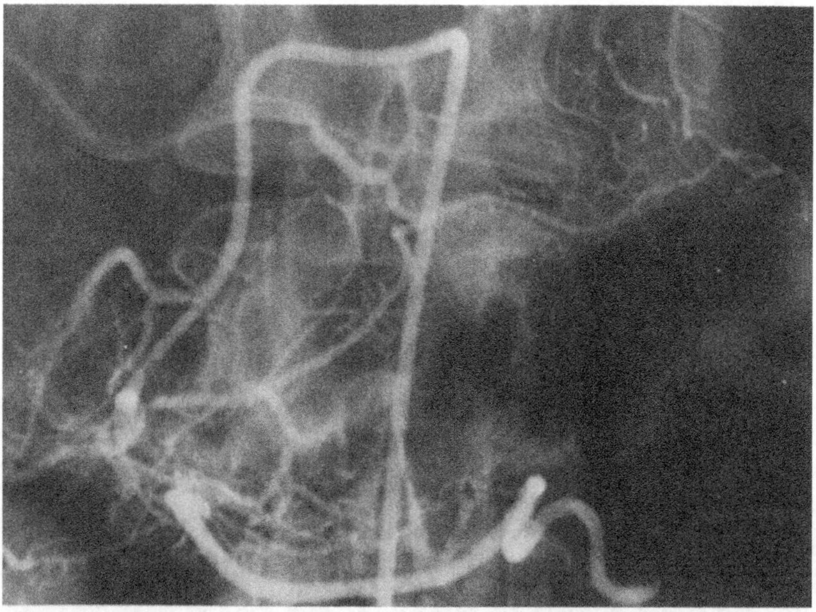

(b)

Figure 5.4 Normal gastro-duodenal angiogram. (a) Control film: there is some opacification of vessels within the pancreas. The transverse pancreatic artery is not completely shown. (b) After prostaglandin: opacification of small vessels is improved and the entire transverse pancreatic artery is shown

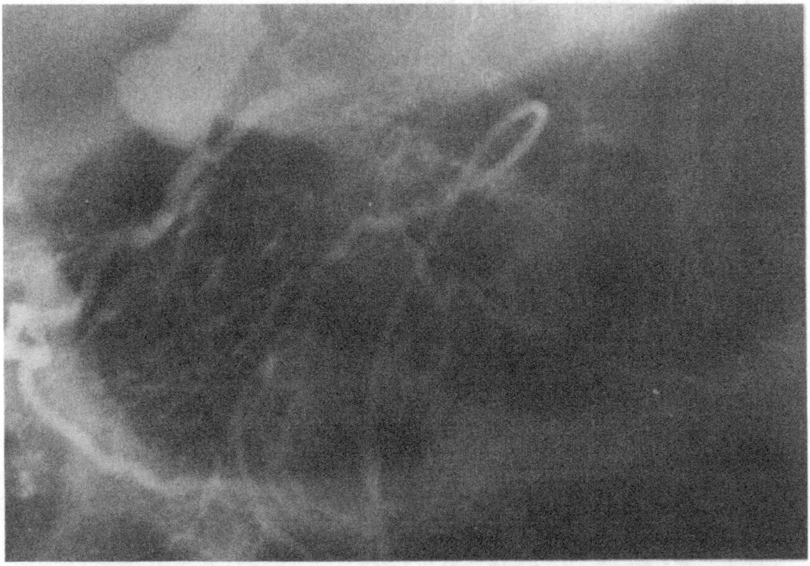

(a)

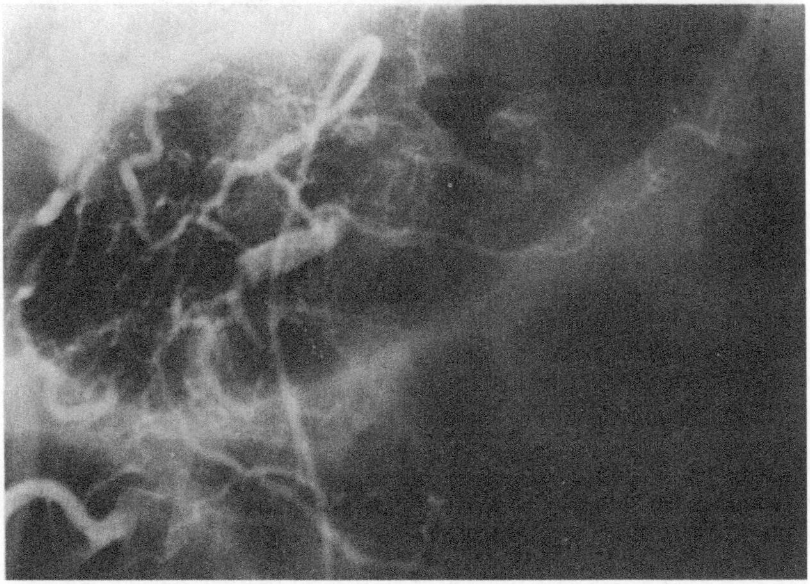

(b)

Figure 5.5 Dorsal pancreatic angiogram on a 61-year-old jaundiced patient with carcinoma of the head of the pancreas. (a) Control study: there is some filling of small vessels within the pancreas. (b) After prostaglandin: increased opacification of the small vessels. These are irregular due to encasement by tumour. Increased flow gives opacification of superior mesenteric artery which is shown to be occluded near its origin by the tumour

5.6 LEFT GASTRIC STUDIES

Injection of 60 μg of $PGF_{2\alpha}$ into the left gastric artery gives an increase in the size of this vessel and improves venous opacification. This allows identification of the left gastric vein draining into the portal vein, thereby establishing that blood flow is towards the liver. In patients with varices the portal vein

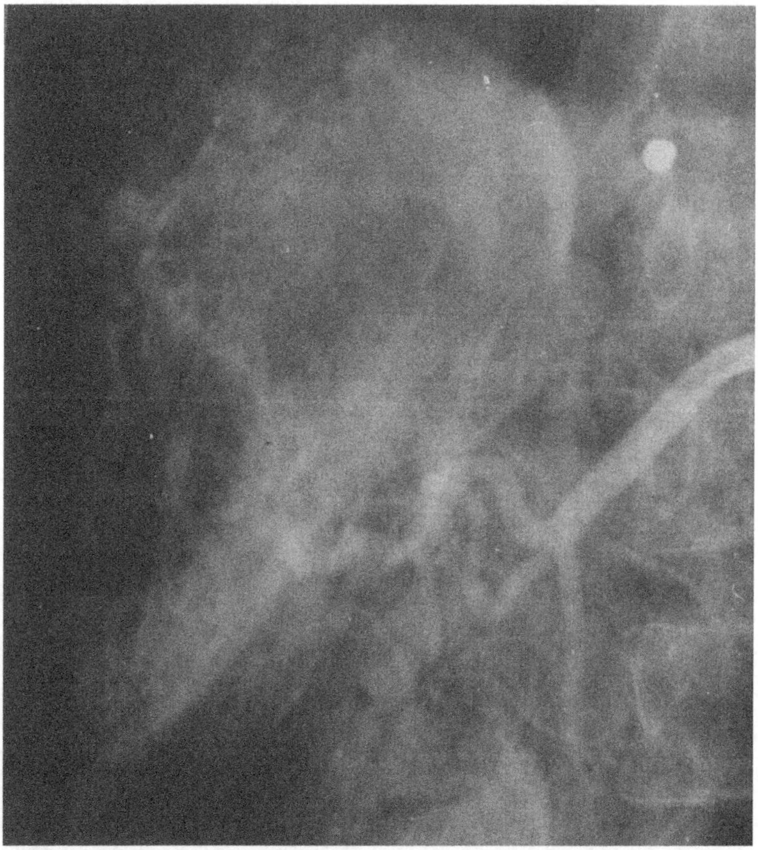

Figure 5.6 Selective hepatic angiogram using prostaglandin in a 65-year-old female with hepatic metastases from carcinoma of the colon. The hepatic parenchyma is densely opacified and large poorly vascularized tumour well demonstrated

cannot be identified since blood flow is away from the liver. Opacification of varices is improved by the use of prostaglandin (Figure 5.8). In cases where the spleen has been removed, left gastric studies may be the only means of demonstrating varices angiographically, and the enhancement of these by prostaglandin may be critical for correct diagnosis (Legge, 1978).

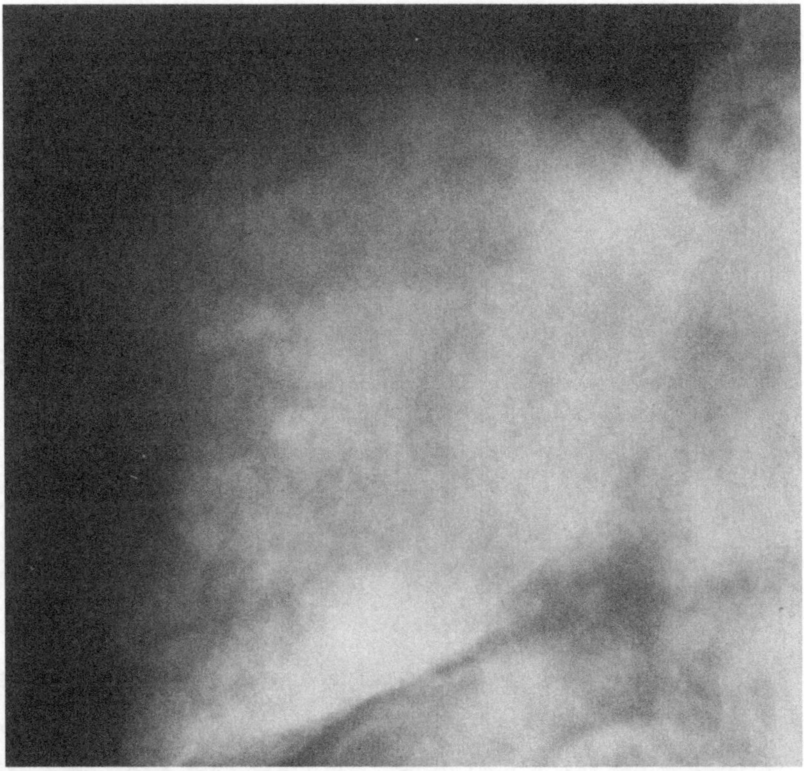

Figure 5.7 Selective hepatic angiogram using prostaglandin in a 67-year-old female with hepatic metastases from carcinoma of the pancreas. Multiple poorly defined metastatic nodules each with a thin vascular rim. These were not shown without prostaglandin

5.7 COMMENTS

The prostaglandins relax vascular smooth muscle, resulting in vasodilatation. This interesting property has been used to advantage for many visceral angiographic studies performed at the Mater Hospital and elsewhere. We have observed no complications from the use of $PGF_{2\alpha}$, whereas other drugs such as tolazoline are known to cause hypotension and bradycardia. Most drugs with vasodilating properties, apart from prostaglandin, impair the quality of the arterial phase of the angiographic study, probably by causing increased vascular permeability.

The effects of prostaglandin in angiography have been documented in experiments using dogs by Davis *et al.* (1975), and by Cho *et al.* (1975). Both investigators injected PGE_1 into the mesenteric circulation of dogs and found

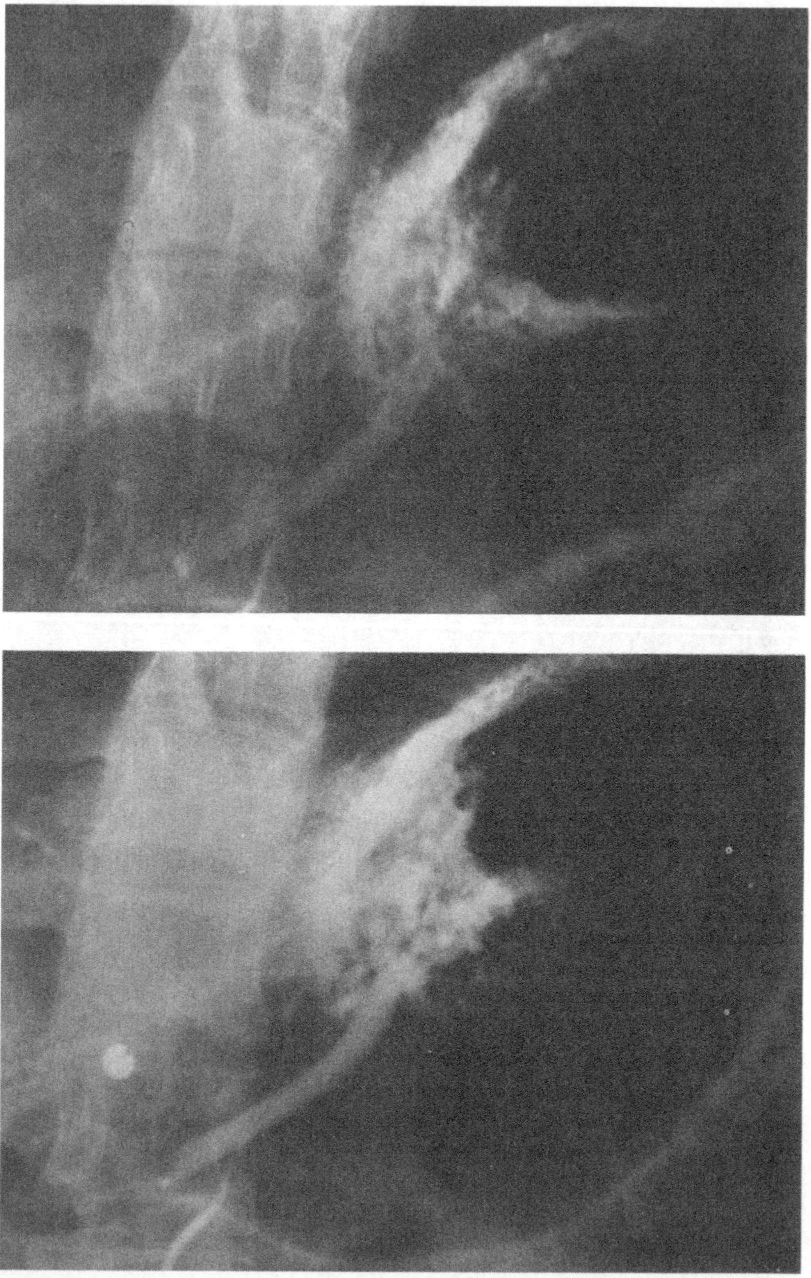

(a)

(b)

Figure 5.8 Venous phase of left gastric angiogram in a 22-year-old female presenting with haematemesis. (a) Control study: left gastric vein and varices within the fundus of the stomach are demonstrated. (b) After prostaglandin: opacification is improved; there is no contrast medium in the portal vein indicating that flow is hepato-fungal increased blood flow of more than 100%. The prostaglandins have only recently been used clinically. Dencker *et al.* (1975) using flow studies in eight patients demonstrated increase in mesenteric circulation of more than 100% with $PGF_{2\alpha}$, and have improved opacification of the venous anatomy in superior mesenteric angiography. $PGF_{2\alpha}$ has been used in more than 200 angiographic studies performed at the Mater Hospital since 1975. It is injected routinely for mesenteric, splenic, left gastric, pancreatic and hepatic studies. Recently Jonsson *et al.* (1977) have used PGE_1 clinically to improve superior mesenteric, hepatic and pancreatic studies. However, the prostaglandins of both E and A series relax most vascular beds and reduce the total vascular peripheral resistance, so may reduce blood pressure (Dencker *et al.*, 1975). $PGF_{2\alpha}$ does not produce any change in blood pressure or heart rate in doses used for angiography.

In the past many drugs with vasodilating properties have been used in an effort to improve angiographic studies. $PGF_{2\alpha}$ gives a consistent response and because it improves both arterial and venous phases of each study, is rapidly metabolized, and is not associated with any significant side-effects. It appears to be an ideal vasodilator for use in a wide range of angiographic studies.

Acknowledgement

Figures 5.5 and 5.8 are reproduced by kind permission of the Editor of *Clinical Radiology*.

References

Cho, K. J., Chuang, V. P. and Reuter, S. R. (1975). Prostaglandin E_1 as a pharmacoangiographic agent for arterial portography. *Radiology*, **116**, 207

Davis, L. J., Anderson, J. H., Wallace, S., Gianturco, C. and Jackson, E. D. (1975). The use of prostaglandin E_1 to enhance the angiographic visualization of the splanchnic circulation. *Radiology*, **114**, 281

Dencker, H., Gothlin, J., Hedner, P., Lunderquist, A., Norryd, C. and Tylen, U. (1975). Superior mesenteric angiography and blood flow following intra-arterial injection of prostaglandin $F_{2\alpha}$. *Am. J. Roentgenol.*, **125**, 111

Jonsson, K., Wallace, S., Jacobson, E. D., Anderson, J. H., Zornoza, J. and Granmayeh, M. (1977). The use of prostaglandin E_1 for enhanced visualization of the splanchnic circulation. *Radiology*, **125**, 373

Legge, D. (1977a). The use of prostaglandin $F_{2\alpha}$ in selective visceral angiography. *Br. J. Radiol.*, **50**, 251

Legge, D. (1977b). The use of prostaglandin $F_{2\alpha}$ in selective hepatic angiography. *Radiology*, **124**, 331

Legge, D. (1978). The use of prostaglandin $F_{2\alpha}$ in selective pancreatic and left gastric angiography. *Clin. Radiol.*, **29**, 285

6
Prostaglandins in Gastro-intestinal Disease

A. ROBERT

6.1 INTRODUCTION

Many prostaglandins (PG) of the E series affect several gastro-intestinal tract functions in laboratory animals. In particular, they inhibit gastric acid secretion, stimulate contraction of the intestinal smooth muscle *in vitro* and *in vivo*, and induce diarrhoea when given in high doses. The latter effect presumably is a result of accumulation of fluid in the small intestine, a phenomenon called enteropooling. In the dog, the gastric antisecretory effect was demonstrated against a variety of stimuli, including histamine, pentagastrin, food, 2-deoxy-D-glucose, carbachol, and reserpine (Robert, Nezamis and Philipps, 1967; Robert, Philipps and Nezamis, 1968; Robert *et al.*, 1976b; Robert, Nezamis and Philipps, 1968). Because of this antisecretory property, these prostaglandins were tested in experimental ulcer models and found to have an anti-ulcer effect. In particular, they prevented the formation of gastric ulcers produced by pylorus ligation (Shay ulcers) (Robert *et al.*, 1968a), serotonin (Ferguson *et al.*, 1973), reserpine (Lee *et al.*, 1973), and by exposure to stress (restraint (Kawarda, *et al.*, 1975), forced exertion (Lee and Bianchi, 1972)). They also inhibited formation of duodenal ulcers produced by administration of gastric secretogogues (histamine, pentagastrin, carbachol (Robert *et al.*, 1971)), cysteamine (Robert *et al.*, 1971, 1975c), propionitrile (Robert *et al.*, 1975b), and by a combination of indomethacin and bile duct ligation (Robert *et al.*, 1975a).

Results of clinical studies obtained with some prostaglandins, especially their effect on gastric secretion and ulcer healing, will be summarized in this review. Other properties of prostaglandins observed in humans, such as their effect on gastro-intestinal motility and as stimuli of enteropooling diarrhoea, will also be discussed.

6.2 GASTRIC SECRETION

The first studies were performed with natural prostaglandins (PGA_1, PGE_1 and PGE_2). They were administered by constant intravenous infusion and found to inhibit acid secretion stimulated with histamine, pentagastrin or tetragastrin (Wilson *et al.*, 1971; Classen *et al.*, 1971; Wada and Ishizawa, 1970; Newman *et al.*, 1975), as well as basal secretion (Wada and Ishizawa, 1970; Classen *et al.*, 1970). The antisecretory dose was approximately 1 (μg/kg)/min. When given orally, PGE_1 failed to inhibit gastric secretion stimulated by pentagastrin (Horton *et al.*, 1968). Similarly, PGE_2 given orally did not affect basal secretion (Karim *et al.*, 1973b). A transient reduction in acid secretion was observed after oral administration of PGA_2, whereas PGA_1 gave inconsistent results (Bhana *et al.*, 1973). As in the case of animals, $PGF_{2\alpha}$ did not produce an antisecretory effect even when administered intravenously (Horton *et al.*, 1968).

Since these natural prostaglandins were orally inactive, had to be injected and had a short duration of action (about 1 h), they were not well suited for chronic administration to humans. Several analogues were therefore prepared. Of special interest are certain analogues with a methyl group at carbon-15 (Yankee *et al.*, 1974; Yankee and Bundy, 1972) or carbon-16 (Magerlein *et al.*, 1973). When administered to animals, they were found to be many times more potent than the corresponding natural prostaglandin, long acting (several hours), and effective orally (Robert *et al.*, 1973; 1976b). Several clinical studies were then performed with these methyl analogues of PGE_2. 15(R)-15-methyl PGE_2 and its methyl ester, administered orally, inhibited both basal and pentagastrin-induced gastric acid secretion (Karim *et al.*, 1973a; Karim *et al.*, 1973b; Carter *et al.*, 1973b; Carter *et al.*, 1973a; Amy *et al.*, 1973; Karim and Fung, 1975; Konturek *et al.*, 1976b). The inhibition of basal acid output was of the order of 70% after a dose of 150 μg, and after a dose of 200 μg in pentagastrin-stimulation secretion. No side-effects were observed. 15(R)-15-methyl PGE_2 also inhibited acid secretion in duodenal ulcer patients (Chen *et al.*, 1977). 15(S)-15-methyl PGE_2 methyl ester was more potent than the 15(R) configuration (Karim *et al.*, 1973b; Konturek *et al.*, 1976b; Robert *et al.*, 1974; Nylander and Andersson, 1974; Nylander, Robert and Andersson, 1974), and in some cases induced nausea at a dose of 50 μg/subject. Meal-induced acid and pepsin secretion was also inhibited by 15(R)-15-methyl PGE_2 methyl ester (Konturek *et al.*, 1976b). Interestingly, 15(R)-15-methyl PGE_2 methyl ester significantly inhibited acid secretion in pregnant women at term, without significant uterine stimulation (Amy *et al.*, 1973).

16,16-Dimethyl PGE_2 and its methyl ester are other potent PGE_2 analogues. They inhibit secretion stimulated by histamine (Wilson *et al.*, 1975), a meal (Konturek *et al.*, 1976b; Ippoliti *et al.*, 1976), pentagastrin (Konturek *et al.*, 1976b; Robert *et al.*, 1974; Nylander and Andersson, 1974; Karim *et al.*, 1973c), as well as basal secretion (Karim *et al.*, 1973c). In general a dose of less than 1 μg/kg given orally inhibited acid secretion by 50% or more. Meal-induced acid secretion was reduced by 60% and 95% with doses of 0.75 μg/kg and 1 μg/kg, respectively, whereas the highest tolerated dose of propantheline bromide reduced acid output by only 35% (Ippoliti *et al.*, 1976). Other studies using either pentagastrin or food as a stimulus showed that 15(S)-15-methyl PGE_2 and 16,16-dimethyl PGE_2 were equipotent in inhibiting acid secretion, whereas 15(R)-15-methyl PGE_2 was approximately half as active (Konturek *et al.*, 1976b). 16,16-Dimethyl PGE_2 was also administered orally in a gelatin capsule containing 127 μg; it inhibited by 60% sub-maximal gastric secretion stimulated by histamine. No side-effects were observed (Wilson *et al.*, 1976).

15(S)-15-Methyl PGE_2 methyl ester and 16,16-dimethyl PGE_2 methyl ester given intravenously also inhibited gastric secretion, either basal (Karim *et al.*, 1973b, 1973c; Carter *et al.*, 1973b, 1973c) or stimulated by pentagastrin

(Karim *et al.*, 1973b, 1973c; Carter *et al.*, 1973a, 1973b, 1973c; Konturek *et al.*, 1976a), histamine (Konturek *et al.*, 1976a) and a meal (Konturek *et al.*, 1976a). Pepsin secretion was also inhibited (Konturek *et al.*, 1976a). On the other hand, intravenous administration of 15(R)-15-methyl PGE_2 methyl ester was ineffective (Karim *et al.*, 1973a, 1973b; Carter *et al.*, 1973b). Subsequent studies explained the lack of activity of 15(R)-15-methyl PGE_2 (or its methyl ester) when given intravenously. It appears that as such the 15(R) configuration has little or no activity. It becomes active when it is epimerized into the 15(S) form. Epimerization is accomplished in an acid medium, such as found in the stomach (Robert and Yankee, 1975).

11-Methyl, 16,16-dimethyl PGE_2 given orally inhibited basal and histamine-induced acid output at doses of 2.5–10 μg/kg, during the first 30 minutes following administration (Wilson and Winter, 1978). The inhibition lasted for 60 minutes. Following a 2-week treatment, three times a day, with either 15(R)-15-methyl PGE_2 methyl ester or 15(S)-15-methyl PGE_2 methyl ester to ulcer patients, the inhibition of acid secretion induced by a maximal dose of histamine was slightly more pronounced than after the first treatment (Gibinski *et al.*, 1977).

$PGF_{2\alpha}$ infused intravenously did not affect basal secretion but produced a transient inhibition of the response to sub-maximal dose of pentagastrin (Newman *et al.*, 1975). Against maximal stimulation, however, $PGF_{2\alpha}$ was inactive.

Conclusion. Prostaglandins of the E series inhibit gastric secretion induced by a variety of stimuli. Addition of methyl groups to C-15 or C-16 of PGE_2 enhances and prolongs this activity, and renders the prostaglandin orally active.

6.3 ULCER HEALING

Certain methyl analogues of PGE_2 were given orally to patients with gastric and duodenal ulcers. Some of these studies were acute (single administration), others were chronic (2 weeks duration).

6.3.1 Acute studies

Oral administration of 15(R)-15-methyl PGE_2 methyl ester (150 μg) relieved typical ulcer (gastric) pain as quickly as an antacid preparation (magnesium triacetate and aluminium hydroxide) (Fung *et al.*, 1974a). This effect is difficult to assess since a group with inert placebo was not included. Gastric juice analysis showed that in patients who experienced pain relief, the pH rose after treatment. In another study, the same prostaglandin was also given orally (150 μg) to six patients with gastritis, one with gastric ulcer and one with antral scarring. The stomach was examined endoscopically before and 1 hour after treatment, and gastric biopsies were taken. In six patients, a viscid mucoid secretion was observed, covering the mucosa, after the prostaglandin had been administered (Fung *et al.*, 1974c). Histologically, the amount of mucin in mucus cells was markedly increased. It was suggested that this increased mucus formation may favour ulcer healing.

6.3.2 Chronic studies

In the following studies, the rate of ulcer healing was assessed by endoscopic measurement of the ulcer size and by the number of patients showing complete cicatrization after treatment with either a prostaglandin or placebo. Evidence of accelerated healing was obtained in gastric ulcer patients treated with 150 μg, four times a day for 14 days, of either 15(R)-15-methyl PGE_2 (Fung and Karim, 1976b) or its methyl ester (Fung *et al.*, 1974b). In another study, 15(R)-15-methyl PGE_2, 15(S)-15-methyl PGE_2 methyl ester and 16,16-dimethyl PGE_2 were given orally, three times a day, to patients with either gastric or duodenal ulcers, at doses of 1.5–2.0 μg/kg for 14 days. Results obtained with the first 77 patients showed that the rate of healing was accelerated during the 2-week treatment (Gibinski *et al.*, 1977). More cases were added and the analysis of a total of 117 patients showed that the methyl analogues accelerated cicatrization of duodenal ulcers but not of gastric ulcers. In another study, oral administration of 1 mg/subject of PGE_2, four times a day for 2 weeks, accelerated the rate of healing of gastric ulcers (Fung and Karim, 1976a; Karim and Fung, 1976).

Conclusion. Prostaglandins of the E series exert anti-ulcer activity in animals. In humans, several studies suggest that certain methyl analogues of PGE_2 promote healing of gastric and duodenal ulcers.

6.4 INTESTINAL SECRETION AND DIARRHOEA

In view of the marked effect of some prostaglandins on gastric secretion, it became of interest to explore their effect on the secretions of the rest of the gastro-intestinal tract. Another reason for exploring this effect was the observation that several prostaglandins, when given at high doses, can induce diarrhoea (Horton *et al.*, 1968; Milton-Thompson *et al.*, 1975), a phenomenon associated with functional changes of the intestine.

Using the technique of jejunal and ileal perfusion, PGE_1 (Matuchansky and Bernier, 1971; Matuchansky and Bernier, 1973; Matuchansky *et al.*, 1972; Matuchansky and Coutrot, 1978), PGE_2 (Newman *et al.*, 1975; Milton-Thompson *et al.*, 1975; Cummings *et al.*, 1973) and $PGF_{2\alpha}$ (Newman *et al.*, 1975; Milton-Thompson *et al.*, 1975: Cummings *et al.*, 1973; Cummings *et al.*, 1974; Newman *et al.*, 1974) were found to increase net secretion of water, sodium and chloride into the lumen of the small intestine. The effect was seen whether the prostaglandin was introduced directly into the intestinal lumen or infused intravenously. Water and ion movements through the colon were not influenced by $PGF_{2\alpha}$, whether it was given intravenously (Milton-Thompson *et al.*, 1975; Cummings *et al.*, 1974) or perfused through the large intestine (Newman *et al.*, 1974).

These studies confirmed earlier findings in dogs which showed that PGA_1, PGE_1 and $PGF_{2\alpha}$ administered into the superior mesenteric artery or into the lumen of the small intestine induced a rapid accumulation of water and electrolytes within the lumen (Greenough *et al.*, 1969; Pierce *et al.*, 1971). This fluid accumulation was later called 'enteropooling', and an assay was developed in rats to quantitate this effect (Roberts *et al.*, 1976a). This assay also determines the diarrhoeogenic potency of a prostaglandin, since diarrhoea occurs with compounds that cause sufficient enteropooling. Prostaglandin-induced diarrhoea appears to result primarily from a rapid and abundant accumulation of fluid in the small intestine. This fluid is transported to the large intestine and eventually eliminated as diarrhoea.

It is of interest that several tumours often associated with diarrhoea have been shown to contain large amounts of prostaglandins of the E and $F_{2\alpha}$ type (Williams *et al.*, 1968; Sandler *et al.*, 1968; Feldman *et al.*, 1974). In certain cases, the blood level of prostaglandins was elevated (Williams *et al.*, 1968; Jaffe *et al.*, 1973). In the case of the medullary carcinoma of the thyroid, the concentration of prostaglandins in the blood draining the tumour was much higher than that of the peripheral blood (Williams *et al.*, 1968).

A case was reported in which certain symptoms developed at a fixed time during menstrual cycle. These included vomiting, abdominal pain and diarrhoea. During these episodes, the blood level of PGE was 60 times higher than normal (Labrum *et al.*, 1976). It was suggested that some of the distress was due to the 'hyperprostaglandinaemia'.

Conclusion. Several prostaglandins produce diarrhoea when given at high doses. This is due to rapid and abundant accumulation of fluid in the small intestine ('enteropooling'). Prostaglandins do not affect water movements in the large intestine.

6.5 GASTRO-INTESTINAL MOTILITY

The effect of prostaglandins on the gastro-intestinal motility in humans is variable. The lower oesophageal sphincter was found to constrict (as shown by increased cardiac sphincter pressure) after intravenous infusion of $PGF_{2\alpha}$ (Dilawari *et al.*, 1975), whereas PGE_2 dilated this sphincter (Goyal *et al.*, 1974). PGE_2, infused intravenously (Dilawari *et al.*, 1975), and 16,16-dimethyl PGE_2, given orally (McCallum *et al.*, 1975), inhibited sphincter contractions elicited by intravenous injections of pentagastrin.

Few studies on the effect of prostaglandins on gastric motility in man have been reported. Intravenous infusion of $PGF_{2\alpha}$ increased antral motility under basal conditions whereas PGE_2 decreased it (Newman *et al.*, 1975). $PGF_{2\alpha}$, however, did not affect the increased contractions caused by pentagastrin, whereas PGE_2 decreased such contractions (Newman *et al.*, 1975). 16,16-Dimethyl PGE_2 given orally (140 μg) accelerated gastric emptying of a barium meal (under radiological observation) (Nylander and Mattson, 1975). However, the same dose inhibited motor activity of the stomach and the duodenum, measured with balloons (Nylander and Mattson, 1975). Another analogue, 15(S)-15-methyl PGE_2 methyl ester, introduced into the duodenum, inhibited its motility (Nylander and Anderson, 1975).

Whereas jejunal and ileal transit was not influenced by intravenous infusion of $PGF_{2\alpha}$, the segmented pressure waves were markedly inhibited (Cummings *et al.*, 1973). On the other hand, intravenous infusion of PGE_2 inhibited segmented pressure waves in the sigmoid colon; $PGF_{2\alpha}$ was without effect (Hunt *et al.*, 1975).

Conclusion. Although many prostaglandins stimulate gastro-intestinal smooth muscle *in vitro*, the *in vivo* effects on motility are not as definite. In general, $PGF_{2\alpha}$ tends to stimulate motility whereas PGE_2 tends to have a relaxant effect.

6.6 CYTOPROTECTION

Cytoprotection is the property of prostaglandins which protects the mucosa of the stomach and the intestine from becoming inflamed and necrotic, when exposed to noxious agents. This property was discovered in animals. An example of gastric cytoprotection is the observation that $PGF_{2\beta}$ and 15(R)-15-methyl $PGF_{2\beta}$ protect the mucosa against the necrotizing effect of orally administered aspirin or of absolute ethanol (Robert, 1975a, 1975b; Robert *et al.*, 1979). Intestinal cytoprotection was shown in studies in which necrotic lesions of the jejunum and the ileum, produced by either indomethacin (Robert, 1975a, 1975b) or prednisolone (Lancaster and Robert, 1978), were prevented by concomitant treatment with 16,16-dimethyl PGE_2.

The concept of cytoprotection by prostaglandins has not been adequately tested in humans. A recent study, however, showed that PGE_2, given orally in doses of 1 mg four times a day to human volunteers, prevented the occurrence of gastric bleeding caused by aspirin (600 mg four times a day) (Cohen, 1978). Occult bleeding was measured by the ^{51}Cr technique. This cytoprotection by PGE_2 was confirmed in arthritic patients treated with indomethacin (50 mg three times a day). PGE_2 prevented occult bleeding produced by indomethacin whereas it did not interfere with its anti-inflammatory activity (Johansson *et al.*, 1979). Since PGE_2 is not antisecretory when given orally, this result is a demonstration of gastric cytoprotection.

Conclusion. In animals, several prostaglandins protect the mucosa of the stomach and the small intestine from damage otherwise produced by noxious agents. In humans, gastric bleeding produced by aspirin is prevented by concurrent administration of PGE_2.

6.7 MECHANISM OF ACTION

The mechanism by which prostaglandins inhibit gastric secretion and exert cytoprotection is not well understood, although more is known of the enteropooling effect.

6.7.1 Antisecretory effect

Prostaglandins seem to inhibit gastric secretion by a mechanism different from that of other agents. They inhibit acid secretion induced by all known stimuli (Robert *et al.*, 1973) except cyclic AMP (Way and Durbin, 1969: Main and Whittle, 1974; Soll, 1978). Whether cyclic AMP is a necessary mediator of the antisecretory effect of prostaglandins is an unsettled issue (Jacobson and Thompson, 1976). Although administration of dibutyryl cyclic AMP increases acid secretion under certain conditions, gastric mucosal levels of cyclic AMP can be raised by inhibitors such as prostaglandin and secretin, as well as by secretogogues such as histamine, depending on the species (Jacobson and Thompson, 1976).

Certain antisecretory prostaglandins reduce gastric mucosal blood flow. However, this is the result of the antisecretory effect, rather than the cause, since the ratio of gastric mucosal blood flow to secretory rate is not reduced (Jacobson, 1970). Finally, antisecretory prostaglandins have no anticholinergic activity nor are they histamine H_2 receptor antagonists.

Several methyl analogues of PGE_2 (15(R)-15-methyl PGE_2, 15(S)-15-methyl PGE_2 and 16,16-dimethyl PGE_2), given orally, were found to inhibit the increase in serum gastrin in response to food (Ippoliti *et al.*, 1976; Konturek *et al.*, 1976a, 1976b). On the other hand, 15(R)-15-methyl PGE_2 methyl ester increased the basal level of gastrin (Adaikan *et al.*, 1974), whereas 16,16-dimethyl PGE_2 reduced histamine-stimulated gastrin level by 80% (Wilson *et al.*, 1975). In another study, 15(S)-15-methyl PGE_2 methyl ester given intravenously did not affect serum gastrin, either under basal conditions or after meal stimulation (Konturek *et al.*, 1976a).

These results suggest that the methyl analogues block the release of gastrin induced by food only when they are administered orally. This inhibitory effect may enhance the antisecretory action of prostaglandins, but is not its cause, since prostaglandins block the secretogogue effect of gastrin itself.

6.7.2 Enteropooling

Enteropooling appears to be due to stimulation of adenyl cyclase activity by prostaglandins (Kimberg *et al.*, 1971). The resulting increase in cyclic AMP in the intestinal mucosa promotes passage of water and electrolytes into the intestinal lumen. The effect is similar to the enteropooling produced by intraluminal application of cholera toxin, an agent that also stimulates formation of cyclic AMP (Pierce *et al.*, 1971).

6.7.3 Cytoprotection

The mechanism of gastric and intestinal cytoprotection is unknown. In the case of mucosal damage produced by non-steroidal anti-inflammatory compounds, such as aspirin and indomethacin, the lesions may result from the prostaglandin deficiency elicited by these drugs, since these compounds block the activity of cyclo-oxygenase, the enzyme responsible for the biosynthesis of prostaglandins (Vane, 1971). Treatment with prostaglandins could exert a protective effect by replacing the missing endogenous prostaglandin. In the case of gastric cytoprotection against such strong agents as absolute ethanol, concentrated acid (0.6 N HCl) or base (0.2 N NaOH), and even boiling water, no such mechanism can be postulated, since these agents kill the epithelium by contact. It appears that pretreatment with a variety of prostaglandins increases the resistance of mucosal cells to necrotizing agents. It has been suggested that prostaglandins may be necessary to maintain cellular integrity (Robert *et al.*, 1979).

6.7.4 Anti-ulcer effect

The anti-ulcer effect of prostaglandins can be due to two factors: inhibition of gastric acid secretion and cytoprotection. In the clinical studies reported above, in which certain methyl analogues of PGE_2 were shown to accelerate ulcer healing, the doses given were antisecretory. Such doses are also cytoprotective, as shown in animal models. Therefore, in these models the resulting beneficial effect could be ascribed to both properties. This conclusion is only tentative since a reduction in the amount of acid present in the stomach can by itself accelerate the rate of healing of duodenal ulcers as was shown for antacids (Peterson *et al.*, 1977). To find out whether peptic ulcer can be healed or its recurrence prevented by a cytoprotective prostaglandin, clinical trials will have to be performed with a prostaglandin that is cytoprotective but devoid of antisecretory effect.

6.8 CONCLUSIONS

Several prostaglandins influence gastro-intestinal function when administered to humans in microgram quantities. Certain prostaglandins of the E series inhibit gastric acid and pepsin secretion, and preliminary studies indicate that they accelerate ulcer healing. It is likely that these prostaglandins, especially certain methyl analogues, will be useful in the treatment of peptic ulcer.

Many prostaglandins tend to stimulate intestinal secretion (enteropooling) and intestinal motility, a dual effect that may explain the development of diarrhoea observed after administration of high doses. These properties may be put to advantage in the management of constipation and post-operative ileus.

The cytoprotective property of prostaglandins that allows the gastro-intestinal mucosa to withstand the presence of noxious substances intraluminally, may have several clinical applications. Prostaglandins, even those devoid of antisecretory activity, may eventually be administered for the treatment of gastritis, ulcers, and inflammatory disease of the bowel. The fact that cytoprotection is shown at very low doses suggests that prostaglandins may exert this action without producing other effects.

References

Adaikan, G. P., Salmon, J. A., Ng, B. K. and Karim, S. M. M. (1974). The effect of 15(R)-15-methyl PGE_2 methyl ester on serum gastrin levels in man. *IRCS*, **2**, 1587

Amy, J. J., Jackson, D. M., Ganesan, P. A. and Karim, S. M. M. (1973). Prostaglandin 15(R)-15-methyl E_2 methyl ester for suppression of gastric acidity in gravida at term. *Br. Med. J.*, **4**, 208

Bhana, D., Karim, S. M. M., Carter, D. C. and Ganesan, P. A. (1973). The effect of orally administered prostaglandins A_1, A_2 and 15-epi-A_2 on human gastric secretion. *Prostaglandins*, **3**, 307

Carter, D. C., Karim, S. M. M., Bhana, D. and Ganesan, P. A. (1973a). The effect of locally administered 15(R)-15-methyl E_2 prostaglandin on basal and pentagastrin-induced acid secretion in man. *Br. J. Surg.*, **60**, 320

Carter, D. C., Karim, S. M. M., Bhana, D. and Ganesan, P. A. (1973b). Inhibition of human gastric secretion by prostaglandin. *Br. J. Surg.*, **60**, 828

Carter, D. C., Karim, S. M. M., Bhana, D. and Ganesan, P. A. (1973c). Inhibition of human gastric secretion by orally or intravenously administered prostaglandin 16,16-dimethyl E_2 methyl ester. *Br. J. Surg.*, **60**, 912

Chen, F. W. K., Teck, H. S. and Karim, S. M. M. (1977). The effect of 15(R)-15-methyl prostaglandin E_2 on gastric acid secretion in duodenal ulcer patients. *Prostaglandins*, **13**, 115

Classen, M., Koch, H., Bickhardt, J., Topf, G. and Demling, L. (1971). The effect of prostaglandin E_1 on the pentagastrin-stimulated gastric secretion in man. *Digestion*, **4**, 333

Classen, M., Koch, H., Deyhle, P., Weidenhiller, S. and Demling, L. (1970). Wirkung von prostaglandin E_1 auf die Basale Magensekretion des Menschen. *Klin. Wochenschr.*, **48**, 876

Cohen, M. M. (1978). Mucosal cytoprotection by prostaglandin E_2. *Lancet*, **ii**, 1253

Cummings, J. H., Milton-Thompson, G. J., Billings, J., Newman, A. and Misiewicz, J. J. (1974). Studies on the site of production of diarrhoea by prostaglandins. *Clin. Sci. Mol. Med.*, **46**, 15p

Cummings, J. H., Newman, A., Misiewicz, J. J., Milton-Thompson, G. J. and Billings, J. A. (1973). Effect of intravenous prostaglandin $F_{2\alpha}$ on small intestinal function in man. *Nature (London)*, **243**, 169

Dilawari, J. B., Newman, A., Poleo, J. and Misiewicz, J. J. (1975). Response of the human cardiac sphincter to circulating prostaglandin $F_{2\alpha}$ and E_2 and to anti-inflammatory drugs. *Gut*, **16**, 137

Feldman, J. M., Plonk, J. W. and Cornette, J. C. (1974). Serum prostaglandin $F_{2\alpha}$ concentration in the carcinoid syndrome. *Prostaglandins*, **7**, 501

Ferguson, W. W., Edmonds, A. W., Starling, J. R. and Wangensteen, S. L. (1973). Protective effect of prostaglandin E_1 (PGE_1) on lysosomal enzyme release in serotonin-induced gastric ulceration. *Ann. Surg.*, **177**, 648

Fung, W. P., Lee, S. K. and Karim, S. M. M. (1974c). Effect of prostaglandin 15(R)-15-methyl-E_2 methyl ester on the gastric mucosa in patients with peptic ulceration – an endoscopic and histological study. *Prostaglandins*, **5**, 465

Fung, W. P. and Karim, S. M. M. (1976a). The effect of prostaglandin E_2 on healing of gastric ulcers: double blind endoscopic trial. *Aust. N.Z. J. Med.*, **6**, 121

Fung, W. P. and Karim, S. M. M. (1976b). Effect of 15(R)-15-methyl prostaglandin E_2 on the healing of gastric ulcers – double blind endoscopic study. *Med. J. Aust.*, **2**, 127

Fung, W. P., Karim, S. M. M. and Tye, C. Y. (1974a). Double-blind trial of 15(R)-15-methyl prostaglandin E_2 methyl ester in the relief of peptic ulcer pain. *Ann. Acad. Med. (Singapore)*, **3**, 375

Fung, W. P., Karim, S. M. M. and Tye, C. Y. (1974b). Effect of 15(R)-15-methyl prostaglandin E_2 methyl ester on healing of gastric ulcers. Controlled endoscopic study. *Lancet*, **ii**, 10

Gibinski, K., Rybicka, J., Mikos, E. and Nowak, A. (1977). Double-blind clinical trial on gastro-duodenal ulcer healing with prostaglandin E_2 analogues. *Gut*, **18**, 636

Goyal, R. K., Mukhopadhyay, A. and Rattan, S. (1974). Effect of prostaglandin E_2 on the lower esophageal sphincter in normal subjects and patients with achalasia. *Clin. Res.*, **22**, 358A

Greenough, W. B., Pierce, N. F., Al Awquati, Q. and Carpenter, C. C. J. (1969). Stimulation of gut electrolyte secretion by prostaglandins, theophylline and cholera exotoxin. *J. Clin. Invest.*, **48**, 32A

Horton, E. W., Main, I. H. M., Thompson, C. J. and Wright, P. M. (1968). Effect of orally administered prostaglandin E_2 on gastric secretion and gastro-intestinal motility in man. *Gut*, **9**, 655

Hunt, R. H., Dilawari, J. B. and Misiewicz, J. J. (1975). The effect of intravenous prostaglandin $F_{2\alpha}$ and E_2 on the motility of the sigmoid colon. *Gut*, **16**, 47

Ippoliti, A. F., Isenberg, J. I., Maxwell, V. and Walsh, J. H. (1976). The effect of 16,16-dimethyl prostaglandin E_2 on meal-stimulated gastric secretion and serum gastrin in duodenal ulcer patients. *Gastroenterology*, **70**, 488

Jacobson, E. D. (1970). Comparison of prostaglandin E_1 and norepinephrine on the gastric mucosal circulation. *Proc. Soc. Exp. Biol. Med.*, **133**, 516

Jacobson, E. D. and Thompson, W. J. (1976). Cyclic AMP and gastric secretion: the illusive second messenger. *Adv. Cyclic Nucleotide Res.*, **7**, 199

Jaffe, B. M., Behrman, H. R. and Parker, C. W. (1973). Radioimmunoassay measurement of prostaglandins E, A and F in human plasma. *J. Clin. Invest.*, **52**, 398

Johansson, C., Kollberg, B., Nordemar, R. and Bergström, S. (1979). Mucosal protection by prostaglandin E_2. *Lancet*, 317

Karim, S. M. M., Carter, D. C., Bhana, D. and Ganesan, P. A. (1973a). Effect of orally and intravenously administered prostaglandin 15(R)-15-methyl E_2 on gastric secretion in man. *Adv. Biosci.*, **9**, 255

Karim, S. M. M., Carter, D. C., Bhana, D. and Ganesan, P. A. (1973b). Effect of orally administered prostaglandin E_2 and its 15-methyl analogues on gastric secretion. *Br. Med. J.*, **1**, 143

Karim, S. M. M., Carter, D. C., Bhana, D. and Ganesan, P. A. (1973c). The effect of orally and intravenously administered prostaglandin 16,16-dimethyl E_2 methyl ester on human gastric acid secretion. *Prostaglandins*, **4**, 71

Karim, S. M. M. and Fung, W. P. (1975). Effect of 15(R)-15-methyl prostaglandin E_2 on gastric secretion and a preliminary study on the healing of gastric ulcers in man. *IRCS Med. Sci.*, **3**, 348

Karim, S. M. M. and Fung, W. P. (1976). Effects of some naturally occurring prostaglandins and synthetic analogues on gastric secretion and ulcer healing in man. *Adv. Prostagland. Thromboxane Res.*, **2**, 529

Kawarada, Y., Lambek, J. and Matsumoto, T. (1975). Pathophysiology of stress ulcer and its prevention. II. Prostaglandin E_1 and microcirculatory responses in stress ulcer. *Am. J. Surg.*, **129**, 217

Kimberg, D. V., Field, M., Johnson, J., Henderson, A. and Gershon, E. (1971). Stimulation of intestinal mucosal adenyl cyclase by cholera enterotoxin and prostaglandins. *J. Clin. Invest.*, **50**, 1218

Konturek, S. J., Oleksy, J., Biernat, J., Sito, E. and Kwiecien, N. (1976a). Effect of synthetic 15-methyl analogue of PGE_2 on gastric acid and serum gastrin response to peptone meal, pentagastrin, and histamine in duodenal ulcer patients. *Am. J. Dig. Dis.*, **21**, 291

Konturek, S. J., Kwiecien, N., Swierczek, J., Oleksy, J., Sito, E. and Robert, A. (1976b). Comparison of methylated prostaglandin E_2 analogues given orally in the inhibition of gastric responses to pentagastrin and peptone meal in man. *Gastroenterology*, **70**, 683

Labrum, A. H., Lipkin, M. and Dray, F. (1976). Hyperprostaglandinemia: A previously unrecognized syndrome. In: B. Samuelsson and R. Paoletti (eds.), *Advances in Prostaglandins and Thromboxane Research*, Vol. II, p. 888 (New York: Raven Press)

Lancaster, C. and Robert, A. (1978). Intestinal lesions produced by prednisolone: prevention (cytoprotection) by 16,16-dimethyl prostaglandin E_2. *Am. J. Physiol.*, **235**, E703

Lee, Y. H. and Bianchi, R. G. (1972). The antisecretory and anti-ulcer activity of a prostaglandin analogue, SC-24665, in experimental animals. *5th Int. Congr. Pharmacol.*, San Francisco, 136 (abstr.)

Lee, Y. H., Cheng, W. D., Bianchi, R. G., Mollison, K. and Hansen, J. (1973). Effects of oral administration of PGE_2 on gastric secretion and experimental peptic ulcerations. *Prostaglandins*, **3**, 29

Magerlein, B. J., DuCharme, D. W., Magee, W. E., Miller, W. L., Robert, A. and Weeks, J. R. (1973). Synthesis and biological properties of 16-alkylprostaglandins. *Prostaglandins*, **4**, 143

Main, I. H. M. and Whittle, B. J. R. (1974). Prostaglandin E_2 and the stimulation of rat gastric acid secretion by dibutyryl cyclic 3′,5′-AMP. *Eur. J. Pharmacol.*, **26**, 204

Matuchansky, C. and Bernier, J. J. (1971). Effects of prostaglandin E_1 on net and undirectional movements of water and electrolytes across jejunal mucosa in man. *Gut*, **12**, 854

Matuchansky, C. and Bernier, J. J. (1973). Effect of prostaglandin E_1 on glucose, water, and electrolyte absorption in the human jejunum. *Gastroenterology*, **64**, 1111

Matuchansky, C. and Coutrot, S. (1978). The role of prostaglandins in the study of intestinal water and electrolyte transport in man. *Biomedicine*, **28**, 143

Matuchansky, C., Mary, J. Y. and Bernier, J. J. (1972). Effect of prostaglandin E_1 on glucose absorption and on transintestinal movements of water and electrolytes in human jejunum. *Biol. Gastroent.* (Paris), **5**, 636C

McCallum, R. W., Ippoliti, A. F. and Sturdevant, R. A. L. (1975). Effect of oral 16,16-dimethyl prostaglandin E_2 (PGE_2) on the lower esophageal sphincter in man. *Gastroenterology*, **68**, 949

Milton-Thompson, G. J., Cummings, J. H., Newman, A., Billings, J. A. and Misiewicz, J. J. (1975). Colonic and small intestinal response to intravenous prostaglandin $F_{2\alpha}$ and E_2 in man. *Gut*, **16**, 42

Newman, A., DeMoraes-Filho, J. P. P., Philippakos, D. and Misiewicz, J. J. (1975). The effect of intravenous infusions of prostaglandins E_2 and $F_{2\alpha}$ on human gastric function. *Gut*, **16**, 272

Newman, A., Milton-Thompson, G., Cummings, J. H., Billings, J. A. and Misiewicz, J. J. (1974). Differential response of the human small and large intestine to prostaglandin $F_{2\alpha}$. *Gastroenterology*, **66**, A-100/754

Nylander, B. and Andersson, S. (1974). Gastric secretory inhibition induced by three methyl analogues of prostaglandin E_2 administered intragastrically to man. *Scand. J. Gastroenterol.*, **9**, 751

Nylander, B. and Andersson, S. (1975). Effect of two methylated prostaglandin E_2 analogues on gastro-duodenal pressure in man. *Scand. J. Gastroenterol.*, **10**, 91

Nylander, B. and Mattsson, O. (1975). Effect of 16,16-dimethyl PGE_2 on gastric emptying and intestinal transit of a barium-food test meal in man. *Scand. J. Gastroenterol.*, **10**, 289

Nylander, B., Robert, A. and Andersson, S. (1974). Gastric secretory inhibition by certain methyl analogues of prostaglandin E_2 following intestinal administration in man. *Scand. J. Gastroenterol.*, **9**, 759

Peterson, W. L., Sturdevant, R. A. L., Franki, H. D., Richardson, C. T., Isenberg, J. I., Elashoff, J. D., Sones, J. Q., Gross, R. A., McCallum, R. W. and Fordtran, J. S. (1977). Healing of duodenal ulcer with an antacid regimen. *N. Engl. J. Med.*, **297**, 341

Pierce, N. F., Carpenter, C. C. J. Jr., Elliot, H. L. and Greenough, W. B. III. (1971). Effects of prostaglandins, theophylline, and cholera exotoxin upon transmucosal water and electrolyte movement in the canine jejunum. *Gastroenterology*, **60**, 22

Robert, A. (1975a). An intestinal disease produced experimentally by a prostaglandin deficiency. *Gastroenterology*, **69**, 1045

Robert, A. (1975b). Antisecretory, anti-ulcer, cytoprotective and diarrheogenic properties of prostaglandins. In: *Advances in Prostaglandin and Thromboxane Research*, p. 507 (New York: Raven Press)

Robert, A., Lancaster, C., Nezamis, J. E. and Badalamenti, J. N. (1973). A gastric antisecretory and anti-ulcer prostaglandin with oral and long-acting activity. *Gastroenterology*, **64**, 790

Robert, A., Nezamis, J. E. and Lancaster, C. (1975a). Duodenal ulcers produced by non-steroidal anti-inflammatory compounds plus bile duct ligation. *Fed. Proc.*, **34**, 442

Robert, A., Nezamis, J. E. and Lancaster, C. (1975b). Duodenal ulcers produced in rats by propionitrile: factors inhibiting and aggravating such ulcers. *Toxicol. Appl. Pharmacol.*, **31**, 201

Robert, A., Nezamis, J. E., Lancaster, C. and Badalamenti, J. N. (1975c). Cysteamine-induced duodenal ulcers: a new model to test anti-ulcer agents. *Digestion*, **11**, 199

Robert, A., Nezamis, J. E., Lancaster, C. and Hanchar, A. J. (1979). Cytoprotection by prostaglandins in rats: prevention of gastric necrosis produced by alcohol, HCl, NaOH, hypertonic NaCl and thermal injury. *Gastroenterology* (In press)

Robert, A., Nezamis, J. E., Lancaster, C., Hanchar, A. J. and Klepper, M. S. (1976a). Enteropooling assay: a test for diarrhoea produced by prostaglandins. *Prostaglandins*, **11**, 809

Robert, A., Nezamis, J. E. and Phillips, J. (1967). Inhibition of gastric secretion by prostaglandins. *Am. J. Dig. Dis.*, **12**, 1073

Robert, A., Nezamis, J. E. and Phillips, J. P. (1968). Effect of prostaglandin E_2 on gastric secretion and ulcer formation in the rat. *Gastroenterology*, **55**, 481

Robert, A., Nylander, B. and Andersson, S. (1974). Marked inhibition of gastric secretion by two prostaglandin analogues given orally to man. *Life Sci.*, **14**, 533

Robert, A., Phillips, J. P. and Nezamis, J. E. (1968). Inhibition by prostaglandin E_1 of gastric secretion in the dog. *Gastroenterology*, **54**, 1263

Robert, A., Schultz, J. R., Nezamis, J. E. and Lancaster, C. (1976b). Gastric antisecretory and anti-ulcer properties of PGE_2, 15-methyl PGE_2, and 16,16-dimethyl PGE_2. Intravenous, oral and intrajejunal administration. *Gastroenterology*, **70**, 359

Robert, A., Stowe, D. F. and Nezamis, J. E. (1971). Prevention of duodenal ulcers by administration of prostaglandin E_2 (PGE_2). *Scand. J. Gastroenterol.*, **6**, 303

Robert, A. and Yankee, E. W. (1975). Gastric antisecretory effect of 15(R)-15-methyl PGE_2 methyl ester and of 15(S)-15-methyl PGE_2 methyl ester. *Proc. Soc. Exp. Biol. Med.*, **148**, 1155

Rybicka, J. and Gibinski, K. (1977). Methyl-prostaglandin E_2 analogues for healing of gastroduodenal ulcers. *Scand. J. Gastroenterol.*, **13**, 155

Sandler, M., Karim, S. M. M. and Williams, E. D. (1968). Prostaglandins in amine-peptide-secreting tumours. *Lancet*, **ii**, 1053

Soll, A. H. (1978). Prostaglandin inhibition of histamine-stimulated aminopyrine uptake and cyclic AMP generation by isolated canine parietal cells. *Gastroenterology*, **74**, 1146

Vane, J. R. (1971). Inhibition of prostaglandin synthesis as a mechanism of action for aspirin-like drugs. *Nature (New Biol.)*, **231**, 232

Wada, T. and Ishizawa, M. (1970). Effects of prostaglandin on the function of the gastric secretion. *Jap. J. Clin. Med.*, **28**, 2465

Way, L. and Durbin, R. P. (1969). Inhibition of gastric acid secretion *in vitro* by prostaglandin E_1. *Nature (London)*, **221**, 874

Williams, E. D., Karim, S. M. M. and Sandler, M. (1968). Prostaglandin secretion by medullary carcinoma of the thyroid. *Lancet*, **i**, 22

Wilson, D. E., Phillips, C. and Levine, R. A. (1971). Inhibition of gastric secretion in man by prostaglandin A_1. *Gastroenterology*, **61**, 201

Wilson, D. E., Quertermus, J., Raiser, M., Curran, J. and Robert, A. (1976). Inhibition of stimulated gastric secretion by an orally administered prostaglandin capsule: a study in normal men. *Ann. Intern. Med.*, **84**, 688

Wilson, D. E., Winnan, G., Quertermus, J. and Tao, P. (1975). Effects of an orally administered prostaglandin analogue (16,16-dimethyl prostaglandin E_2) on human gastric secretion. *Gastroenterology*, **69**, 607

Wilson, D. E. and Winter, S. L. (1978). The effects of 11-methyl 16,16-dimethyl prostaglandin E_2 on gastric acid secretion in man. *Prostaglandins*, **16**, 127

Yankee, E. W., Axen, U. and Bundy, G. L. (1974). Total synthesis of 15-methyl prostaglandins. *J. Am. Chem. Soc.*, **96**, 5865

Yankee, E. W. and Bundy, G. L. (1972). 15(S)-15-methyl prostaglandins. *J. Am. Chem. Soc.*, **94**, 3651

7
Prostaglandins and their Synthesis Inhibitors in Bartter's Syndrome

M. FICHMAN

7.1 INTRODUCTION

Pronove, McCardle and Bartter (1960), and Bartter *et al.* (1962) originally described the syndrome characterized by hypokalaemic alkalosis, with renal potassium wasting, elevated plasma renin activity and aldosterone levels, normal or low blood pressure, resistance to the pressor effect of angiotensin and norepinephrine, and juxtaglomerular cell hyperplasia. Other characteristics of many patients with this syndrome include growth retardation and polyuria, both presumably the result of hypokalaemia (Bryan *et al.*, 1966).

Bartter *et al.* (1974) also described excessive delivery of proximal tubular fluid to the distal nephron, with impairment in generation of free water at the diluting site. While the majority of over 60 patients reported were children (e.g. 31/37 by Fanconi *et al.*, 1971), this syndrome also occurs in adults without evidence of growth retardation. Indeed, Barbour and Day (1978) reported an asymptomatic 63-year-old patient with all the cardinal manifestations of this syndrome. A number of the childhood cases (Arant *et al.*, 1970; Sutherland *et al.*, 1970; Trygstad, 1969; and Bourke and Delaney, 1977) are familial and associated with other tubular defects and progressive renal failure attributed to pathological findings of glomerulonephritis and interstitial nephritis. Previous treatment of Bartter's syndrome has in general been unsatisfactory (see editorial in *Lancet*, 1976). Potassium loading or attempted blockade of distal tubular secretion of potassium by triamterene or spironolactone have produced only minimal increase in serum potassium level. Bilateral adrenalectomy was also unsuccessful in correcting hypokalaemia (Trygstad *et al.*, 1969).

7.2 PATHOGENESIS OF BARTTER'S SYNDROME

Previous theories on the pathogenesis of Bartter's syndrome are summarized by Vaisrub (1978), Stein (1978), and Bartter (1977), and in an editorial in *Lancet* (1976).

7.2.1 Angiotensin resistance

Bartter *et al.* (1962) postulated that the basic defect in the syndrome is a vascular insensitivity to the pressor effect of angiotensin, leading to a decrease in vascular resistance and renal hypoperfusion, and a secondary stimulation of the renin–angiotensin system and aldosterone.

7.2.2 Volume depletion due to renal sodium wasting

The possibility that underlying extracellular fluid volume depletion, resulting from increased fractional sodium excretion observed in many patients with this syndrome was originally suggested by Cannon *et al.* (1968). Goodman *et al.* (1969), also Beilin *et al.* (1967), Bourke and Delaney (1977), White (1972), Solomon and Brown (1975) and Tomko *et al.* (1976) all showed that infusion of albumin or saline tended to suppress the elevated levels of plasma renin activity and aldosterone and restore pressor sensitivity to angiotensin towards normal. Chan *et al.* (1975) and Tomko *et al.* (1976) proposed that a leak in the reabsorption of sodium in the proximal tubule was present in this syndrome leading to increased distal delivery of sodium. Measurements of the sum of C_{Na} and C_{H_2O} were used as an estimate of distal delivery from the proximal tubule. Nielson *et al.* (1973) also demonstrated defective renal sodium conservation in response to sodium restriction.

Chaimowitz *et al.* (1973) on the other hand localized the site of tubular rejection of sodium to the ascending limb of the loop of Henle.

The resultant extracellular fluid contraction could then lead to stimulation of the renin–angiotensin aldosterone system, renal potassium wasting, and hypovolaemia-induced resistance to the pressor effect of angiotensin. Norby *et al.* (1976), Bartter *et al.* (1962), and Bryan *et al.* (1966) however noted normal renal conservation of sodium in response to sodium restriction in several patients with this syndrome. Furthermore, Beilin *et al.* (1967), Erkelens and von Epps (1973), and James *et al.* (1975) obtained measurements of plasma volume using RISA in their patients which were normal.

7.2.3 Glomerular–distal tubular shunts

Biava *et al.* (1969) demonstrated histologically glomerulo-distal tubular shunts in renal biopsies from patients with Bartter's syndrome which could account for the enhanced delivery of sodium to the distal tubule bypassing proximal tubular and ascending limb resorptive sites.

7.2.4 Impaired chloride reabsorption in the ascending limb of the loop of Henle

Kurtzman and Gutierrez (1975) originally proposed that the basic defect in Bartter's syndrome was an impairment in active chloride transport out of the thick ascending limb. This would lead secondarily to an increased chloride and therefore sodium and potassium delivery to the distal nephron, acceleration of distal tubular sodium–potassium exchange, and resultant renal sodium, chloride and potassium loss.

Cannon *et al.* (1968) and Sutherland *et al.* (1970) had previously demonstrated defective chloride reabsorption in Bartter's syndrome.

Gill and Bartter (1978) showed a more marked impairment in distal fractional chloride reabsorption (calculated as $C_{H_2O}/(C_{H_2O}+C_{Cl})$) in five patients with Bartter's syndrome compared to five patients with hypokalaemic alkalosis due to psychogenic vomiting (Figure 7.1). Since urinary dilution is dependent on ascending limb chloride reabsorption, maximal free-water clearance was impaired in all the patients with Bartter's syndrome. Increased distal delivery of proximal tubular fluid ($(C_{H_2O}+C_{Cl})/C_{inulin}$) was present only in those patients with Bartter's syndrome with low glomerular filtration rate.

7.2.5 Cell membrane sodium–potassium transport defect

A cell membrane sodium transport defect leading to decreased extrusion of sodium from erythrocytes and an increase in intracellular sodium concentration were demonstrated by Gardner *et al.* (1972) in six out of eight patients with Bartter's syndrome as well as in their otherwise normal siblings. Gall *et al.* (1971), and Oliver *et al.* (1978) on the other hand found an increase in sodium influx in five siblings with Bartter's syndrome, leading to increased erythrocyte sodium concentration. They postulated that hypokalaemia *per se* accounted for the increased sodium influx. Potassium content was normal.

Haljamae *et al.* (1975) showed a reduction in potassium concentration of skeletal muscle cells and increased erythrocyte ATPase activity in patients with Bartter's syndrome compared to controls.

Delaporte *et al.* (1978) analysed muscle biopsies for electrolyte content by neutron activation in six children with Bartter's syndrome. Muscle potassium was decreased and whole muscle sodium increased compared to normal subjects. Following therapy with spironolactone and potassium chloride, intracellular potassium still remained below normal.

7.2.6 Primary magnesium depletion

A low serum magnesium has occasionally been found in patients with Bartter's syndrome (Sutherland *et al.*, 1970; Barbour and Day, 1978; Donker *et al.*, 1977; and Zipser *et al.*, 1978).

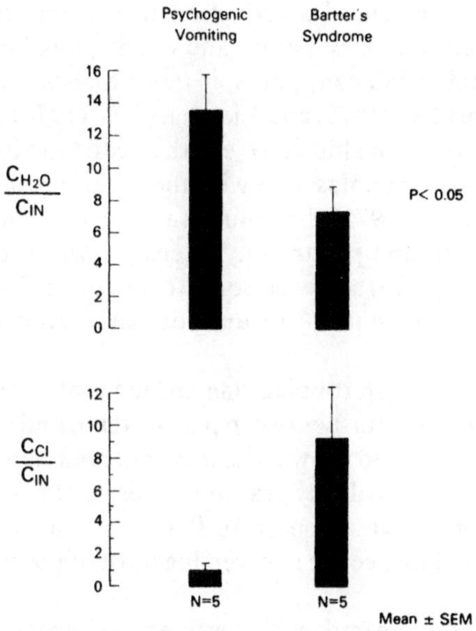

Figure 7.1 Fractional clearance of free water (C_{H_2O}/C_{in}) and fractional clearance of chloride (C_{Cl}/C_{in}) during water diuresis in patients with psychogenic vomiting and in patients with Bartter's syndrome.

Reprinted by permission of authors and *Am. J. Med.* from Gill, J. R. and Bartter, F. C. (1978). *Am. J. Med.* **65**, 769, Figure 5

A congenital renal magnesium wasting hypomagnesaemic syndrome with secondary hypokalaemia and renal potassium wasting has been described by Gittelman *et al.* (1966), which is distinct from Bartter's syndrome. Aguilera *et al.* (1978) showed that magnesium increases sodium transport across the toad bladder probably by increasing the activity of the sodium pump. By analogy, magnesium depletion may interfere with tubular sodium reabsorption leading to enhanced distal sodium delivery and potassium loss. Magnesium repletion in the hypomagnesaemic patient studied by Zipser *et al.* (1978), and Barbour and Day (1978) failed to raise serum potassium. These findings as well as the normal serum magnesium in most reported patients with Bartter's syndrome suggest that the occasional finding of hypomagnesaemia is likely to be the result rather than a cause of Bartter's syndrome.

7.2.7 β-adrenergic stimulation of renin–angiotensin-induced natriuresis

Modlinger *et al.* (1973) postulated that renal sodium and potassium wasting in Bartter's syndrome resulted from β-adrenergic mediated increase in renin release which produced a natriuretic effect in these patients by activating angiotensin. They administered propranolol (as a β-adrenergic blocker of renin release) which produced a reduction in plasma renin activity, aldosterone, and initiated sodium retention and weight gain, but failed to improve serum potassium unless concomitant spironolactone was employed.

Schwartz and Cornfeld (1975) and Fichman *et al.* (1976) showed an increase in plasma renin activity and aldosterone with a reduction in urine sodium, but no improvement in serum potassium with the use of propranolol in Bartter's syndrome. Tomko *et al.* (1976) also found an increase in plasma renin activity with sodium retention and postural hypotension with propranolol therapy. Solomon and Brown (1975) achieved some reduction in elevated plasma renin activity and aldosterone, but not serum potassium even with high doses of propranolol.

With the addition of spironolactone, serum potassium rose, but propranolol did not prevent a further rise in plasma renin and aldosterone. Norby *et al.* (1976) likewise failed to show a rise in serum potassium or normalization of plasma renin activity with propranolol. Clearly the angiotensin-induced natriuresis theory of the pathogenesis of Bartter's syndrome was invalid and the use of propranolol ineffective in reversing most of the manifestation of the syndrome.

The possibility that increased angiotensin was a primary cause rather than a compensatory response to volume depletion in Bartter's syndrome was refuted by the findings of Sasaki *et al.* (1976) that saralisin, a competitive inhibitor of angiotensin, produced a profound reduction in blood pressure in a patient with Bartter's syndrome.

7.2.8 Abnormalities in the kallikrein–kinin system

Vinci *et al.* (1978) suggested the possibility that the vasodilator effects of the kallikrein–kinin system may play a role in the angiotensin resistance and natriuresis in Bartter's syndrome.

Seven female patients aged between 9 and 46 years with Bartter's syndrome had high levels of plasma bradykinin (a potent vasodilator) and urinary kallikrein (which generates bradykinin from precursor kininogen). Increased urinary kallikrein may in part be due to the stimulant effect of increased

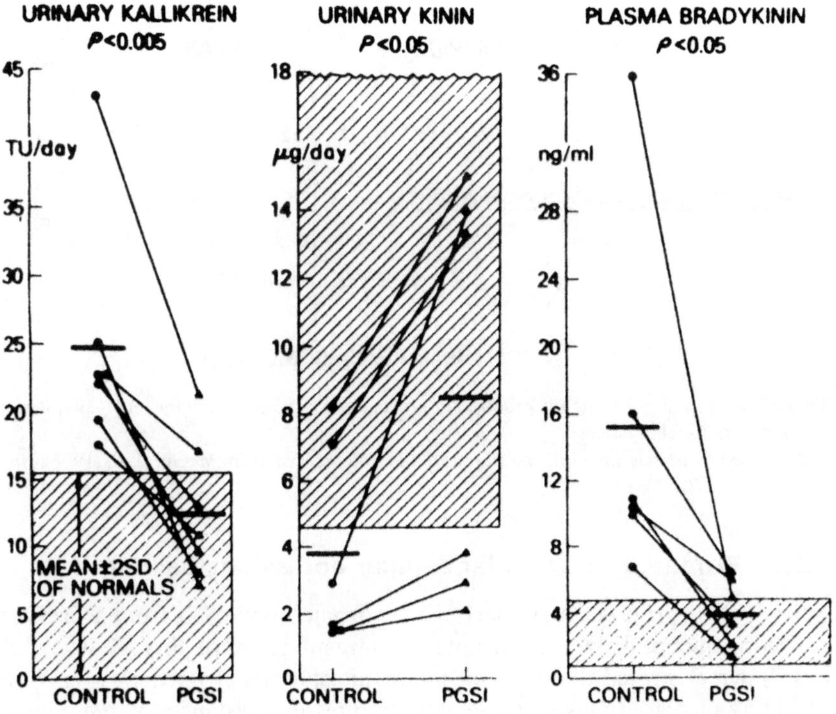

Figure 7.2 Effect of prostaglandin synthetase inhibition (PGSI) on urinary kallikrein excretion ($U_{ka}V$), on urinary kinin secretion ($U_{ki}V$) and on mean plasma bradykinin (PBK) by the 7th day of treatment in six patients with Bartter's syndrome. The shaded area is the mean ±2 SD for normal subjects fed 109 mmol sodium. Horizontal bars represent mean for each group.

Reprinted by permission of the authors and *J. Clin. Invest.* from Vinci, J. M. *et al.* (1978). *J. Clin. Invest.*, **61**, 1677, Figure 3

aldosterone in Bartter's syndrome. Urinary kinins on the other hand were reduced which probably reflected decreased secretion of unmetabolized bradykinin from distal tubule (Figure 7.2). Plasma pre-kallikrein levels were normal, so that the high levels of bradykinin may be due to decreased destruction rather than increased production. Halusha *et al.* (1977) also report

5–10 fold higher than normal levels of urinary kallikrein in two female children with Bartter's syndrome.

McGiff (1977) postulated that Bartter's syndrome may result from an imbalance of the inter-relationships between three vasoactive hormone systems: kallikrein–kinin, renin–angiotensin and prostaglandin (Figure 7.3).

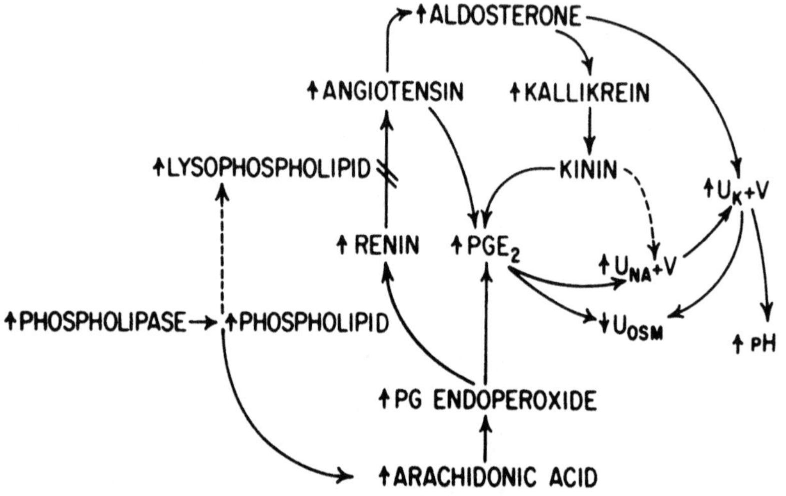

Figure 7.3 Relations among the products of prostaglandin synthesis and the renin–angiotensin and kinin–kallikrein systems.

Reprinted by permission of the authors and *Ann. Intern. Med.* from McGiff, J. C. (1977). *Ann. Intern. Med.*, **87**, 370, Figure 1

7.2.9 Primary renal tubular cellular potassium wasting

Ferris (1978) proposed that Bartter's syndrome may result from a primary collecting duct or distal tubular potassium wasting abnormality. Galvez *et al.* (1977) demonstrated that most of the manifestations of Bartter's syndrome including increased plasma renin activity, pressor resistance to angiotensin, and increase in urinary PGE excretion occurred with severe potassium depletion in dogs. However, these animals had marked sodium retention, increased body weight and plasma volume in response to potassium depletion and no increase in plasma aldosterone, all of which are contrary to what is observed in Bartter's syndrome in man.

7.3 ROLE OF PROSTAGLANDINS IN THE PATHOGENESIS OF BARTTER'S SYNDROME–RATIONALE

Fichman *et al.* (1976) and Verberkmoes *et al.* (1976) originally proposed that increased renal prostaglandin production may mediate the manifestations of

Bartter's syndrome. The observed properties of renal medullary prostaglandins interrelate with several of the aforementioned theories of the pathogenesis of this disorder.

(1) Prostaglandin A has a vasodepressor effect in man (Lee, 1971) and antagonizes the vasopressor response to angiotensin (Golub *et al.*, 1975). More important, PGE_2 which has conclusively been shown by Danon *et al.* (1975) to be the major product of renal medullar prostaglandin synthesis antagonizes the vasoconstrictor effect of angiotensin on renal cortical blood flow (Vane and McGiff, 1975; and Lonigro *et al.*, 1973).

(2) Vander (1968) showed that prostaglandins increased renin release possibly by increasing sodium chloride delivery past the macula densa. PGE_2 failed to increase renin release from renal medullar slices (Weber *et al.*, 1976). However, arachidonic acid and the cyclic endoperoxide PGG_2 did increase renin release. Other prostaglandins such as prostacyclin (PGI_2) which is synthesized in the renal cortical blood vessels and glomerulae (Terragno *et al.*, 1978) may stimulate renin release from rabbit cortical slices (Whorton *et al.*, 1977). Also, PGD_2 which is produced in the renal medulla and cortex stimulates plasma renin activity when infused into the renal vein of the dog (Bolger *et al.*, 1977).

(3) PGA_1 has been shown by Fichman *et al.* (1972, 1973) to increase plasma aldosterone in normal and anephric man. This is independent of effects on plasma renin, sodium or potassium balance.

(4) Infusion of PGE and PGA compounds in animals and man produced a natriuretic response which may be accounted for by renal cortical vasodilation (Itzkovitz *et al.*, 1974). Furthermore, micropuncture studies by Stokes and Kokko (1976) demonstrated that PGE_2 inhibits sodium reabsorption from the isolated rabbit collecting tubule.

(5) Increased renomedullar prostaglandins could account for the polyuria observed in Bartter's syndrome, in view of the antagonistic effect of PGE on the hydro-osmotic effect of vasopressin originally demonstrated by Granthum and Orloff (1968).

(6) Vane and McGiff (1975) demonstrated that angiotensin II is a potent stimulator of prostaglandin production. Likewise, bradykinin which is also elevated in plasma in Bartter's syndrome can stimulate renal vein PGE levels 10–50 times when infused into animals (McGiff *et al.*, 1972b).

Angiotensin II and bradykinin also stimulate prostaglandin biosynthesis by rabbit renal medullary interstitial cells (Zusman and Keiser, 1977).

(7) Evidence supporting a role for prostaglandins as inhibitors of ascending limb chloride reabsorption was derived by Higashihara *et al.* (1978) who demonstrated that inhibition of prostaglandin synthesis by meclofenemate in

rat renal papillae increased water reabsorption and interstitial chloride concentration. Reduction in chloride reabsorption from the thick ascending limb by prostaglandins would fit the hypothesis of Kurtzman and Gutierrez (1975) that inhibition of ascending limb chloride reabsorption is the cause of Bartter's syndrome.

(8) Galvez *et al.* (1977) demonstrated a 10-fold rise in urinary PGE in dogs due to severe potassium depletion. Dusing *et al.* (1978) showed an inverse correlation between production of PGE_2 from arachidonic acid, and media potassium concentration in the rabbit, and human renal medullary and papillary slices. Human medullary PGE_2 content doubled when media potassium was reduced from 9 to 0 mmol/l. Radfar *et al.* (1978) showed that potassium depletion due to psychogenic vomiting or Bartter's syndrome was associated with a rise in urinary PGE, plasma renin activity, and resistance to the pressor effect of norepinephrine and angiotensin. Potassium repletion reduced plasma renin activity and normalized the pressor response to both angiotensin II and norepinephrine. Thus enhanced PGE production secondary to a primary renal potassium wasting defect could mediate the manifestation of Bartter's syndrome.

(9) The sodium retention and weight gain observed by Modlinger *et al.* (1973) following administration of propranolol to a patient with Bartter's syndrome could not be explained by suppression of renin release, since Schwartz and Cornfeld (1975), Fichman *et al.* (1976) and Tomko *et al.* (1976) demonstrated sodium retention with actually a rise in plasma renin activity following propranolol. Conceivably the sodium retaining action of propranolol in Bartter's syndrome could be due to β-adrenergic blockade interfering with adrenergic stimulation of prostaglandin production (McGiff *et al.*, 1972a; Berl *et al.*, 1978).

7.4 MEASUREMENT OF PROSTAGLANDINS IN BARTTER'S SYNDROME

The hypothesized role of prostaglandins in the pathogenesis of Bartter's syndrome has been verified by measurements of prostaglandins in blood or urine and determining the response to prostaglandin synthetase inhibitors in patients with Bartter's syndrome. The interpretation of measured levels of prostaglandins is hampered by the uncertain validity of most assay procedures, and the variety of influences such as sodium balance, potassium balance and urine volume on prostaglandin generation.

Fichman *et al.* (1976) found elevated levels of immunoreactive PGA in whole blood: 1396 and 945 pg/ml in their 28-year-old male patient with Bartter's syndrome, compared to normal values of 546 ± 307 (SD) pg/ml. Urinary PGE measured by radioimmunoassay in the same patient was also elevated to 0.91 μg/day (normal males 0.50 ± 0.20 (SD)) (Zipser *et al.*, 1978). In a 29-year-old male who was the second patient from the same study, urinary PGE was also increased to a level of 1.40 μg/day. This patient had a horseshoe kidney with a right renal vein blood level of PGE of 634 pg/ml and

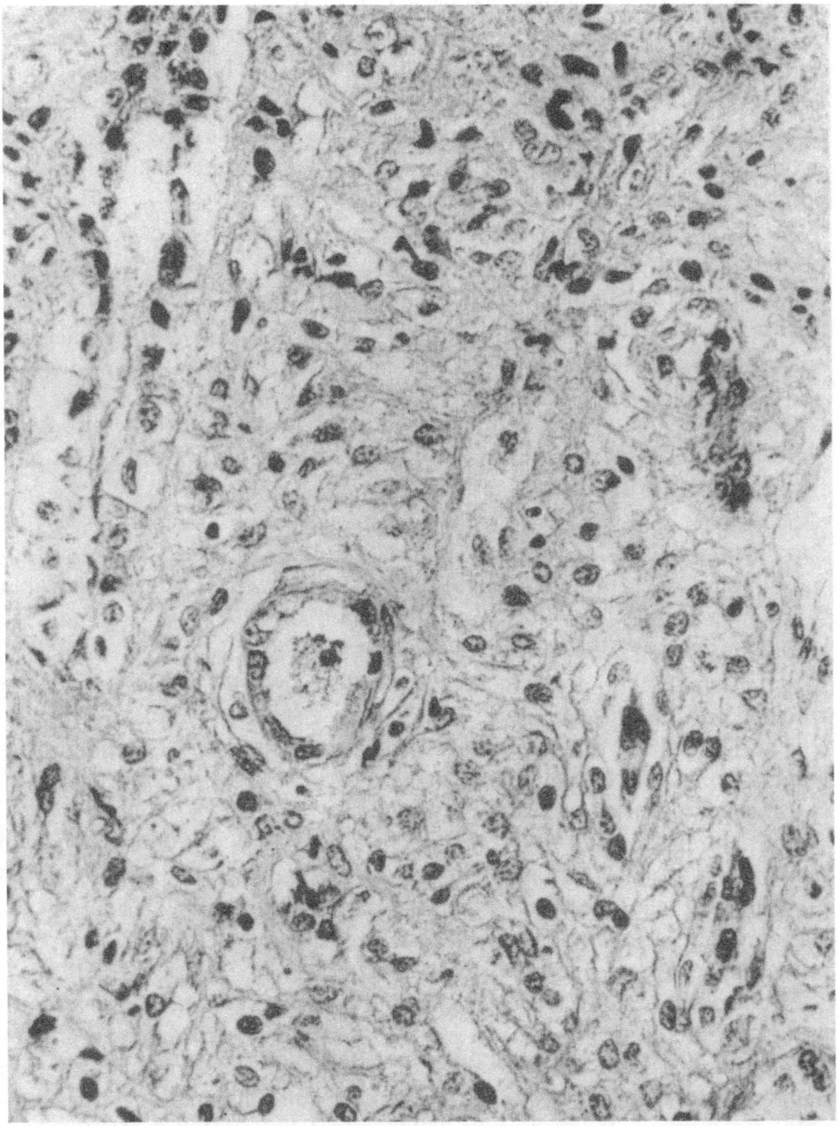

Figure 7.4 Hyperplasia of renomedullary interstitial cells ($\times 310$).
Reprinted by permission of the authors and *Kidney Int.* from Verberkmoes, R. *et al.* (1976). *Kidney Int.* **9**, 305, Figure 5

left renal vein level of 229 pg/ml compared to an inferior vena caval level of 90 pg/ml. Verberkmoes *et al.* (1976) reported a patient with Bartter's syndrome who had on renal biopsy not only juxtaglomerular cell hyperplasia, but hyperplasia of the renal medullary interstitial cells (Figure 7.4). Renal medullary interstitial cells are one of the primary sites of renal PGE production in tissue cultures (Muirhead *et al.*, 1972).

Gill *et al.* (1976) measured urinary PGE_2 and $PGF_{2\alpha}$ by gas chromatography–mass spectrometry and PGE-like material by radioimmunoassay (PGE-M) in four female patients aged between 14 and 46 years with Bartter's syndrome. $PGF_{2\alpha}$ and PGE-M were normal in three out of four and elevated in one patient; PGE_2 was elevated in all with a mean value of 640 ± 314 ng/day compared to normal values of 185 ± 81 SD.

According to Bartter *et al.* (1976), urinary PGE-M reflects total body production of PGE_1 and PGE_2 while urinary PGE_2 reflects renal synthesis. Two additional cases (including one male patient) with elevated urinary PGE_2 were reported. The male subject excreted 5700 ng/day of PGE_2 (normal range 68–935 ng/day in male subjects), and also had medullary interstitial cell hyperplasia on renal biopsy.

Norby *et al.* (1976) reported immunoreactive urinary PGE of 225 ± 56 (SE) ng/day and plasma PGE of 293 ± 69 (SE) pg/ml in a 22-month female with all of the manifestations of Bartter's syndrome.

Schwarz *et al.* (1977, 1978) reported bilaterally elevated renal venous (465 and 281 pg/ml) and peripheral plasma (124 pg/ml) PGE_2 measured by radioimmunoassay in a 50-year-old male patient with Bartter's syndrome. Normal plasma levels of PGE_2 by this method are 39 ± 18 (SD) pg/ml.

Donker *et al.* (1977) reported the finding of renal medullary interstitial cell hyperplasia on renal biopsy in a 38-year-old patient with Bartter's syndrome who had previously been reported by Erkelens and Statius von Epps (1973) to have polycythaemia and a 10-fold normal erythropoetin level. Renal prostaglandin overproduction in Bartter's syndrome may be a stimulatory factor in erythropoetin generation (Mujovic and Fisher, 1974).

Bourke and Delaney (1977) reported a family group of six siblings with Bartter's syndrome, who demonstrated juxtaglomerular cell hyperplasia but no renal medullary interstitial cell hyperplasia on renal biopsy. Urinary PGE_2 was markedly elevated (1500–3000 ng/day) in two female subjects compared to their normal range in females of 410–700 ng/day.

Littlewood, Lee and Meadow (1978) found markedly elevated levels of both urinary PGE_2 (up to 809 ng/24 h) and $PGF_{2\alpha}$ (up to 933 ng/24 h) measured by radioimmunoassay in a 3-year-old male patient with Bartter's syndrome on no therapy between periods of treatment with anti-inflammatory drugs.

In studies carried out in eight children and seven adults with Bartter's syndrome by Dray (1978), plasma levels of PGE_2 and PGF_2 measured by radioimmunoassay were normal. In the pre-pubertal children with Bartter's syndrome on no therapy, urinary PGE was elevated (0.99 ± 0.28 nmol/24 h) compared to normal children (0.24 ± 0.07 nmol/24 h), and urinary $PGF_{2\alpha}$ was also about three times the value in normal children. Surprisingly urinary PGE_2 and $PGF_{2\alpha}$ in adult patients with Bartter's syndrome were not significantly different from normal. Four out of seven adult patients studied were males but did not have higher values of urinary PGE_2 than females. Mean value of urinary PGE_2 was 1.06 ± 0.22 (SE) nmol/24 h in adult patients with Bartter's syndrome versus 0.99 ± 0.24 nmol/24 h in normal adults and 0.24 ± 0.07 nmol/24 h in normal children.

Elevated urinary PGE_2 was not only found in children with Bartter's syndrome, but also in those with renal tubular acidosis by Guesry *et al.* (1978). Barbour and Day (1978) reported an enormously elevated value of urinary PGE of 25 134 ng/24 h (normal 1275 ng/24 h) in a 63-year-old patient with Bartter's syndrome, in contrast to the normal value in adults with Bartter's syndrome reported by Dray (1978).

Haloshka *et al.* (1977) found 10-fold higher urinary immunoreactive PGE levels in a 6½-year-old female and three times higher values in a 12½-year-old female with Bartter's syndrome compared to levels in age-matched normal females (normal 345 ± 35 ng/24 h for normal children; 843 ± 99 ng/24 h for normal female adults).

Simatupang *et al.* (1978) found in a 32-year-old male with familial Bartter's syndrome, elevated plasma PGE_2 of 39 pg/ml (normal 5.5 ± 0.8 pg/ml), plasma PGA of 241 pg/ml (normal 94 ± 15 pg/ml), urinary PGE_2 of 138 ng/24 h (normal 9–12 ng/24 h) and PGA of 205 ng/24 h (normal 71–94 ng/24 h). All were measured by radioimmunoassay. The reported normal values from this study are much lower than reported by others.

Bowden *et al.* (1978) reported increased levels of urinary PGE measured by radioimmunoassay in five out of seven female patients with Bartter's syndrome with a mean value of 60 ± 19 (SD) ng/h, compared to normal values for adult females of 29 ± 10 (SD) ng/h (Figure 7.5). The two patients with Bartter's syndrome with normal urinary PGE included a 9-year-old child whose level was 45 ng/h which was four-fold greater than found in normal children of the same age. The other patient was an adolescent. In one patient followed for 2 years, urinary PGE on no therapy measured intermittently throughout this period remained elevated between 87 and 100 ng/h (approx. 2–3 μg/24 h).

Sasaki *et al.* (1977) found markedly elevated levels of serum PGE, 41.9 pg/ml (normal 1.38 ± 0.77 pg/ml) and $PGF_{2\alpha}$, 20.2 pg/ml (normal 0.90 ± 0.55 pg/ml) measured by radioimmunoassay in a 24-year-old female patient with Bartter's syndrome.

O'Regan *et al.* (1978) observed a defect in epinephrine-induced platelet aggregation in three patients with Bartter's syndrome which they attributed to high circulating plasma levels of prostaglandins since epinephrine-induced platelet aggregation was normal when the platelets were studied in plasma from a normal subject.

In summary, in the majority of both childhood and adult cases of both sexes with Bartter's syndrome, blood and urine levels of prostaglandins, in particular PGE, have been elevated above normal values. The finding of renal medullary interstitial cell hyperplasia in several of the biopsy cases, suggests a possible anatomical source of increased prostaglandin production in this

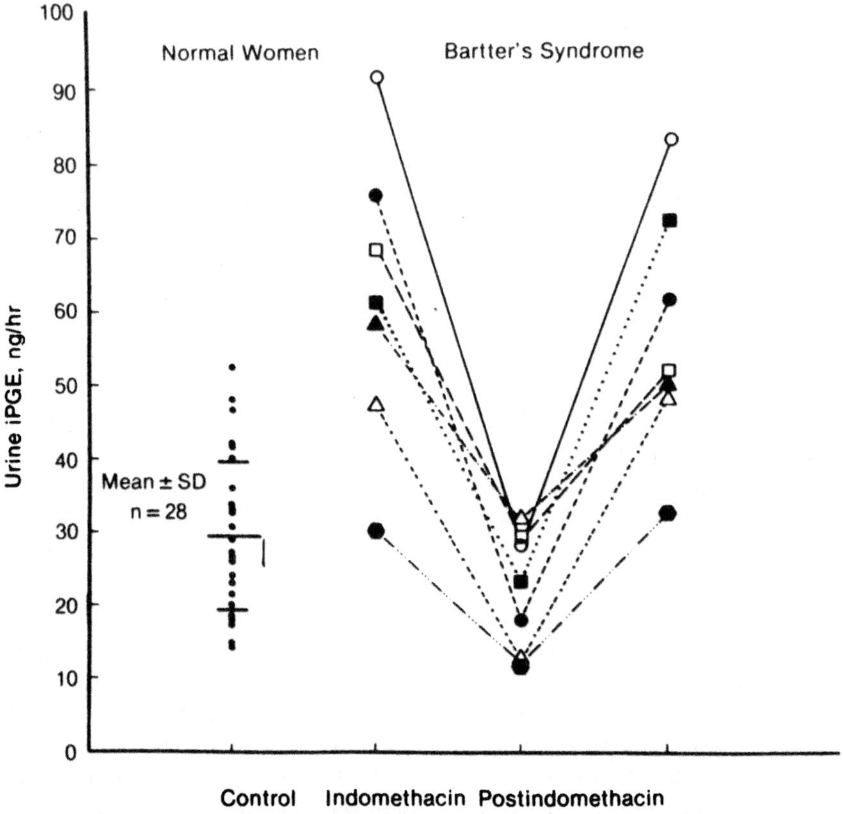

Figure 7.5 Excretion of urinary immunoreactive prostaglandin E (iPGE) before, during and after indomethacin therapy in seven patients with Bartter's syndrome compared to 28 normal women.

Reprinted by permission of the authors and *J. Am. Med. Assoc.* from Bowden, R. E. *et al.* (1978). *J. Am. Med. Assoc.* **239**, 118, Figure 2

syndrome. The finding of erythrocytosis in one case and defects in platelet aggregation in others may be attributed to the effects of increased circulating prostaglandins. Even in those subjects with normal urinary PGE levels, it is conceivable that increased renal production of other prostaglandins such as PGG_2, PGD_2, PGA_2, or PGI_2 could be mediating the manifestations of Bartter's syndrome.

7.5 RESPONSE TO PROSTAGLANDIN SYNTHESIS INHIBITORS

7.5.1 Effects on major manifestations of Bartter's syndrome in adults

The most convincing evidence supporting a role for prostaglandins in the pathogenesis of Bartter's syndrome has been the reversal of most of the manifestations of this disorder with inhibitors of prostaglandin synthesis at the cyclo-oxygenase step. Vane (1971) proposed this mechanism as the mode of action of non-steroidal anti-inflammatory drugs.

Fichman *et al.* (1976) initially demonstrated reversal or improvement of the following manifestations of Bartter's syndrome with indomethacin (200 mg daily) in their 28-year-old patient: (1) sodium retention with a reduction in urine sodium to less than 11 mmol/24 h with a 5 kg increase in body weight during the first 4 days of treatment (Figure 7.6). (2) Isotopically determined

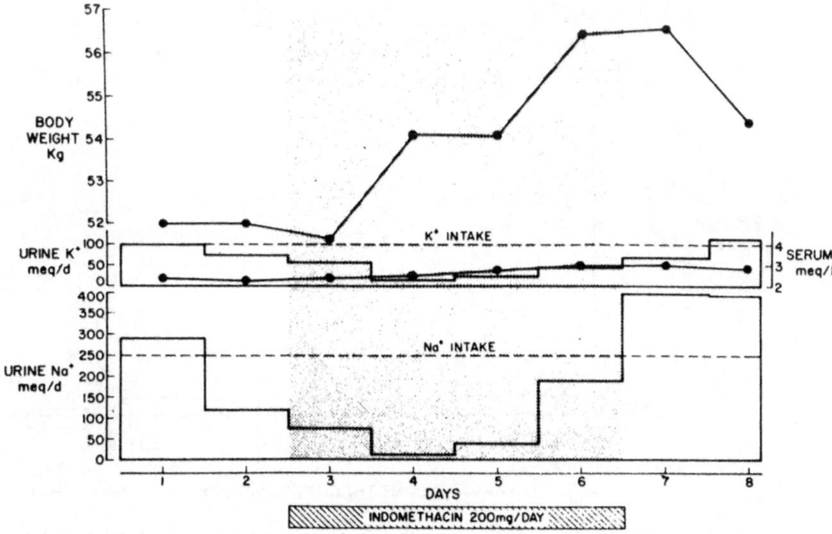

Figure 7.6 Sodium and potassium retention with indomethacin in Bartter's syndrome. Reprinted by permission of the authors and *Am. J. Med.* from Fichman, M. P. *et al.* (1976). *Am. J. Med.* **60**, 791, Figure 10

plasma volume and exchangeable sodium which were less than predicted on no therapy increased to slightly greater than predicted value with indomethacin treatment. (3) Restoration of elevated supine plasma renin activity of 55 (ng/ml)/h to normal, 4.3 (ng/ml)/h, and elevated plasma aldosterone of 74.1 ng/100 ml to normal value of 3.6 ng/100 ml. Indeed by the fourth day of indomethacin treatment even the postural rise in plasma renin activity and aldosterone was abolished (Figure 7.7). (4) Elevated levels of blood PGA and urine PGE (Zipser *et al.*, 1978) were reduced to normal. (5) Marked resistance to the pressor effect of infused angiotensin was normalized (Figure 7.8). (6) Urinary potassium initially decreased to as low as 16 mmol/24 h, paralleling the reduction in urine sodium, and serum potassium rose from 2.4 to 3.0 mmol/l. Exchangeable potassium increased from 2260 mmol to 2579 mmol (2850 mmol was the predicted normal value). (7) There was an initial rise in the patient's BUN from 11 to 28 mg/100 ml and a decrease in creatinine clearance from 90 to 70 ml/min. (8) This patient has remained on

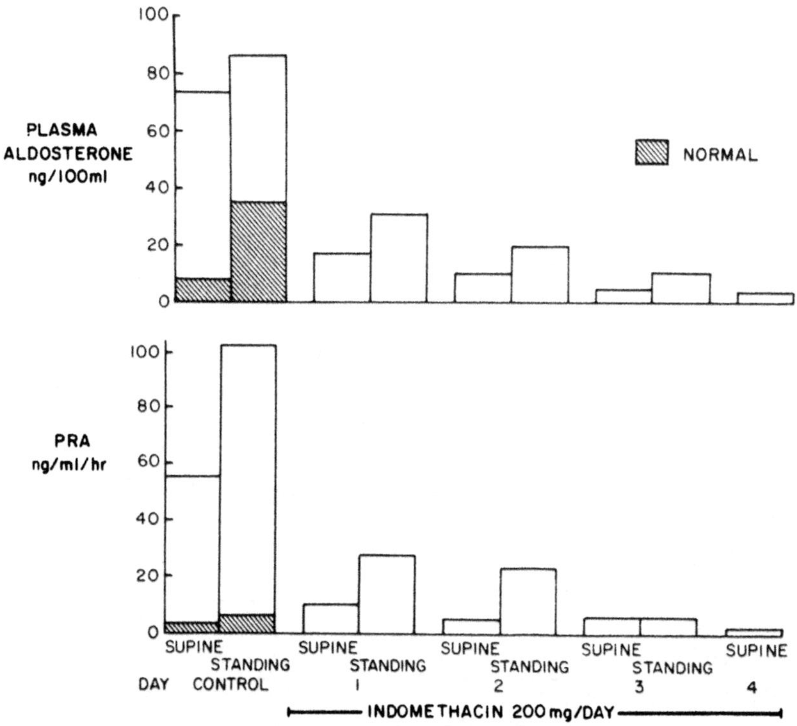

Figure 7.7 Reduction of plasma renin activity (PRA) and plasma aldosterone with indomethacin in Bartter's syndrome.

Reprinted by permission of the authors and *Am. J. Med.* from Fichman, M. P. *et al.* (1976). *Am. J. Med.*, **60**, 792, Figure 11

therapy with indomethacin (200 mg/daily) either alone or in combination with spironolactone or triamterene for the last 4 years. The serum potassium has ranged between 3.0 mmol/l and 3.6 mmol/l on indomethacin treatment alone and from 3.4–3.8 mmol/l with the combination of indomethacin and potassium retaining diuretics. On previous massive doses of spironolactone plus triamterene therapy alone his serum potassium ranged from 2.0–2.8 mmol/l.

Ibuprofen therapy in this patient produced similar changes. Thus, administration of indomethacin to this patient with Bartter's syndrome corrected all the manifestations of this disorder with the exception of the hypokalaemia which improved marginally.

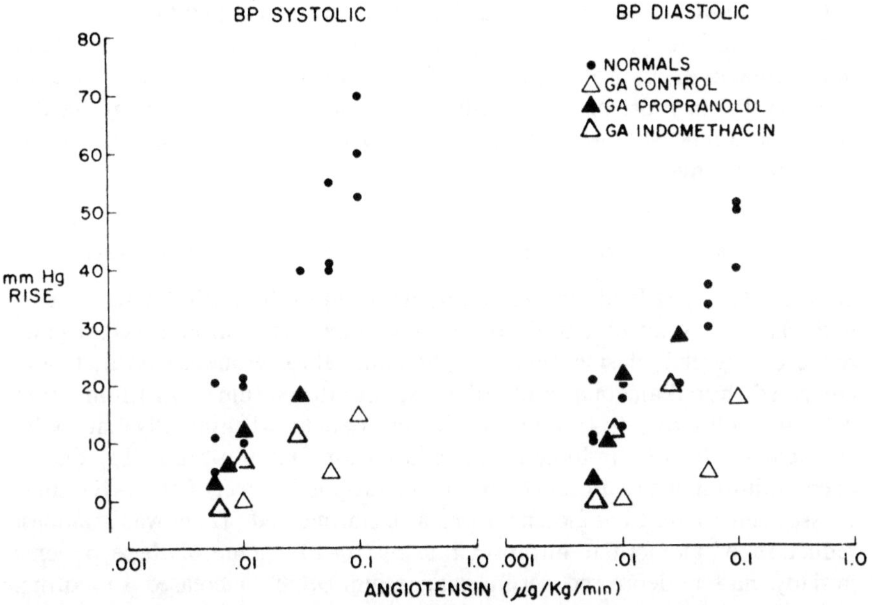

Figure 7.8 Reversal of angiotensin resistance following propranolol or indomethacin therapy in Bartter's syndrome.

Reprinted by permission of the authors and *Am. J. Med.* from Fichman, M. P. *et al.*, (1976). *Am. J. Med.*, **60**, 790, Figure 7

In a 25-year-old patient reported by Verberkmoes *et al.* (1976), administration of indomethacin produced similar results: sodium retention and weight gain, suppression of elevated plasma renin activity and aldosterone to normal, and normalization of the pressor response to angiotensin. In this patient who had medullary interstitial cell hyperplasia (Figure 7.4) however, resultant renal potassium conservation took place and serum potassium rose to a low normal level. The depressed erythrocyte potassium content on no therapy increased to normal after indomethacin treatment.

Gill *et al.* (1976) observed similar effects with indomethacin therapy in three adult and one adolescent female patient with Bartter's syndrome: (1) Reduction in elevated urinary PGE by 69–74% to normal levels. (2) Reduction of elevated supine and upright plasma renin activity to normal. (3) Reduction of elevated urinary aldosterone to normal. (4) Sodium retention and weight gain. (5) A decrease in creatinine clearance by a mean of 22%. (6) Potassium retention and increase in serum potassium from 2.0–2.5 mmol/l to

3.0–3.4 mmol/l in all except one patient whose serum potassium rose to 4.0 mmol/l. In most instances serum potassium eventually declined, but was still higher than on no therapy. (7) Reversion of all of these parameters to abnormal levels prior to therapy when indomethacin treatment was discontinued.

Bartter *et al.* (1976) showed that ibuprofen produced qualitatively similar effects to indomethacin in two patients with this syndrome, and either indomethacin or ibuprofen normalized the sensitivity to the pressor effect of angiotensin. In most of the patients treated with indomethacin by Bartter (1977), serum potassium remained higher than on no therapy, but still below the normal range.

7.5.2 Effects in Bartter's syndrome with hypomagnesaemia

Donker *et al.* (1977) administered indomethacin to three adult male patients with Bartter's syndrome and produced sodium retention and weight gain, reduced elevated plasma renin activity and aldosterone to normal, and corrected hypokalaemia and alkalosis in all (serum potassium from 2.2–2.4 mmol/l to 3.6–4.2 mmol/l). In one patient who initially had polycythaemia (Hct 63), indomethacin reduced the Hct to 48 possibly due to haemodilution or to suppression of the erythropoetic effect of prostaglandins. Pressor sensitivity to angiotensin was also normalized. There was a modest reduction of glomerular filtration rate by 10–20%. One of these patients initially had a depressed serum magnesium which increased to normal (1.2–1.7 mmol/l).

Indomethacin also decreased urinary calcaemia and phosphate excretion and increased serum phosphate which implies that prostaglandins may be inhibiting proximal tubular reabsorption of magnesium, calcium and phosphate as well as sodium.

Zipser *et al.* (1978) found that while indomethacin or ibuprofen normalized elevated urinary PGE, plasma renin activity and plasma aldosterone, and restored pressor sensitivity to angiotensin in a hypomagnesaemic patient with Bartter's syndrome confirmed by renal biopsy, serum potassium rose from 2.1 to only 3.1 mmol/l but serum magnesium remained depressed at 1 mmol/l.

Schwarz *et al.* (1978) administered a high dose of indomethacin (300 mg/day) to a 52-year-old patient with Bartter's syndrome. Elevated plasma renin activity, plasma aldosterone and plasma PGE_2 levels were all markedly reduced by indomethacin, and pressor sensitivity to angiotensin was restored. Sodium retention, weight gain, and potassium retention with increase in serum potassium to the low normal range of 3.4–3.8 mmol/l occurred during indomethacin therapy. There was a 350 mmol positive balance of potassium and 450 mmol positive balance of sodium over 10 days. Plasma and urine catecholamines and pressor sensitivity to norepinephrine were unaltered by treatment but were initially normal. Plasma PGE_2 was highly correlated with both plasma renin activity and plasma aldosterone levels with and without indomethacin. Plasma volume and exchangeable sodium were normal with no therapy. Their patient also had a markedly reduced serum magnesium but no mention was made of the response of serum potassium to magnesium repletion or serum magnesium to indomethacin, and in the absence of renal biopsy it is conceivable that their patient had a primary magnesium wasting abnormality rather than true Bartter's syndrome.

Barbour and Day (1978) also reported a 63-year-old patient with all the manifestations of Bartter's syndrome plus hypomagnesaemia (1.1 mmol/l) with renal magnesium wasting of 7 mmol/24 h. However, no renal biopsy was performed so conceivably this case also might not have been classical Bartter's syndrome. Elevated plasma renin activity, aldosterone and urinary PGE were normalized with indomethacin as was restoration of normal pressor sensitivity to angiotensin. There was a 48-hour period of sodium and potassium retention following indomethacin therapy with a 1.6 kg weight gain. However, indomethacin failed to increase serum potassium or serum magnesium. Magnesium loading of 20 mmol/daily for 2 weeks failed to raise the serum potassium.

Kornerup *et al.* (1978) described a 41-year-old male patient with all the characteristics of Bartter's syndrome plus hypomagnesaemia (1.1 mmol/l), with the exception that there was no evidence of juxtaglomerular cell hyperplasia on two renal biopsies. Indomethacin therapy reduced elevated plasma renin activity and aldosterone to normal. The slightly depressed pressor sensitivity to angiotensin was normalized following indomethacin treatment. Serum potassium was 2.0–2.5 mmol/l on no therapy and potassium influx studies in lymphocytes were normal. Indomethacin plus 120 mmol/daily potassium supplement, raised serum potassium slightly to 2.8–3.0 mmol/l. Since the patient had only a slight angiotensin resistance and no apparent juxtaglomerular cell hyperplasia and hypomagnesaemia, it is probable that this was not a true case of Bartter's syndrome.

7.5.3 Effects in childhood Bartter's syndrome

Norby *et al.* (1976) first used aspirin to treat Bartter's syndrome in a 22-month-old girl with growth retardation, muscle weakness and polyuria. After 10 weeks of therapy, serum potassium increased from 2.9 to 3.6 mmol/l. Elevated levels of plasma renin activity and urinary aldosterone were suppressed to normal while high levels of plasma and urine PGE were decreased by 90%, and of plasma and urinary $PGF_{2\alpha}$ by 50%. The patient gained weight, had improved appetite and activity, and muscle weakness and polyuria resolved.

Littlewood *et al.* (1978) also treated an infant with the manifestations of Bartter's syndrome at 33 months of age with indomethacin for 12 months followed by treatment with a possibly less toxic prostaglandin synthetase inhibitor, ketoprofen. Elevated plasma renin activity and plasma aldosterone and urinary prostaglandin (E_2 and $F_{2\alpha}$) were partially suppressed by both drugs. There was a marked improvement in growth rate, well-being, and reduction in polyuria. During the changeover period on no therapy the patient's polyuria and polydipsia recurred with a rise in urinary prostaglandins and plasma renin activity. Serum potassium remained below 3.0 mmol/l despite therapy with either indomethacin or ketoprofen.

Zancan *et al.* (1976) treated an 11-year-old male patient with Bartter's syndrome with indomethacin, which produced a reduction in plasma renin activity to normal by the fourth day of treatment and a rise in serum potassium from 2.5–2.8 mmol/l to 3.1–3.5 mmol/l. Treatment with propranolol and spironolactone had previously been ineffective.

Konomi *et al.* (1978) described the development of pseudotumour cerebri in a 10-year-old girl with Bartter's syndrome 8 weeks after treatment with indomethacin. There was bilateral papilloedema and abducens palsy with a cerebro-spinal fluid pressure of 350 mmHg. These signs and symptoms subsided 3 weeks after discontinuation of indomethacin. Presumably, the increased intracerebral pressure was related to the salt and water retaining effects of indomethacin.

7.5.4 Comparison of the effects of indomethacin with other anti-inflammatory drugs in Bartter's syndrome

Bowden *et al.* (1978) made a comparison of tolerance and effectiveness of indomethacin, aspirin and ibuprofen in the treatment of seven patients with Bartter's syndrome. With a dosage of 150 mg daily, indomethacin caused a 65% decrease in mean urinary PGE to the normal range, 22% decrease in urinary potassium, 40% rise in serum potassium (from 2.35 to 3.3 mmol/l), a 37% decrease in urine sodium, a 71% decrease in plasma renin activity and 11% decrease in urinary aldosterone with a 2% increase in body weight and an 18% decrease in creatinine clearance. However, four patients treated with indomethacin had headaches or gastric irritation and therefore three of these patients were switched to ibuprofen 1600 mg/daily and one to aspirin 2.7 g/daily. Ibuprofen produced significantly less decrease in urinary PGE (mean of 43%) than did indomethacin (mean of 68%). However, ibuprofen decreased creatinine clearance by a mean of only 4% compared to a decrease by 23% with indomethacin. Mean serum potassium increased insignificantly with ibuprofen or aspirin. There was less sodium retention, weight gain, reduction in urinary potassium, or fall in plasma renin activity with ibuprofen than with indomethacin. However, there were no significant side-effects with ibuprofen or aspirin. There was a correlation between the capacity of indomethacin to produce a greater reduction in urinary PGE than ibuprofen or aspirin and the degree of correction of the abnormalities of Bartter's syndrome and the degree of reduction of creatinine clearance and side-effects.

The greater potency of indomethacin in suppressing prostaglandins would lead to greater renal vasoconstriction, fall in glomerular filtration rate, sodium retention and secondarily to more potassium conservation.

In this adult trial study aspirin was ineffective (in contrast to the paediatric case of Norby *et al.*, 1976). While ibuprofen alone or spironolactone alone produced only a minimal increase in serum potassium (2.8 mmol/l) the combination of ibuprofen 1600 mEq/daily and spironolactone 150 mEq/daily produced a normal serum potassium. Katz and Bortz (1978) showed that another prostaglandin synthesis inhibitor, naproxen, produced a dose-dependent therapeutic effect in a 31-year-old female with Bartter's syndrome. A dosage of 250 mg three times a day resulted in a decrease in plasma renin activity from 7.1–29.0 (ng/ml)/h to 3.6 (ng/ml)/h, and in urine aldosterone from 22–69 μg/24 h to 8 μg/24 h while serum potassium increased from 2.7–3.2 mmol/l to 3.4–3.7 mmol/l. These differences in potency may be related to the relative potencies of various prostaglandin synthesis inhibitors on renal medullary PGE production.

Gafni *et al.* (1978) showed that indomethacin and meclofenamic acid were equipotent in inhibiting PGE synthesis by rabbit renal medullary homogenates *in vitro* while aspirin was much weaker. Effects on PGE synthesis *in vivo* showed that indomethacin was the most potent inhibitor, meclofenamate intermediate and aspirin the weakest.

Bourke and Delaney (1977) studied six siblings with biopsy confirmed Bartter's syndrome demonstrating juxtaglomerular cell hyperplasia but no renal medullary interstitial cell hyperplasia. Prior to therapy there was greater than three-fold increase in fractional sodium excretion compared to controls. Administration of indomethacin or meclofenamate to two females in this group reduced elevated urinary PGE and plasma renin activity to normal, reduced angiotensin pressor insensitivity and restored elevated fractional sodium excretion to normal, and increased serum potassium from 2.4 to 3.0 mmol/l. It is of great interest that administration of a phospholipase inhibitor, mepacrine, by contrast, reduced urinary PGE to normal but failed to decrease plasma renin activity or raise serum potassium.

Simatupang *et al.* (1978) compared the effects of propranolol and potassium retaining diuretics with that of prostaglandin synthesis inhibitors in a patient with Bartter's syndrome. Spironolactone and amiloride both markedly increased plasma renin activity and increased the resistance to the pressor activity of angiotensin. Aldosterone secretion rate increased markedly with amiloride while spironolactone decreased plasma volume and extracellular fluid volume. Urinary potassium decreased with treatment for 48 hours then returned to pretreatment levels. In contrast, therapy with indomethacin decreased plasma renin activity, plasma aldosterone and potassium clearance, and allowed a rise in serum potassium. Ibuprofen produced a less dramatic decrease in plasma renin activity and failed to alter potassium clearance.

7.5.5 Effects on other manifestations or mechanisms of Bartter's syndrome by prostaglandin synthesis inhibitors

Rado *et al.* (1978) showed that despite polyuria on *ad lib.* fluids in a patient with familial Bartter's syndrome, DDAVP produced a highly concentrated urine of 924 mosmol/kg. With indomethacin treatment, urinary concentrating ability was enhanced to a maximum urine osmolality of 1169 mosmol/kg coincident with a decrease in urinary PGE to a value 40% of that on no therapy. Thus, despite the presence of hypokalaemic nephropathy renal concentrating ability remained intact and the response to DDAVP was potentiated by prostaglandin synthesis inhibition.

Gill and Bartter (1978) demonstrated that administration of indomethacin in four and ibuprofen in one patient with Bartter's syndrome in doses sufficient to decrease urinary PGE failed to alter the estimated abnormally elevated distal fractional chloride reabsorption (Figure 7.9). Their results

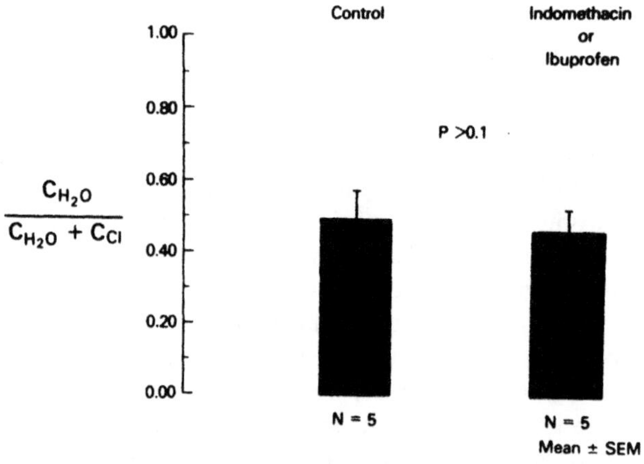

Figure 7.9 Distal fractional reabsorption of chloride ($C_{H_2O}/C_{H_2O}+C_{Cl}$) in patients with Bartter's syndrome before and during treatment with indomethacin or ibuprofen.

Reprinted by permission of the authors and *Am. J. Med.* from Gill, J. G. and Bartter, F. C. (1978). *Am. J. Med.*, **65**, 770, Figure 7

would imply that while impaired ascending chloride reabsorption was the primary defect in Bartter's syndrome, this abnormality was not mediated by increased prostaglandin production.

Vinci *et al.* (1978) found that treatment of seven patients with Bartter's syndrome with indomethacin or ibuprofen decreased elevated immunoreactive PGE excretion by 67%, plasma renin activity by 80%, plasma bradykinin by 25%, and urinary kallikrein excretion by 50%. Mean urinary kinin excretion increased from 3.8 to 8.5 μg/24 h and plasma kallikrein was unchanged (Figure 7.2). Thus, all of the kallikrein–kinin system abnormalities in Bartter's syndrome reverted to normal with the inhibition of prostaglandin synthesis.

These results suggest that prostaglandins mediate the high plasma bradykinin and low urinary kinins found in Bartter's syndrome and that the urinary kallikrein is aldosterone dependent (Figure 7.2). The high plasma bradykinin could account for the angiotensin resistance in this syndrome and could also be responsible for stimulating renal PGE production.

Halusha *et al.* (1977) also showed in two children with Bartter's syndrome that indomethacin reduced elevated urinary PGE, urinary kallikrein, and plasma renin activity, and increased angiotensin sensitivity and serum potassium to normal. Urinary kallikrein and PGE excretion were highly correlated both on and off indomethacin. Indomethacin produced sodium retention and weight gain but no significant reduction in urinary chloride or potassium. Also, atypically, urinary aldosterone did not decrease with indomethacin. Thus, the inhibitory effect of indomethacin on urinary kallikrein must have been due to decreased prostaglandins rather than diminished aldosterone.

Sasaki *et al.* (1977) described a patient with Bartter's syndrome who had a hypotensive response to an angiotensin II antagonist (1-sar-8-ile-angiotensin II) in association with elevated plasma renin activity and aldosterone levels. With indomethacin therapy elevated plasma renin activity and aldosterone, and plasma PGE and $PGF_{2\alpha}$, returned towards normal. There was a 2 kg weight gain, sodium and potassium retention, and increase in serum potassium from 2.0 mmol/l to 3.1 mmol/l. Pressor sensitivity to angiotensin was restored to normal. While blood pressure had fallen from 105/48 to 78/35 with the angiotensin antagonist on no therapy, with indomethacin therapy there was a paradoxical rise in blood pressure from 98/35 to 139/50 showing an agonist effect of this compound in the renin suppressed state. These results suggest that angiotensin II receptors are not impaired in Bartter's syndrome and play a compensatory role possibly to volume depletion in maintaining blood pressure. The response to the angiotensin antagonist depends upon the level of circulating angiotensin II which is elevated in the untreated state, and suppressed with indomethacin.

Silverberg *et al.* (1978) found that in five patients with Bartter's syndrome plasma norepinephrine levels while supine and after 2.5, 5 and 10 minutes standing were elevated above normal whereas plasma epinephrine levels were in the normal range. They also found (as was originally described by Bartter *et al.*, 1962) a resistance to the pressor effect of infused norepinephrine although the metabolic response was normal. With indomethacin administration pressor responsiveness to infused norepinephrine and the response of plasma norepinephrine to standing were normalized. These data suggested that Bartter's syndrome is a hyperadrenergic state and conceivably the adrenergic system (as suggested by Fichman *et al.*, 1976) stimulates renal prostaglandin production and the response to propranolol is due to adrenergic blockade.

More likely, however, the resistance to the pressor effect of norepinephrine or angiotensin II and its correction by indomethacin is related to alterations in extracellular fluid volume.

O'Regan *et al.* (1978) showed that aspirin actually improved the platelet dysfunction noted in their patient with Bartter's syndrome. This was attributed to an inhibition of prostaglandin synthesis.

In summary, administration of prostaglandin synthesis inhibitors to patients with Bartter's syndrome reverses most of the manifestations of this disorder including: (1) suppression of elevated plasma renin activity, (2) suppression of elevated plasma and urinary aldosterone, (3) sodium retention and weight gain, (4) normalization of pressor sensitivity to angiotensin and norepinephrine, (5) suppression of elevated urinary PGE, and (6) suppression of elevated plasma bradykinin and urinary kallikrein.

In the majority of cases reported, however, while there is some reduction in urinary potassium and increase in serum potassium, a sustained increase in serum potassium to normal does not usually take place. When there is accompanying magnesium wasting, no improvement in serum magnesium occurs with therapy. Also, there is some reduction in glomerular filtration rate, salt retention and increase in body weight with indomethacin therapy and to a lesser degree with other less potent anti-inflammatory drugs. Subnormal fractional chloride reabsorption in the ascending limb is not corrected by indomethacin. These findings suggest that while prostaglandins play an important role in the pathogenesis of Bartter's syndrome, inhibitors of prostaglandin synthesis do not totally reverse all manifestations of this syndrome.

7.6 POSSIBLE MECHANISMS OF INCREASED URINE PGE AND RESPONSE TO PROSTAGLANDIN INHIBITION IN BARTTER'S SYNDROME

7.6.1 Stimulation of prostaglandins by primary potassium wasting defect

Since hypokalaemia is the major manifestation of Bartter's syndrome that fails to be fully corrected by inhibition of prostaglandin synthesis, Ferris (1978) proposed that a primary distal tubular potassium wasting state might be the primary cause of hyperprostaglanduria in Bartter's syndrome. Galvez *et al.* (1977) had previously shown that severe potassium depletion in dogs increases urinary PGE excretion 10-fold, and increases plasma renin activity and pressor resistance to angiotensin. These changes were all reversed by indomethacin. However, these potassium depleted dogs developed sodium retention, weight gain and a reduction in aldosterone in contrast to the findings in Bartter's syndrome.

Dusing *et al.* (1978) showed that removal of potassium from the bathing media increased PGE_2 production by renal medullary slices. Radfar *et al.* (1978) showed that potassium depletion in Bartter's syndrome or psychogenic vomiting increased urinary PGE, plasma renin activity and induced pressor resistance to angiotensin. Potassium repletion restored plasma renin activity and pressor sensitivity to angiotensin II to normal.

Weber *et al.* (1978) showed that rats on a low potassium intake had higher levels of urinary PGE than when on a high potassium diet. Elevated urinary PGE production due to hypokalaemia might also explain the concentrating defect in polyuria seen in hypokalaemic nephropathy due to Bartter's syndrome in view of the antagonist effect of PGE to vasopressin.

Zipser *et al.* (1978), on the other hand, found that potassium loading for 3–6 days in two patients with Bartter's syndrome not only failed to suppress elevated urinary PGE, but actually produced a 2–7-fold rise in urinary PGE associated with a positive potassium balance of 400–1000 mmol and a rise in serum potassium from 2.3–2.8 mmol/l to 3.0–3.1 mmol/l.

7.6.2 Role of hypomagnesaemia

In the same study, in a hypomagnesaemic patient with Bartter's syndrome, Zipser *et al.* (1978) found that magnesium loading failed to correct the hypokalaemia and increased rather than decreased elevated levels of urinary PGE.

7.6.3 Role of sodium depletion

The relationship of urinary PGE and renal prostaglandin production to sodium balance remains very uncertain. Different studies have shown either a rise, a depression or no change in urinary PGE in relation to alterations in sodium balance. Thus, while sodium depletion in Bartter's syndrome could conceivably stimulate prostaglandin production, there is no uniform evidence to support this concept.

Lifschitz *et al.* (1978) showed no relationship between urinary PGE and sodium intake in rabbits. Weber *et al.* (1978) showed that sodium chloride loading decreased urinary PGE in rats on a high potassium intake but had an opposite effect in animals on a low potassium intake.

7.6.4 Role of chloride reabsorptive defect

While it is attractive to postulate that the primary defect in Bartter's syndrome is prostaglandin-mediated inhibition of ascending limb chloride reabsorption, the lack of change in chloride clearance with indomethacin administration in Bartter's syndrome appears to contradict this hypothesis.

7.6.5 Role of angiotensin

Since angiotensin has been shown to be a potent stimulator of prostaglandin production *in vitro* (Vane and McGiff, 1975) a primary inhibition of proximal tubular reabsorption of sodium or ascending limb reabsorption of chloride could lead to salt depletion and stimulation of the renin angiotensin system which could then lead to enhanced renal prostaglandin production.

7.6.6 Role of kallikrein–kinin system

A primary overproduction of plasma bradykinin which is found in Bartter's syndrome could increase renal prostaglandin production as shown by McGiff *et al.* (1972b). However, reversion of the elevated bradykinin levels with indomethacin implies that increased bradykinin is the result of rather than the cause of increased PGE in Bartter's syndrome.

7.6.7 Role of adrenergic nervous system

As described by Silverberg *et al.* (1978) a hyperadrenergic state with elevated norepinephrine levels might increase renal PGE production. Since these changes are reversed by indomethacin, it would appear that adrenergic overactivity is not the primary cause of increased renal PGE production.

7.6.8 Renal medullary interstitial cell hyperplasia

The findings of renal medullary interstitial cell hyperplasia in several patients with Bartter's syndrome (as originally described by Verberkmoes *et al.*, 1976) suggested an anatomical source of increased urinary PGE production. In the majority of cases of Bartter's syndrome however, medullary interstitial cell hyperplasia was not found on renal biopsy.

7.6.9 Role of urine volume

Since Bartter's syndrome is generally associated with polyuria presumably as a result of hypokalaemic nephropathy, the possibility that the increased urinary PGE is due to increased urine volume *per se* was entertained by Zipser *et al.* (1978). To test this hypothesis fluid intake was varied to produce alterations in urine volume from 1550 ml/24 h to 7550 ml/24 h.

Urinary PGE increased serially with increase in urine volume and a high degree of correlation between urine volume and urinary PGE was observed. Indeed, at lower urine volumes of 2000 ml/24 h or less, urinary PGE was in the normal range. The possibility that urinary PGE is in part volume flow dependent must therefore be considered. Elevated urinary PGE has also been found in other polyuric states including central and nephrogenic diabetes insipidus (Fichman *et al.*, 1978). Furthermore, both urinary PGE and urine volume were reduced by indomethacin or ibuprofen in nephrogenic diabetes insipidus and by DDAVP in diabetes insipidus.

7.7 ACTION OF PROSTAGLANDIN SYNTHESIS INHIBITORS IN STATES SIMULATING BARTTER'S SYNDROME

Although Bartter's syndrome has been recognized more frequently in the last few years because of the possible role of prostaglandins in this disorder, it still remains a rare disease. The correction of the manifestations of Bartter's syndrome by indomethacin and other anti-inflammatory drugs has also been observed in more commonly recognized high renin states such as cirrhosis, renal vascular hypertension, and in patients receiving diuretics.

7.7.1 Diuretics

Rumpf *et al.* (1975) observed in man and Larsson *et al.* (1974) in the rabbit that indomethacin decreases basal plasma renin activity. Furthermore, the normal rise in plasma renin activity while standing or following furosemide is inhibited by indomethacin. This inhibitory response was observed without significant alterations in sodium balance and therefore was a consequence of a direct inhibitory effect on prostaglandins and in turn renin production.

Virtually all the manifestations of Bartter's syndrome may be simulated by the use of loop diuretics such as furosemide or ethacrynic acid. Diuretics produce a fall in blood pressure, increase in renal sodium, chloride, and potassium wasting, cause salt depletion, stimulate renin and aldosterone, and would presumably induce a state of resistance to the pressor effect of angiotensin as a result of volume depletion. Indomethacin (just as in Bartter's syndrome) markedly blunts the vasodepressor natriuretic and stimulatory effect on plasma renin activity and aldosterone induced by furosemide in normal and hypertensive man (Patak *et al.*, 1975). Indeed, the action of loop diuretics may be mediated by prostaglandins. Furosemide and ethacrynic acid are inhibitors of the prostaglandin metabolizing enzyme 15-OH-PG-dehydrogenase (Angaard, 1974; Paulsrud and Miller, 1974).

Rosenblum *et al.* (1977) described a 29-year-old man with normal blood pressure, serum potassium 1.7 mmol/l, plasma renin activity elevated to 22.8 (ng/ml)/h, urinary aldosterone at 97 mg/24 h, and resistance to the pressor effect of angiotensin. Plans for renal biopsy were cancelled, however, when urinary thiazide was detected spectrophotometrically.

7.7.2 Vomiting

Chronic vomiting may also induce a syndrome which may simulate Bartter's syndrome with hypokalaemic alkalosis, high plasma aldosterone and plasma renin activity, and even elevated urinary PGE.

Tarm *et al.* (1973) described an 18-year-old female patient who had many of the manifestations of Bartter's syndrome including hypokalaemic alkalosis (serum potassium 1.6 mmol/l), high plasma renin activity and aldosterone, and juxtaglomerular cell hyperplasia on renal biopsy. This patient had self-induced vomiting and when observed several years later she was normokalaemic and admitted to having previously taken diuretics surreptitiously. Thus, vomiting and/or diuretics may account for all of her symptoms and the juxtaglomerular cell hyperplasia. Undoubtedly, the overwhelming preponderance of patients presenting with such cardinal manifestations of Bartter's syndrome including hypokalaemic alkalosis and possibly including juxtaglomerular cell hyperplasia are surreptitiously ingesting diuretics or have self-induced vomiting rather than the much rarer true Bartter's syndrome.

7.7.3 Effects of prostaglandin synthesis inhibitors on renal function

Donker *et al.* (1976) showed that indomethacin produced salt and water retention and a decrease in glomerular filtration rate in patients with impaired renal function especially when placed on sodium restriction. While indomethacin counteracts the sodium wasting, potassium wasting, renin and aldosterone elevation found in Bartter's syndrome, and in patients receiving diuretics, these effects may be accompanied by some decrease in renal function. Presumably, inhibition of prostaglandins leads to a decrease in renal cortical blood flow.

Kimberly *et al.* (1978b) found elevated levels of urinary PGE in seven patients with lupus nephritis (42.7 ± 6.4 (SE) ng/h) compared to normal subjects (29.0 ± 1.9 (SE) ng/h). Administration of aspirin produced a mean of 18% decrease in creatinine clearance, 14% decrease in inulin clearance and 29% decrease in *p*-aminohippurate clearance which was closely correlated with a fall in urinary PGE of 45%. There was also sodium and water retention. The latter were attributed to the enhancement of the effects of antidiuretic hormone by inhibition of prostaglandin synthesis. In three of these patients, Kimberly *et al.* (1978a) demonstrated that ibuprofen, naproxen, and fenoprofen produced similar effects. Plasma renin activity, plasma aldosterone, and urinary PGE were all reduced by each of the anti-inflammatory drugs. In the patient receiving ibuprofen, serum creatinine rose from 0.9 mg% to 3.0 mg% and potassium from 4.7 mmol/l to 6.1 mmol/l. In the patient receiving naproxen, creatinine clearance decreased initially from 106 to 42 ml/min, then rose after 10 days to 73 ml/min and serum potassium rose from 3.8 mmol/l to 4.3 mmol/l. In the patient receiving fenoprofen, creatinine clearance decreased from 60 to 35 ml/min and serum potassium rose from 3.7 to 4.2 mmol/l. It appears therefore that prostaglandin synthesis inhibition by indomethacin and other anti-inflammatory drugs in susceptible patients with renal disease such as lupus nephritis or diabetes may produce a state opposite to that of Bartter's syndrome.

Tan *et al.* (1977) described a patient with glomerulonephritis who had suppression of plasma renin activity and urinary PGE_2 and aldosterone with a rise in serum potassium from 4.1 to 6.5 mmol/l when treated with indomethacin. Prostaglandin synthesis inhibition therefore induced a state similar to hyporeninaemic hypoaldosteronism seen in many patients with diabetic nephropathy. Indeed it has been proposed that the latter disorder is due to 'anti-Bartter', that is a deficiency of renal prostaglandins.

Farese and Rodriguez (1978) failed to find a decrease in urinary PGA in patients with hyporeninaemic hypoaldosteronism. However, Norby *et al.* (1976) showed that PGA infusion increased plasma renin activity, plasma aldosterone, and lowered serum potassium from 6.5 mmol/l to 5.2 mmol/l in such a patient. Urinary PGE was low–normal.

7.8 CONCLUSION

(1) Bartter's syndrome in most instances is associated with an increase in plasma and urinary PGE.

(2) Treatment of patients with this disorder with non-steroidal anti-inflammatory drugs reverses most of the manifestations of this syndrome including elevated plasma renin activity, plasma aldosterone, urinary PGE, renal sodium wasting, and angiotensin and norepinephrine pressor insensitivity, and elevated plasma bradykinin and urinary kallikrein.

(3) The hypokalaemia and renal potassium wasting usually improves but generally is not fully corrected by indomethacin, but a combination of anti-inflammatory drug with spironolactone or triamterene will usually fully correct the hypokalaemia.

(4) Increased fractional chloride excretion in Bartter's syndrome does not appear to be reversed by prostaglandin synthesis inhibition although there is evidence that prostaglandins may inhibit ascending limb chloride transport.

(5) Magnesium wasting when present is not generally reversed by indomethacin.

(6) Excessive renal production of prostaglandins probably plays a crucial though not a primary role in the pathogenesis of Bartter's syndrome.

(7) Prostaglandin synthesis inhibition may cause sodium, chloride, potassium and water retention, and a decrease in glomerular filtration rate not only in patients with Bartter's syndrome but also in other renal disorders such as lupus nephritis.

(8) While Bartter's syndrome is a rare disorder the discovery of the role of prostaglandins in the pathogenesis of Bartter's syndrome has far-reaching implications in enhancing our understanding of the interrelationship between

the renin angiotensin, kallikrein–kinin and prostaglandin generating systems, and the renal handling of sodium, chloride and potassium.

(9) Paralleling the action of prostaglandin synthetase inhibitors in Bartter's syndrome, these drugs also inhibit the therapeutic action of loop diuretics which may be prostaglandin mediated, and may induce deterioration of renal function, salt and water retention, and hyperkalaemia in patients with other renal disorders.

References

Aguilera, A. J., Kirk, K. L. and DiBona, G. F. (1978). Effect of magnesium on sodium transport in toad urinary bladder. *Am. J. Physiol.*, **3**, F192

Angaard, E. (1974). In: M. Robinson and J. R. Vane (eds.), *Prostaglandin Synthetase Inhibitors*, p. 77 (New York: Raven Press)

Arant, B. S., Brackett, W. C., Young, R. B. and Still, W. J. S. (1970). Case studies of siblings with juxtaglomerular hyperplasia and secondary aldosteronism associated with severe azotermia and renal rickets – Bartter's syndrome or disease. *Pediatrics*, **46**, 344

Barbour, G. L. and Day, J. O. (1978). Asymptomatic Bartter's syndrome in a 63-year-old man. *S. Med. J.*, **71**, 1341

Bartter, F. C. (1977). Bartter's syndrome. *Urol. Clin. North Am.*, **4**, 253

Bartter, F. C., Delea, C. S., Kawasaki, T. and Gill, J. R. (1974). The adrenal cortex and the kidney. *Kidney Int.*, **6**, 272

Bartter, F. C., Gill, J. R., Frolich, J. C., Bowden, R. E., Hollifield, J. W., Radfar, N., Keiser, M. R., Oates, J. A., Seyberth, M. and Taylor, A. A. (1976). Prostaglandins are overproduced by the kidneys and mediate hyperreninemia in Bartter's syndrome. *Trans. Assoc. Am. Physicians*, **39**, 72

Bartter, F. C., Pronove, P., Gill, J. R. and McCardle, R. C. (1962). Hyperplasia of the juxtaglomerular complex with hyperaldosteronism and hypokalemic alkalosis. A new syndrome. *Am. J. Med.*, **33**, 811

Beilin, C. J., Schiffman, N., Crane, M. and Nelson, D. M. (1967). Hypokalaemic alkalosis and hyperplasia of the juxtaglomerular apparatus without hypertension or edema. *Br. Med. J.*, **4**, 327

Berl, T., McDonald, R. M., Hyde, D. A. and Schrier, R. W. (1978). On the mechanism of renin secretion during beta-adrenergic stimulation; the role of prostaglandins. In: *VII International Congress of Nephrology*, p. R-10 (Montreal, Canada)

Biava, C. G., Desjardins, R., Bravo, E. and Bartter, F. C. (1969). Glomerular changes with glomerulo-disto-tubular shunts in patients with Bartter's syndrome. *Lab. Invest.*, **20**, 575

Bolger, D. M., Eisner, G. M., Terez Shea, P., Ramwell, P. and Slotkoff, L. M. (1977). Effects of prostaglandin D_2 on canine renal function. *Nature (London)*, **267**, 628

Bourke, E. and Delaney, V. (1977). Pathogenesis of Bartter's syndrome: a family study. *Kidney Int.*, **11** (Abst.), 447

Bowden, R. E., Gill, J. R. and Radfar, N. (1978). Prostaglandin synthetase inhibitors in Bartter's syndrome: effect on immunoreactive prostaglandin E excretion. *J. Am. Med. Assoc.*, **239**, 117

Bryan, G. T., McCardle, R. C. and Bartter, F. C. (1966). Hyperaldosteronism, hyperplasia of the juxtaglomerular complex, normal blood pressure, and dwarfism: report of a case. *Pediatrics*, **37**, 43

Cannon, P. J., Leeming, J. M., Sommers, S. C., Winters, R. W. and Laragh, J. M. (1968). Juxtaglomerular cell hyperplasia and secondary hyperaldosteronism (Bartter's syndrome): a re-evaluation of the pathophysiology. *Medicine (Baltimore)*, **47**, 107

Chaimowitz, C., Levi, J., Better, O. S., Oslander, L. and Benderli, A. (1973). Studies on the site of renal salt loss in a patient with Bartter's syndrome. *Pediatr. Res.*, **7**, 89

Chan, J. C. M., Maleksadeh, M. and Anand, S. (1975). Bartter's syndrome defect in renal tubular sodium reabsorption. *Clin. Proc. Child. Hosp. Nat. Med. Cent.*, **31**, 67

Danon, A., Chang, L. C. T., Sweetman, B. J., Nies, A. S. and Oates, J. A. (1975). Synthesis of prostaglandins by the rat renal papilla *in vitro*. Mechanism of stimulation by angiotensin II. *Biochem. Biophys. Acta*, **388**, 71

Delaporte, C., Stulzaft, J., Loirat, C. and Broyer, M. (1978). Muscle electrolytes and fluid compartments in six children with Bartter's syndrome. *Clin. Sci. Mol. Med.*, **54**, 223

Donker, A. J. M., Arisz, L. and Brentjens, J. R. M. (1976). The effect of indomethacin on kidney function and plasma renin activity in man. *Nephron*, **17**, 288

Donker, A. J. M., deJong, P. E., Statius von Epps, L. W., Brentjens, J. R. M., Bakker, K. and Dorrenbos, H. (1977). Indomethacin in Bartter's syndrome. *Nephron*, **19**, 200

Dray, F. (1978). Bartter's syndrome: contrasting patterns of prostaglandin excretion in children and adults. *Clin. Sci. Mol. Med.*, **54**, 115

Dusing, R., Atallah, A. A., Prezyna, A. P. and Lee, J. B. (1978). Renal biosynthesis of prostaglandin E_2 and $F_{2\alpha}$ dependence on extracellular potassium. *J. Lab. Clin. Med.*, **92**, 669

Editorial. (1976). Bartter's syndrome. *Lancet*, **ii**, 721

Erkelens, D. W. and Statius von Epps, L. W. (1973). Bartter's syndrome and erythrocytosis. *Am. J. Med.*, **55**, 711

Fanconi, A., Schnaechenmann, G., Nussli, R. and Prader, A. (1971). Chronic hypokalemia with growth retardation, normotensive hyperrenin hyperaldosteronism (Bartter's syndrome) and hypercalciuria. *Helv. Paed. Acta*, **26**, 144

Farese, R. V. and Rodriguez, M. E. (1978). Urinary prostaglandin levels in diabetic hyporeninemic hypoaldosteronism. *Clin. Res.*, **26** (Abst.), 305

Ferris, T. F. (1978). Prostaglandin, potassium and Bartter's syndrome. *J. Lab. Clin. Med.*, **92**, 663

Fichman, M. P., Littenburg, G., Brooker, G. and Horton, R. (1972). Effect of prostaglandin A_1 on renal and adrenal function in man. *Circ. Res.*, **31** (Suppl. II), 19

Fichman, M., Littenburg, G., Woo, J. and Horton, R. (1973). The effect of prostaglandin PGA_1 on adrenal function in man. *Adv. Biosci.*, **9**, 313

Fichman, M. P., Telfer, N., Zia, P., Speckart, P., Golub, M. and Rude, R. (1976). Role of prostaglandins in pathogenesis of Bartter's syndrome. *Am. J. Med.*, **60**, 785

Fichman, M., Zipser, R., Kaye, Z., Lee, A. and Zia, P. (1978). Antidiuresis with suppression of elevated urinary prostaglandin E by ibuprofen in nephrogenic diabetes insipidus and DDAVP in primary diabetes insipidus. In: *VII International Congress of Nephrology*, p. Q-2 (Montreal, Canada)

Gafni, Y., Schwartzman, M. and Raz, A. (1978). Prostaglandin biosynthesis in rabbit kidney medulla. Inhibition *in vitro* vs. *in vivo* by aspirin, indomethacin and meclofenamic acid. *Prostaglandins*, **15**, 759

Gall, G., Waitukaitis, J., Haddow, J. E. and Klein, R. (1971). Erythrocyte Na^+ flux in a patient with Bartter's syndrome. *J. Clin. Endocrinol. Metab.*, **32**, 562

Galvez, O. G., Bay, W. M., Roberts, B. W. and Ferris, T. F. (1977). The hemodynamic effects of potassium deficiency in the dog. *Circ. Res.*, **40** (Suppl. I), 11

Gardner, J. D., Simopoulos, A. P. and Shibolet, S. (1972). Altered membrane sodium transport in Bartter's syndrome. *J. Clin. Invest.*, **51**, 1565

Gill, J. R. and Bartter, F. C. (1978). Evidence for a prostaglandin independent defect in chloride reabsorption in the loop of Henle as a proximal cause of Bartter's syndrome. *Am. J. Med.*, **65**, 766

Gill, J. R., Frolich, J. C., Bowden, R. E., Taylor, A. A., Keiser, H. R., Seyberth, H. W., Oates, J. A. and Bartter, F. C. (1976). Bartter's syndrome: a disorder characterized by high urinary prostaglandins and dependence of hyperreninemia on prostaglandin synthesis. *Am. J. Med.*, **61**, 43

Gittelman, H. J., Graham, J. B. and Welt, L. G. (1966). A new familial disorder characterized by hypokalemia and hypomagnesemia. *Trans. Assoc. Am. Physicians*, **79**, 221

Golub, M., Speckart, P. and Horton, R. (1975). Prostaglandin A_1 (PGA_1) and angiotensin II interaction on aldosterone. *Clin Res.*, **23** (Abst.), 128

Goodman, A. D., Vagnucci, A. M. and Hartroft, P. M. (1969). Pathogenesis of Bartter's syndrome. *N. Engl. J. Med.*, **281**, 1435

Granthum, J. J. and Orloff, J. (1968). Effect of prostaglandin E_1 on the permeability response of the isolated collecting tubule to vasopressin, adenosine 3′-5′ renophosphate and theophylline. *J. Clin. Invest.*, **47**, 1154

Guesry, P., Dray, F., Lenoir, G., Gagnadoux, M. F. and Broyer, M. (1978). Specificity of hyperprostaglandinemia in Bartter's syndrome. In: *VII International Congress of Nephrology*, p. D-34 (Montreal, Canada)

Haljamae, H., Enger, E. and Sigstrom, L. (1975). Cellular potassium transport and ATPase activity in Bartter's syndrome. *Scand. J. Clin. Lab. Invest.*, **35**, 53

Halusha, P. V., Wohltman, M., Privitera, P. J., Horwitz, G. and Margolius, H. S. (1977). Bartter's syndrome: urinary prostaglandin E like material and kallikrein: indomethacin effects. *Ann. Intern. Med.*, **87**, 281

Higashihara, M., Stokes, J., DuBose, T. and Kokko, J. (1978). Segmental chloride transport in Munich Wistar rats: effect of prostaglandin inhibition. In: *VII International Congress of Nephrology*, p. C-7 (Montreal, Canada)

Itskovitz, H. D., Terragno, N. A. and McGiff, J. C. (1974). Effect of a renal prostaglandin on distribution of blood flow in the isolated canine kidney. *Circ. Res.*, **34**, 770

James, T., Holland, N. M. and Preston, P. (1975). Bartter's syndrome: typical facies and normal plasma volume. *Am. J. Dis. Child.*, **129**, 1205

Katz, F. M. and Bortz, A. I. (1978). Treatment of Bartter's syndrome with naproxen. *N. Engl. J. Med.*, **299**, 100

Kimberly, R. P., Bowden, R. E., Keiser, H. R. and Plotz, P. H. (1978a). Reduction of renal function by newer non-steroidal anti-inflammatory drugs. *Am. J. Med.*, **64**, 804

Kimberly, R. P., Gill, J. R., Bowden, R. E., Keiser, H. R. and Plotz, P. M. (1978b). Elevated urinary prostaglandins and the effects of aspirin on renal function in lupus erythematosis. *Ann. Intern. Med.*, **89**, 336

Konomi, M., Imai, M. and Nihei, K. (1978). Indomethacin causing pseudotumor cerebri in Bartter's syndrome. *N. Engl. J. Med.*, **268**, 855

Kornerup, H. J., Pedersen, E. B. and Posborg Petersen, P. (1978). Bartter's syndrome without hyperplasia of the juxtaglomerular apparatus treated with indomethacin. *Acta Med. Scand.*, **204**, 235

Kurtzman, N. A. and Gutierrez, L. F. (1975). Pathophysiology of Bartter's syndrome. *J. Am. Med. Assoc.*, **237**, 758

Larsson, C., Weber, P. and Angaard, E. (1974). Arachidonic acid increases and indomethacin lowers plasma renin activity in the rabbit. *Eur. J. Pharmacol.*, **28**, 391

Lee, J. B. (1971). Prostaglandin A_1: antihypertensive and renal effects. *Ann. Intern. Med.*, **74**, 703

Lifschitz, M. D., Patek, R. V., Fadeum, S. Z. and Stein, J. H. (1978). Chronic changes in renal sodium excretion and renal prostaglandin E production in the rabbit. In: *VII International Congress of Nephrology*, p. U-8 (Montreal, Canada)

Littlewood, J. M., Lee, M. R. and Meadow, S. R. (1976). Treatment of childhood Bartter's syndrome with indomethacin. *Lancet*, **ii**, 795

Littlewood, J. M., Lee, M. R. and Meadow, S. R. (1978). Treatment of Bartter's syndrome in early childhood with prostaglandin synthetase inhibitors. *Arch. Dis. Child.*, **53**, 43

Lonigro, A. V., Terragno, W. A., Malik, K. U. and McGiff, J. C. (1973). Differential inhibition by prostaglandin of the renal action of pressor stimuli. *Prostaglandins*, **3**, 595

McGiff, J. C. (1977). Bartter's syndrome results from an imbalance of vasoactive hormones. *Ann. Intern. Med.*, **87**, 369

McGiff, J. C., Crowshaw, K., Terragno, N. A. and Lonigro, A. J. (1970). Renal prostaglandins: possible regulators of the renal actions of pressor hormones. *Nature (London)*, **227**, 1255

McGiff, J. C., Crowshaw, K., Terragno, N. A., Malik, K. U. and Lonigro, A. J. (1972a). Differential effects of nor-adrenaline and renal nerve stimulation on vascular resistance in the dog kidney and the release of prostaglandin E-like substance. *Clin. Sci.*, **42**, 223

McGiff, J. C., Terragno, N. A., Malik, K. U. and Lonigro, A. J. (1972b). Release of a prostaglandin E-like substance from canine kidney by bradykinin. *Circ. Res.*, **31**, 36

Meadow, S. R., Littlewood, J. M. and Lee, M. R. (1977). Prostaglandin synthetase inhibitors in the treatment of Bartter's syndrome. *Kidney Int.*, **11** (Abst.), 447

Modlinger, R. S., Nicolis, G. L., Krakoff, L. R. and Gabrilove, J. L. (1973). Some observations on the pathogenesis of Bartter's syndrome. *N. Engl. J. Med.*, **239**, 1022

Muirhead, E. E., Germain, G., Leach, B. E., Pitcock, J. A., Stephenson, P., Brooks, B., Brosius, W. L., Daniels, E. G. and Hinman, J. W. (1972). Production of renomedullary prostaglandins by renomedullary interstitial cells grown in tissue culture. *Circ. Res.*, **31** (Suppl. II), 161

Mujovic, V. M. and Fisher, J. W. (1974). The effects of indomethacin on erythropoetin production in dogs following renal artery constriction. I. The possible role of prostaglandins in the generation of erythropoetin by the kidney. *J. Pharmacol. Exp. Ther.*, **191**, 575

Nakada, T., Momose, G., Yoshida, T., Tateno, Y., Shigematsu, H. and Saito, T. (1974). Renin angiotensin–aldosterone system of a woman with Bartter's syndrome: juxtaglomerular cell hyperplasia without hypertension. *Int. Urol.*, **112**, 293

Nielsen, I., Jacobsen, J. G. and Olesen, K. H. (1973). On the pathogenesis of the secondary hyperaldosteronism of the Bartter's syndrome. *Clin. Sci. Mol. Med.*, **48**, 301

Norby, L., Flamenbaum, W., Lentz, R. and Ramwell, P. (1976). Prostaglandins and aspirin therapy in Bartter's syndrome. *Lancet*, **ii**, 604

Norby, L., Mark, A. L. and Kaloyanides, G. J. (1976). On the pathogenesis of Bartter's syndrome: report of studies in a patient with this disorder. *Clin. Nephrol.*, **6**, 404

Norby, L. M., Weidig, J., Ramwell, P., Slotkoff, L. and Gagnon, J. (1976). Role of prostaglandins in selective hypoaldosteronism. *Kidney Int.*, **10** (Abst.), 534

Oliver, J. F., Delaney, V. B. and Bourke, E. (1978). Increased erythrocyte sodium permeability in patients with Bartter's syndrome. *Min. Elect. Metab.*, **1**, 225

O'Regan, S., Rivard, G. E., Robitaille, P. O. and Mongeau, J. G. (1978). Aspirin improves platelet dysfunction in Bartter's syndrome. In: *VII International Congress of Nephrology*, p. P-1 (Montreal, Canada)

Patak, R. B., Mookerjee, B. K., Bentzel, C. J., Hysert, P. E., Babej, M. and Lee, J. B. (1975). Antagonism of the effects of furosemide by indomethacin in normal and hypertensive man. *Prostaglandins*, **10**, 649

Paulsrud, J. R. and Miller, O. N. (1974). Inhibition of 15-OH prostaglandin dehydrogenase by several diuretic drugs. *Fed. Proc.*, **33**, 590

Pronove, P., McCardle, R. C. and Bartter, F. C. (1960). Aldosteronism, hypokalemia, and a unique renal lesion in a 5-year-old boy. *Acta Endocrinol.* (Suppl. 5), 167

Radfar, N., Gill, J. R., Bartter, F. C., Bravo, E., Taylor, A. A. and Bowden, R. E. (1978). Hypokalemia in Bartter's syndrome and other disorders produce resistance to vasopressors via prostaglandin overproduction. *Proc. Soc. Biol. Med.*, **158**, 502

Rado, J. P., Simatupang, T., Boer, P. and Dorhout Mees, E. J. (1978). Pharmacologic studies in Bartter's syndrome: effect of DDAVP and indomethacin on renal concentrating operation. *Int. J. Clin. Pharmacol.*, **16**, 22

Rosenblum, M., Simpson, D. F. and Evenson, M. (1977). Factitious Bartter's syndrome. *Arch. Intern. Med.*, **137**, 1244

Rumpf, K. W., Frenzel, S., Lowitz, H. D. and Scheler, F. (1975). The effect of indomethacin on plasma renin activity in man under normal conditions and after stimulation of the renin–angiotensin system. *Prostaglandins*, **10**, 641

Sasaki, M., Oklumura, M., Asano, T. and Arakawa, K. (1977). Response to angiotensin II antagonist before and after treatment with indomethacin in Bartter's syndrome. *Br. Med. J.*, **2**, 995

Sasaki, M., Okumura, M., Ikeda, M., Kawashi, T. and Fukiyma, K. (1976). Hypotensive response to angiotensin II analogue in Bartter's syndrome. *N. Engl. J. Med.*, **294**, 611

Schwartz, G. J. and Cornfeld, D. (1975). Bartter's syndrome: clinical study of its treatment with salt loading and propranolol. *Clin. Nephrol.*, **4**, 45

Schwarz, H. A., Weidman, P., Messerli, F. M., Zia, P. K., Flammer, J. and Reubi, F. C. (1977). Erhohte renale prostaglandin E_2 secretion bei Bartter-syndrome. *Schweiz. Med. Wochenschr.*, **107**, 1872

Schwarz, H. A., Weidmann, P., Messerli, F. M., Zia, P. K., Flammer, J. and Reubi, F. C. (1978). Increased levels of renal venous and peripheral prostaglandin E-like activity in Bartter's syndrome. *Min. Elect. Metab.*, **1**, 288

Silverberg, A. B., Mennes, P. A. and Cryer, R. E. (1978). Resistance to endogenous norepinephrine in Bartter's syndrome. Reversion during indomethacin administration. *Am. J. Med.*, **64**, 231

Simatupang, T. A., Rado, J. P., Boer, P., Geyskes, G. G., Vos, J. and Dorhout Mees, E. J. (1978). Pharmacologic studies in Bartter's syndrome. Opposite effects of treatment with antinatiuretic and antiprostaglandin drugs. *Int. J. Clin. Pharmacol.*, **16**, 14

Solomon, R. J. and Brown, R. S. (1975). Bartter's syndrome. New insights into pathogenesis and treatment. *Am. J. Med.*, **59**, 575

Stein, J. M. (1978). Prostaglandins and Bartter's syndrome. *Resident and Staff Physicians*, p. 73

Stokes, J. B. and Kokko, J. P. (1976). Effects of prostaglandin E_2 on Na^+ transport across the rabbit cortical collecting tubule. *Kidney Int.*, **10** (Abst.), 600

Sutherland, L. E., Hartcroft, P., Baylis, J. O., Bailey, J. D. and Lynch, M. J. (1970). Bartter's syndrome: a report of four cases including three in one sibship with comparative histological evaluation of juxtaglomerular apparatus and glomerulae. *Acta Paediatr. Scand.*, **201** (Suppl.), 2

Tan, S. Y., Shapiro, R., Franco, R., Stockard, H. and Mulrow, P. J. (1977). Indomethacin-induced prostaglandin inhibitor with hyperkalemia: a reversible cause of hyporeninemic hypoaldosteronism. *Clin. Res.*, **25** (Abst.), 598

Tarm, F., Juncos, L. L., Anderson, C. F. and Donadio, J. V. (1973). Bartter's syndrome: an unusual presentation. *Mayo Clin. Proc.*, **48**, 280

Terragno, N. A., McGiff, J. C. and Terragno, A. (1978). Prostacyclin (PGI_2) production by renal blood vessels: relationship to an endogenous prostaglandin synthesis inhibitor. *Clin. Res.*, **26** (Abst.), 545

Tomko, D. J., Yeh, B. P. Y. and Falls, W. F. (1976). Study of a 52-year-old man with evidence for a defect in proximal tubular sodium reabsorption and comments on therapy. *Am. J. Med.*, **61**, 111

Trygstad, C. W., Mangos, J. A., Bloodworth, J. M. P. Jr. and Labeck, C. C. (1969). A sibship with Bartter's syndrome: failure of total adrenalectomy to correct the potassium wasting. *Pediatrics*, **44**, 234

Vaisrub, S. (1978). Bartter's syndrome – limelight on prostaglandins. *J. Am. Med. Assoc.*, **239**, 137

Vane, J. R. (1971). Inhibition of prostaglandin synthesis as a mechanism of action for aspirin-like drugs. *Nature (New Biol.)*, **231**, 232

Vane, J. R. and McGiff, J. C. (1975). Possible contributions of endogenous prostaglandins to the control of blood pressure. *Circ. Res.*, **37** (Suppl. 1), 68

Vander, A. J. (1968). Direct effects of prostaglandin on renal function and renin release in anesthetized dog. *Am. J. Physiol.*, **214**, 218

Verberkmoes, R., van Damme, B., Clement, J., Amery, A. and Michielson, P. (1976). Bartter's syndrome with hyperplasia of renomedullary interstitial cells. Successful treatment with indomethacin. *Kidney Int.*, **9**, 302

Vinci, J. M., Gill, J. R., Bowden, R. E., Pisano, J. U., Izzo, J. L., Radfar, N., Taylor, A. A., Zusman, R. M., Bartter, F. C. and Keiser, H. R. (1978). The kallikrein–kinin system in

Bartter's syndrome and its response to prostaglandin synthetase inhibition. *J. Clin. Invest.*, **61**, 1671

Weber, P., Larsson, C., Angaard, E., Hamburg, M., Corey, E. J., Nicolaou, K. C. and Samuellson, B. (1976). Stimulation of renin release from rabbit renal cortex by arachidonic acid and prostaglandin endoperoxides. *Circ. Res.*, **39**, 868

Weber, P. C., Scherer, B. and Schnermann, J. (1978). Effect of sodium and potassium chloride intake on urinary prostaglandin excretion in the rat. *Clin. Res.*, **26** (Abst.), 478

White, M. G. (1972). Bartter's syndrome. *Arch. Intern. Med.*, **124**, 41

Whorton, A. R., Misono, K., Hollifield, J., Frolich, J. C., Inagumi, T. and Oates, J. A. (1977). Prostaglandins and renin release: I. Stimulation of renin release from rabbit renal cortical slices by PGI_2. *Prostaglandins*, **14**, 1095

Zancan, L., Zacchello, F. and Mantero, F. (1976). Indomethacin for Bartter's syndrome. *Lancet*, **ii**, 1354

Zipser, R., Rude, R., Zia, P., Singer, F. and Fichman, M. (1978). Stimulation of renal prostaglandins by potassium and by magnesium in Bartter's syndrome. *Clin. Res.*, **26** (Abst.), 480

Zusman, R. M. and Keiser, H. R. (1977). Prostaglandin biosynthesis by rabbit renomedullary interstitial cells in tissue culture, stimulation by angiotensin II, bradykinin, and arginine vasopressin. *J. Clin. Invest.*, **60**, 215

8
Prostaglandins and their Synthesis Inhibitors in Migraine

J. VARDI, J. M. RABEY and M. STREIFLER

8.1 INTRODUCTION

There is a general agreement that migraine is primarily an expression of vascular disturbance. A number of vasoactive substances including catecholamines, histamine, serotonin, kinins and prostaglandins have been implicated in migraine attacks. Dalessio (1978) has summarized the roles of different vasoactive substances in migraine.

8.2 VASOACTIVE SUBSTANCES IN MIGRAINE ATTACK

8.2.1 Tyramine

Tyramine, a pressor amine found in certain foods, is known to induce migraine attacks in susceptible subjects. A defect in the conjugation and inactivation of tyramine has been reported in patients with migraine (Smith *et al.*, 1970). Tyramine also liberates noradrenaline from tissues. Temporal arteries removed from subjects during the painful stage of migraine have an increased capacity for noradrenaline uptake. On the other hand, noradrenaline administered intravenously has also been used to treat migraine (Ostfeld and Wolff, 1955).

8.2.2 Serotonin

Serotonin levels in plasma fall at the onset of migraine attack (Lance *et al.*, 1967) and platelets from patients during migraine attack aggregate more readily than from controls when incubated with serotonin (Hilton and Cumings, 1971). Serotonin has also been shown to constrict human scalp arteries (Sicuteri, 1966). An increase in 5-hydroxyindole acetic acid (the major metabolite of serotonin) has been demonstrated in urine during migraine attack (Curzon *et al.*, 1966).

8.2.3 Histamine

Histamine levels in whole blood increase in patients with cluster headache (believed to be related to migraine) at the onset of attack (Anthony and Lance, 1971). Histamine and other vasodilators injected into susceptible subjects can provoke cluster headache.

8.2.4 Kinins

Local accumulation of a bradykinin-like vasodilator polypeptide at the subsurface of vessel walls in patients with migraine has been reported by Chapman *et al.* (1960).

8.2.5 Prostaglandins

Prostaglandins might be involved in migraine. However attempts to detect these substances either in venous blood or in cerebro-spinal fluid during a migrainous episode have not been successful (Sandler, 1972). Carlson *et al.* (1968) noted that intravenous infusion of PGE_1 resulted in a headache in 10 out of 11 healthy subjects. Two had visual symptoms, similar to those occurring in migraine. Administration of PGE_1 to monkeys increased external carotid blood flow and reduced external carotid vascular resistance

(Spira *et al.*, 1978; Welch *et al.*, 1974b). These authors have suggested that migraine headache is induced by PGE_1 released locally in the external carotid artery in response to nervous or biochemical stimulation. They have also demonstrated a specific vasodilator action of PGE_1 on the external carotid artery. The resulting increase in external carotid blood flow leads to a reduction in internal carotid flow through a steal mechanism and may be a cause of the neurological deficit occurring during migraine attack.

In their animal model, Spira *et al.* (1978) demonstrated that small amounts of directly injected PGE_1, although only slightly raising its *normal* concentration, produced a marked vasodilatation in the external carotid artery.

Welch *et al.* (1974a) attribute the pathophysiology of migraine to a hereditary hypersensitivity of the external carotid artery to PGE_1.

$PGF_{2\alpha}$ has been shown to constrict arterioles in the internal carotid system (Denton *et al.*, 1972; Pennick *et al.*, 1972; Rosenbaum, 1975; Allen *et al.*, 1974) and may produce attacks of migraine by this mechanism.

Arachidonic acid, a natural precursor of prostaglandins, stimulates platelet aggregation. Furlow and Bass (1975) have shown that intra-carotid injection of arachidonic acid in rats induces platelet hyperaggregation with temporary arterial thrombus formation in the brain. Catalysed by the enzyme cyclo-oxygenase, this fatty acid is converted to prostaglandins G_2 and H_2. PGH_2 causes platelets to release their granule contents and to aggregate. It is then converted to thromboxane A_2 (TXA_2); a highly unstable compound with potent aggregatory and vasoconstrictor properties (Hamberg *et al.*, 1975). A similar effect with an increase in blood and plasma levels of free fatty acids (FFA) has been reported (Fieshi, 1975) during migraine attack. The combined effects of prostaglandins on platelet aggregation and vasoconstriction in the internal carotid system may in fact explain the pathophysiology of the migraine 'aura' and the neurological manifestations of migraine. These phenomena have previously been ascribed to serotonin and adrenaline (Kalendovsky and Austin, 1975; Rosenbaum, 1975) which also promote the endogenous production of prostaglandins (Welch *et al.*, 1974b).

It thus appears that increased biosynthesis of endogenous prostaglandins from arachidonic acids or stimulated by serotonin and histamine may play an important role in the development of migraine.

8.3 PROSTAGLANDIN SYNTHESIS INHIBITORS IN THE TREATMENT OF MIGRAINE

Non-steroidal anti-inflammatory drugs, such as aspirin, indomethacin and fenamates are potent inhibitors of prostaglandin synthesis (Vane, 1971; Flower and Vane, 1972). These drugs also reduce the levels of prostaglandins in cerebro-spinal fluid (Feldberg, 1973). In addition they inhibit platelet aggregation and thrombus growth (Kadatz, 1975).

The fenamates are unique in that they inhibit not only the biosynthesis of prostaglandins, but also some of the actions of exogenous prostaglandins (Collier and Sweatman, 1968; Levy and Lindner, 1971; Zor *et al.*, 1973; Lindner *et al.*, 1974).

Theoretical considerations, as outlined above, led us to examine the effects of flufenamic acid and mefenamic acid in the treatment of migraine.

Since different factors appear to be involved in the pathogenesis of migraine attacks (Figure 8.1) treatment with a single drug with a specific mode of action

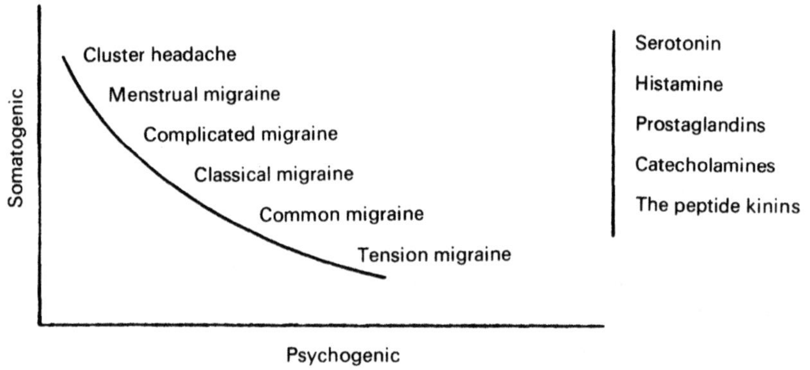

Figure 8.1 Nosological classification of migraine and vasoactive substances implicated in migraine attacks

cannot be expected to be effective in all patients. This open trial was conducted in ambulatory patients and hence was subject to methodological limitations. Furthermore, there are no valid methods for objective grading of headache pain and allied symptoms.

The study was carried out in 51 patients (40 women and 11 men). Clinical characteristics are summarized (Table 8.1). Pregnant women and patients

Table 8.1 Clinical characteristics of patients with migraine

Sex	*No. of patients*	*Positive familial history*	*Dysmenorrhoea concomitant with migraine*	*Type of migraine*		*Frequency of attacks*	
				Typical	*Atypical*	*≥1 per month*	*<1 per month*
F	40	13	31	20	20	25	15
M	11	5	—	2	9	7	4

with abnormal neurological, clinical or laboratory findings were excluded. After discontinuing all previous antimigraine drugs the patients received flufenamic acid or mefenamic acid for a period of 1 year.

An initial dose of 250–500 mg of flufenamic acid or mefenamic acid was administered at the onset of migraine attack. Additional doses of 250 mg were given at 1½ hourly intervals if needed, up to a total of 1500 mg per attack. The effect of fenamate treatment on migraine attack during 1 year of treatment was compared with conventional migraine therapy (Table 8.2) for a similar period in the same patients. The results are summarized in Tables 8.2 and 8.3.

Table 8.2 Comparison between the efficacy of fenamates and conventional antimigraine drugs

Drug used	*Intensity of migraine during treatment (No. of patients)*				*Side-effects*
	Abolished	*Slight*	*Moderate*	*Severe*	
*Conventional antimigraine drugs (n = 51)	8	12	19	12	dyspepsia drowsiness weakness dizziness 38˙
Fenamates (n = 51)	13	20	11	7	slight dyspepsia, cessation of treatment due to severe GI symptoms 19

*The drugs used were Temigran, Teva, Jerusalem (containing: ergotamine tartrate, chlorocyclizine, caffeine, codein phosphate and dipyrone), Migristene, Specia, Paris (dimetiotazine), Deseril, Sandoz, Basle (methysergide), Tegretol, Geigy, Basle (carbamazepine), Migranol, Zori, Tel-Aviv (containing: ergotamine tartrate, meclizine HCl and caffeine), Percodan, Taro, Haifa (containing: dihydrohydroxycodeinone terephthalate, homatropine terephthalate, acetylsalicyclic acid, phenacetin, and caffeine), Valium, Hoffman-La Roche, Basle (diazepam), Optalgin, Teva, Jerusalem (dipyrone), aspirin, Bayer, A.G., Frankfurt (acetylsalicyclic acid), Deralin, Teva, Jerusalem (propranolol)
n = No. of patients

Table 8.3 Effect of fenamates on severity of migraine attacks

Drug used	*Abolished*	*Slight headache persisted*
Fenamates (n = 560)	144 (25.6%)	164 (29%)
Common antimigraine drugs (n = 560)	90 (16%)	132 (23.5%)

n = No. of attacks

For evaluating the efficacy of fenamates, we took into consideration 560 migrainous attacks from a total score of 615. This 'framework' was chosen for the purpose of comparison with 560 migraine attacks previously treated with common antimigraine drugs. Every patient acted as his own control and identical number of attacks were treated with common antimigraine drugs and fenamates. All the antimigraine drugs or fenamates were administered at the onset of the attack.

Fenamates abolished 144 migraine attacks in 13 patients whereas conventional therapy resulted in alleviation of 90 attacks in eight patients. In an

Table 8.4 Ophthalmoplegic migraine

Sex	*Age*	*Family history of migraine*	*Frequency of attacks/ months*	*Neuro-logical findings*	*Four vessels angiog-raphy*	*Lumbar puncture protein* mg%	*Brain scan*	*EEG*	*Coagula-tion factors*	*Thrombo-cytes aggre-gability*
F	28	+	1/2	3 nerve palsy in-complete right eye	negative	normal	negative	normal	normal	hyper-aggregation
F	35	+	1/3–4	3 nerve palsy complete right eye	negative	normal	negative	normal	normal	hyper-aggregation
M	23	–	1/3–4	3 nerve palsy in-complete left eye	negative	60	negative	diffuse slowness	normal	hyper-aggregation
F	35	+	1/1	3 nerve palsy in-complete right eye	negative	normal	negative	normal	normal	hyper-aggregation
F	18	–	1/3–4	3 nerve palsy in-complete left eye	negative	normal	negative	normal	normal	hyper-aggregation

additional 20 patients with a total of 164 migraine attacks treated with fenamates, slight headache persisted. Slight headache also persisted in 12 patients (132 migraine attacks) treated with conventional drugs. Thus fenamates were effective in 55% of migraine attacks compared to conventional therapy in 40%.

Five out of 51 patients in this study suffered from recurrent ophthalmoplegic migraine. Their clinical characteristics and investigatory findings are summarized (Table 8.4). The only positive and constant finding was hyperaggregation of platelets during migraine attack. Four-vessel angiography and coagulation factors were normal.

During a 1-year control period in which the patients used ergot derivatives only at the onset of the headache, they had 30 attacks of migraine. Nineteen of them were accompanied by an oculomotor nerve palsy, which lasted for 1–4 weeks. Eleven attacks were successfully treated and the patients did not suffer from third nerve palsy. The same patients were treated with flufenamic or mefenamic acid given at the beginning of the attack, during the following year. These five patients suffered from 25 attacks of migraine. Twenty-two of these were successfully treated with fenamates, and have not experienced oculomotor palsy. In two patients (one attack each) the migraine was accompanied by a third nerve palsy. One patient suffered from a severe headache but without any neurological deficit. The high rate of platelet aggregation encountered during the control (ergot treatment) period was reduced during treatment with fenamates.

Table 8.5 Effect of fenamates on ophthalmoplegic migraine (1-year trial)

Patient No.	*Migraine attacks*		*Ophthalmoplegic events*		*Successful treatment of migraine attacks*	
	Control (year)	*Fenamate (year)*	*Control (year)*	*Fenamate (year)*	*Control (year)*	*Fenamate (year)*
1	10	8	6	1	5	7
2	6	4	3	0	3	4
3	4	4	2	0	1	3
4	3	3	3	1	0	3
5	7	6	5	0	2	5
Total	30	25	19	2	11	22

The most common side-effects associated with fenamate treatment were dyspepsia, heartburn with belching and gastric bleeding. Since prostaglandin synthesis inhibitors may interfere with the production of prostacylin (PGI_2) in the stomach (Vergroesen, 1978) and are known to be ulcerogenic in laboratory animals, the use of such drugs in patients with peptic ulcers is contraindicated.

The results of this study suggest that fenamates are effective in relieving the symptoms of the migraine attack (see Table 8.5).

It should be emphasized that the best results were obtained in women suffering from migraine attacks related to their menstrual period. This may be due to the increased rate of prostaglandin release during menstruation (Pickles *et al.*, 1965; Schwartz *et al.*, 1974; Anderson *et al.*, 1976; see Chapter 12 by Toppozada).

In patients suffering from ophthalmoplegic migraine, increased platelet aggregability during the events suggests that some pro-aggregatory prostaglandins possibly play an aetiologically important role by causing thrombus formation and vascular constriction in the affected area. The amelioration of the headache and the prevention of neurological complications by fenamates may support this hypothesis.

Although prostaglandins have been identified in brain (Holmes and Horton, 1968) and they impair cerebral vascular autoregulation (Welch *et al.*, 1974b) their role in the chain of events leading to a migraine attack is not firmly established. The favourable observations in the therapeutic trial may support the view that release of prostaglandins plays a role in the mechanism and possibly also the aetiology of migraine. Other products of arachidonic acid metabolism may also be involved in migraine by producing vasoconstriction and platelet aggregation.

8.4 COMMENTS

Prostaglandins released locally or from other organs appear to be involved in migraine (Sandler, 1972) by selectively acting on the carotid artery system. These substances are released from vascular tissues in response to nervous and chemical stimulation. 5-Hydroxytryptamine (serotonin) and histamine, which are such stimulants, also have a direct effect on blood vessels and may be independently involved in migraine. This may explain the inconsistent therapeutic response to antagonists of these drugs and to prostaglandin synthesis inhibitors in migraine.

PGE_1 and possibly other prostaglandins are thought to be involved in migraine. Fenamates which inhibit the biosynthesis and some actions of prostaglandins were found effective in alleviating migraine attacks in some patients. Increased levels of prostaglandins in circulation or in cerebro-spinal fluid in association with migraine attack have so far not been demonstrated. However, an increased local vascular sensitivity to certain prostaglandins could provoke migraine attack.

References

Allen, G. S., Henderson, L. M., Chou, S. N. and Gold, L. H. (1974). Cerebral arterial spasm: 1. *In vitro* contractile activity of vasoactive agents on canine basilar and middle cerebral arteries. *J. Neurosurg.*, **40**, 433

Anderson, A. B. M., Haynes, P. J., Guillebaud, F. and Turnbul, A. C. (1976). Reduction of menstrual blood-loss by prostaglandin-synthetase inhibitor. *Lancet*, **i**, 774

Anthony, M. and Lance, J. W. (1971). Histamine and serotonin in cluster headache. *Arch. Neurol.*, **25**, 225

Carlson, L. A., Ekelund, L. G. and Oro, L. (1968). Clinical and metabolic effects of different doses of prostaglandin E_1 in man. *Acta Med. Scand.*, **183**, 423

Collier, H. O. J. and Sweatman, W. J. F. (1968). Antagonism by fenamates of prostaglandin $F_{2\alpha}$ and of slow-reacting substance on human bronchial muscle. *Nature*, **219**, 864

Curzon, G., Theaker, P. and Phillips, B. J. (1966). Excretion of 5-hydroxyindole acetic acid in migraine. *J. Neurol. Neurosurg. Psychiatry*, **29**, 85

Chapman, L. F., Ramos, P. O., Goodell, H. and Wolf, H. G. (1960). Neurokinine: a polypeptide formed during neuronal activity in man. *Trans. Am. Neurol. Assoc.*, **85**, 42

Dalessio, D. J. (1978). Mechanisms of headache. In: A. P. Friedman (ed.), *Symposium on Headaches and Related Pain Syndromes. The Medical Clinics of North America*, pp. 424–442 (Philadelphia, London, Toronto: W. B. Saunders Company)

Denton, J. C. Jr., White, K. P. and Roberston, J. T. (1972). The effect of prostaglandins E_1, A_1 and $F_{2\alpha}$ on the cerebral circulation of dogs and monkeys. *J. Neurosurg.*, **36**, 34

Feldberg, W., Gupta, K. P., Milton, A. S. and Shaligram, S. U. (1973). Effect of pyrogen and antipyretic on prostaglandin activity in cisternal cerebrospinal fluid of unanaesthetized cat. *J. Physiol.*, **234**, 279

Fieshi, C. (1975). Experimental and clinical observation on platelet aggregability in focal brain ischemia. In: Summary of the International Round Table Conference of Platelet Aggregation in the Pathogenesis of Cerebrovascular Disorders. *Stroke*, **6**, 239

Furlow, T. W. Jr. and Bass, N. H. (1975). Stroke in rats produced by carotid injection of sodium arachidonate. *Science*, **187**, 258

Flower, R. and Vane, R. J. (1972). Inhibition of prostaglandin synthetase in brain explains the antipyretic activity of paracetamol (4-acetamidophenol). *Nature*, **240**, 410

Greeberg, S., Kordovitz, P. J. and Diecke, F. P. J. (1973). Effect of prostaglandin $F_{2\alpha}$ on arterial and venous contractility and ^{45}Ca uptake. *Arch. Int. Pharmacodyn Ther.*, **205**, 381

Hamberg, M., Svensson, J. and Samuelsson, B. (1975). Thromboxanes: A new group of biologically active compounds derived from prostaglandin endoperoxides. *Proc. Natl. Acad. Sci.*, **72**, 2994

Hilton, B. P. and Cunnings, J. M. (1971). An assessment of platelet aggregation induced by 5-hydroxytryptamine. *J. Clin. Pathol.*, **24**, 250

Holmes, S. W. and Horton, E. W. (1968). The identification of four prostaglandins in the dog brain and their regional distribution in the central nervous system. *J. Physiol. (London)*, **195**, 731

Kadatz, R. (1975). Inhibition of platelet thrombus formation by pharmacological agents. In: Summary of the International Round Table Conference of Platelet Aggregation in the Pathogenesis of Cerebrovascular Disorders. *Stroke*, **6**, 239

Kalendovsky, Z. and Austin, J. H. (1975). Complicated migraine; its association with increased platelet aggregability and abnormal plasmo-coagulation factors. *Headaches*, **15**, 18

Lance, J. W., Anthony, M. and Ginski, A. (1967). Serotonin, the carotid body, and cranial vessels in migraine. *Arch. Neurol.*, **16**, 553

Levy, B., Lindner, H. R. (1971). Selective blockade of the vasodepressor response to prostaglandin $F_{2\alpha}$ in the anaesthetized rabbit. *Br. J. Pharmacol.*, **43**, 236

Lindner, H. R., Zor, U. and Bauminger, S. (1974). Use of prostaglandin synthetase inhibitors in analysing the role of prostaglandin in reproductive physiology. In: H. Y. Robinson and R. J. Vane (eds.), *Prostaglandin Synthetase Inhibitors*, pp. 271–287 (New York: Raven Press)

Nachman, R. L. (1975). The platelet as an inflammatory cell. In: Summary of the International Round Table Conference of Platelet Aggregation in the Pathogenesis of Cerebrovascular Disorders. *Stroke*, **6**, 239

Ostfeld, A. M. and Wolff, H. G. (1955). Studies on headache: Arterenol (norepinephrine) and vascular headache of the migraine type. *Arch. Neurol. Psychiatry*, **74**, 131

Pennick, M., White, R. P., Crockarell, J. T. and Robertson, J. T. (1972). Role of prostaglandin $F_{2\alpha}$ in the genesis of experimental vasospasm. *J. Neurol.*, **37**, 398

Pickles, V. R., Hall, W. J., Best, F. A. and Smith, G. N. (1965). Increased production of prostaglandins during menses. *J. Obstet. Gynaecol. Br. Cmnwlth.*, **72**, 185

Rosenbaum, W. J. (1975). Constriction of pialarterioles produced by prostaglandin $F_{2\alpha}$. *Stroke*, **6**, 273

Sandler, M. (1972). Migraine: A pulmonary disease. *Lancet*, **i**, 618

Schwartz, A., Zor, U., Lindner, H. R. and Naor, S. (1974). Primary dysmenorrhea: alleviation by an inhibitor of prostaglandin synthesis and action. *Obstet. Gynecol.*, **44**, 709

Sicuteri, F. (1966). Vasoneuroactive substances in migraine. *Headache*, **6**, 109

Smith, I., Kellow, A. H. and Hanington, E. (1970). A clinical and biochemical correlation between tyramin and migraine headache. *Headache*, **10**, 43

Spira, P. J., Mylecharane, E. J., Misbach, J., Duckworth, J. W. and Lance, J. W. (1978). Internal and external carotid vascular responses to vasoactive agents in the monkey. *Neurology (Minneap.)*, **28**, 162

Vane, J. R. (1971). Inhibition of prostaglandin synthesis as a mechanism of action for aspirin-like drug. *Nature (New Biol.)*, **231**, 232

Vergroesen, A. J. (1978). Linoleic acid, its prostaglandins and atherosclerotic C.V.D. *Prostagl. Ther.*, **4**, 1

Welch, K. M. A., Knowles, L. and Spira, P. (1974a). Local effect of prostaglandins on cat pial arteries. *Eur. J. Pharmacol.*, **25**, 155

Welch, K. M. A., Spira, P. J., Knoules, L. and Lance, J. W. (1974b). Effects of prostaglandin on the internal and external carotid blood flow in the monkey. *Neurol. (Minneap.)*, **24**, 705

Welch, K. M. A., Spira, P. J. and Lance, J. W. (1975). Letters to the editor. *Neurol. (Minneap.)*, **25**, 33A

Zor, U., Bauminger, S., Lamprecht, S. A. and Lindner, H. R. (1973). Stimulation of cyclic AMP production in the rat ovary by luteinizing hormone: Independence of prostaglandin mediation. *Prostaglandins*, **4**, 499

9
Prostaglandins and Cancer

A. BENNETT

Some aspects of this topic have been reviewed previously (Jaffe, 1974; Karim and Rao, 1976; Bennett, 1976a; Easty and Easty, 1976). There is now substantial evidence of relationships between prostaglandins and cancer, but since cancer comprises a heterogeneous group of diseases, uniform relationships would not be expected. As described later in detail, many tumours can synthesize substantial amounts of prostaglandins, and these may affect tumour growth, spread and response to treatment, or give rise to conditions such as diarrhoea or hypercalcaemia. Prostaglandins may be released by agents used to treat cancer, and so contribute to the side-effects of treatment. In animals, drugs which inhibit prostaglandin synthesis can reduce tumour growth, increase survival time and increase the response to radiotherapy and chemotherapy. In breast cancer patients, survival time after mastectomy correlates inversely with amounts of prostaglandin which the tumours can synthesize *in vitro*. The reasons for continuing to study prostaglandins in cancer are therefore compelling.

No previous review has extensively cited the available literature on prostaglandins and cancer. Some early papers are more of historical than of scientific value, but they are discussed briefly here to provide a full background to the subject. Almost all studies have concerned PGE and PGF compounds, but future studies can be expected to involve thromboxanes, prostacyclin and other potentially important prostanoids. In most cases the extracted prostaglandins have not been rigorously identified, and should therefore be referred to as 'prostaglandin-like' even though the authors may not have done so. The term 'prostaglandin' is used in this chapter for simplicity, even in the absence of rigorous identification.

9.1 PROSTAGLANDINS EXTRACTED FROM TUMOURS

Data on extracted prostaglandins have to be interpreted cautiously. Prior to extraction the tissue must be homogenized, but different types of solution can yield different amounts of prostaglandins. Solutions which inhibit enzyme activity indicate the 'basal' quantities in tissues, but this value is unlikely to be a true basal amount since prostaglandins may be formed while the tissue is being prepared for homogenization, or in the brief period during homogenization before enzyme activity is inhibited. When tissue is homogenized in an aqueous solution which does not inhibit enzyme activity, endogenous precursors are released and prostaglandin synthesis usually occurs. The amounts of material present in these homogenates represent 'basal' quantities plus material newly formed from released precursors, less any degradation (usually slight) which may occur.

Tumours consist of neoplastic cells together with host cells, inflammatory cells, etc. all of which may contribute to the total prostaglandin production. The proof that malignant cells in whole tumours release prostaglandins is therefore difficult. Bennett *et al.* (1977a) considered that human malignant breast cells produce high amounts of prostaglandins because there was no relationship between the quantities of prostaglandin extracted from the tumours and the numbers of non-malignant cells seen histologically. This is far from ideal, since non-malignant cells contribute by an unknown extent to the total prostaglandin. In the human head-and-neck cancers, discussed later, where an attempt was made to kill malignant cells with X-irradiation and cytotoxic drugs prior to excision, prostaglandin formation by the residual tumour was related to the degree of inflammation and the amounts of granulation and fibrous tissue present (A. Bennett, R. L. Carter and B. Tanner, unpublished). A direct demonstration that malignant cells produce prostaglandin should therefore come from cell culture studies, but this is difficult to do with human tumours, and there is also the problem of contamination with other cells.

9.1.1 Prostaglandins extracted from human endocrine tumours and released into the blood stream

Much of the early work concerned human cancers. The endocrine tumours considered here are those of classical endocrine glands, and also various 'endocrine-like' tumours arising from cells of the APUD system (Pearse, 1966) and classified as apudomas (Welbourn, 1977).

9.1.1.1 *Medullary carcinoma of the thyroid*

Williams *et al.* (1968) reported that some human medullary carcinomas of the thyroid contained higher amounts of PGE_2 and $PGF_{2\alpha}$ than did normal thyroid tissue, and Grimley *et al.* (1969) found that monolayer cultures of a medullary carcinoma synthesized PGE_2 and $PGF_{2\alpha}$ The former authors reported raised amounts of PGE_2 and $PGF_{2\alpha}$ in peripheral venous blood of two patients, and very high prostaglandin concentrations in the blood draining the tumour of one patient. Raised peripheral plasma PGE was found in the three patients studied by Kaplan *et al.* (1973), possibly in the patient examined by Isaacs *et al.* (1974), in the patients described by Jaffe *et al.* (1973) and Jaffe (1974), and in 18 out of 19 cases studied by Jaffe and Condon (1976). Others have not confirmed this (van Dorp, 1971; Melvin *et al.*, 1972; Ménagé *et al.*, 1975), but the sensitivity of the assay used by Melvin *et al.* may have been too low. Bennett (1976b) reported that only one of five patients had clearly raised blood prostaglandin levels. This patient was the subject of a paper by Barrowman *et al.* (1975) and was the only case with pulmonary metastases. Inactivation of PGE and PGF compounds during passage through the pulmonary circulation would reduce the amount reaching the peripheral circulation from the thyroid. Perhaps the pulmonary metastases released prostaglandin into the circulation distal to the site of pulmonary inactivation.

Because of pulmonary inactivation, measurement of prostaglandins in the peripheral blood may often be inappropriate. However, some prostaglandins are not broken down in the lung, and the rate of inactivation in man may be less than in laboratory animals. Golub *et al.* (1975) found that almost 70% of injected PGE_1 is cleared in a single passage through the human lung, compared with 90–95% in rabbit and dog (Ferreira and Vane, 1967), but they did not study PGE_2 or PGF compounds. More recent attempts to overcome this problem have involved the measurement of prostaglandin metabolites in the blood (see later), but they have rarely been applied to endocrine tumours.

9.1.1.2 *Carcinoid tumours*

Sandler *et al.* (1968) found that an extract of a bronchial carcinoid tumour contained substantial amounts of PGE_2 and $PGF_{2\alpha}$, whereas only an unidentified hydroxy fatty acid was detected in the two cases of ileal carcinoid. Extracts of one caecal carcinoid contained only small amounts of prostaglandin (Bennett *et al.*, 1977). Elevated plasma PGE was found in some patients by Kaplan *et al.* (1973) and Jaffe (1974). Feldman and Plonk (1974) measured serum $PGF_{2\alpha}$ and its 13,14-dihydro-15-keto-metabolite in 12 patients with carcinoid tumours. Levels of both substances were raised in one patient, $PGF_{2\alpha}$ was raised in another, and the amount of metabolite was increased in a third patient. Jaffe and Condon (1976) found elevated plasma PGE levels in 18 out of 22 patients, but there was no correlation with diarrhoea.

9.1.1.3 *Phaeochromocytomas*

Sandler *et al.* (1968) found PGE_2 and $PGF_{2\alpha}$ in extracts of some phaeochromocytomas, and Papanicolau *et al.* (1975) also extracted substantial amounts of PGE and PGF from four phaeochromocytomas.

9.1.1.4 *Neural tumours*

Substantial amounts of prostaglandins have been extracted from ganglioneuromas, neuroblastomas, and a ganglioneuroblastoma (Sandler *et al.*, 1968; Papanicolau *et al.*, 1975). In the one patient studied by Jaffe and Condon (1976), the plasma PGE level was normal, but the PGF level was elevated.

9.1.1.5 *Other endocrine tumours*

Sandler *et al.* (1968) found PGE_2 and $PGF_{2\alpha}$ in a pancreatic α-cell tumour but not in a β-cell tumour. Jaffe and Condon (1976) studied patients with various diseases. They found raised blood prostaglandin levels in some patients with Verner–Morrison syndrome (watery diarrhoea, hypokalaemia and hypochlorhydria) due to non-β islet-cell tumours, adrenal tumours, islet cell hyperplasias, or histologically undiagnosed causes. Many of these patients had elevated concentrations of vasoactive intestinal peptide in the blood, and some had elevated levels of PGE. Only two of 29 patients with the Zollinger–Ellison syndrome had significantly increased plasma PGE levels. Blood prostaglandins were not generally elevated in the various non-endocrine diarrhoeas they studied, and this reinforces the suggestion of Williams *et al.* (1968) that high peripheral blood prostaglandins do not arise as a result of the diarrhoea.

Some lung tumours secrete amines, and lung cancers were discussed together with other amine-peptide secreting tumours by Sandler *et al.* (1968), but these are presented later under 'non-endocrine' tumours.

9.2 HUMAN NON-ENDOCRINE TUMOURS

9.2.1 Tumours removed post-mortem

These are discussed because historically they include the first tumours to be extracted for prostaglandins, but obviously the relevance of the data must be in some doubt. Williams *et al.* (1968) found prostaglandins in an extract of oesophageal carcinoma, but did not detect prostaglandins in extracts of a malignant melanoma, a prostatic cancer or a gastric cancer. Brereton *et al.* (1974) studied metastases from a renal cell adenocarcinoma. Amounts of PGE and PGF extracted from liver metastases were several times greater than from normal liver, whereas amounts from lung metastases were about half those from normal lung.

Drut and Cusminsky (1975) reported that PGE_1 and PGE_2 were present in an extract of one human renal tumour, but no prostaglandin was found in a case of renal clear-cell carcinoma. Robertson *et al.* (1975) extracted liver metastases from a renal cell carcinoma. The amounts of PGE, PGF and PGA were substantially higher than from normal liver. Robertson *et al.* (1976) found elevated amounts of PGE in extracts of liver metastases from hypercalcaemic patients with various cancers.

9.2.2 Human tumours removed at operation

9.2.2.1 *Kaposi's sarcoma*

Bhana *et al.* (1968) extracted PGE and PGF from this sarcoma and found that the tumour metabolized exogenous arachidonic acid to PGE and PGF compounds.

9.2.2.2 *Colonic carcinoma*

Jaffe *et al.* (1971, 1972) found that human colonic malignant cells in organ culture produced substantially more PGE than did normal mucosa from the same specimen. Bennett *et al.* (1977b) extracted prostaglandins from tumours homogenized in an acid–ethanol solution to indicate 'basal' amounts of prostaglandin, and in an aqueous solution to indicate ability to synthesize prostaglandin. In almost all of the cancers the 'basal' prostaglandin was higher than in normal mucosa from the same specimen, and in most cases the synthetic capacity of cancers was higher. No statistically significant relationships were found between prostaglandins and tumour type, size, location, stage, degree of differentiation, mucin production, cellular infiltration, amount of fibrous tissue, numbers of involved regional lymph nodes or the degree of sinus histiocytosis in the lymph nodes.

9.2.2.3 *Kidney carcinoma*

Zusman *et al.* (1974) extracted PGA, PGE and PGF from a renal cell carcinoma. Atkins *et al.* (1977) obtained PGE release from fragments of human renal cortical carcinoma in culture; the amount was increased by the phosphodiesterase inhibitor theophylline and reduced by the cyclo-oxygenase inhibitor indomethacin.

9.2.2.4 *Breast carcinoma*

Bennett *et al.* (1975, 1976, 1977a) showed that homogenates of malignant breast tumours contained more prostaglandins than did those of benign tumours or normal tissue. Furthermore, those patients whose malignant tumours produced most prostaglandin had the highest incidence of bone metastases at the time of surgery as indicated by skeletal scintigraphy. This may be related to the potent ability of some prostaglandins to resorb bone (see Section 9.12). 'Basal' amounts of prostaglandin tended to be highest in tumours showing histological evidence of spread from the primary tumour. Thin layer chromatography indicated the presence of various prostaglandins and suggested an association between tumour PGF production and bone metastases. More recent data (Bennett *et al.*, 1979a) show that those patients whose excised tumours can produce most prostaglandin die soonest of cancer following surgical removal of the tumour.

Dowsett *et al.* (1976a), Robinson (1976) and Easty *et al.* (1977) reported that incubated slices of breast cancer release substantially more PGE and PGF than does normal breast tissue. However, Dowsett *et al.* (1976b) and Robinson (1976) also found that incubated benign breast tumours (fibroadenomas) released large amounts of PGE and PGF, whereas Bennett *et al.* (1975, 1976, 1977a) obtained only low amounts from homogenized benign tumours. The explanation is probably the difference in methodology. Further experiments have shown that fibroadenomas yielded low amounts of prostaglandins when homogenized in aqueous solution but high amounts when slices were incubated. Malignant tumours yielded large amounts with either method (A. Bennett, M. Harris, D. J. F. Rowe, I. F. Stamford and J. E. Wright, unpublished). Perhaps the difference was due to metabolism of prostaglandins released during homogenization of benign tumours but not of malignant tumours; the supernatant from homogenized normal rabbit lung or kidney metabolized PGE_2 whereas that from a VX2 tumour did not (Seyberth *et al.*, 1977). Greaves (1978) reported that homogenates of malignant breast tumours and, to a lesser extent, benign tumours contained substantial amounts of PGE and some PGF. However, he did not wash the tissue after cutting it finely prior to homogenization so that the procedure is to some extent a combination of incubation and homogenization. Bockman and Laird Myers (1977) also demonstrated the release of PGE from incubated slices of breast cancer, but using a bone assay Jenkins *et al.* (1976) considered that only a few malignant and benign breast lesions released prostaglandins. When bone is incubated with breast tumour, resorption usually takes place due, in part, to prostaglandin released by the tumour (Dowsett *et al.*, 1976a). Jenkins *et al.* (1976) did not incubate the tumour directly with bone. Instead, they first cultured it for 2 days, diluted the culture medium and then incubated this with bone. With the small amount of tissue they used, and the inactivation of released prostaglandin during culture, they would have needed a very high release of prostaglandin (many μg PGE_2/g tissue) to obtain bone resorption. Thus their failure to detect prostaglandin release by every tumour is not surprising.

9.2.2.5 *Lung carcinoma*

Sandler *et al.* (1968) found PGE_2 and $PGF_{2\alpha}$ in extracts of bronchial carcinomas. We have extracted prostaglandins from lung tumours, but in some cases the amount was less than from the normal region of the lung. Thin-layer chromatography has indicated that several prostaglandins are present (A. Bennett, M. A. Carroll and I. F. Stamford, unpublished).

9.2.2.6 *Head and neck carcinoma*

We have extracted 42 squamous carcinomas which mostly arose in the tongue, floor of the mouth, or larynx. Following radiotherapy and chemotherapy in an attempt to destroy the malignant cells, the residual tumours were excised and homogenized. The amounts of extracted prostaglandins correlated with the degree of inflammation and the amounts of granulation and fibrous tissue (A. Bennett, R. L. Carter and B. Tanner, unpublished).

9.2.2.7 *Pancreatic carcinoma*

Sandler *et al.* (1968) found PGE_2 in an extract of a pancreatic exocrine tumour.

9.2.2.8 *Uterine carcinoma*

The amounts of PGE_2 and $PGF_{2\alpha}$ extracted from endometrial carcinoma were several times higher than amounts obtained from healthy women during the proliferative phase of the menstrual cycle (Willman *et al.*, 1976).

9.3 HUMAN CELLS IN CULTURE

Jaffe *et al.* (1971, 1972), studied various human neoplastic and normal tissues maintained in organ or cell culture for up to 1 year. They found release of PGE, but not its 15-keto-metabolite, into the medium, with highest amounts from epithelial neoplasms (colon carcinomas, carcinoid, oesophageal and duodenal carcinomas, medullary and papillary carcinomas of the thyroid, and an insulinoma). Lower amounts were found in cultures of a lymphosarcoma, a liposarcoma, and four fibroblast lines. One colon tumour released eight times the amount of prostaglandin more than did normal epithelium from the same colon; addition of dibutyryl cAMP appeared to decrease prostaglandin release by about one-third. They thought that prostaglandin production was not related only to the rate of cell division, since L cells (see Section 9.4), fibroblasts and sarcomas were dividing at least as rapidly as some of the sarcomas.

HeLa cells (human cervical cancer cells) in culture did not yield detected amounts of prostaglandin in the studies of Levine *et al.* (1972) or Tashjian *et al.* (1972), but did so in the experiments of Thomas *et al.* (1974a, 1974b), and of Cohen and Jaffe (1973) who found in addition that HeLa cells and HEp-2 cells converted added arachidonic acid into PGE_2 and some $PGF_{2\alpha}$. Thomas *et al.* (1974a) found also that HT-29 cells derived from a human adenocarcinoma produced PGE. The amounts released by the HT-29 cells, which had a rapid doubling time, were small compared with HeLa, HEp-2 and L cells. Dibutyryl cAMP 1 mM inhibited proliferation and increased PGE production, whereas 10 nM indomethacin had the reverse effect.

Cells aspirated from the bone marrow of patients with myeloma produced bone-resorbing material thought to be osteoclast activating factor, but no PGE was detected (Mundy *et al.*, 1974).

9.4 RELEASE OF PROSTAGLANDINS INTO THE BLOOD STREAM FROM HUMAN NON-ENDOCRINE TUMOURS

Those experiments in which prostaglandin levels in blood draining the tumour are higher than in peripheral blood, suggest that the tumour is the source of the prostaglandin. However, it could be that the tumour releases material which stimulates prostaglandin release from other sites, or sensitizes the blood cells so that they more readily form prostaglandins during sampling or processing the blood sample. In experiments where peripheral blood levels were measured it can only be presumed that raised amounts were due to prostaglandin release by the tumour.

Bhana *et al.* (1968) found no evidence for prostaglandin release into the blood draining a Kaposi's sarcoma, although peripheral blood levels may have been elevated in some cases.

No PGE or PGF (less than 100 pg/ml) was detected in blood from the right atrium of a patient with liver and lung metastases from a previously resected renal cell adenocarcinoma (Brereton *et al.*, 1974). However, Zusman *et al.* (1974) found elevated levels of PGA, but not PGE or PGF, in the plasma of a patient with a renal tumour; following tumour excision the level of PGA fell. Unfortunately, they did not give the details of sampling and extraction. Cummings *et al.* (1975) reported higher amounts of PGE and PGA in renal venous blood than in peripheral venous blood from a patient prior to surgery for a renal tumour. Dindogru *et al.* (1975) studied one patient with a renal cell carcinoma and bone metastases, and four with multiple myeloma. They stated that serum prostaglandin levels in two unspecified patients were not elevated, but no other details were given.

Benvenisti and Goldberg (1975) extracted PGE and PGF from the plasma of a patient with a squamous cell lung carcinoma, but they too did not say how the plasma was obtained or the measurements made.

PGE was measured in the peripheral plasma from 79 patients with various solid malignant tumours (Demers *et al.*, 1977). Hypercalcaemia was present in 14 patients, and 11 of these had elevated amounts of plasma PGE (greater than 100 pg/ml). Four out of 21 normocalcaemic cancer patients with bone metastases also had PGE levels greater than 100 pg/ml. In patients with various types of cancer, Robertson *et al.* (1976) found elevated PGE levels in the peripheral blood of four out of 11 hypercalcaemic cases and one out of 10 who were normocalcaemic. Bockman and Laird Myers (1977) found raised amounts of PGE in the serum of some patients with breast cancer.

Mortel *et al.* (1977) studied patients with endometrial adenocarcinomas or cervical squamous cell carcinomas. During surgery they withdrew blood from the internal iliac artery and vein, prior to clamping the uterine vessels. They reported no significant arterio-venous difference in prostaglandin levels, and they claimed that no significant difference occurred between the blood prostaglandin levels in these patients and five controls undergoing surgery for non-malignant gynaecological disease. However, since the blood was collected from the internal iliac vein, much of it must have come from non-uterine sources. Although there was clearly no consistent arterio-venous difference in patients with squamous cell carcinomas, the venous prostaglandin level was higher in three of the four patients with endometrial adenocarcinoma, and equal to the arterial level in the remaining patient. Another criticism is their use of a parametric statistical test on data that are not normally distributed. The Mann–Whitney U-test shows significantly higher venous prostaglandin levels in the patients with malignant disease compared with benign disease ($p = 0.0174$), whereas the arterial prostaglandin levels were similar in both groups ($p = 0.46$). Thus these tumours may release prostaglandin into the blood. The amounts may be small since only one of the values was above their normal range of 100 pg/ml, but this could be due to dilution with blood from non-uterine sources.

Powles *et al.* (1977) found elevated amounts of the 13,14-dihydro-15-keto-PGE_2 metabolite in the plasma of some patients with breast cancer, and at operation we found significantly higher prostaglandin levels in blood draining breast tumours compared with peripheral blood (A. Bennett, J. MacIntyre and I. F. Stamford, unpublished). Seyberth *et al.* (1975) had previously reported elevated levels of PGE_2 metabolite in the urine of patients with various solid tumours and hypercalcaemia. Slightly elevated levels occurred in the urine of normocalcaemic patients with solid tumours. This data does not identify the source of the prostaglandins, but presumably at least some originated in the primary tumours.

9.5 PROSTAGLANDINS EXTRACTED FROM ANIMAL CANCERS OR TRANSFORMED CELLS, OR RELEASED DURING CULTURE

Numerous animal cancers have now been studied with respect to prostaglandin 'content' and synthesis, so that not all references will be given. Those tumours that have been most extensively studied are dealt with first.

Mouse HSMD fibrosarcoma cells in culture produce PGE_2, whereas control cell lines including mouse fibroblasts do not; this PGE_2 production is inhibited by indomethacin, aspirin, eicosatetraynoic acid, or hydrocortisone (Levine *et al.*, 1972; Tashjian *et al.*, 1972, 1974, 1975). Methylcholanthrene-transformed mouse BALB/3T3 fibroblasts in culture release mostly PGE_2 with some $PGF_{2\alpha}$, but yield less in the presence of indomethacin (Howell *et al.*, 1976; Pong *et al.*, 1976; Pong *et al.*, 1977; Tam *et al.*, 1977). The latter authors found that transformation of 3T3 mouse fibroblasts by methylcholanthrene, simian virus 40, polyoma virus, or spontaneous change, resulted in a higher PGE_2 production, whereas radiation-transformed cells produced about the same amount as untransformed cells. Microsomal prostaglandin synthetase activity from methylcholanthrene-transformed cells was higher than that from untransformed cells, but arachidonic acid release from both types was similar. The higher prostaglandin production was therefore considered to result from an increased prostaglandin synthetase activity. Lynch *et al.* (1978) found that a methylcholanthrene-induced fibrosarcoma from C3H mice produced substantial amounts of PGE_2.

The VX_2 carcinoma in rabbits produces mainly PGE_2 with a little PGD_2 and $PGF_{2\alpha}$ (identified by mass spectrometry) which seem to be partly involved in bone destruction by the tumour (Voelkel *et al.*, 1975; Galasko and Bennett, 1976 and unpublished; Seyberth *et al.*, 1977). Release of prostaglandins into the blood, and bone destruction, are discussed later (Sections 9.6 and 9.7.7).

There are numerous other examples of prostaglandin formation by tumours, many being the subject of only one publication. Some are discussed briefly below in chronological order.

Jaffe *et al.* (1971) obtained predominantly the release of PGE, but not of 15-keto-PGE, from a dog renal cell carcinoma in culture, and a lower release from L cells. They also measured PGE release from the human cell lines discussed in Section 9.3.

Levine *et al.* (1972) did not detect prostaglandin release from cultured murine neuroblastoma 41A3, rat C6 glioma or mouse adrenal AT10 cells.

Sykes and Maddox (1972) identified PGE_2 by mass spectrometry in extracts of mouse $BP8/P_1$ and mouse S180 tumours, but no $PGF_{2\alpha}$ was found. Indomethacin *in vivo* reduced tumour prostaglandin formation. Extracts of similar tumours from a different source were said to contain little or no prostaglandin, but details were not given. The $BP8/P_1$ ascites tumour cells in the presence of reduced glutathione and hydroquinone converted 10% of added arachidonic acid to PGE_2, but omission of either co-factor resulted in negligible conversion.

Apps and Cater (1973) found evidence of prostaglandin release from minced incubated mouse BP8 ascites tumours as well as from rat hepatoma 233 and various dog tumours.

Cohen and Jaffe (1973) obtained formation of PGE_2 from added arachidonic acid by disrupted L cells, but the amounts were small compared with those from the cultured HeLa cells discussed previously.

Hammarström *et al.* (1973) found a considerable increase in PGE_2 synthesis (identified by mass spectrometry) by baby-hamster kidney fibroblasts transformed by polyoma virus, compared with control cells.

Hamprecht *et al.* (1973) and Jaffe *et al.* (1973) obtained PGE release from three cultured cell lines (mouse N4 neuroblastoma, rat C6 glioma, and a mutant L cell line B82). The output of PGE was increased by dibutyryl cAMP and inversely related to the rate of cell growth. Formation of PGA and PGF was low.

Humes and Strausser (1974), Humes *et al.* (1974) and Strausser and Humes (1974) found that PGE, cAMP, and to a lesser extent PGF, were higher in mouse tumours induced by injection of Maloney sarcoma virus compared with tissue from the non-injected leg. Indomethacin reduced the amounts of prostaglandins but did not significantly affect the amounts of cAMP or cGMP.

Tan *et al.* (1974) reported that homogenates of dimethyl benzanthracene-induced rat mammary tumours and normal tissue contained mostly PGE_2, and sometimes PGF. The tumours were generally more active than normal tissue in converting labelled precursors into prostaglandins.

Strausser and Humes (1974) found that the PGE_2 content of tumours induced by Maloney sarcoma virus increased markedly as the tumour grew, and fell as the tumour spontaneously regressed. By contrast, the amount of prostaglandin extracted from Cloudman S91 melanomas was similar to that from control tissues.

Thomas *et al.* (1974a, 1974b) studied L cells in culture, and reported that PGE production was inversely related to growth rates. Addition of dibutyryl cAMP increased PGE output and inhibited replication.

Ritzi and Stylos (1976) found that production of PGE_2, and to some extent PGE_1 and $PGF_{2\alpha}$, by BALB/3T3 fibroblasts was increased by transformation with simian virus 40. In contrast, Ishikawa *et al.* (1976) obtained decreased prostaglandin production by SV40 transformed WI-38 cells, and attributed this to lower prostaglandin synthetase activity.

Santoro *et al.* (1976) showed that B-16 melanoma cells in culture synthesized PGE, and this was inhibited by indomethacin or hydrocortisone.

Burstein *et al.* (1977) showed that in the presence of added arachidonic acid epithelial cell cultures from spontaneous mammary tumours in C3H female mice yielded PGE and PGF, and the cAMP content increased. Since the effect on cAMP was inhibited by the prostaglandin synthesis inhibitor naproxen, a metabolite of arachidonic acid was presumably involved. However, the rise in cAMP was faster than that of prostaglandins, so that PGE_2 may not be the primary stimulant of cAMP formation.

Bennett *et al.* (1978, 1979b) extracted substantial amounts of prostaglandin from homogenates of mouse NC carcinoma, a syngeneic transplanted tumour originally arising spontaneously in mouse mammary gland, and Kibbey *et al.* (1978) found that four rat mammary carcinomas produced PGE_2.

Levine (1977) found that many chemical carcinogens stimulate MDCK cells from a normal dog kidney to produce PGE and PGF. In general, the most active carcinogens caused the highest output of prostaglandins. Benzo(a)pyrene was the most potent stimulant. These MDCK cells are particularly sensitive to several chemical carcinogens, aflatoxin B and epidermal growth factor, but fibroblasts from man (D-550) or mouse (3T3), or methylcholanthrene-transformed mouse fibroblasts (MC5-5) seem little affected (Ohuchi and Levine, 1978a). The latter authors observed that cycloheximide but not hydrocortisone inhibited the stimulation of prostaglandin synthesis and morphological change induced in MDCK cells by two phorbol esters; indomethacin inhibited only the prostaglandin synthesis (Ohuchi and Levine, 1978b).

9.6 RELEASE OF PROSTAGLANDINS INTO THE BLOOD STREAM FROM ANIMAL TUMOURS

Several studies have been made with the VX_2 tumour in rabbits. Voelkel *et al.* (1975) found that PGE_2 was released into the peripheral blood, with highest concentrations in the blood draining the tumour. Tashjian *et al.* (1977a, 1977b) and Voelkel *et al.* (1978) showed that the concentration of the metabolite 13,14-dihydro-15-keto-PGE_2 was raised in the peripheral blood. Seyberth *et al.* (1977), using mass spectrometry, found that the 13,14-dihydro-15-keto-PGE_2 levels in blood rose 25-fold by the end of the 2nd week after implantation with VX_2 carcinoma and rose 256-fold at the 4th week. The $PGF_{2\alpha}$ metabolite rose in parallel but to a lesser degree. The output of the major urinary PGE_2 metabolite was also elevated 2 weeks after tumour implantation and rose until the 5th week. Indomethacin treatment lowered the plasma levels of 13,14-dihydro-15-keto-PGE_2.

Raised PGE_2 metabolite levels also occurred in the plasma of mice carrying the SAI spindle cell sarcoma or the SaD2 fibrosarcoma, and continued to increase with time after transplantation (Levine, 1977). In the same study, normal plasma levels of PGE_2 metabolite occurred in mice carrying a transplantable anaplastic carcinoma (15091 AK), lymphatic leukaemia (AW5147), two mammary adenocarcinomas (CAD 1 and CAD 2), myeloid leukaemia (C1498), or a hepatoma (BW7756).

9.7 TUMOUR GROWTH

The involvement of prostaglandins in tumour growth is not clear, and some of the data appear contradictory. Inhibition of growth occurred in many cell culture studies with added PGE compounds, and also in many *in vivo* studies using drugs which inhibit prostaglandin synthesis. It has already been stressed that cancer comprises a heterogeneous group of diseases, and it would be surprising if differences in response did not occur. Although some of the contradictions may be more apparent than real, part of the answer may be the difference between *in vitro* and *in vivo* studies. Tumour growth *in vivo* is particularly complex and involves many events which may be influenced by prostaglandins.

9.7.1 Prostaglandins, cell proliferation and cyclic AMP

PGE compounds potently stimulate adenyl cyclase in many cells and so increase their cAMP content. In a review of this subject MacManus and whitfield (1974) wrote 'The field of endeavour concerning cyclic AMP, cell proliferation and cancer is very confusing to say the least . . . the use of high concentrations and indiscriminate use of analogues are probably the cause . . .'.

Furthermore, because of the difficulties of measuring cAMP it is probably better to measure adenyl cyclase activity. Some *in vitro* studies suggest that low intracellular amounts of cAMP are associated with the growth of malignant cells (Sheppard, 1971; Ryan and Heidrick, 1974; Pastan *et al.*, 1975), but there are many exceptions (Chlapowski *et al.*, 1975). Adenyl cyclase activity and/or the cAMP content of tumours may be low (Allen *et al.*, 1971; De Rubertis *et al.*, 1973), normal (Boyd *et al.*, 1974) or raised (Chayoth *et al.*, 1973; Humes *et al.*, 1974; Hunt *et al.*, 1978). Therefore most of what follows must be treated with caution. This discussion is presented firstly as evidence mainly favouring an inhibitory role of prostaglandins and then secondly some contradictory data are given.

Jaffe *et al.* (1971) considered that prostaglandin production was not related to the rate of cell division, since cells which produced low amounts of prostaglandin divided at least as fast as carcinomas which produced more prostaglandin. Later work from these authors, cited subsequently, shows an inverse relationship between cell division and prostaglandin production.

Johnson and Pastan (1971, 1972) slowed the growth of mouse 3T3 fibroblasts in culture by adding dibutyryl cAMP or PGE_1. Cellular cAMP was increased both by the addition of PGE_1 and when the cells reached confluency (Otten *et al.*, 1972). These authors, and many others, believe that cAMP mediates the contact inhibition of growth of various cell types. However, Sheppard (1972) did not find a rise in cAMP at cell confluency with 3T3 mouse fibroblasts or the lines transformed spontaneously (3T6) or virally (py3T3), although PGE_1, but not $PGF_{1\alpha}$, increased the cAMP content of these cells.

Hamprecht *et al.* (1973) studied N4TG3 (mutant of mouse neuroblastoma clone), C6-BU-1 (mutant of rat glioma) and B82 (mutant L-line) cells in culture. Dibutyryl cAMP retarded cell growth and increased the calculated output of PGE per cell; no release of PGA or PGF was detected.

Jaffe *et al.* (1973) found that at confluency of mouse N4 neuroblastoma cells the rate of PGE production abruptly and markedly increased. Dibutyryl cAMP 1 mM inhibited proliferation of three cell lines (N4 neuroblastoma, B82, and rat C6 glioma), and stimulated PGE production. Naseem and Hollander (1973) suppressed the growth of a murine plasma cell tumour (MPC-11) by 12–300 μM cAMP, 0.1–10 μg/ml PGE_1 or to a lesser extent by PGE_2; $PGF_{2\alpha}$ was virtually ineffective. Thomas *et al.* (1974a, 1974b) showed that the rates of cell proliferation of HEp-2, L, and HeLa cells were inversely related to PGE production. Dibutyryl cAMP 1 mM increased PGE production and inhibited cell replication, whereas indomethacin inhibited PGE production and stimulated proliferation.

Sonis *et al.* (1977) found that methylcholanthrene-induced mouse fibrosarcoma cells in culture released PGE which, when added to cultures of mouse EL-4 lymphoma cells, inhibited their growth. PGE_2 1–100 μg/ml similarly inhibited proliferation as shown by a reduced incorporation of thymidine.

With mouse B-16 melanoma PGE_1 1 μg/ml inhibited cell replication by cells in culture, and *in vivo*, 16,16-dimethyl-PGE_2 methyl ester 5 μg injected subcutaneously at the site of tumour cell injection reduced tumour growth (Santoro *et al.*, 1976). Previously, Stein-Werblowsky (1974a) studied a cell suspension of a chemically-induced tumour made up in very high concentrations (1 mg/ml, presumably +10% ethanol) of PGA_2, PGE_2 or $PGF_{2\alpha}$. She found that addition of a prostaglandin, especially PGA_2, resulted in small or absent tumours compared with controls given tumours suspended in vehicle. At 6 days, histological examination of the controls showed proliferating tumour cells surrounded by only a few lymphocytes and immunoblasts. In mice also given prostaglandin, there were large numbers of immunoblasts traversing the capillary walls to migrate towards the tumour, and few morphologically intact tumour cells were seen. This was interpreted as inhibition of implantation. However, tumours injected in prostaglandin grew at sites of 'immunological privilege', i.e. in striated muscle or in neonatal subcutaneous tissue. Concentrations of prostaglandin less than 1 mg/ml were ineffective, and this diminishes the interest of the work, although the prostaglandin was administered only at the time of injecting the tumour cells. Perhaps the prostaglandin altered the responsiveness to white cells, possibly by a detergent action. This work has formed part of the evidence for Stein-Werblowsky's theory (1974b) that tumours secrete a prostaglandin antagonist.

Somewhat in contrast, Abraham and Rao (1976) found that feeding mice with corn oil (which contains linoleate, an essential fatty acid needed for arachidonate synthesis) caused a 3–4 times increase in the weight of mammary adenocarcinomas which developed after transplantation of hyperplastic alveolar nodules. Hydrogenated oils did not have this effect. Since eicosatetraynoic acid, an inhibitor of cyclo-oxygenase and lipoxygenase, reduced tumour growth regardless of diet, Abraham and Rao thought that prostaglandin synthesis may be important for tumour growth, but the absence of effect in their preliminary experiments referred to in Section 9.7.5 argue against this view.

Although tumours induced in mice by Maloney sarcoma virus produce prostaglandins, including PGE_2, administration of indomethacin did not affect the cAMP or cGMP contents (Humes *et al.*, 1974). A reduction of cAMP production would be expected if its stimulation involved mainly PGE_2, but indomethacin alters the production of other prostaglandins and of substances formed by the lipoxygenase pathway, and it can also inhibit phosphodiesterase (Kuehl *et al.*, 1974).

MacManus and Whitfield (1974) showed that PGE_1 or PGA_1, but not $PGF_{1\alpha}$ or $PGF_{2\alpha}$, increase cell proliferation and the amount of intracellular cAMP. They concluded that an increase in cAMP occurs in thymic lymphocytes or rat liver as the cells enter a cell cycle. The authors also pointed out that when the extracellular calcium concentration was raised from 0.5 to 1 mM, PGE_1 could still increase cAMP levels and initiate DNA synthesis, but the cells did not enter mitosis.

Human 1321N1 astrocytoma cells in culture showed a marked increase in cAMP content with 30 nM–10 μM PGE_1, but there was no change in growth rate. Low concentrations of PGE_1 (3–100 nM) reduced the responsiveness of the cells even to concentrations of PGE_1 that normally caused maximal accumulation of cAMP. This effect seemed to be due to a selective desensitization of PGE_1-activated adenyl cyclase (Leichtling *et al.*, 1976).

$PGF_{2\alpha}$ 10–400 ng/ml added to mouse quiescent 3T3 fibroblasts in culture initiated DNA synthesis and cell proliferation in a small proportion of cells. This was associated with an increase in cellular cGMP and a small fall in cAMP. The effect with PGE_1 (0.2–0.4 μg/ml) was less than 10% that with $PGF_{2\alpha}$, and PGB_1 was ineffective. However, with SV40-transformed 3T3 fibroblasts $PGF_{2\alpha}$ 100 ng/ml did not increase the number of cells (de Asua *et al.*, 1975). PGE_2 and $PGF_{2\alpha}$ can enhance carcinogenesis in methylcholanthrene-induced murine skin tumours, possibly by stimulating DNA, RNA and protein synthesis (Lupulescu, 1977).

Lynch *et al.* (1978) cite unpublished work that PGE_2 1.5 μg intraperitoneally each day *in vivo* lessened the antitumour effect of indomethacin on a (presumably) mouse methylcholanthrene-induced fibrosarcoma.

9.7.2 Cell morphology and differentiation

This picture too is confused as shown by just three examples. Prasad (1972) found that PGE_1 or PGE_2, but not $PGF_{2\alpha}$, induced irreversible morphological differentiation of mouse neuroblastoma cells in culture, as shown by axon formation. Cells treated with PGE_1 also showed greater adhesion to the glass surface. Studies with actinomycin D and cycloheximide suggested that PGE_1-induced axon formation required synthesis of new protein but not of new RNA. Schwannona cells in culture treated with cAMP analogues or PGE_1 undergo shape changes, but the meaning of this is not clear (Sheppard *et al.*, 1975). In contrast, however, PGE_1 3 nM–3 μM added to human 1321N1 astrocytoma cells in culture had no effect on the morphology (Leichtling *et al.*, 1976).

9.7.3 Stimulation of tumour cell replication in culture by inhibitors of prostaglandin synthesis

Thomas *et al.* (1974a) found that indomethacin 0.1–100 nM increased the replication of HEp-2, L and HeLa cells; the effect was reversed by adding PGE_1 1 μg/ml to the culture. However, a higher concentration of indomethacin (1 μM) did not significantly alter growth and surprisingly had less effect than the lower concentrations on PGE accumulation.

Santoro *et al* (1976) enhanced the growth of mouse B-16 melanoma *in vitro* with indomethacin or hydrocortisone. Replication of methylcholanthrene-induced fibrosarcoma cells from C3H mice were not significantly affected by 0.1 μg/ml indomethacin, but the high concentration of 20 μg/ml caused a 2.5-fold increase in thymidine uptake (Lynch *et al.*, 1978).

9.7.4 Inhibition of cell replication in culture by inhibitors of prostaglandin synthesis

Hial *et al.* (1977) studied the proliferation of rat hepatoma and human fibroblasts in culture. They said that indomethacin, aspirin or sodium salicylate reversibly inhibited growth of both cell lines but only data on rat hepatoma cells are presented. They point out the high concentrations needed to cause a reduction in growth (zero effect at 1–10 μM indomethacin, but approximately 20% inhibition with 0.1 mM, and 80% inhibition with 0.5 mM). The amounts are higher than those needed to inhibit prostaglandin synthesis but are within the blood concentrations reached with therapeutic doses. These drugs and meclofenamate, salicylamide, phenylbutazone and phenacetin also inhibited protein and nucleic acid synthesis, except for low concentrations of the salicylates which caused a stimulation.

9.7.5 Lack of effect on tumour growth *in vitro* by inhibitors of prostaglandin synthesis

Sykes and Maddox (1972) stated that indomethacin 5 mg/kg intraperitoneally each day in mice reduced the weight of $BP8/P_1$ tumours, but the effect was not statistically significant. No further details were given except that PGE_2 formation by the tumour was reduced by 66%. Perhaps this is not sufficient to achieve an effect on tumour growth. Powles *et al.* (1973) injected rats with Walker carcinosarcoma cells intra-aortically, and gave the animals a mixture of aspirin and indomethacin daily. There was no significant difference from controls in the amount of soft tissue tumour 2 weeks after inoculation with tumour cells, but bone destruction was prevented or greatly reduced. The experiments by Galasko and Bennett (1976) yielded somewhat similar results. In rabbits injected with VX_2 tumour cells into a thigh muscle or tibia, and given indomethacin 7.5 mg/kg by mouth daily, there was a non-significant tendency for an increase in the number of pulmonary metastases, but bone destruction was greatly reduced. Since the development of metastases depends on many factors such as the movement of cells out of the blood stream or lymphatics, and their ability to survive and flourish, these experiments may not measure only tumour growth.

Abraham and Rao (1976) cite their unpublished preliminary data that in mice fed 15% corn oil (containing linoleate which is an essential fatty acid needed for arachidonate synthesis) aspirin 0.4 mg/g diet did not retard the growth of adenocarcinomas.

9.7.6 Reduction of tumour growth *in vivo* by inhibitors of prostaglandin synthesis

Several groups have shown reduction of tumour growth by non-steroidal inhibitors of prostaglandin synthesis *in vivo* but all the studies are in mice.

Tashjian *et al.* (1973) studied the $HSDM_1$ fibrosarcoma in mice given 100–125 μg indomethacin daily in their normal diet. There was a highly significant reduction of 27% in tumour weight in the treated group, even though indomethacin *in vitro* had no significant effect on the growth of cultured $HSDM_1$ cells (Levine *et al.*, 1972).

Using BALB/c mice inoculated with Maloney sarcoma virus, Humes *et al.* (1974) found that indomethacin 50 μg subcutaneously on alternate days delayed the onset of the tumour growth and approximately halved the eventual size. They considered that this was due to the reduction of inflammation which was observed histologically in indomethacin-treated mice.

Treatment of mice with antilymphocyte serum at the time of virus injection accelerated and enhanced tumour growth. Indomethacin was still able to suppress tumour growth, but less so than in mice not given the antilymphocyte serum. Thus, even though the immune system may be important for tumour regression, some of the action of indomethacin may be through a different mechanism.

In the experiments reported by Strausser and Humes (1975) indomethacin 50 μg subcutaneously on alternate days completely suppressed the growth of mouse tumours induced by Maloney sarcoma virus. They commented on the greater effect in this experiment using 6-week-old mice compared with the results of Humes *et al.* (1974) in which the mice were 20 days old at the time of virus injection. However, they did not comment on the use of another mouse strain (male DBA/1J mice in addition to the male BALB/cJ strain used by Humes *et al.*, 1974). Strausser and Humes (1975) also reported that indomethacin inhibited bone destruction by the virus-induced tumour.

Plescia *et al.* (1975) measured the growth of a transplanted methylcholanthrene-induced mouse fibrosarcoma (MC-16), and gave the mice indomethacin 125 μg/day intraperitoneally for the first 10 or 14 days. The tumours from the indomethacin-treated mice were consistently smaller by approximately 50%. These authors suggested that indomethacin acted by removing a prostaglandin-induced inhibition of the immune system (see Section 9.8). Indomethacin might therefore prevent the development of strongly antigenic tumours, and retard the development of weakly antigenic tumours. Hial *et al.* (1976) treated mice bearing a transplanted mast-cell ascites tumour (P185) or Lewis lung carcinoma with aspirin 150 mg/kg twice daily by mouth for several days. The growth of both tumours was substantially inhibited. Indomethacin 3 or 5 mg/kg substantially inhibited the ascites tumour growth; with the higher dose no tumour growth was observed in half the animals, but signs of drug toxicity appeared. Aspirin treatment reduced the number of cells and appeared to alter the rate of appearance of the tumour, but it did not alter the size or number of ascites cells per unit volume of tumour.

When drug treatment was begun 24 hours after implantation of ascites tumour, indomethacin 5 mg/kg twice daily, but not aspirin, decreased the growth; no tumour was found in 22% of the indomethacin-treated mice. The aspirin was prepared every 3 days as an aqueous suspension, and stored at 4 °C, so that a substantial amount may have been hydrolysed.

Several reports have appeared regarding the NC carcinoma in WHT/Ht mice. This tumour originally arose spontaneously in a mouse mammary gland and has been transplanted subcutaneously in the same strain. The prostaglandin synthesis inhibitor flurbiprofen given orally once or twice a day in raspberry syrup (total daily dosage 5 mg/kg) reduced tumour growth by about 50% over several weeks (Bennett *et al.*, 1978, 1979b; Leaper *et al.*, 1978a, 1978b). Since the tumour seems to have low immunogenicity (Hewitt, 1976), the main effect of flurbiprofen may not involve the immune system. However, the histology of tumours from flurbiprofen-treated mice was similar to controls except that lymphocytic infiltration in and around tumours from treated mice tended to be greater. These findings do not explain the reduction of tumour growth by flurbiprofen, although the drug might enhance a host immunological response (D. J. Leaper, B. French and A. Bennett, unpublished).

In a paper packed with information, Lynch *et al.* (1978) studied the growth of a methylcholanthrene-induced fibrosarcoma of C3H mice transplanted subcutaneously. In their first experiment they added indomethacin 20 μg/ml to the drinking water so that each mouse received 80–120 μg daily, or they gave indomethacin 50 or 100 μg intraperitoneally. Other animals received either aspirin 1 mg/ml in the drinking water, the phosphodiesterase inhibitor theophylline orally, or hydrocortisone. Indomethacin or aspirin in the drinking water from day 7 to 49 after tumour transplantation reduced the mean tumour diameters at day 46 by 51% and 42% respectively; the reductions of 24% and 21% with hydrocortisone and theophylline respectively were not statistically significant. Indomethacin was effective despite the absence of inhibition in cell culture described in Section 9.7.3. As discussed later, indomethacin, aspirin or hydrocortisone increased survival time. The reduction of tumour growth was presumably underestimated since they measured tumour diameters when the majority of the controls had died. Since many controls died earlier, it seems that some measurements were made on tumours that had less time to grow. In their second experiment with indomethacin in the drinking water, the reduction of tumour growth was even more striking, and the initial growth was followed by complete and lasting tumour regression in most animals. In this experiment there was no effect with theophylline 40 μg injected intraperitoneally twice weekly, or with heparin. The authors cite work of Lynch and Salamon (in press) that indomethacin exerts little effect on tumour growth until the tumours reach diameters of about 1 cm, and they cite unpublished work that 1.5 μg PGE_2 intraperitoneally each day significantly reduces the antitumour effect of indomethacin. Intramuscularly implanted tumour destroyed the tibia, but this was diminished by orally administered indomethacin. Lynch *et al.* (1978)

considered that the reduction of tumour size with indomethacin was not due to a restoration of a depressed immune system (see Section 9.9).

Prednisolone 2–32 mg/kg in Wistar rats decreased the survival of Yoshida ascites sarcoma cells which were sensitive to alkylating agents. The effect on cells resistant to alkylating agents was less (Harrap *et al.*, 1977).

With regard to human cancer, Stoll (1973) reported that a woman with metastatic breast cancer showed regression of secondary skin nodules when she was treated with indomethacin.

The findings that PGE compounds *in vitro* usually inhibit cell proliferation, and indomethacin sometimes stimulates proliferation, seem to conflict with the reduction of tumour growth with prostaglandin synthesis inhibitors *in vivo*. However, non-steroidal inhibitors of prostaglandin synthesis reduce not only the synthesis of PGE compounds, but also the formation of all prostanoids resulting from the action of cyclo-oxygenase on prostaglandin precursor fatty acids. In addition, the inhibitors divert released precursors into metabolism by lipoxygenase. The corticosteroids also block the formation of prostanoids and of products resulting from the action of lipoxygenase, since they inhibit the release of fatty acids precursors. Thus perhaps indomethacin and similar drugs are effective *in vivo* because they increase the formation of a lipoxygenase product which inhibits cell growth, or block the formation of a prostanoid which stimulates cell growth. This might be $PGF_{2\alpha}$ (de Asua *et al.*, 1975) or possibly endoperoxides, thromboxanes or prostacyclin. Administered PGE itself might alter endogenous prostaglandin metabolism. The finding that indomethacin sometimes stimulates proliferation in cultures of cancer cells, but has the reverse effect *in vivo*, may mean that prostaglandin formation by host cells in the tumour is important.

9.7.7 The role of prostaglandins in destruction of bone by tumours, and in the formation of skeletal metastases

This section, which was the subject of a *Lancet* leading article (1976), relates to the previous section (9.7.6) on reduction of tumour growth by inhibitors of prostaglandin synthesis. However, it is dealt with separately because of its special nature. Several human and animal tumours cause bone destruction. Those in man may arise in the bone or, more commonly, are metastases from a variety of primary tumours such as those in the lung or breast. Hypercalcaemia in the absence of demonstrated bone destruction will be discussed in Section 9.12.

PGE_1 and PGE_2 were first shown to be potent bone-resorbing agents by Klein and Raisz (1970). Several groups have confirmed this observation and shown that some other prostaglandins and their metabolites are potent bone resorbing agents (see Section 9.12) which act by stimulating osteoclasts. There is some dispute about potency of PGF compounds, but $PGF_{2\alpha}$ seems capable of causing bone resorption in man (Kuppe and Wetter, 1974). Recently prostacyclin has been shown to have potent bone-resorbing activity *in vitro* (Ali *et al.*, 1979).

Powles *et al.* (1973) showed that Walker carcinoma cells and some human breast tumours *in vitro* cause osteolysis which can be blocked by inhibitors of prostaglandin synthesis. They administered 30 mg aspirin and 0.1 mg indomethacin daily to rats 3 days before injecting Walker tumour cells intra-aortically; after another 7 days the doses were doubled. All the control animals had widespread tumour deposits in bone and many had hypercalcaemia. No bone deposits were detected in the treated animals, and there was no hypercalcaemia. In another experiment, delay of treatment with indomethacin until 7 days after inoculation with tumour cells still prevented the appearance of destructive bone deposits, although malignant cells enter the bone and grow when drug treatment is stopped (T. J. Powles, personal communication).

Strausser and Humes (1974) observed tibial pocking and sponginess in mice injected locally with Maloney sarcoma virus, and found that the effect paralleled the tumour prostaglandin content. Osteoclastic activity occurred on the side of the bone adjacent to the tumour, with extensive osteoblastic activity on the opposite side. These tumours show a normal regression, and when this happens the prostaglandin content diminishes and the bone changes disappear. Treatment with indomethacin 50 μg/mouse on alternate days prevented the bone damage.

Galasko and Bennett (1976) found markedly raised numbers of osteoclasts in rabbits injected with VX_2 tumour into a tibia. The number of osteoclasts was reduced by about 53% in rabbits given indomethacin 7.5 mg/kg daily in the drinking water, but were still substantially greater than normal. Radiographs indicated that indomethacin markedly reduced, but did not prevent, the bone destruction. These data provide evidence for the involvement of both prostaglandins and a non-prostaglandin osteoclast activating substance, possibly osteoclast activating factor (Horton *et al.*, 1972). However the production of osteoclast activating factor by human activated peripheral blood leukocytes seem to require prostaglandins (Yoneda and Mundy, 1979). Galasko (1976) showed that osteoclasts are involved in the initial stages of bone destruction by tumour, but they subsequently disappear despite continued destruction. Eilon and Mundy (1978) obtained direct resorption of bone by human breast cancer cells *in vitro*.

Galasko and Bennett (unpublished) have shown that the timing of indomethacin administration to rabbits with VX_2 tumour is important for the reduction of damage to bone. Doses of 4 mg/kg and above started prior to, or 1 week after, tumour implantation reduced osteoclast proliferation and bone destruction. Indomethacin 8 mg/kg did not significantly reduce osteoclast proliferation or bone destruction when it was started 2 or more weeks after tumour implantation.

In their study of a methylcholanthrene-induced C3H mouse fibrosarcoma, Lynch *et al.* (1978) showed that intramuscularly injected tumour cells caused hypercalcaemia and substantial destruction of the tibia, both of which were diminished by giving indomethacin.

Bennett *et al.* (1975, 1976, 1977a) found a relationship between the amount of prostaglandin extracted from homogenates of human breast carcinomas and the incidence of bone metastases as indicated by skeletal scanning near to the time of breast surgery. Those tumours which yielded most prostaglandin tended to be associated with bone metastases, and the association seemed even stronger when the data were expressed in terms of 'PGF'. Since PGE and PGF are largely inactivated in the pulmonary circulation, it seems unlikely that these prostaglandins released from breast tumours survive in sufficient amounts to affect the bone. However, some PGE metabolites are potent bone-resorbing agents, and prostacyclin survives passage through the pulmonary circulation. Another possibility is that tumour cells which become trapped in bone release prostaglandins and so cause bone resorption which allows a metastasis to develop. In addition, there tends to be a relationship between tumour 'basal' prostaglandin and the invasiveness as judged by the appearance of malignant cells in the blood vessels, lymphatics and lymph nodes. Thus higher amounts of tumour prostaglandins might result in more malignant cells entering the circulation, and this could contribute to, or explain, the increased incidence of bone metastases in patients whose tumours produce most prostaglandin. In a pilot study, 12 breast cancer patients with bone-scan evidence of bone metastases have been treated with the prostaglandin synthesis inhibitor flurbiprofen. The preliminary data seem to indicate that the drug slowed down the progression of the bone metastases (D. J. Leaper and A. Bennett, unpublished).

Powles *et al.* (1976) and Easty *et al.* (1977) found that the *in vitro* osteolytic activity of human malignant breast tumours correlated with the presence or subsequent development of bone metastases and hypercalcaemia. Aspirin usually reduced, but did not prevent, the *in vitro* osteolysis, indicating the presence of other bone-resorbing material. Dowsett *et al.* (1976a) found that incubated slices of breast carcinomas release PGE, PGF and non-dialysible–non-prostaglandin osteolytic material. Perhaps the material is osteoclast activating factor. None of the extracts for neutral lipids contained significant osteolytic activity. This excludes the participation of vitamin D metabolites, but some breast tumours contain osteolytic sterols (Gordan *et al.*, 1966; Day *et al.*, 1969). Dowsett *et al.* (1976a) also obtained evidence that the tumours produce material which stimulates bone to produce prostaglandins.

9.8 TUMOUR SPREAD TO NON-SKELETAL SITES

Cancer kills usually as a result of its spread to distant sites. Platelet aggregation may be important in the formation of metastases (see review by

Hilgard and Thornes, 1976), and reduction of aggregation may be a mechanism by which inhibitors of prostaglandin synthesis exert their effects. However, this is disputed (Wood, 1972; Powles *et al.*, 1973). As with the inhibition of tumour growth by non-steroidal prostaglandin synthesis inhibitors (Section 9.7.6), experiments showing reduction of metastatic spread are all in mice. Kolenich *et al.* (1972) injected the adenocarcinoma BW10232 subcutaneously in C57B1/6Jax mice. Aspirin 75 mg/kg daily administered at the time of implantation reduced the incidence of animals with pulmonary metastases at the time of death. Unfortunately, the authors did not say why the mice died. Gasic *et al.* (1972) injected mice with MCA2 ascites tumour cells or T241 tumour cells intravenously, or T241 cells into the muscle of a hind leg. Aspirin 0.625 mg/ml in the drinking water for 6–13 days starting 2 days before inoculation with tumour significantly reduced the formation of lung 'metastases' from the MCA2 tumour, and from the T241 tumour given intramuscularly. In their subsequent full paper the authors say that MCA6 ascites tumour was used, but gave the results previously obtained with MCA2 tumour. They found in addition that aspirin prevented the formation of lung metastases in mice bearing a transplanted mammary tumour. This occurred even though treatment with aspirin was stopped at least 35 days before the animals were killed, and there was no reduction of primary tumour growth. The prevention of lung metastases was not accompanied by appearance of metastases elsewhere. This fascinating paper showed that thrombocytopenia reduced the number of metastases produced by a wide variety of murine tumours, particularly those capable of aggregating platelets.

Pelus and Strausser (1976) performed experiments on C3H/HeJ mice bearing the syngeneic C3HBA adenocarcinoma. Indomethacin 75 μg intraperitoneally on alternate days, starting the day after inoculation with tumour, markedly decreased the incidence of metastasis to liver and stomach.

We have studied in WHT/Ht mice with transplanted NC carcinomas referred to in Section 9.7.6. This tumour metastasizes particularly to the lungs, mediastinum and viscera. In the work by Bennett *et al.* (1979b) the mice were given 5 mg/kg flurbiprofen orally each day starting the day before tumour transplantation. The primary tumours were excised with a narrow rim of tissue 3 weeks after transplantation. There was a tendency for a reduction in local recurrence but the difference was not statistically significant. However, when a distinction was made between scar recurrences and local satellite metastases the incidence and volume of satellite metastases was less but scar recurrences were unaffected (Leaper *et al.*, 1978b). When a wide excision was made around the tumour it was not possible to distinguish between satellite metastases and scar recurrences. In mice given chemotherapy (melphalan and methotrexate), additional treatment with flurbiprofen 2.5 mg twice daily reduced local recurrence (Berstock *et al.*, 1979). In two other experiments with different species, aspirin and/or indomethacin did not reduce tumour spread. Powles *et al.* (1973) found no difference in the soft tissue metastases in rats with Walker tumours given aspirin and indomethacin, and with regard to lung metastases Wood (1972) found a non-significant tendency for a decrease with aspirin in rabbits with VX_2 tumours, and Galasko and Bennett (1976) found a non-significant tendency for an increase with indomethacin. These data argue against a role of platelets in the formation of metastases.

In the human breast carcinomas the 'basal' amounts of prostaglandin extracted from tumour homogenates tended to correlate ($p = 0.052$) with the 'invasiveness' as judged histologically by the appearance of malignant cells in the blood vessels, lymphatics and lymph nodes (Bennett *et al.*, 1977a). Two of the tumours with no histological evidence of spread were from patients who had bone scans indicative of skeletal metastases. If there are included with tumours showing histological evidence of spread, the correlation between tumour 'basal' prostaglandin and invasiveness increases to $p = 0.019$. However, Kibbey *et al.* (1978) found that three non-metastasizing rat mammary tumours (MTWA, B, D) produced substantial amounts of PGE_2, whereas the metastasizing and rapidly growing SMT-2A tumour produced much less PGE_2. Unfortunately, the authors did not say how they extracted the prostaglandin, but the high values seem unlikely to represent 'basal' amounts. They also did not comment on the immunogenicity of their tumours (see Section 9.9), or the site to which the SMT-2A tumour metastasized.

9.9 TUMOUR IMMUNOLOGY

The importance of immunology with regard to cancer in man is a highly complex and controversial issue. The degree of immunogenicity will help determine the importance of immunological defence by the host against the tumour. Many cancers produced in animals, such as some induced by chemicals, are highly immunogenic. These might resemble chemically induced human carcinomas, for example some tumours in bladder and lung. Other cancers, such as in the breast, are presumably more 'spontaneous' in origin and possibly less immunogenic.

Tumours can produce material which depresses the immune system, and a substantial amount of evidence suggests that prostaglandins are involved. Plescia *et al.* (1975) showed that mice bearing tumours induced by chemicals or viruses became decreasingly responsive immunologically to sheep erythrocytes as the tumour grew. Addition of tumour cells to cultures of spleen cells and sheep erythrocytes caused suppression of the antibody response. The effect was inhibited by indomethacin or aspirin *in vitro*, and PGE_2 also caused immunosuppression. As reported in Section 9.7.6, aspirin and indomethacin reduced tumour growth *in vivo*.

Strausser and Humes (1975) found that growth of tumours induced in BALB/cJ mice by Maloney sarcoma virus was prevented by indomethacin. In mice given antilymphocyte serum the tumours grew larger; indomethacin inhibited the growth by only about one-third, presumably because of increased activity of the residual immune system and/or because of an unrelated mechanism.

Pelus and Strausser (1976) studied mice with a methylcholanthrene-induced fibrosarcoma (MC-16) or a syngeneic mammary adenocarcinoma. 'Spleen' cells showed a suppressed mitogenic responsiveness to phytohaemagglutinin, but indomethacin given to the animals or added to spleen cell cultures overcame the suppression.

The prostaglandin synthesis inhibitors may act on 'suppressor' cells. Webb and Osheroff (1976) showed that in mice injected with sheep erythrocytes, indomethacin *in vivo* increased the appearance of splenic cells which formed antibody against the erythrocytes. Similarly, indomethacin *in vitro* enhanced the immune response to sheep red blood cells. The drug also increased spleen DNA synthesis, but the effect was much less when the spleen cells were depleted of those cells (including mitogen-activated T-suppressor cells) which adhered to glass wool. They considered that prostaglandins play an important role in controlling interactions between T and B lymphocytes.

Lymphocytes from patients with Hodgkin's disease showed a depressed incorporation of thymidine and an increased output of PGE_2 in response to phytohaemagglutinin (Goodwin *et al.*, 1977). Addition of indomethacin restored thymidine incorporation to normal. A population of lymphocytes which adhered to glass wool was found to contain the suppressor cells responsible for the depressed response to phytohaemagglutinin.

Not all authors have thought that indomethacin reduces tumour growth by an action involving the immune system. Lynch and Salomon (1977) found no diminution of the serum IgG_1 and IgE titres against ovalbumin in tumour-bearing mice. In untreated mice with MeC3-1 tumours, Lynch *et al.* (1978) found no evidence of a generalized immunosuppression, but an enhanced response against sheep erythrocytes. They found the MeC3-1 tumour to be only weakly antigenic, and that animals whose tumours disappeared on treatment with indomethacin showed no immunity on re-administration of tumour. The authors drew attention to the possibility (Winchurch *et al.*, 1974) that aspirin and indomethacin inhibit lymphocyte-mediated cytotoxicity. Nevertheless, Lynch *et al.* believe that inhibition of prostaglandin synthesis is the basis of the reduction of tumour growth by indomethacin, partly because daily intraperitoneal injection of 1.5 μg PGE_2 inhibited the effect.

In contrast, Loose and DiLuzio (1973) produced evidence that PGE_1 stimulated the immune system. In mice injected intravenously with PGE_1, the formation of haemagglutinin to sheep erythrocytes was enhanced. The graft-versus-host reaction was greater in mice receiving spleen cells from PGE_1-treated mice. There did not seem to be alterations in the primary immune response or phagocytosis.

Harvey *et al.* (1977) found no relationship between blood PGE levels and the depression of immunological responsiveness of normocalcaemic patients with various malignancies as judged by various skin tests. However, they point out that this does not exclude a local action of prostaglandins.

9.10 EFFECT OF INHIBITORS OF PROSTAGLANDIN SYNTHESIS ON ANIMAL SURVIVAL TIME

Survival time is closely linked with tumour spread since it is usually metastatic growth that kills. Many factors are involved such as the release of malignant cells from the primary tumour, their entrance first into lymphatics or blood vessels and then into secondary sites at which they must survive, establish themselves and grow.

9.10.1 Absence of effect on survival

Strausser and Humes (1975) found that indomethacin reduced the growth of tumours induced by Maloney sarcoma virus in BALB/c male mice treated with antilymphocyte serum, but indomethacin did not alter survival time. Hial *et al.* (1976) studied the transplantable P815 ascites tumour line in CD_{f1} mice. Although twice daily administration of aspirin 150 mg/kg or indomethacin 3 or 5 mg/kg reduced tumour growth it did not alter survival time. The animals died with widespread bleeding into the abdominal cavity. Presumably this contributed to the death, but perhaps the ability to cause bleeding depends more on the length of contact than on the rate of tumour growth.

Wistar rats injected intraperitoneally on day 0 with a chemoresistant variant of Walker tumour died on day 9; those given indomethacin 7 mg/kg subcutaneously three times daily on days 0, 1 and 2 died on days 9 and 10. Rats given this dose of flurbiprofen died on days 9–13, but the increase in survival time was not statistically significant (Powles *et al.*, 1978). However, it should be stressed that the prostaglandin synthesis inhibitors were given for only 3 days, that the cause of death was not stated, and that perhaps the high dosages of indomethacin and flurbiprofen were themselves somewhat toxic.

Galasko and Bennett (1976) cite unpublished data that survival time in rabbits bearing VX_2 tumours was not significantly altered by 7.5 mg/kg indomethacin daily given in the drinking water.

9.10.2 Prolongation of survival

Bennett *et al.* (1978, 1979b) and Leaper *et al.* (1978a) administered flurbiprofen 5 mg/kg daily in raspberry syrup to mice, starting the day prior to inoculation with NC carcinoma. After 3 weeks the primary tumours were excised, and the survival of the mice measured. The flurbiprofen-treated group survived significantly longer than controls, but there was no significant effect when treatment with flurbiprofen was started at the time of tumour excision. The prolongation of survival with early drug administration may have been due to the reduction of primary tumour growth by flurbiprofen, although in untreated mice metastatic spread occurs within a few days of implantation. Survival in relation to the administration of conventional anticancer treatment is discussed in Section 9.11.

In their studies of C3H mice injected subcutaneously with a methylcholanthrene-induced MeC3-1 fibrosarcoma, Lynch *et al.* (1978) found that indomethacin 10 μg/ml or aspirin 1 mg/ml in the drinking water, or hydrocortisone 10 μg/ml + 200 μg subcutaneously twice a week, significantly prolonged survival. However, only indomethacin or aspirin reduced tumour growth. They cited the work of Schechter and Feldman (1977) and suggested that hydrocortisone may have acted by eliminating the precursors of suppressor cells. Survival time was not significantly affected by theophylline or heparin.

9.11 RESPONSE TO CONVENTIONAL CANCER THERAPY

Bennett *et al.* (1978, 1979b) and Leaper *et al.* (1978), in their experiments with subcutaneously injected mouse NC tumour, found that low doses of radiotherapy, or chemotherapy (melphalan + methotrexate) or flurbiprofen 5 mg/kg orally each day, started 25 *days* after tumour transplantation, had no significant effect on tumour size. However, in mice given combined treatment with flurbiprofen 5 mg/kg and radiotherapy the tumours were about half the size of controls. When the three treatments of radiotherapy, chemotherapy and flurbiprofen were given to each mouse, the tumours were about one-third the size of controls.

Berstock *et al.* (1979) used this NC tumour model and excised the primary tumours 10–24 days after implantation. The mice were then treated with chemotherapy (melphalan and methotrexate) and/or flurbiprofen 2.5 mg twice daily. Those mice receiving the combined treatment lived significantly longer than untreated mice or those receiving only one type of treatment. Aspirin and similar drugs can displace methotrexate from its binding sites on plasma proteins and this may contribute to the increased effect. However, this argument does not apply to the enhanced response to radiotherapy. In the gastro-intestinal tract prostaglandins protect against damage by a mechanism (cytoprotection, Robert, 1977) which is not totally understood. Perhaps inhibitors of prostaglandin synthesis remove a protection of malignant cells to damaging agents. Powles *et al.* (1978) injected rats intraperitoneally with Walker ascites tumour cells made resistant to chlorambucil. Administration of chlorambucil had no effect on survival, but flurbiprofen or indomethacin 7 mg/kg subcutaneously three times daily for 3 days starting at the time of inoculation with tumour frequently caused a dramatic increase of survival following a single dose of chlorambucil. Three patients with metastatic breast cancer responded better when flurbiprofen was administered with the chemotherapy, but no further details were given (Powles *et al.*, 1978)

When Wistar rats with Yoshida ascites tumour were treated with 10 mg/kg chlorambucil, the effectiveness was increased by administering prednisolone 10 mg/kg 4 h later. Similarly, the antitumour effect of prednimustine (a prednisolone ester of chlorambucil) was potentiated by a subsequent administration of prednisolone. The timing of the prednisolone dose seems to be important (Harrap *et al.*, 1977). However, in male BALB/c mice the Ehrlich ascites tumour, which is intrinsically resistant to alkylating agents, did not respond to large doses of chlorambucil and prednisolone given alone or together. Although phenylbutazone inhibits prostaglandin synthesis, the potentiation of the effect of chlorambucil on P388 tumours in mice was accompanied by an increase in toxicity. The phenybutazone appeared to act by displacing chlorambucil from plasma protein binding sites (Schiffman *et al.*, 1978).

Tamoxifen is an antioestrogen drug used in the treatment of human breast cancer. The drug is a relatively potent inhibitor of prostaglandin synthesis (Ritchie, 1977), and it is intriguing to think that this may contribute to its efficacy, including the relief of bone pain. Female sex hormones can themselves stimulate prostaglandin synthesis (El Attar, 1976).

It is also relevant to point out the work cited in Section 9.2.2.4 that the ability of human breast tumours to produce prostaglandin during homogenization correlates inversely with the patient survival time.

9.12 HYPERCALCAEMIA

Hypercalcaemia in malignant disease has been the subject of several reviews (e.g. Seyberth *et al.*, 1978) and will not be dealt with in depth here. The problem may be related to bone metastases, but this is by no means always the case. Various prostaglandins and their metabolites can resorb bone *in vitro* by stimulating osteoclast activity (Klein and Raisz, 1970; Tashjian *et al.*, 1972; Harris *et al.*, 1973; Dietrich *et al.*, 1975; Dowsett *et al.*, 1976; Raisz *et al.*, 1977; Tashjian *et al.*, 1977; Ali *et al.*, 1979). The latter authors showed that prostacyclin potently resorbs bone. PGE_2 is probably the most potent, but whereas some consider the PGF compounds to be much less active (e.g. Dietrich *et al.*, 1975) others do not agree (Dowsett *et al.*, 1976a; D. J. F. Rowe, M. Harris, N. N. Ali and A. Bennett, unpublished), and $PGF_{2\alpha}$ given intravenously in man can cause hypercalcaemia (Kuppe and Wetter, 1974).

Tashjian *et al.* (1972) showed that mouse $HSDM_1$ fibrosarcoma resorbed bone *in vitro* by releasing PGE_2, and caused hypercalcaemia *in vivo*. Voelkel *et al.* (1975) obtained similar results with the VX_2 carcinoma in rabbits. Powles *et al.* (1973) showed that rats with Walker tumours underwent bone destruction and sometimes developed hypercalcaemia, both of which were inhibited by giving the rats aspirin and indomethacin. Other aspects relating to bone destruction by tumour are given in Section 9.7.7. Brereton *et al.* (1974) obtained the first indication that prostaglandins might mediate hypercalcaemia in human malignancy, since indomethacin reduced the blood calcium level in a patient with a renal cell adenocarcinoma. Seyberth *et al.* (1975) produced an impressive paper showing that urinary excretion of a PGE_2 metabolite was increased in patients with various solid tumours and hypercalcaemia, both of which were reduced by giving aspirin or indomethacin.

Some patients do not respond to indomethacin (e.g. those with breast cancer in the paper by Coombes *et al.* (1976), so that non-prostaglandin mechanisms are presumably involved, such as parathyroid hormone, osteoclast activating factor (Mundy *et al.*, 1974) or direct resorption of bone by tumour (Galasko, 1976; Eilon and Mundy, 1978). It seems unlikely that PGE or PGF compounds released into the blood stream reach the bone in sufficient amounts to cause substantial bone destruction, but some prostaglandin metabolites, and prostacyclin which is stable in the pulmonary circulation, might be contributory factors. Another possibility is that prostaglandins are released in bone by material produced by the tumour.

9.13 A RÉSUMÉ OF POSSIBLE MECHANISMS BY WHICH PROSTAGLANDIN SYNTHESIS INHIBITORS REDUCE TUMOUR GROWTH

The reasons why anti-inflammatory drugs reduce tumour growth *in vivo* but tend to have the opposite effect *in vitro* are not clear. Possibilities for the *in vivo* effect include a reduction of inflammation (Strausser and Humes, 1975; Hial *et al.*, 1977), which may mean that the bulk of the tumour is reduced because inflammatory cells disappear, or that inflammation enhances the establishment and/or growth of some tumours (Van den Brenk *et al.*, 1974). However, Lynch *et al.* (1978) did not obtain a significant reduction of tumour size with the anti-inflammatory steroid hydrocortisone although indomethacin was effective, and a reduction of inflammation would not explain the complete regression of tumours sometimes obtained by Lynch *et al.* (1978). At least in some tumours non-steroidal anti-inflammatory drugs seem to act by removing an inhibition of the immune system by prostaglandins (see Section 9.9). With regard to tumours which resorb bone, Strausser and Humes (1975) cited work of Whitfield *et al.* (1973) and suggested that indomethacin reduces tumour growth by restricting the amount of calcium available to the tumour cells. PGE_1 may act as a calcium ionophore (Kirtland and Baum, 1972). Indomethacin is also a phosphodiesterase inhibitor (Flores and Sharp, 1972) and this action may lead to an increase in cAMP which affects cell growth. However, theophylline did not alter the growth of MeC3-1 tumours in mice

(Lynch *et al.*, 1978) and even has antitumour effects in some systems (Webb *et al.*, 1972).

Non-steroidal anti-inflammatory drugs have various other actions which may be unrelated to their ability to inhibit prostaglandin synthesis. These actions might explain why high concentrations of non-steroidal anti-inflammatory drugs inhibit cell proliferation *in vitro* (see Section 9.7.4, and Hial *et al.*, 1976).

9.14 PROSTAGLANDIN RELEASE BY CANCER THERAPY, AND THE SIDE-EFFECTS OF DRUGS

Alexander *et al.* (1955) found that sodium salicylate protected 50% of mice from the lethal effect of X-irradiation. Salicylate is only a weak inhibitor of prostaglandin synthesis (Vane, 1971), but this action might have contributed to the protection. The authors thought that hydroperoxy-radicals are important for X-ray-induced lethality, and suggested that protective drugs compete for this radical. Inhibitors of prostaglandin synthesis block the formation of the hydroperoxy-PGG compounds. Kuehl *et al.* (1977) believe that damage in inflammation involves PGG_2. Mennie and Dally (1973) and Mennie *et al.* (1975) studied patients with cervical cancer treated with irradiation. These patients frequently develop diarrhoea which is resistant to conventional therapy, but which responds to aspirin. Presumably, the radiation causes incidental damage to the intestine, and releases prostaglandins which cause or contribute to the diarrhoea. In mice exposed to a single dose of whole-body X-irradiation the amount of prostaglandin extracted from the lungs and spleen increased at day 4, whereas amounts from the brain, blood and seminal vesicles showed little or no change. The splenic tissue from mice exposed to X-irradiation 4 days earlier showed a depressed ability to inactivate PGE_1 (Eisen and Walker, 1976).

The inflammation caused by X-irradiation in treating cancers of the head and neck can be severe enough to delay treatment, thus preventing optimum therapy. For many years, the mucositis has been treated by giving the patients aspirin mucilage. It is of interest that the blood levels of prostaglandin in these patients correlate with the degree of mucositis (B. Tanner and A. Bennett, unpublished). Side-effects of chemotherapy may also involve prostaglandins, since Ohuchi and Levine (1978a) found that anticancer drugs can stimulate PGE release from tumour cells.

Harrap *et al.* (1977) found that a single dose of chlorambucil 32 mg/kg subcutaneously to rats caused some deaths within 2 or 3 days. This did not happen when prednisolone 10 mg/kg was given 4 h after the chlorambucil, but prednisolone gave no protection when it was administered at the same time as the chemotherapeutic drug. In mice, prednisolone 64 mg/kg administered at the same time as chlorambucil 64 mg/kg actually increased the toxicity, but gave protection when administered 4 h later. The protection with delayed prednisolone administration may be because maximal subcellular binding of chlorambucil occurs at about 4 h. Perhaps prednisolone given together with the chemotherapeutic drug was no longer active at the time chlorambucil maximally exerted its damage. The authors did not say why the animals died. Perhaps co-administration of chlorambucil and prednisolone caused toxic effects on one organ (for example, the gastro-intestinal mucosa) which masked the increase in survival due to protection against damage at another site. Such reasoning seems plausible, since corticosteroids and chemotherapeutic drugs are said to damage the gastro-intestinal tract. However, experiments with non-steroidal anti-inflammatory drugs run contrary to this idea. Powles *et al.* (1978) gave indomethacin 1.75 mg/kg three times daily for 3 days to CBA mice, starting the day before a single intraperitoneal injection of melphalan 20 mg/kg. Treatment with the indomethacin halved the mortality due to necrosis of the small-intestinal mucosa. Similarly, indomethacin protected bone-marrow stem cells from damage by whole-body irradiation with 900 R gamma-rays or, to a lesser extent, by the alkylating agent busulphan.

Aspirin 60 mg orally in Wistar rats causes gastric mucosal damage. Administration of melphalan 0.7 or 2.8 mg/kg and methotrexate 1 or 4 mg/kg daily for 4 days did not cause gastric mucosal damage, but the chemotherapeutic drugs greatly reduced the damage by aspirin, possibly by stimulating prostaglandin synthesis and gastric mucus production (A. Bennett, D. A. Berstock, G. J. Frank and I. F. Stamford, unpublished).

These results, together with the improved therapeutic effect when flurbiprofen is combined with radiotherapy and/or chemotherapy (Section 9.11), indicate that inhibitors of prostaglandin synthesis may be valuable adjuncts to the treatment of cancer.

References

Abraham, S. and Rao, G. A. (1976). Lipids and lipogenesis in a murine mammary neoplastic system. In: W. E. Criss *et al.* (eds.), *Control Mechanisms in Cancer*, pp. 363–378 (New York: Raven Press)

Alexander, D., Bacq, Z. M., Cousens, S. F., Fox, M., Herve, A. and Lazar, J. (1955). Mode of action of some substances which protect against the lethal effects of X-rays. *Radiat. Res.*, **2**, 392

Allen, D. O., Munshower, J., Morris, H. P. and Weber, G. (1971). Regulation of adenyl cyclase in hepatomas of different growth rates. *Cancer Res.*, **31**, 557

Apps, M. C. P. and Cater, D. B. (1973). Production of histamine-like and prostaglandin-like substances from human serum incubated with rat, dog, mouse or human tumours. *Br. J. Exp. Pathol.*, **54**, 203

Atkins, D., Ibbotson, K. J., Hillier, K., Hunt, N. H., Hammonds, J. C. and Martin, T. J. (1977). Secretion of prostaglandins as bone resorbing agents by renal cortical carcinoma in culture. *Br. J. Cancer*, **36**, 601

Barrowman, J. A., Bennett, A., Hillenbrand, P., Rolles, K., Pollock, D. J. and Wright, J. T. (1975). Diarrhoea in medullary carcinoma of the thyroid: evidence for the role of prostaglandins and the therapeutic effect of nutmeg. *Br. Med. J.*, **3**, 11

Bennett, A. (1976a). Prostaglandins and the alimentary tract. In: S. M. M. Karim (ed.), *Prostaglandins: Physiological, Pharmacological and Pathological Aspects*, pp. 247–276 (Lancaster: MTP Press)

Bennett, A. (1976b). Prostaglandins as factors in diseases of the alimentary tract. In: B. Samuelsson and R. Paoletti (eds.), *Advances in Prostaglandin and Thromboxane Research*, Vol. 2, pp. 547–555 (New York: Raven Press)

Bennett, A., Berstock, D. A., Raja, B. and Stamford, I. F. (1979a). Survival time after surgery is inversely related to the amounts of prostaglandins extracted from human breast cancers. *Br. J. Pharmacol.* (In press)

Bennett, A., Charlier, E. M., McDonald, A. M., Simpson, J. S. and Stamford, I. F. (1976). Bone destruction by breast tumours. *Prostaglandins*, **11**, 461

Bennett, A., Charlier, E. M., McDonald, A. M., Simpson, J. S., Stamford, I. F. and Zebro, T. (1977). Prostaglandins and breast cancer. *Lancet*, **ii**, 124

Bennett, A., del Tacca, M., Stamford, I. F. and Zebro, T. (1977). Prostaglandins extracted from tumours of human large bowel. *Br. J. Cancer*, **35**, 881

Bennett, A., Houghton, J., Leaper, D. J. and Stamford, I. F. (1978). Tumour growth and response to treatment: beneficial effect of the prostaglandin synthesis inhibitor flurbiprofen. *Br. J. Pharmacol.*, **63**, 356P

Bennett, A., Houghton, J., Leaper, D. J. and Stamford, I. F. (1979b). Cancer growth, response to treatment and survival time in mice: beneficial effect of the prostaglandin synthesis inhibitor flurbiprofen. *Prostaglandins*, **17**, 179

Bennett, A., McDonald, A. M., Simpson, J. S. and Stamford, I. F. (1975). Breast cancer, prostaglandins and bone metastases. *Lancet*, **i**, 1218

Bennett, A., Stamford, I. F. and Unger, W. G. (1973). Prostaglandin E_2 and gastric acid secretion in man. *J. Physiol.*, **229**, 349

Benvenisti, D. and Goldberg, H. (1975). Prostaglandins, indomethacin and hypercalcemia in neoplastic disease. *N. Engl. J. Med.*, **292**, 1189

Berstock, D. A., Houghton, J. and Bennett, A. (1979). Improved anticancer effect by combining cytotoxic drugs with an inhibitor of prostaglandin synthesis. *Cancer Treat. Rev.* (In press)

Bhana, D., Hillier, K. and Karim, S. M. M. (1971). Vasoactive substances in Kaposi's sarcoma. *Cancer*, **27**, 233

Bockman, R. S. and Myers, W. P. L. (1977). Osteotropism of human breast cancer. In: S. B. Day *et al.* (eds.), *Cancer Invasion and Metastasis: Biologic Mechanisms and Therapy*, pp. 431–450 (New York: Raven Press)

Boyd, H., Louis, C. J. and Martin, T. J. (1974). Activity and hormone responsiveness of adenyl cyclase during induction of tumours in rat liver with 3′-methyl-4-dimethylaminoazobenzene. *Cancer Res.*, **34**, 1720

Brereton, H. D., Halushka, P. V., Alexander, R. W., Mason, D. M., Keiser, H. R. and De Vita, V. T. (1974). Indomethacin-responsive hypercalcemia in a patient with renal-cell adenocarcinoma. *N. Engl. J. Med.*, **291**, 83

Burstein, S., Gagnon, G., Hunter, S. A. and Maudsley, D. V. (1976). Prostaglandin biosynthesis and stimulation of cyclic AMP in primary monolayer cultures of epithelial cells from mouse mammary gland. *Prostaglandins*, **11**, 85

Burstein, S., Gagnon, G., Hunter, S. A. and Maudsley, D. V. (1977). Elevation of prostaglandin and cyclic AMP levels by arachidonic acid in primary epithelial cell cultures of C3H mouse mammary tumours. *Prostaglandins*, **13**, 41

Carpenter, M. P., Thuy, L. P. and Robinson, R. D. (1977). Prostaglandin metabolism in normal and neoplastic rat mammary gland. *Prostaglandins*, **13**, 1010

Chayoth, R., Epstein and Field, J. B. (1973). Glucagon and prostaglandin E_1 stimulation of cyclic adenosine 3′,5′-monophosphate levels and adenylate cyclase activity in benign hyperplastic nodules and malignant hepatomas of ethionine-treated rats. *Cancer Res.*, **33**, 1970

Chlapowski, F. J., Kelly, L. A. and Butcher, R. W. (1975). Cyclic nucleotides in cultured cells. *Adv. Cyclic Nucleotide Res.*, **6**, 245

Cohen, F. and Jaffe, B. M. (1973). Production of prostaglandins by cells *in vitro*: radioimmunoassay measurement of the conversion of arachidonic acid to prostaglandin E_2 and prostaglandin $F_{2\alpha}$. *Biochem. Biophys. Res. Commun.*, **55**, 724

Coombes, R. C., Neville, A. M., Bondy, P. K. and Powles, T. J. (1976). Failure of indomethacin to reduce hydroxyproline excretion or hypercalcaemia in patients with breast cancer. *Prostaglandins*, **12**, 1027

Cummings, K. B., Wheelis, R. F. and Robertson, R. P. (1975). Prostaglandin: increased production by renal cell carcinoma. *Surg. Forum*, **26**, 572

Day, E. A., Malcolm, G. T. and Beeler, M. F. (1969). Tumor sterols. *Metabolism*, **18**, 646

De Asua, L. J., Clingan, D. and Rudland, P. S. (1975). Initiation of cell proliferation in cultured mouse fibroblasts by prostaglandin $F_{2\alpha}$. *Proc. Natl. Acad. Sci.*, **72**, 2724

Demers, L. M., Allegra, J. C., Harvey, H. A., Lipton, A., Luderer, J. R., Mortel, R. and Brenner, D. E. (1977). Plasma prostaglandins in hypercalcemic patients with neoplastic disease. *Cancer*, **39**, 1559

De Rubertis, F. R., Chayoth, R. and Field, J. B. (1973). The content and metabolism of cyclic adenosine 3′,5′-monophosphate and cyclic guanosine 3′,5′-monophosphate in adenocarcinoma of the human colon. *J. Clin. Invest.*, **57**, 641

Dietrich, J. W., Goodson, J. M. and Raisz, L. G. (1975). Stimulation of bone resorption by various prostaglandins in organ culture. *Prostaglandins*, **10**, 231

Dindogru, A., Gailani, S., Henderson, F. S., Wallace, H. J. and Fitzpatrick, J. (1975). Indomethacin and hypercalcaemia. *Lancet*, **ii**, 365

Dorp, D. A. van (1971). Recent developments in the biosynthesis and the analyses of prostaglandins. *Ann. N.Y. Acad. Sci.*, **180**, 181

Dowsett, M., Easty, G. C., Powles, T. J., Easty, D. M. and Neville, A. M. (1976a). Human breast tumour-induced osteolysis and prostaglandins. *Prostaglandins*, **11**, 447

Dowsett, M., Gazet, J. C., Powles, T. J., Easty, G. C. and Neville, A. M. (1976b). Benign breast lesions and osteolysis. *Lancet*, **i**, 970

Drut, R. and De Cusminsky, B. S. (1975). Prostaglandins en sarcoma renal humano. Probable sarcoma de celulas reno-medulares intersticiales. *Medicina (B. Aires)*, **35**, 154

Easty, G. C., Dowsett, M., Powles, T. J., Easty, D. M., Gazet, J. C. and Neville, A. M. (1977). Hypercalcaemia in malignant disease. *Proc. R. Soc. Med.*, **70**, 191

Easty, G. C. and Easty, D. M. (1976). Prostaglandins and cancer. *Cancer Treat. Rev.*, **3**, 217

Eilon, G. and Mundy, G. R. (1978). Direct resorption of bone by human breast cancer cells *in vitro*. *Nature*, **276**, 726

Eisen, V. and Walker, D. I. (1976). Effect of ionizing radiation on prostaglandin-like activity in tissues. *Br. J. Pharmacol.*, **57**, 527

El Attar, T. M. A. (1976). Prostaglandin E_2 in human gingiva in health and disease and its stimulation by female sex steroids. *Prostaglandins*, **11**, 331

Feldman, J. M., Plonk, J. W. and Cornette, J. C. (1974). Serum prostaglandin F_2 alpha concentration in the carcinoid syndrome. *Prostaglandins*, **7**, 501

Ferreira, S. H. and Vane, J. R. (1967). Prostaglandins: their disappearance from and release into the circulation. *Nature*, **216**, 868

Flores, A. G. A. and Sharp, G. W. G. (1972). Endogenous prostaglandins and osmotic water flow in the toad bladder. *Am. J. Physiol.*, **223**, 1392

Galasko, C. S. B. (1976). Mechanisms of bone destruction in the development of skeletal metastases. *Nature*, **263**, 507

Galasko, C. S. B. and Bennett, A. (1976). Relationship of bone destruction in skeletal metastases to osteoclast activation and prostaglandins. *Nature*, **263**, 508

Gasic, G. J., Gasic, T. B., Galanti, N., Johnson, T. and Murphy, S. (1973). Platelet–tumor–cell interactions in mice. The role of platelets in the spread of malignant disease. *Int. J. Cancer*, **11**, 704

Gasic, G. J., Gasic, T. B. and Murphy, S. (1972). Anti-metastic effect of aspirin. *Lancet*, **ii**, 932

Golub, M., Zia, P., Metsuno, M. and Horton, R. (1975). Metabolism of prostaglandins A_1 and E_1 in man. *J. Clin. Invest.*, **56**, 1404

Goodwin, J. S., Messner, R. P., Bankhurst, A. D., Peake, G. T., Saiki, J. H. and Williams, R. C. (1977). Prostaglandin-producing suppressor cells in Hodgkin's disease. *N. Engl. J. Med.*, **297**, 963

Gordan, G. S., Cantino, T. J., Erhardt, L., Hansen, J. and Lubich, W. (1966). Osteolytic sterol in human breast cancer. *Science*, **151**, 1226

Greaves, M. (1978). The measurement of prostaglandins E and F by radioimmunoassay and its application to the study of malignant and inflammatory diseases. MD Thesis, University of Sheffield

Grimley, P. M., Dettos, L. J., Weeks, J. R. and Robson, A. S. (1969). Growth *in vitro* and ultrastructure of cells from medullary carcinoma of the human thyroid gland: Transformation by simian virus 40 and evidence of thyrocalcitonin and prostaglandins. *J. Natl. Cancer Inst.*, **42**, 663

Hammarström, S., Claesson, H. K. and Lindgren, J. A. (1977). Arachidonic acid metabolism and adenosine 3′:5′-monophosphate levels in mouse 3T3 fibroblasts. *Prostaglandins*, **13**, 1009

Hammarström, S., Samuelsson, B. and Bjursell, G. (1973). Prostaglandin levels in normal and transformed baby-hamster-kidney fibroblasts. *Nature (New Biol.)*, **243**, 50

Hamprecht, B., Jaffe, B. M. and Philpott, G. (1973). Prostaglandin production by neuroblastoma, glioma and fibroblast cell lines: Stimulation by N^6,O^2-dibutyryl adenosine 3′:5′-cyclic monophosphate. *FEBS Lett.*, **36**, 193

Harrap, K. R., Riches, P. G., Gilby, E. D., Sellwood, S. M., Wilkinson, R. and Konyves, I. (1977). Studies on the toxicity and antitumour activity of prednimustine, a prednisolone ester of chlorambucil. *Eur. J. Cancer*, **13**, 873

Harris, M., Jenkins, M. V., Bennett, A. and Willis, M. R. (1973). Prostaglandin production and bone resorption by dental cysts. *Nature*, **245**, 213

Harvey, H. A., Allegra, J. C., Demers, L. M., Luderer, J. R., Brenner, D. E., Trautlein, J. J., White, D. S., Gillin, M. A. and Lipton, A. (1977). Immunosuppression and human cancer: role of prostaglandins. *Cancer*, **39**, 2362

Hewitt, H. B., Blake, E. R. and Walder, A. S. (1976). A critique of the evidence for active host defence against cancer, based on personal studies of 27 murine tumours of spontaneous origin. *Br. J. Cancer*, **33**, 241

Hial, V., de Mello, M. C. F., Horakova, Z. and Beaven, M. A. (1977). Antiproliferative activity of anti-inflammatory drugs in two mammalian cell culture lines. *J. Pharmacol. Exp. Ther.*, **202**, 446

Hial, V., Horakova, Z., Shalf, R. E. and Beaven, M. A. (1976). Alteration of tumor growth by aspirin and indomethacin: studies with two transplantable tumors in mice. *Eur. J. Pharmacol.*, **37**, 367

Hilgard, P. and Thornes, R. D. (1976). Anticoagulants in the treatment of cancer. *Eur. J. Cancer*, **22**, 755

Hong, S.-C. L., Polsky-Cynkin, R. and Levine, L. (1976). Stimulation of prostaglandin biosynthesis by vasoactive substances in methylcholanthrene transformed mouse BALB/3T3. *J. Biol. Chem.*, **251**, 776

Hong, S. L., Wheless, C. M. and Levine, L. (1977). Elevated prostaglandin synthetase activity in methylcholanthrene-transformed mouse BALB/3T3. *Prostaglandins*, **13**, 271

Horton, J. E., Raisz, L. G., Simmons, H. A., Oppenheim, J. J. and Mergenhagen, S. E. (1972). Bone resorbing activity in supernatant fluid from cultured human peripheral blood leucocytes. *Science*, **177**, 793

Humes, J. L., Cupo, J. J. and Strausser, H. R. (1974). Effects of indomethacin on Moloney sarcoma virus-induced tumours. *Prostaglandins*, **6**, 463

Humes, J. L. and Strausser, H. R. (1974). Prostaglandins and cyclic nucleotides in Maloney sarcoma tumors. *Prostaglandins*, **5**, 183

Hunt, N. H., Shortland, J. R., Michelangelo, V. P., Hammonds, J. C., Atkins, D. and Martin, T. J. (1978). Adenylate cyclase activity of renal cortical carcinoma and its relation to histology and ultrastructure. *Cancer Res.*, **38**, 23

Isaacs, P., Whittaker, S. M. and Turnberg, L. A. (1974). Diarrhoea associated with medullary carcinoma of the thyroid. *Gastroenterology*, **67**, 521

Ishikawa, Y., Ciosek, C. P., Fahey, J. V. and Newcombe, D. S. (1976). Prostaglandin synthetase activity and hormone responsiveness in normal and SV40 transformed WI-38 fibroblasts. *J. Cyclic Nucleotide Res.*, **2**, 115

Ito, H., Sanada, T., Katayama, T. and Shimazaki, J. (1975). Indomethacin-responsive hypercalcemia. *N. Engl. J. Med.*, **293**, 558

Jaffe, B. M. (1974). Prostaglandins and cancer: an update. *Prostaglandins*, **6**, 454

Jaffe, B. M. and Condon, S. (1976). Prostaglandins E and F in endocrine diarrheagenic syndromes. *Ann. Surg.*, **184**, 516

Jaffe, B. M., Parker, C. W. and Philpott, G. W. (1971). Immunochemical measurement of prostaglandin or prostaglandin-like activity from normal and neoplastic tissues in culture. *Surg. Forum.*, **22**, 90

Jaffe, B. M., Philpott, G. W., Hamprecht, B. and Parker, C. W. (1973). Prostaglandin production by cells *in vitro*. *Adv. Biosci.*, **9**, 129

Jenkins, M. V., Polanska, N. and Wills, M. R. (1976). Bone resorption by breast cancer tissue. *Lancet*, **i**, 1186

Johnson, G. S. and Pastan, I. (1971). Change in growth and morphology of fibroblasts by prostaglandins. *J. Natl. Cancer Inst.*, **47**, 1357

Johnson, G. S. and Pastan, I. (1972). Role of 3′,5′-adenosine monophosphate in regulation of morphology and growth of transformed and normal fibroblasts. *J. Natl. Cancer Inst.*, **48**, 1377

Kaplan, E. L., Sizemore, G. W., Peskin, G. W. and Jaffe, B. M. (1973). Humoral similarities of carcinoid tumors and medullary carcinomas of the thyroid. *Surgery*, **74**, 21

Karim, S. M. M. and Rao, B. (1976). Prostaglandins and tumours. In: S. M. M. Karim (ed.), *Prostaglandins: Physiological, Pharmacological and Pathological Aspects*, pp. 303–325 (Lancaster: MTP Press)

Kibbey, W. E., Brown, D. G. and Minton, J. P. (1978). Prostaglandins and metastasis. *Lancet*, **i**, 101

Kirtland, S. J. and Baum, H. (1972). Prostaglandin E_1 may act as a 'calcium ionophore'. *Nature (New Biol.)*, **236**, 47

Klein, D. C. and Raisz, L. G. (1970). Prostaglandins: stimulation of bone resorption in tissue culture. *Endocrinology*, **86**, 1436

Kolenich, J. J., Mansour, E. G. and Flynn, A. (1972). Haematological aspects of aspirin. *Lancet*, **ii**, 714

Kuehl, F. A., Humes, J. L., Egan, R. W., Ham, E. A., Beveridge, G. C. and van Arman, C. G. (1977). Role of prostaglandin endoperoxide PGG_2 in inflammatory processes. *Nature*, **265**, 170

Kuppe, G. and Wetter, O. (1974). Prostaglandins, bone resorption and hypercalcaemia (cont.). *Lancet*, **i**, 230

Leading Article (1976). Osteolytic metastases. *Lancet*, **ii**, 1063

Leaper, D. J., Bennett, A., Charlier, E. M. and Stamford, I. F. (1978a). The enhancement of radiotherapy and chemotherapy on a murine tumour using the prostaglandin synthetase inhibitor flurbiprofen. *Br. J. Surg.*, **65**, 369

Leaper, D. J., Bennett, A., Houghton, J. and Stamford, I. F. (1978b). Tumour growth and survival time; effect of a prostaglandin synthetase inhibitor. *Clin. Oncol.*, **4**, 388

Leichtling, B. H., Drotar, A. M., Ortmann, R. and Perkins, J. P. (1976). Growth of astrocytoma cells in the presence of prostaglandin E_1: effect of regulation of cyclic AMP metabolism. *J. Cyclic Nucleotide Res.*, **2**, 89

Levine, L. (1977). Levels of 13,14-dihydro-15-keto-PGE_2 in some biological fluids as measured by radioimmunoassay. *Prostaglandins*, **14**, 1125

Levine, L. (1977). Chemical carcinogens stimulate canine kidney (MDCK) cells to produce prostaglandins. *Nature*, **268**, 447

Levine, L. and Hassid, A. (1977). Effects of phorbol-12,13-diesters on prostaglandin production and phospholipase activity in canine kidney (MDCK) cells. *Biochem. Biophys. Res. Commun.*, **79**, 477

Levine, L., Hinkle, P. M., Voelkel, E. F. and Tashjian, A. H. (1972). Prostaglandin production by mouse fibrosarcoma cells in culture: Inhibition by indomethacin and aspirin. *Biochem. Biophys. Res. Commun.*, **47**, 888

Loose, L. D. and DiLuzio, N. R. (1973). Effect of prostaglandin E_1 on cellular and humoral immune responses. *J. Reticuloendothelial Soc.*, **13**, 70

Lupulescu, A. (1978). Enhancement of carcinogenesis by prostaglandins. *Nature*, **272**, 634

Lynch, N. R., Castes, M., Astoin, M. and Salomon, J. C. (1978). Mechanism of inhibition of tumour growth by aspirin and indomethacin. *Br. J. Cancer*, **38**, 503

Lynch, N. R. and Salomon, J. C. (1977). Tumour-associated inhibition of immediate hypersensitivity reactions in mice. *Immunology*, **32**, 645

MacManus, J. P. and Whitfield, J. F. (1974). Cyclic AMP, prostaglandins and the control of cell proliferation. *Prostaglandins*, **6**, 475

Melvin, K. E. W., Tashjian, A. H. and Miller, A. A. (1972). Studies in familial (medullary) thyroid carcinoma. *Rec. Progr. Horm. Res.*, **28**, 399

Ménagé, J. J., Besnard, J. C., Guilmot, J. L., Vandooren, M. and Neel, J. L. (1975). Preuves de l'absence de sécrétion de prostaglandines par un carcinome médullaire de la thyroide avec diarrhée motrice. *Dir. N. Presse Med.*, **4**, 2862

Mennie, A. T. and Dalley, V. (1973). Aspirin in radiation-induced diarrhoea. *Lancet*, **i**, 1131

Mennie, S. A. T., Dalley, V., Dinneen, L. C. and Collier, H. O. J. (1975). Treatment of radiation-induced gastrointestinal distress with acetylsalicylate. *Lancet*, **ii**, 942

Mortel, R., Allegra, J. C., Demers, L. M., Harvey, H. A., Trautlein, J., Nahhas, W., White, D., Gillin, M. A. and Lipton, A. (1977). Plasma prostaglandins across the tumour bed of patients with gynaecologic malignancy. *Cancer*, **39**, 2201

Mundy, G. R., Luben, R. A., Raisz, L. G., Oppenheim, J. J. and Buell, D. N. (1974). Bone resorbing activity in supernatants from lymphoid cell lines. *N. Engl. J. Med.*, **290**, 867

Naseem, S. M. and Hollander, V. P. (1973). Insulin reversal of growth inhibition of plasma cell tumor by prostaglandin or adenosine 3',5'-monophosphate. *Cancer Res.*, **33**, 2909

Ohuchi, K. and Levine, L. (1978a). Stimulation of prostaglandin synthesis by tumor-promoting phorbol 12,13-diesters in canine kidney (MDCK) cells. *J. Biol. Chem.*, **253**, 4783

Ohuchi, K. and Levine, L. (1978b). Stimulation of prostaglandin production, deacylation of lipids and morphological changes by tumor-promoting phorbol-12,13-diesters and adriamycin in MDCK cells: effect of cycloheximide, indomethacin and hydrocortisone on these stimulations. *Prostaglandins*, **15**, 723

Otten, J., Johnson, G. S. and Pastan, I. (1972). Regulation of cell growth by cyclic adenosine 3',5'-monophosphate. Effect of cell density and agents which alter cell growth on cyclic adenosine 3',5'-monophosphate levels in fibroblasts. *J. Biol. Chem.*, **247**, 7082

Papanicolaou, N., Mountokalakis, Th., Tcherdakoff, Ph., Bariety, J. and Milliez, P. (1975). Prostaglandins in neural-crest tumours. *Prostaglandins*, **10**, 405

Pastan, I. M., Johnson, G. S. and Anderson, W. B. (1975). Role of cyclic nucleotides in growth control. *Annu. Rev. Biochem.*, **44**, 491

Pearse, A. G. E. (1966). 5-Hydroxytryptophan uptake by dog thyroid 'C' cells and its possible significance in polypeptide hormone production. *Nature*, **211**, 598

Pelus, L. M., Strausser, H. R. (1976). Indomethacin enhancement of spleen-cell responsiveness to mitogen stimulation in tumorous mice. *Int. J. Cancer*, **18**, 653

Plescia, O. J., Smith, A. H. and Grinwick, K. (1975). Subversion of immune system by tumor cells and role of prostaglandins. *Proc. Natl. Acad. Sci. USA*, **72**, 1848

Powles, T. J., Alexander, P. and Millar, J. L. (1978). Enhancement of anti-cancer activity of cytotoxic chemotherapy with production of normal tissues by inhibition of prostaglandin synthesis. *Biochem. Pharmacol.*, **27**, 1389

Powles, T. J., Clark, S. A., Easty, D. M., Easty, G. C. and Neville, A. M. (1973). The inhibition by aspirin and indomethacin of osteolytic tumour deposits and hypercalcaemia in rats with Walker tumour, and its possible application to human breast cancer. *Br. J. Cancer*, **28**, 316

Powles, T. J., Coombes, R. C., Neville, A. M., Ford, H. T., Gazet, J. C. and Levine, L. (1977). 15-keto-13,14-dihydroprostaglandin E_2 concentrations in the serum of patients with breast cancer. *Lancet*, **ii**, 138

Powles, T. J., Dowsett, M., Easty, G. C., Easty, D. M. and Neville, A. M. (1976). Breast cancer osteolysis, bone metastases and anti-osteolytic effect of aspirin. *Lancet*, **i**, 608

Prasad, K. N. (1972). Morphological differentiation induced by prostaglandin in mouse neuroblastoma cella in culture. *Nature (New Biol.)*, **236**, 49

Raisz, L. G., Dietrich, J. W., Simmons, H. A., Seyberth, H. W., Hubbard, W. and Oates, J. A. (1977). Effect of prostaglandin endoperoxides and metabolites on bone resorption *in vitro*. *Nature*, **267**, 532

Ritchie, G. A. F. (1977). The direct inhibition of prostaglandin synthetase of human breast cancer tissue by 'Novaldex'. Paper presented at the ICI Symposium on Breast Cancer, Cambridge, 1977

Ritzi, E. M. and Stylos, W. A. (1976). Prostaglandin production in cultures of BALB/3T3 and SV3T3 mouse fibroblasts. *J. Natl. Cancer Inst.*, **56**, 529

Robert, A. (1977). Effect of prostaglandins on gastro-intestinal functions. In: F. Berti, B. Samuelsson and G. P. Velo (eds.), *Prostaglandins and Thromboxanes*, pp. 287–313 (New York: Plenum Press)

Robertson, R. P., Baylink, D. J., Marini, J. J. and Adkinson, H. W. (1975). Elevated prostaglandins and suppressed parathyroid hormone associated with hypercalcemia and renal cell carcinoma. *J. Clin. Endocrinol. Metab.*, **41**, 164

Robertson, R. P., Baylink, D. J., Metz, S. A. and Cummings, K. B. (1976). Plasma prostaglandin E in patients with cancer with and without hypercalcemia. *J. Clin. Endocrinol. Metab.*, **43**, 1330

Robinson, D. R. (1976). Studies on the role of prostaglandins in mammary gland neoplasia. Contract research summary. Breast cancer task force program and related projects, p. 63, Division of Cancer Biology and Diagnosis, US National Cancer Institute

Ryan, W. L. and Heidrick, M. L. (1974). Role of cyclic nucleotides in cancer. *Adv. Cyclic Nucleotide Res.*, **4**, 81

Sandler, M., Karim, S. M. M. and Williams, E. D. (1968). Prostaglandins in amine-peptide secreting tumours. *Lancet*, **ii**, 1053

Santoro, M. G., Philpott, G. W. and Jaffe, B. M. (1976). Inhibition of tumour growth *in vivo* and *in vitro* by prostaglandin E. *Nature*, **263**, 777

Schechter, B. and Feldman, M. (1977). Hydrocortisone affects tumor growth by eliminating precursors of suppressor cells. *J. Immunol.*, **119**, 1563

Schiffman, F. J., Yehara, Y., Fisher, J. M. and Robinovitz, M. (1978). Potentiation of chlorambucil activity by phenylbutazone. *Cancer Lett.*, **4**, 211

Seyberth, H. W., Hubbard, W. C., Oelz, O., Sweetman, B. J., Watson, J. T. and Oates, J. A. (1977). Prostaglandin mediated hypercalcemia in the VX_2 carcinoma-bearing rabbit. *Prostaglandins*, **14**, 319

Seyberth, H. W., Raisz, L. G. and Oates, J. A. (1978). Prostaglandins and hypercalcemic states. *Ann. Res. Med.*, **29**, 23

Seyberth, H. W., Segre, G. V., Morgan, J. L., Sweetman, B. J., Potts, J. T. and Oates, J. A. (1975). Prostaglandins as mediators of hypercalcemia associated with certain types of cancer. *N. Engl. J. Med.*, **293**, 1278

Sheppard, J. R. (1971). Restoration of contact-inhibited growth to transformed cells by dibutyryl adenosine 3',5'-cyclic monophosphate. *Proc. Natl. Acad. Sci. USA*, **68**, 1316

Sheppard, J. R. (1972). Difference in the cyclic adenosine 3',5'-monophosphate levels in normal and transformed cells. *Nature (New Biol.)*, **236**, 14

Sheppard, J. R., Hudson, T. H. and Larson, J. R. (1975). Adenosine 3',5'-monophosphate analogs promote a circular morphology of cultured Schwannoma cells. *Science*, **187**, 179

Sonis, S. T., Stelos, P., Stylos, W. A. and Wilson, R. E. (1977). Inhibition of lymphoma cell proliferation by supernatant from fibrosarcoma cultures: preliminary evidence that the inhibitory material is prostaglandin E. *Prostaglandins*, **13**, 89

Stein-Werblowsky, R. (1974a). The effect of prostaglandin on tumour implantation. *Experientia*, **30**, 957

Stein-Werblowsky, R. (1974b). Prostaglandin and cancer. *Oncology*, **30**, 169

Stoll, B. A. (1973). Indomethacin in breast cancer. *Lancet*, **ii**, 384

Strausser, H. and Humes, J. (1975). Prostaglandin synthesis inhibition: Effect on bone changes and sarcoma tumour induction in BALB/c mice. *Int. J. Cancer*, **15**, 724

Sykes, J. A. C. and Maddox, I. S. (1972). Prostaglandin production by experimental tumours and effects of anti-inflammatory compounds. *Nature (New Biol.)*, **237**, 59

Tam, S., Hong, S.-C. L. and Levine, L. (1977). Relationships among the steroids of anti-inflammatory properties and inhibition of prostaglandin production and arachidonic acid release by transformed mouse fibroblasts. *J. Pharm. Exp. Ther.*, **203**, 162

Tan, W. C., Privett, O. S. and Goldyne, M. E. (1974). Studies of prostaglandins in rat mammary tumors induced by 7,12-dimethylbenz(a)anthracene. *Cancer Res.*, **34**, 3229

Tashjian, A. H., Tice, J. E. and Sides, K. (1977a). Biological activities of prostaglandin analogues and metabolites in bone organ culture. *Nature*, **266**, 645

Tashjian, A. H., Voelkel, E. F., Goldhaber, P. and Levine, L. (1973). Successful treatment of hypercalcemia by indomethacin in mice bearing a prostaglandin-producing tumor. *Prostaglandins*, **3**, 515

Tashjian, A. H., Voelkel, E. F., Goldhaber, P. and Levine, L. (1974). Prostaglandins, calcium metabolism and cancer. *Fed. Proc.*, **33**, 81

Tashjian, A. H., Voelkel, E. F. and Levine, L. (1977a). Plasma concentrations of 13,14-dihydro-15-keto-prostaglandin E_2 in rabbits bearing the VX_2 carcinoma: effects of the hydrocortisone and indomethacin. *Prostaglandins*, **14**, 309

Tashjian, A. H., Voelkel, E. F. and Levine, L. (1977b). Effects of hydrocortisone on the hypercalcemia and plasma levels of 13,14-dihydro-15-keto-prostaglandin E_2 in mice bearing the $HSDM_1$ fibrosarcoma. *Biochem. Biophys. Res. Commun.*, **74**, 199

Tashjian, A. H., Voelkel, E. F., Levine, L. and Goldhaber, P. (1972). Evidence that the bone resorption stimulating factor produced by mouse fibrosarcoma cells is prostaglandin E_2. *J. Exp. Med.*, **136**, 1329

Tashjian, A. H., Voelkel, E. F., McDonough, J. and Levine, L. (1975). Hydrocortisone inhibits prostaglandin production by mouse fibrosarcoma cells. *Nature*, **258**, 739

Thomas, D. R., Philpott, G. W. and Jaffe, B. M. (1974a). Prostaglandin E control of cell replication *in vitro*. *J. Surg. Res.*, **16**, 463

Thomas, D. R., Philpott, G. W. and Jaffe, B. M. (1974b). The relationship between concentration of prostaglandin E and rates of cell replication. *Exp. Cell Res.*, **84**, 40

Van den Brenk, H. A. S., Stone, M., Kelly, H., Orton, C. and Sharpington, C. (1974). Promotion of growth of tumour cells in acutely inflamed tissues. *Br. J. Cancer*, **30**, 246

Voelkel, E. F., Tashjian, A. H., Franklin, R., Wasserman, E. and Levine, L. (1975). Hypercalcemia and tumor prostaglandins: The VX_2 carcinoma model in the rabbit. *Metabolism*, **24**, 973

Webb, D., Braun, W. and Plescin, O. J. (1972). Antitumor effects of polynucleotides and theophylline. *Cancer Res.*, **32**, 1814

Webb, D. R. and Jamieson, A. T. (1976). Control of mitogen-induced transformation: characterization of a splenic suppressor cell and its mode of action. *Cell. Immunol.*, **24**, 45

Webb, D. R. and Osheroff, P. L. (1976). Antigen stimulation of prostaglandin synthesis and control of immune responses. *Proc. Natl. Acad. Sci. USA*, **73**, 1300

Welbourn, R. B. (1977). Apudomas of the gut. *Am. J. Surg.*, **133**, 13

Whitfield, J. R., Rixon, R. H., MacManus, J. P. and Balk, D. S. (1973). Calcium, cyclic adenosine 3′,5′-monophosphate and the control of cell proliferation. A review. *In Vitro*, **8**, 257

Willman, E. A., Collins, W. P. and Clayton, S. G. (1976). Studies in the involvement of prostaglandins in uterine symptomatology and pathology. *Br. J. Obstet. Gynaecol.*, **83**, 337

Williams, E. D., Karim, S. M. M. and Sandler, M. (1968). Prostaglandin secretion by medullary carcinoma of the thyroid. A possible cause of the associated diarrhoea. *Lancet*, **i**, 22

Winchurch, R. A., Foschi, G. V. and Watz, D. T. (1974). Inhibition of the lymphocyte-mediated cytotoxic reaction by anti-inflammatory drugs. *J. Reticuloendothelial Soc.*, **15**, 112

Wood, S. and Hilgard, P. (1972). Aspirin and tumour metastasis. *Lancet*, **ii**, 1416

Yoneda, T. and Mundy, G. R. (1979). Prostaglandins are necessary for osteoclast activating factor (OAF) production by activated peripheral blood leukocytes. *J. Exp. Med.*, **149**, 297

Zusman, R. M., Snider, J. J., Cline, A., Caldwell, B. V. and Speroff, L. (1974). Antihypertensive function of a renal-cell carcinoma. *N. Engl. J. Med.*, **290**, 843

10
Veterinary Uses of Prostaglandins

M. J. COOPER, D. HAMMOND and R. H. SCHULTZ

10.1 INTRODUCTION

Considerable progress has been made in the development of prostaglandin application in veterinary science, and their early promise as agents capable of affecting the breeding and treatment of infertility in larger domestic species has to some extent been fulfilled. Since the preparation of a similar chapter (Cooper and Walpole, 1975) both natural prostaglandin $PGF_{2\alpha}$[1] and cloprostenol[2] are commercially available in many parts of the world, and have established an important position for themselves in animal health markets. Fluprostenol[3] and the 15-methyl prostaglandin analogue[4] are now also available for the treatment of infertility in mares.

In veterinary practice the importance of luteolytic prostaglandins has already been confirmed. However, their major potential use is in the control of bovine oestrous cycle and the consequent exploitation of the well-established benefits of artificial insemination (AI). Since the first report by Christian and Casida (1948) that repeated injections of progesterone could result in some synchronization of oestrous cycles in cattle, the control of the cycle and predetermined timing of ovulation has been a clearly defined research objective for many animal science laboratories. In spite of this, only recently has detailed consideration been given to the practical and managemental implications of ovulation control. After 2 or 3 years field experience it is becoming obvious that these go far beyond the simple exploitation of AI.

Early experience with the long-term administration of progesterone and progestins was discouraging for research workers and expensive for the pharmaceutical industry. The oestrus following such a treatment, although well synchronized, was of lower than normal fertility (Trimburger and Hansel, 1955; Nellor and Cole, 1956). Consequently, during early studies too much attention was paid to the effect on the fertility of the oestrus following prostaglandin treatment, and the versatility of the luteolytic activity was to some extent neglected. As previously described (Cooper and Walpole, 1975), random bovine cycles can be controlled by two injections of either cloprostenol or $PGF_{2\alpha}$ 10–12 days apart. Less precise synchronization follows single injections of these substances administered at an appropriate stage in the cycle. It is now well established that fertility following either double-spaced injections (Leaver *et al.*, 1975; Hafs and Manns, 1975; Karg *et al.*, 1976; Trounson *et al.*, 1976; Schultz *et al.*, 1977; Fulka *et al.*, 1978) or single injection (Lauderdale *et al.*, 1974; Eddy, 1978) is normal.

In most markets prostaglandins were first available for use in mares, since

---

[1] 'Lutalyse' (Upjohn Ltd.)
[2] 'Estrumate' and 'Planate' (Imperial Chemical Industries Ltd.)
[3] 'Equimate' (Imperial Chemical Industries Ltd.)
[4] 'Synchrocept' (Syntex Pharmaceuticals Ltd.)
All Trade Marks

milk and tissue residue investigations are usually unnecessary in this species. It is therefore not surprising that a wealth of data now exists to show that the fertility of this animal is unaffected by prostaglandin administration (Allen and Rowson, 1973; Allen *et al.*, 1974; Oxender *et al.*, 1974; Brand *et al.*, 1975a, 1975b).

In parallel with field investigations to confirm the fertility of the synchronized heat, various detailed studies have been performed to demonstrate that the induced heat is physiologically normal, and that the associated endocrine changes are similar or identical to those accompanying a spontaneous heat.

Following treatment with either $PGF_{2\alpha}$ or cloprostenol changes in plasma concentrations of progesterone, oestradiol-17β and luteinizing hormone are similar to those occurring physiologically (Oxender *et al.*, 1974; Cooper and Rowson, 1975; Cooper *et al.*, 1974). It is perhaps important to point out that, in contrast to clinical applications of prostaglandins in the human, only the luteolytic activity is being exploited in veterinary medicine. If other pharmacological actions of prostaglandins are important, then this has not yet become obvious except perhaps in a recent report on the efficacy of fluprostenol in the induction of parturition in mares (Jeffcot and Rossdale, 1977).

The induction of parturition in pigs has received considerable attention and the potential of this development to the pig industry has now been clarified (Bichard *et al.*, 1976). Both cloprostenol (under the trade name 'Planate') and $PGF_{2\alpha}$ have been investigated, developed and marketed for this purpose. This aspect will be considered in detail in Section 10.3.

As has been pointed out, prostaglandins have become established not only as useful drugs in clinical veterinary practice but also as a significant tool in the management of cattle and horse breeding. This chapter is therefore concerned less with physiological and pharmacological aspects of prostaglandin activity and more with the practical applications of these drugs. The conditions necessary to obtain best results from controlled breeding in cattle are discussed together with the important applications of prostaglandins in the treatment of bovine infertility and the induction of parturition. The treatment of infertility in mares has been comprehensively discussed previously (Cooper and Walpole, 1975).

10.2 USE OF PROSTAGLANDINS TO CONTROL OVULATION IN CATTLE

10.2.1 Controlled breeding of heifers

Artificial breeding of heifers is never easy. In both dairy and beef herds, replacement heifers tend to be inaccessible and therefore difficult to detect when in heat. However, on any farm with a coherent breeding programme, the heifer should be the best genetic material in the herd and therefore the most appropriate animal for artificial insemination. Since heifers are not under any form of production stress other than growth, they tend to cycle normally and regularly and have better fertility than their adult counterparts. They are therefore good candidates for the double-spaced injection regime described by Cooper (1974) and have been the subject of extensive field investigations. Studies with both cloprostenol and $PGF_{2\alpha}$ have shown that heifers inseminated twice, at around 72 h and 96 h after the second injection of prostaglandin, produce pregnancy rates which are the same or closely comparable to contemporary controls inseminated once at spontaneous heat (Hafs *et al.*, 1975; Deletang, 1975; Cooper *et al.*, 1976; Fulka *et al.*, 1978). Some reports indicate that a single insemination at 72 h also gives normal fertility (Leaver *et al.*, 1975), and reference to physiological data leaves little doubt that 72 h is the correct time for a single AI (Cooper *et al.*, 1974; Cooper and Rowson, 1975; Britt *et al.*, 1978).

In spite of some reports to the contrary, it has been shown that when single and double AI are directly compared (Cooper, 1975) two inseminations invariably result in higher pregnancy rates, both in beef and in dairy heifers. Using over 700 beef heifers, Cooper (1975) has shown a difference in conception rate of 15% between a single and double insemination.

Similar results have been recorded in dairy heifers (Cooper, 1977) and it would appear that the higher the control or background fertility, the wider this margin is likely to be. There are several different regimes of treatment with prostaglandins which can be used on the farm and some of these alternatives may be used in heifers. However, their inaccessibility usually demands two injections of prostaglandin and two fixed-time inseminations as the method of choice. It is important when selecting a regime to note that the heat and ovulation response in heifers following the second of two spaced injections is more prompt and better synchronized than that following a single injection given at the appropriate stage of the cycle (Cooper, 1974; Leaver *et al.*, 1976; Johnson, 1978). The reason for this is not clear but Johnson (1978) has shown that animals treated once, on day 8 of the cycle, showed a similar pattern of heat onset to those treated twice with cloprostenol at an interval of 11 days. Heifers treated at other times in the luteal phase showed a more scattered and delayed response. It is well known that there is some follicular activity in the bovine ovary at this stage of the cycle (Rajakoski, 1960) and it is likely that these follicles will mature and ovulate if the developing luteal tissue is inhibited. It is likely that fixed-time inseminations will be more successful following two spaced injections than following a single injection. This point is illustrated by the well-synchronized pattern of LH release following the second injection of cloprostenol when compared to that following the first (Cooper and Rowson, 1975).

Whatever the technique used and whatever the class of stock employed, both trials and early field usage have left no doubt that adequate nutrition is essential if best results are to be obtained. Using a different synchronizing technique (norgestamet implants) Drew *et al.* (1976) have shown that feeding a supplement which provides an extra 20 MJ of metabolizable energy per day for 6 weeks before and after the synchronized inseminations results in about 15% improvement in conception rate over unsupplemented controls.

With early breeding of heifers in many modern intensive dairy herds, it is more important than ever to ensure that sufficient rate of growth and maturation is allowed by a carefully planned feeding policy. However, given a careful and informed approach to the controlled breeding of heifers, it is fair to say that the results from 3 years of field usage leave little cause for concern. Insemination figures from a recent survey (Waters and Ball, 1978) by the British Milk Marketing Board showed an overall conception rate of 57.9% in 3597 synchronized heifers. Apart from the desirability of artificially inseminating heifers, there are considerable benefits to be derived from feeding and managing in-calf heifers in batches and from knowing precisely when such heifers are due to enter the main herd for milking.

10.2.2 Controlled breeding of dairy cows

In most areas of the world where dairy cow production is on a reasonably modern or intensive basis, artificial insemination is an accepted and established method of breeding. Dairy cows are under regular supervision and heat detection is therefore a practical procedure. In spite of this, much of the early commercial use of prostaglandins has been in this class of stock because they provide the veterinarian and the farmer with an important management tool.

The importance of maintaining a regular optimum calving interval of 365 days (or a good calving to conception interval of 85–90 days) in dairy cows is well established. A recent calculation (R. J. Esslemont, 1979, personal communication) has shown that in the UK, failure to maintain this interval costs approximately £1.15 per day in lost profits. The most common cause of not maintaining optimum calving intervals is failure to inseminate the cow at the right time because of the difficulty of detecting heat at the correct post-partum interval. This applies particularly to large dairy units in the UK and USA where animals are managed in yard and parlour systems and supervised by a very small staff.

Control of ovulation in dairy cows may be applied to batches or to individual animals. The treatment of individual cows or small groups for non-detected heat is discussed in Section 10.2.3. Controlled breeding may be contemplated not only for the maintenance of good calving intervals, but also, in larger groups of cattle, for establishing and maintaining a particular calving pattern. This can be important in countries like the UK where milk prices vary with the season.

There are two main regimes of prostaglandin treatment for the synchronization of oestrus in batches of cows. The first is the classical two injection and two insemination regime described by Cooper (1974) and by Hafs *et al.* (1975).

As with heifers, fertility following this regime appears to be normal under commercial conditions (Christie and Medcalf, 1976; Weaver and Schultz, 1977; Esslemont *et al.*, 1977) although some reservations have been expressed about fertility in dairy cows (Leaver *et al.*, 1976).

Lamming and Bulman (1976), using a radioimmunoassay of progesterone in milk found that only approximately 7% of cows are unlikely to be cycling or will be cycling irregularly at around 50 days post-partum. These animals will be unable to respond in the expected manner. Baiyshya (1977) found a much higher incidence of abnormality in his small population of cows and prostaglandin treatment resulted in unacceptably low fertility. However, informed use of the drug in dairy practice produces good results (Eddy, 1978) (as with heifers), if careful attention is paid to nutrition. It is to be expected that the proportion of animals cycling irregularly (and therefore not responding properly) will be higher than in heifers since cows are often under considerable production stress.

The second regime used (and perhaps now preferred) has been described by Cooper (1978), Eddy (1978) and Weaver and Schultz (1977). The first injection of prostaglandin is given and cows are then inseminated as they come into heat over the next few days. Animals not detected in heat receive a second injection at 11 days and are inseminated twice, 72 h and 96 h later. This regime also provides a normal pregnancy rate and has the added benefit of requiring less prostaglandin and inseminations. The method is now commonly used in the UK for controlled breeding of both heifers and cows, and for the treatment of individuals or small groups which have not been detected in heat. In some areas of the world and under some circumstances of management (e.g. in New Zealand) the proportion of cows not cycling properly may be unacceptably high.

In order to avoid a wastage of drug and semen on animals which are unlikely to respond, a regime has been described involving several days heat detection and prostaglandin treatment only of those animals known to be cycling. The method may prove to be important where the breeding season is very short but artificial insemination is still considered essential.

Prostaglandins have proved versatile enough to be of use in the dairy cow under widely differing circumstances of management. It is encouraging to note that in the UK at least they are now an accepted part of dairy herd management and herd owners consider them an essential aid to profitable production.

10.2.3 Controlled breeding of beef cows

Heat detection in suckler beef cows, particularly those kept on extensive or ranching systems, is difficult or impossible. However, the desirability of using AI in such cows, to improve both the herd and quality of the offspring, is beyond doubt. It is for these reasons that the beef animal has always represented the primary target for controlled breeding techniques and they were used for much of the early trial work with $PGF_{2\alpha}$ and cloprostenol.

As with dairy cows, the benefits of controlled breeding go beyond the simple exploitation of artificial insemination, and there are considerable managemental benefits to be obtained from a successful programme. These include benefits of a tightly controlled calving pattern, batch rearing and marketing of high quality (genetically improved) calves, and a facility to feed the cows economically and to best effect. It is not easy to quantify these advantages since profitability in beef enterprises (in the UK at least) is the result of an interaction of a number of complex factors, including market fluctuations. Bailie and Dury (1976), however, have prepared a sophisticated computer model which has enabled them to calculate the financial benefits of controlled breeding in UK beef herds. The model has also enabled them to determine the level of success which is necessary to obtain a profit from synchronization and circumstances under which the exercise should not be considered. A similar model is in preparation to evaluate the benefits to the dairy herd (Bailie, 1979, personal communication). On the whole, however, commercial use of prostaglandins by beef farmers and ranchers has been disappointingly low. The slump in international beef prices in recent years has given little incentive for herd improvement.

Early work once again showed the need for proper nutrition (Cooper, 1975; Lauderdale, 1978). In many parts of the world good or even adequate feeding is not a feature of extensive beef management. As with heifers, inadequate feeding coupled with the stress or stimulus of suckling leads not only to low fertility following AI but also to ovarian inactivity in an unacceptably high propertion of animals. Such animals are clearly poor candidates for prostaglandin treatment.

Extensive field trials with both cloprostenol (Cooper *et al.*, 1976; Schultz *et al.*, 1977; Wilson, 1978) and $PGF_{2\alpha}$ (Hafs and Manns, 1975; Hafs *et al.*, 1978) have shown that, when handled correctly, the double injection, double insemination treatment yields normal fertility. However, in many beef herds normal or control fertility has been disappointingly low (Bailie *et al.*, 1977). A single insemination at 72 h following two prostaglandin injections has been reported to give consistently lower fertility (Cooper *et al.*, 1976), but attempts to tighten up the synchronization with oestradiol (Nancarrow, 1976; Peters *et al.*, 1977; Holness and Hurrell, 1977) or with GnRH (Hartl, 1974; Hoffman *et al.*, 1975a, 1975b) have not improved conception rate. Bailie and Dury (1976) have stated that controlled breeding in the UK is not economically viable in the beef herd under existing conditions unless the conception rate in the herd is at least 40%. Most herd owners would probably demand substantially more than this as recompense for their time, trouble and investment. Cooper *et al.* (1976) reported an average conception rate of 44% in trials involving 3810 beef cows. Similar results have recently been achieved in the USA using both cloprostenol (Wilson, 1978) and $PGF_{2\alpha}$ (Lauderdale, 1978).

It is therefore of great importance to ensure that controlled breeding programme in a beef herd is carried out with utmost care and is not attempted in situations where it is unlikely to succeed.

10.2.4 General considerations

A number of important points are worth considering if best results are to be obtained from any controlled breeding exercise.

(1) It is essential that the veterinarian and his client should discuss in detail the proposed programme to ensure that the most appropriate treatment regime is selected and that the objectives of the exercise are precisely clarified.

(2) It is important that the farmer should have a realistic appreciation of the results he is likely to obtain for his investment. Extensive trial work with controlled breeding techniques has given us a better appreciation of the true fertility of various classes of stock. The results likely to be achieved in terms of pregnancy rate or calving pattern must be clearly understood and must be capable of fulfilling the agreed objectives.

(3) No controlled breeding can succeed without careful attention to detailed planning. Trial experience and results have shown that such factors as the quality of semen and inseminators used, the stress on both inseminators and cattle, correct selection of cattle, provision of adequate staff and facilities and management of the cattle during controlled breeding period may all play a part in achieving optimum results. The acute importance of good nutritional planning and management has already been discussed and cannot be over-emphasized.

(4) Lastly, herd owners should be prepared to consider the benefits of controlled breeding over a number of years, and not expect a single programme to produce long-term objectives instantly.

When careful attention is paid to all these points, control of oestrus with prostaglandins can indeed profoundly benefit cattle breeding both at a local and a national level.

The major problem is a lack of ovarian cyclicity in the post-partum beef and dairy cow. It has been suggested (Roche, 1976) that combinations of short-term progesterone or progestagen treatments may be effective in overcoming this difficulty. Progesterone releasing intravaginal device (PRID, Abbott) is now on the market in some countries for the treatment of anoestrus. However, there is yet no good evidence that the technique is effective.

It would also be desirable to refine the timing of ovulation following prostaglandin treatment more precisely, so that only one insemination is required for normal fertility. Experience with GnRH or HCG is not promising and at present all our controlled breeding techniques rely for their efficacy upon the fact that follicular growth and maturation, and the appearance of heat and ovulation are a consistently timed and well-ordered series of biological events. Interference with this sequence does not appear to be a satisfactory method of increasing the precision of synchronization.

10.3 INDUCTION OF PARTURITION IN THE SOW

10.3.1 Introduction

The benefits of controlled farrowing in commercial pig breeding arise from the ability to farrow sows during normal working hours and to group these births on pre-determined days of the week. Piglet deaths in the pre-weaning period are a source of considerable economic loss to the industry and prediction of farrowing allows more convenient and detailed supervision during the critical peri-natal period. Piglets born in the foetal membranes can be attended immediately on delivery, small or weak piglets can be placed under a heat source to assist in drying out and prevent crushing by the sow. These can then be assisted to suckle and obtain the colostrum which is essential to protect them from neonatal disease. Sows likely to savage their young and dystocia can also be attended to more promptly and therefore to better effect.

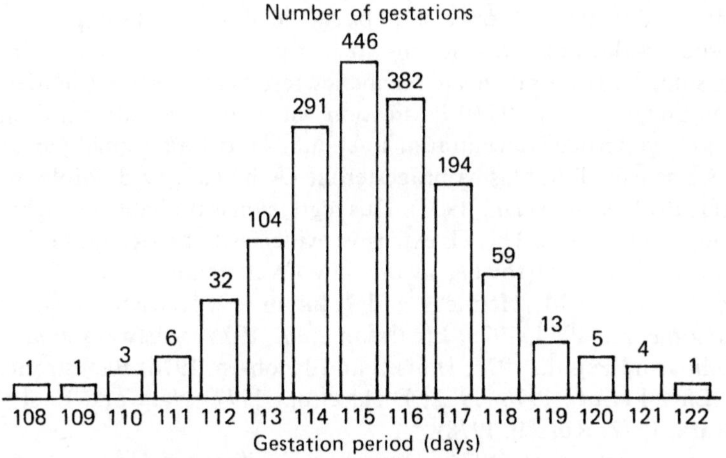

Figure 10.1 Frequency distribution of gestation period

Interfostering of piglets of similar weights and ages is facilitated, as is the performance of routine tasks such as injections, teeth and tail clipping, and cleaning and disinfection of farrowing accommodation. The grouping of farrowings can be timed to coincide with the requirements of the stockman and experienced personnel can be allocated to supervise farrowing. To the smaller farmer with an alternative enterprise, the convenience of this may be valued highly but to the large breeder it will provide better utilization of available labour.

To make optimal use of high-cost specialized buildings and equipment, a system of management has been evolved in modern pig farming in which sows are grouped together in batches for breeding and farrowing. The variation in gestation length presents problems for successful functioning of such a system. This variation is dependent not only upon breed but also upon managemental influences (Musson, 1951; Joubert, 1958; Cox, 1964a, 1964b; Bichard *et al.*, 1976). Figure 10.1 shows the distribution of gestation on a typical commercial pig farm (English *et al.*, 1977a).

The repeatability of gestation length is low (Musson, 1951; Cox, 1964a; Bichard *et al.*, 1976) and it is impossible to predict accurately when a sow will farrow by examining her previous records of gestation length. Neither are the signs of impending parturition in the sow easy to assess clinically, even by the most experienced stockman. Some control of farrowing is therefore desirable to facilitate more efficient management.

10.3.2 Physiological responses and results

During early pregnancy in the sow, plasma progesterone concentrations are high (Guthrie *et al.*, 1972) but fall to slightly lower levels during late gestation (Short, 1960). The progesterone is principally of ovarian origin although some placental and foetal synthesis cannot be excluded (Ash and Heap, 1975). The latter sources, however, provide insufficient progesterone to maintain pregnancy, since ovariectomy in late pregnancy results in abortion (du Mesnil du Buisson and Dauzier, 1957). Parturition will only occur after a decline in plasma progesterone concentrations. About 24 h before normal parturition, there is a sharp fall in plasma progesterone (Ash *et al.*, 1973; Molokwu and Wagner, 1973; Killian *et al.*, 1973). This regression is probably brought about by endogenous $PGF_{2\alpha}$. There is extensive evidence that exogenous $PGF_{2\alpha}$ will successfully induce farrowing in the sow (Wettemann *et al.*, 1974, 1977; Hallford *et al.*, 1974; Henricks and Handlin, 1974; Diehl *et al.*, 1974a; Robertson *et al.*, 1974, 1978; Einarsson *et al.*, 1975; Sugawara *et al.*, 1976; Wierzchos and Pejsak, 1976; Hansen and Jacobsen, 1976; Backström *et al.*, 1976; Envall *et al.*, 1976, 1977; Diehl *et al.*, 1977; Nara and First, 1977; Sugawara, 1977; Russell, 1978).

However, Diehl *et al.* (1974b), found no significant change in the time to onset of farrowing in animals receiving either 0, 5, or 10 mg of $PGF_{2\alpha}$ on day 111 or 112 of gestation.

Analogues of $PGF_{2\alpha}$ have also been successfully used to induce farrowing. Cloprostenol (ICI 80996) was shown to be effective at doses from 150 to 175μg (Bosc *et al.*, 1975; Bosc and Martinat-Botte, 1976; Hammond and Carlyle, 1976; Kostov *et al.*, 1977; Bosc *et al.*, 1977; Cerne and Nikolic, 1977; Walker, 1977; Herak *et al.*, 1977; Cerne, 1977; English *et al.*, 1977b; Einarsson *et al.*, 1978; Bonte, 1978, Herak *et al.*, 1978; Hammond, 1978a; Kostov *et al.*, 1978; Hansen, 1978). Other analogues have also been used (Ash and Heap, 1973; Downey *et al.*, 1976; Diallo, 1976).

Figure 10.2 shows the distribution of farrowing following a single injection of 175 μg of cloprostenol given to sows 1, 2, 3 or 4 days before term or expected farrowing date (Hammond, 1978b). Following injection, the peak time of onset of farrowing was around 26 h and 73% of animals commenced farrowing during the period 24 ± 5 h.

Fonda *et al.* (1977) compared the activity of 8 mg $PGF_{2\alpha}$, oestradiol

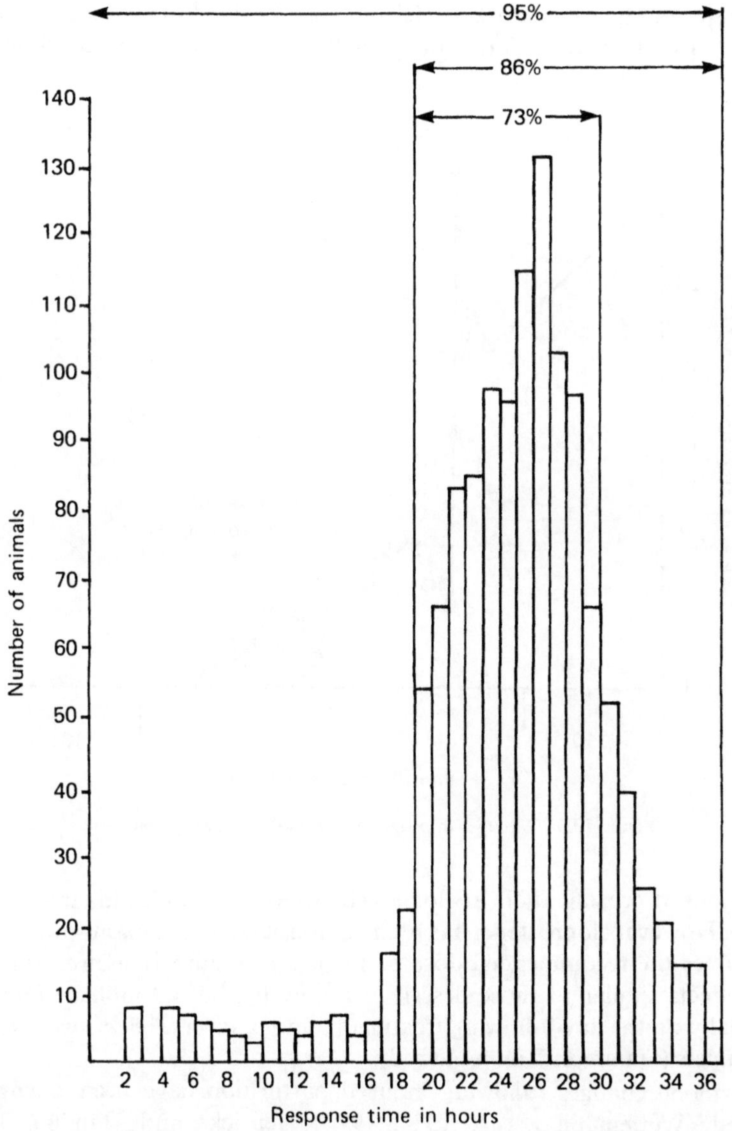

Figure 10.2 Distribution of farrowing: treated T-1, T-2, T-3 or T-4. Total 1355 animals

cypionate + $PGF_{2\alpha}$, and 175 μg cloprostenol, and found that cloprostenol was the most effective. Similarly, Bonte *et al.* (1978) compared 15 or 20 mg $PGF_{2\alpha}$ with 175 μg cloprostenol and showed that cloprostenol produced more predictable onset of farrowing. No side-effects were noted following cloprostenol injection. However, $PGF_{2\alpha}$-treated sows experienced side-effects of diarrhoea and behavioural changes such as scratching with the forelegs, biting and high excitation. Similar side-effects within 1 h of injection of $PGF_{2\alpha}$ have been reported by other workers (Diehl *et al.*, 1974a; Robertson *et al.*, 1974, 1978; Russell, 1978). Transient side-effects have been noted following

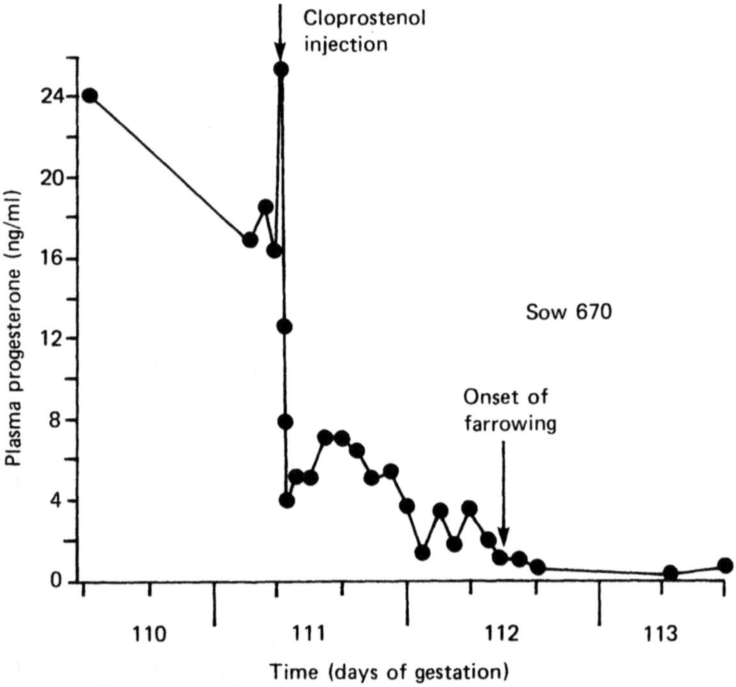

Figure 10.3 Changes in progesterone levels following treatment

injections of prostaglandin analogues (Downey *et al.*, 1976; Einarsson *et al.*, 1978). However cloprostenol has been administered to pregnant sows at up to 160 times the recommended dose of 175 μg. The animals showed transient side-effects similar to those described for $PGF_{2\alpha}$ but all animals farrowed normally on the day following treatment and no adverse effects were seen in the piglets (Hammond, unpublished).

Hormone changes following induced parturition have been extensively studied (Wettemann *et al.*, 1974, 1977; Henricks and Handlin, 1974; Gustafsson *et al.*, 1976b; Diehl *et al.*, 1974; Bonte *et al.*, 1978).

All authors report a rapid fall in plasma progesterone concentrations following injection of $PGF_{2\alpha}$ or its analogue in those sows which were successfully induced. Figure 10.3 shows the changes in plasma progesterone following intramuscular injection of 175 μg of cloprostenol to a sow on day 111 of gestation (Furr and Hammond, unpublished). Progesterone concentrations declined very sharply following injection and the sow commenced farrowing 28 h later when the progesterone had fallen to around 1 ng/ml.

Induction of parturition with prostaglandins does not increase the incidence of dystocia or uterine inertia and induced farrowings appear to follow the normal pattern. However, several workers have reported higher than normal piglet mortality (Hammond and Carlyle, 1976; Downey *et al.*, 1976; Bosc and Martinat-Botte, 1976; Walker, 1977; Einarsson *et al.*, 1978). The conclusions to be drawn from these data and the results of world-wide trials using cloprostenol (Hammond, unpublished) are that sows can be treated with prostaglandin within 48 h of the expected farrowing date without adverse effect on piglet survival. However, if parturition is induced outside these limits, higher piglet mortality may occur under some management conditions. The limiting factor in this may be the birth weight of the piglets. Several authors report a decrease in piglet birth weight following induction of parturition (Bosc and Martinat-Botte, 1976; Einarsson *et al.*, 1978).

Einarsson *et al.* (1978) reported that serum protein concentrations in induced piglets were as high as in piglets born naturally. It would therefore appear that uptake of colostrum is not affected by the piglets' slight prematurity. Following induced parturition there is no adverse effect on the subsequent breeding performance of the treated sow.

There is some evidence to suggest that a reduction in the incidence of mastitis, metritis, agalactia syndrome (MMA) may occur in herds in which parturition is induced routinely (Einarsson *et al.*, 1975; Backström *et al.*, 1976). However other workers did not find any significant effect of treatment (Hansen and Jacobsen, 1976; Hansen, 1978).

10.3.3 Conclusions

The demands of different management systems and herd sizes will vary considerably. It may be considered strategic to allow most sows to farrow normally and only induce those expected at the weekend, or it may be preferable to induce batches of sows on two or three predetermined days of each week. Prostaglandins offer the pig farmer a flexibility of approach and an important aid to his management and organization which was not previously available.

The dangers of inducing parturition at the wrong time or under sub-optimal conditions have been emphasized. As with the use of prostaglandins in cattle, best results and most financial benefit will only be obtained where herd records are good and herd management is of a high standard.

10.3.4 Prostaglandins and the cyclical porcine corpus luteum

In the domestic sow the corpora lutea are insensitive to the luteolytic action of prostaglandins for the first 10–12 days of the oestrous cycle. Diehl and Day (1974) found that 2 or 5 mg of prostaglandin $PGF_{2\alpha}$ injected into the uterus on day 10, or by intramuscular injection on day 12, had no significant effect on luteal function in gilts, as judged by progesterone changes and the interval to oestrus following treatment. Hallford *et al.* (1975) administered four injections of 20 mg $PGF_{2\alpha}$ in gilts at 12 h intervals starting on day 4 or 12 of the oestrous cycle and found that plasma progesterone was not affected in those gilts treated on day 4. However in gilts treated on day 12 the decline in the plasma progesterone level was more rapid than in untreated gilts, and the oestrous cycle was shortened by about 1½ days. This suggests that treatment with prostaglandin on days 12 and 13 of the oestrous cycle will hasten luteal regression. Connor *et al.* (1975, 1976) also showed that the oestrous cycle could be shortened by an average of 1.7 days in gilts given a single intramuscular injection of 20 mg $PGF_{2\alpha}$ on day 12 of the cycle, while treatment on day 9 or day 10 caused only a temporary decrease in progesterone levels. Side-effects, including increased respiratory rate, defaecation, shivering and other signs of discomfort were observed in these animals soon after treatment. Gleeson (1974a) obtained a temporary reduction in plasma progesterone concentration following treatment of gilts with 20 mg $PGF_{2\alpha}$ on day 9 or day 12 but oestrous cycle lengths were not altered by treatment. Douglas and Ginther (1975) treated gilts with 10 mg or 20 mg $PGF_{2\alpha}$ on day 12 of the oestrous cycle and, at necropsy on day 16 of the oestrous cycle, the weights of corpora lutea from treated gilts were significantly less than those of untreated gilts.

Krzymowski *et al.* (1978) found histological changes in the corpora lutea and reduced plasma progesterone levels following infusion of 1.5 mg of $PGF_{2\alpha}$ into the anterior uterine vein of sows over a 10 h period. Infusion on day 6 inhibited the normal growth of corpora lutea and prevented the rise in plasma progesterone usually observed at this stage of the cycle. Progesterone levels in sows treated on days 8 and 10 decreased only slightly, but fell rapidly in sows treated on days 12, 14 and 15 of the cycle. Synthetic analogues of $PGF_{2\alpha}$ have also been used to induce oestrus. Guthrie and Polge (1976a) using ICI 79 939 were unable to induce oestrus in gilts treated before day 11. Oestrus could be induced in some gilts given 0.25 mg or 0.5 mg on day 12 and in all gilts given 0.5 mg on day 12 and again on day 13. Temporary decreases in plasma progesterone were observed in gilts given multiple doses of 0.5 mg starting on day 8 of the cycle. In gilts treated on days 12 and 13, plasma progesterone fell rapidly during the first 24 h.

It is apparent from most of the work outlined above that porcine corpora lutea will not regress in response to exogenous prostaglandins until days 11–12 of the cycle. The effective period of sensitivity is therefore too short for prostaglandins to be used alone to control the porcine cycle.

Attempts have been made to synchronize oestrus by treating gilts in which the life-span of the corpus luteum has been prolonged by daily injections of oestrogen (Kraeling *et al.*, 1975; Guthrie, 1975) and by treating gilts with accessory corpora lutea induced by gonadotrophic hormones (Guthrie and Polge, 1976b). More recently, a short-term progestagen (norethandrolone) regime followed by cloprostenol injection has been described (Martinat-Botte *et al.*, 1977a, 1977b) with promising results on fertility. However, none of these regimes can at present be considered of practical value.

Further work is needed to define more clearly the changes which must occur in the pig's corpus luteum late in the cycle or during early pregnancy (Diehl and Day, 1974; Kraeling and Rampacek, 1977; Guthrie and Polge, 1978) which make it sensitive to prostaglandins known to be luteolytic in other species.

10.4 THERAPEUTIC APPLICATIONS IN CATTLE

10.4.1 Non-detected oestrus (sub-oestrus, anoestrus)

The terms non-detected oestrus (NDO) or non-visible oestrus (NVO) are used to describe the condition of any cow not inseminated by the desired post-partum interval. A small proportion of these animals (Bulman and Lamming, 1976) may lack ovarian activity but the great majority usually have regular cyclical ovarian activity, but have not been seen in heat. The terms 'sub-oestrus' or 'silent heat' are also used, suggesting that in some animals the symptoms of oestrus may be very mild or absent. The incidence of abnormally prolonged persistence of the corpus luteum in the cow, without uterine abnormalities or palpable contents in the uterus is very low (Zemjanis *et al.*, 1969). Bulman and Lamming (1976) found only 1.5% incidence of prolonged luteal activity in 300 non-pregnant lactating dairy cattle. Thus, the primary problem appears to be failure to detect heat in normal cycling cattle. Many factors contributing to this failure have been reviewed (Zemjanis *et al.*, 1969; King *et al.*, 1976; Williamson *et al.*, 1972) and these reports indicate that the incidence of this problem may be as high as 40–50% in some herds.

Various treatments and management schemes have been used to combat this problem, including hormone therapy (oestrogens and FSH), heat mount detectors, tail painting, constant observation, nutritional supplementation, and marker bulls. These have provided varying degrees of success. Although prostaglandins of the $F_{2\alpha}$ series can be used for several indications, exploitation of their luteolytic properties for the purpose of solving the problem of non-detected oestrus probably represents the greatest value of this drug for the dairy herd owner.

Cooper *et al.* (1976) and Jackson and Cooper (1976) reported that 84.5% of 232 cows which had not been detected in oestrus responded within 7 days following treatment with cloprostenol. Prior to treatment a corpus luteum was detected by rectal palpation. Cooper *et al.* (1976) also reported a conception rate of 57% in the animals detected in oestrus and inseminated following treatment. DeKruif and Brand (1976) reported similar results in 111 out of 150 (74%) sub-oestrous cows detected and bred following prostaglandin treatment. In this study either 500 μg cloprostenol or 25 mg $PGF_{2\alpha}$ was used. The average interval from treatment to breeding in the treated group was 8.8 days. Brand *et al.* (1976) suggested that the rather long interval may reflect a marginal dose of $PGF_{2\alpha}$ when used in lactating animals. The conception rate for the animals bred following treatment was normal.

Eddy (1977) found that 169 out of 253 (66.8%) cows given 500 μg cloprostenol for non-visible oestrus were detected in oestrus within 8 days of treatment. Of these, 159 were inseminated and 87 (54.7%) conceived. Thus, 36.5% of the treated animals became pregnant after induced oestrus. Kupfer (1977) reported similar results, 54% of cows treated for non-detected oestrus responded within 2–6 days and 65% of these conceived, yielding a pregnancy rate of 35% of those treated. In the study reported by Leidl *et al.* (1977) 81% of 98 treated cows responded within 4 days following 500 μg cloprostenol treatment. Of these 29 out of 54 (53.7%) conceived.

Seguin *et al.* (1978) compared 500 μg cloprostenol with a placebo in the treatment of unobserved oestrus. In the cloprostenol group 66% and 13% in the placebo group were detected in oestrus within 5 days after treatment. Both groups had 44% conception rate yielding 31% and 5% pregnancies, respectively.

All these studies confirm that induced oestrus is not easier to detect than a non-induced oestrus. Thus, the success of treatment still depends to a large extent on the ability of the herdsman to detect oestrus. Too many of the induced heat periods were still missed.

Table 10.1 Reproductive performance of cattle treated for sub-oestrus with saline (control) and cloprostenol (ICI 80 996)

	I *Saline control*	*II* *Cloprostenol and bred at oestrus*	*III* *Cloprostenol and bred at 72 h and 96 h*
Number on trial (5 days)	122	454	177
Number inseminated in 5 days	23 (18.9%)*	333 (73.3%)*	177 (100%)
Number pregnant in 5 days	12	151	89
Conception rate (5 days)	52.2% NS	45.3% NS	50.3%
Per cent of trial animals pregnant in 5 days	9.8%*	33.3%*	50.3%

* Statistically significant ($p < 0.001$)
NS = Not statistically significant

Cooper *et al.* (1976) treated 17 silent heat animals with 500 μg cloprostenol and bred them at fixed times of 72 h and 96 h after the injection; 10 (59%) became pregnant. Seguin *et al.* (1978) used cows classed as 'sub-oestrous' and treated with 500 μg cloprostenol to compare breeding at the induced oestrus with fixed-time breeding at 72 h and 96 h. The number pregnant within 5 days post-treatment was in favour of the fixed-time bred group (59% vs. 40%). More semen was used for the double-insemination group but this was offset by savings in days to first service and number pregnant. Schultz (1978) expanded the numbers with multilocation trials using the same trial plan. The results are given in Table 10.1.

Another approach which is being commonly employed by practitioners, particularly in the United Kingdom (Eddy, 1978; Cooper, 1978) is to treat non-detected animals (provided they have a palpably mature corpus luteum) with prostaglandin, observe them closely, and breed those detected in oestrus.

Eleven days later animals not detected and bred are re-treated with a second prostaglandin injection and bred at fixed times of 72 h and 96 h. This regime is the same as used in controlled breeding programmes for both beef and dairy cattle (Weaver and Schultz, 1977; Cooper, 1978).

It must be recognized that successful use of prostaglandins for the treatment of non-detected oestrus requires accurate diagnosis of the condition. This involves intelligent study of reproductive records, accurate rectal palpation and good scientific judgement. It is especially important to determine that the animal is not pregnant since prostaglandins are potent abortifacient drugs. Used properly, they are very effective in the management of this condition.

10.4.2 Pyometra (chronic purulent endometritis)

Damage to the reproductive tract at calving or post-partum retention of the placenta frequently leads to infection and inflammation of the uterus. Acute or sub-acute endometritis occurring within 3 weeks of parturition may require both local and systemic antibiotic treatment which often results in resolution of the condition. However, under certain circumstances, the endometritis may resist routine treatment and progress until the uterus becomes distended with purulent material. This is referred to as chronic endometritis or pyometra and is usually accompanied by persistence of the corpus luteum probably caused by a failure of the normal luteolytic mechanism.

Persistently elevated plasma progesterone concentrations associated with prolonged life of the corpus luteum render the uterus more susceptible to infection and damage (Rowson *et al.*, 1953). The condition may be characterized by intermittent purulent discharge but usually there is a closed cervix with no visible discharge. The affected animals are obviously anoestrous and upon rectal palpation, a variable amount of fluid can be detected in the uterus. This is occasionally confused with a normal pregnancy.

The logical approach to therapy is to induce an oestrus. This causes relaxation of the cervix and contractions of the uterine muscle which in turn result in emptying of the uterus. Manual enucleation of the corpus luteum has been employed with some success. However, the persistent corpus luteum is often very difficult to express and attempts to do so may result in haemorrhage leading to salpingitis, adhesions, and reduced fertility. Oestrogens have been used with variable success, but often lead to cystic ovaries.

In cases of pyometra, prostaglandins of the $F_{2\alpha}$ series have proven effective in causing regression of the persistent corpus luteum, induction of oestrus, emptying of the uterus and resolution of the problem. Several reports describing prostaglandin therapy for pyometra have appeared in the literature during the past 3 years. All have demonstrated high rates of efficacy. Cooper *et al.* (1976) reported a response rate of 91% in 43 cases treated intramuscularly with 500 μg cloprostenol.

Jackson and Cooper (1976) reported similar success (93% of 82 cases) as more numbers were treated. Gustafsson *et al.* (1976a) reported a success rate of 84.6% using doses of 5, 12, 15, and 25 mg $PGF_{2\alpha}$ THAM salt. Wenkoff (1978) successfully treated all of 16 cases with 500 μg cloprostenol, and Coulson (1978) treated 55 cases using 25 mg $PGF_{2\alpha}$ THAM salt with 76.4% responding. More recently, Schultz (1978) reported results from eight trials in the United States in which 500 μg cloprostenol was compared to conventional treatment (usually oestrogen). The results are shown in Table 10.2.

Table 10.2 Prostaglandin treatment of bovine pyometra

	Conventional treatment	*500 μg cloprostenol i.m.*
Number on trial	69	200
Number of complete responses*	41 (59.4%)‡	176 (88.0%)
Number of partial responses†	11 (15.9%) NS	12 (6.0%)
Number of failures	17 (24.6%)‡	12 (6.0%)

* Uterus was completely empty and of normal consistency when re-examined
† Fluid was almost always gone but uterus was slow in returning to normal consistency
‡ Statistically significantly different ($p < 0.001$)
NS = Not statistically significantly different ($p > 0.05$)
Pregnancy rates following treatment have been normal or near normal indicating good recovery of the reproductive tract

10.4.3 Unwanted pregnancy and induction of abortion in the 'feedlot' heifer

In the bovine the corpus luteum is necessary for the maintenance of pregnancy until an ill-defined stage of 150–210 days (Cooper and Walpole, 1975). Destruction or removal of the corpus luteum prior to this time results in abortion. Since prostaglandins are potent luteolytic agents, they are very effective for induction of abortion in cattle prior to 150 days. The abortion is usually accomplished with ease and without complications.

The most frequent indication for induction of abortion in dairy cattle is when young heifers are accidentally served by a neighbour's bull. Most are too young and underdeveloped to carry the calf to term and normal delivery. Alternatively the heifer (or cow) may be accidentally bred to a bull not desired for that particular mating.

In the beef industry the pregnant heifer entering the feedlot is a well-recognized cause of economic loss. These losses are related to a reduction in the price paid by purchasers for heifers in advanced pregnancy. The heifers may spend from 90 to 180 days or longer in the feedlot before they are ready for slaughter. Thus, some may calve in the feedlot which leads to many difficulties including dystocia, retained placenta, acute metritis, and peritonitis which may result either in death or a severe setback in the feeding of the animal. Also, it is generally accepted that pregnant heifers don't fatten as well as non-pregnant heifers. In North America this indication for induction of abortion is of considerable economic importance.

Lauderdale (1972) reported that injection of $PGF_{2\alpha}$ THAM salt in doses of 45 or 150 mg invariably induced an abortion in cattle while three of six cows aborted when treated with 15 or 30 mg. Lamond *et al.* (1973) produced abortion in two cows infused with 16.8 mg or 28 mg $PGF_{2\alpha}$ directly into the uterine artery. Brand *et al.* (1975b) aborted 10 out of 10 heifers (2–5 months pregnant) with intramuscular injections of 12.5 mg or 25 mg $PGF_{2\alpha}$ on 2 consecutive days. Millar (1974) aborted 15 heifers (29 to 52 days pregnant) with subcutaneous injections of 15 or 30 mg $PGF_{2\alpha}$ while Refsal *et al.* (1976) produced abortion in 20 heifers (35 to 80 days pregnant) with a single intramuscular dose of 20 or 40 mg $PGF_{2\alpha}$.

Using 500 µg cloprostenol, Jackson and Cooper (1976) reported 100% successful induction of abortion within 7 days in 32 animals treated prior to 150 days of gestation. At gestation between 150 and 200 days, 12 out of 33 (37%) aborted within 7 days, 20 took longer than 7 days, and one did not abort. Similar results have been reported by Jackson (1977a).

Fields *et al.* (1977) treated Brahman crossbred heifers at 60, 90 and 120 days of gestation with 250, 375, or 500 µg cloprostenol. A total of 100 out of 107 animals aborted; those in the 60-day gestation stage aborting earlier and developing new corpora lutea sooner than animals at 90 and 120 days. All abortions were uncomplicated. Youngquist *et al.* (1977) found cloprostenol to be effective in feedlot heifers at a dose of 250 µg up to 120 days of gestation whereas 500 µg was required from 120–150 days of gestation. They also made an interesting suggestion that concomitant treatment with 0.5 (mg/head)/day melgenestrol acetate reduced the efficacy of the cloprostenol.

In further dose titration work with cloprostenol using feedlot heifers 50–150 days pregnant Copeland *et al.* (1978) found single doses of 375 and 500 µg cloprostenol significantly more effective (in 94.2% and 96.8%) than doses of 62.5, 125 and 250 µg (in 59.3%, 63.3% and 76%) regardless of stage of gestation. Subsequent work (Schultz, unpublished) has suggested that efficacy of cloprostenol for induction of abortion may be affected by the concomitant treatments and stress which is typical in animals entering feedlots. Further, Schultz and Wilson (1978) using heifers (with known breeding dates) between 114 and 140 days pregnant found concomitant treatment with 375 μg cloprostenol with intranasal vaccination for IBR and PI_3, intramuscular vaccination with Pasteurella bacterin, intramuscular vitamins A, D, and E and treatment with coumaphos insecticide did not reduce the abortifacient efficacy of cloprostenol. However, a reduced efficacy was seen when coumaphos was administered 7 days prior to cloprostenol.

Kelley *et al.* (1978a) have reported both reduced efficacy and increased complications with 500 μg cloprostenol as an abortifacient in cows more than 5 months pregnant.

Seguin *et al.* (1978) reported similar findings in animals in the second trimester of pregnancy (although they also found cloprostenol more effective than oestrogen at this stage of gestation) while Day (1977) found a dramatic reduction in efficacy of cloprostenol in heifers over 150 days of gestation. In late pregnancy (245 days) he found increased efficacy in animals that had been treated with dexamethasone 8–11 days previous to cloprostenol treatment. It appears that after the 250th day of gestation, abortion (or parturition induction) is possible using prostaglandins, although this is not so between the 150th and 250th days. Whether increased dosage or repeated treatment will enhance the efficacy during this period has not been adequately studied.

10.4.4 Parturition induction in cattle

It is speculated that an effective means for induction of parturition could result in a reduction in calving loss and labour costs by making the calving period shorter and more predictable (Henricks *et al.*, 1977). Further indications include the induction of early or prompt calving in large breeds or crosses (to avoid distocias), and early calving (as in New Zealand) to utilize a short grass season for the production of cheap milk. Most of the work in the induction of parturition has been carried out with adrenal corticoids and their analogues. A consistent problem has been an increased incidence of retained placenta leading to lowered fertility.

Henricks *et al.* (1977) found that 30 mg $PGF_{2\alpha}$ THAM salt significantly reduced the gestation length in Hereford heifers treated on day 267 of pregnancy. Again, an increase in the incidence of retained placenta was noted as well as dystocia and reduced udder development. Zerobin *et al.* (1973) have suggested that prostaglandins do not induce sufficient myometrial contractions for normal labour.

Seguin *et al.* (1978) reported variable success using 500 μg cloprostenol at 273 and 277 days of gestation. The incidence of retained placenta was 57% and 42% respectively. Kelley *et al.* (1978b, 1978c) reported more consistent results but also encountered retained placenta as a sequela of the treatment. Further investigations into the mechanisms of parturition and the role prostaglandins play are necessary before their full potential for this indication is realized. An excellent review of the topic has been published by First (1978).

10.4.5 Other therapeutic indications

Although not frequently encountered, the mummified or macerated foetus has been a problem for the veterinary practitioner. Such cases have been traditionally treated with oestrogens with variable success. For successful treatment of this condition 30 mg $PGF_{2\alpha}$ or 500 μg cloprostenol appears to be effective (Brand *et al.*, 1976; Jackson and Cooper, 1976; Jackson, 1977b; Wenkoff, 1978; Schultz, 1978; Uwland, 1978). The success rate reported by these authors is high with good fertility subsequent to treatment. Frequently, the mummified foetus will be forced into the vaginal canal and moderate traction is required to complete delivery.

Cystic ovarian degeneration in the cow takes several forms. Cysts may be singular and thick walled, with luteal tissue (luteal cysts), or multiple with varying degree of luteal tissue in the wall of the cyst (follicular cysts). The luteal tissue produces progesterone which results in a high incidence of anoestrus associated with the condition. Regression of the luteal tissue with prostaglandins can be expected to resolve the problem in many cases.

Using 500 μg cloprostenol, Jackson and Cooper (1976) reported a response in 78 out of 91 cases treated. These included both luteal and follicular cysts as determined by rectal palpation and reproductive history. Eddy (1977) treated 16 cases of luteinized ovarian cysts with 500 μg cloprostenol. Thirteen were detected in oestrus in 8 days, 12 of which were bred and seven conceived. In total, 14 out of the 16 conceived with a mean interval from treatment to conception of 19.4 days. Schultz (1978) found that 17 out of 18 animals with a luteal cyst responded to 500 μg cloprostenol.

References

Allen, W. R. and Rowson, L. E. A. (1973). Control of the mare's oestrous cycle by prostaglandins. *J. Reprod. Fertil.*, **33**, 539

Allen, W. R., Stewart, F., Cooper, M. J., Crowhurst, R. C., Simpson, D. J., McEnery, R. J., Greenwood, R. E. S., Rossdale, P. D. and Ricketts, S. W. (1974). Further studies on the use of synthetic prostaglandin analogues for inducing luteolysis in mares. *Equine Vet. J.*, **6**, 31

Ash, R. W., Banks, P., Bailes, G., Broad, S. and Heap, R. B. (1973). Plasma oestrogen, progesterone and corticoid concentrations in the pregnant, parturient and lactating sow. *J. Reprod. Fertil.*, **33**, 359

Ash, R. W. and Heap, R. B. (1973). The induction and synchronization of parturition in sows treated with ICI 79 939, an analogue of prostaglandin $F_{2\alpha}$. *J. Agric. Sci.*, **81**, 365

Ash, R. W. and Heap, R. B. (1975). Oestrogen, progesterone and corticosteroid concentrations in peripheral plasma of sows during pregnancy, parturition, lactation and after weaning. *J. Endocrinol.*, **64**, 141

Backström, L., Einarsson, S., Gustafsson, B. and Larsson, K. (1976). Prostaglandin $F_{2\alpha}$-induced parturition for prevention of the agalactia syndrome in the sow. *Proc. 4th Congr. Int. Pig. Vet. Soc.* Iowa, 22–24 June

Bailie, J. H. and Dury, N. S. (1976). The economic implications of the use of 'Estrumate' (ICI 80996, cloprostenol) in the control of the bovine oestrous cycle – the beef suckler herd. *Proc. 8th Int. Congr. Animal Reproduction and A.I.* Krakow, 12–16 July

Bailie, J. H., Dury, N. S. and Norman, J. A. (1977). The significance of herd conception rate in the economics of beef suckler cow management. *Anim. Prod.*, **24** (Abstr.), 130

Baiyshya, N. (1977). Ph.D. Thesis, Reading University

Bichard, M., Stork, M. G., Rickatson, S. and Pease, A. H. R. (1976). The use of synchronized farrowing in large pig units. *Winter Mtg. British Soc. Anim. Prod.* Harrogate, 16 March

Bonte, P. (1978). A parturition programme to everyone's liking. *Sterility Committee Conference.* Ghent, 19 May

Bonte, P., Coryn, M. and Spincemaille, J. (1978). Induction of parturition in multiparous sows: Clinical and endocrinological aspects. *Vl. Diergeneesk. Tijd.*, **47**, 188

Bosc, M. J., Martinat-Botte, F. and Duchene, P. (1975). Induction de la mise bas de la truie par un analogue de la prostaglandine $F_{2\alpha}$. *Ann. Zootech.*, **24**, 661

Bosc, M. J. and Martinat-Botte, F. (1976). Induction de la parturition chez la truie au moyen de prostaglandines. *Econ. Med. Anim.*, **17**, 235

Bosc, M. J., Martinat-Botte, F., Grouzelle, G. and Hurault, B. (1977). Use of prostaglandins at the time of parturition in the sow. Results in field conditions. *Ann. Zootech.*, **26**, 445

Brand, A., DeBois, C. H. W., Kommerij, R. and DeJong, M. P. (1975b). Induction of abortion in cattle with prostaglandin $F_{2\alpha}$ and estradiol valerate. *Tijd. Diergeneesk.*, **100**, 432

Brand, A., DeBois, C. H. W. and Vandenhende, R. (1975a). Indications for prostaglandins in the field of reproduction in farm animals. *Tijd. Diergeneesk.*, **100**, 191

Brand, A., Trounson, A. O. and Straver, G. M. (1976). The use of prostaglandins in animal breeding. II. Clinical indications for the use of prostaglandins in cattle and pigs. *Diergeneesk. Memo.*, **23 (516)**, 163

Britt, J. H., Hafs, H. D. and Stevenson, J. S. (1978). Oestrus in relation to time of administration of $PGF_{2\alpha}$ to heifers. *J. Dairy Sci.*, **61**, 513

Bulman, D. C. and Lamming, G. E. (1976). Diagnosis of sub-fertility in lactating cows by measurement of milk progesterone levels. *Proc. 8th Int. Congr. Animal Reproduction and A.I.* Krakow, 12–16 July

Cerne, F. (1977). Induction of farrowing with cloprostenol in a commercial pig breeding farm. *Vet. Rec.*, **101**, 17 September (Abstr.), 238

Cerne, F. and Nikolic, P. (1977). Primena sintetickog prostaglandina-cloprostenola u indukciji I sinhronizaciji partusa krmaca. *Vet. Glasnik.*, **7**, 499

Christian, R. E. and Casida, L. E. (1948). The effects of progesterone in altering the oestrous cycle of the cow. *J. Anim. Sci.*, **7** (Abstr.), 540

Christie, E. H. L. and Medcalf, J. D. (1976). Observations on the use of cloprostenol in a large diary herd in Cheshire. *Vet. Rec.*, **99**, 272

Chupin, D., Pelot, J. and Mauleon, P. (1977). Control of oestrus and ovulation in dairy cows. *Theriogenology*, **7**, 339

Connor, L., Phillips, G. D. and Palmer, W. M. (1975). Effect of prostaglandin $F_{2\alpha}$ on the cycling gilt. *Can. J. Anim. Sci.*, **55**, 788

Connor, L., Phillips, G. D. and Palmer, W. M. (1976). Effects of prostaglandin $F_{2\alpha}$ on the oestrous cycle and hormone levels in the gilt. *Can. J. Anim. Sci.*, **56**, 661

Cooper, M. J., Dobson, H. and Furr, B. J. A. (1974). Endocrine changes in Friesian heifers during luteolysis and oestrus synchronization with ICI 80996, a synthetic analogue of $PGF_{2\alpha}$. *J. Steroid Biochem.*, **5** (Abstr. 449), 403

Cooper, M. J. (1974). Control of oestrous cycles of heifers with a synthetic prostaglandin analogue. *Vet. Rec.*, **95**, 200

Cooper, M. J. (1975). Synchronization of oestrous and ovulation in cattle. Ph.D Thesis. C.N.A.A./University of Liverpool

Cooper, M. J. and Rowson, L. E. A. (1975). Control of the oestrous cycle in Fresian heifers with ICI 80 996, a synthetic prostaglandin analogue structurally related to PGF_2. *Ann. Biol. Anim. Biochim. Biophys.*, **15**, 427

Cooper, M. J. and Walpole, A. L. (1975). Practical applications of prostaglandins in animal husbandry. In: S. Karim (ed.), *Adv. Prostaglandin Res. Prostaglandins and Reproduction*, p. 310

Cooper, M. J., Hammond, D., Harker, D. B. and Jackson, P. S. (1976). Control of the bovine oestrous cycle with ICI 80 996 (cloprostenol). Field results in 3810 beef cattle. *Proc. 8th Int. Congr. Animal Reproduction and A.I.* Krakow, 12–16 July

Cooper, M. J. (1977). Ovulation control in the cow. In: D. B. Crighton, N. B. Haynes, G. R. Forcroft and G. E. Lamming (eds.), *Control of Ovulation* (London: Butterworth)

Cooper, M. J. (1978). Application of proprostenol and synthetic prostaglandin analogue in the management of the post-partum dairy cow. *Proc. 10th Int. Conf. Buiatrics.* Mexico City. Abstract

Copeland, D. D., Schultz, R. H. and Kemtrup, M. E. (1978). Induction of abortion in feedlot heifers with cloprostenol (a synthetic analogue of prostaglandin $F_{2\alpha}$): A dose response study. *Can. Vet. J.*, **19**, 29

Coulson, A. (1978). Treatment of metritis in cattle with prostaglandin $F_{2\alpha}$. *Vet. Rec.*, **103**, 359

Cox, D. F. (1964a). Genetic variation in the gestation period of swine. *J. Anim. Sci.*, **23**, 746

Cox, D. F. (1964b). Relation of litter size and other factors to the duration of gestation in the pig. *J. Reprod. Fertil.*, **7**, 405

Day, A. M. (1977). Cloprostenol for termination of pregnancy in cattle. *N.Z. Vet. J.*, **25**, 136

DeKruif, A. and Brand, A. (1976). Behandeling van suboestrus bij runderen met prostaglandinen. *Tijd. Diergeneesk.*, **101**, 169

Deletang, F. (1975). Synchronization of oestrus in cattle using a progestogen (SC21009) and synthetic analogue of $PGF_{2\alpha}$ (cloprostenol). *Vet. Rec.*, **97**, 453

Diallo, T. (1976). Clinical experiences in the induction of parturition in the pig by means of a prostaglandin analogue. *Congr. Phys. Pathol. Reprod. Domest. Anim.* Hanover, 19–20 February

Diehl, J. R. and Day, B. N. (1974). Effect of prostaglandin $F_{2\alpha}$ on luteal function in swine. *J. Anim. Sci.*, **39**, 392

Diehl, J. R., Godke, R. A., Killian, D. B. and Day, B. N. (1974a). Induction of parturition in swine with prostaglandin $F_{2\alpha}$. *J. Anim. Sci.*, **38**, 1229

Diehl, J. R., Dziuk, P. J. and Baker, D. H. (1974b). Induced parturition in gilts with $PGF_{2\alpha}$ (THAM salt). *J. Anim. Sci.*, **39**, 988

Diehl, J. R., Baker, D. H. and Dzuik, P. J. (1977). Effect of $PGF_{2\alpha}$ on sow and litter performance during and following parturition. *J. Anim. Sci.*, **44**, 89

Douglas, R. H. and Ginther, O. J. (1975). Effects of prostaglandin $F_{2\alpha}$ on oestrus cycle or corpus luteum in mares and gilts. *J. Anim. Sci.*, **40** (3), 518

Downey, B. R., Conlon, P. D., Irvine, D. S. and Baker, R. D. (1976). Controlled farrowing programme using a prostaglandin analogue AY24655. *Can. J. Anim. Sci.*, **56**, 655

Drew, B., Wishart, D. F. and Thomason, D. (1976). The effect of nutrition on the fertility of dairy heifers. *Anim. Prod.*, **22** (Abstr. 20), 145

Eddy, R. G. (1977). Cloprostenol as treatment for no visible oestrus and cystic ovarian disease in dairy cows. *Vet. Rec.*, **100**, 62

Eddy, R. G. (1978). Therapeutic use of prostaglandins in dairy practice. *Proc. 10th World Congr. Buiatrics.* Mexico

Einarsson, S., Gustafsson, B. and Larsson, K. (1975). Prostaglandin-induced parturition in swine with some aspects on prevention of the MMA (Metritis, Mastitis, Agalactia) syndrome. *Nord. Vet. Med.*, **27**, 429

Einarsson, S., Envall, R. and Andren, B. (1978). Induced parturition in sows: effects upon serum protein patterns in the neonate. *5th World Congr. Hyology and Hyoiatrics.* Zagreb, 12–16 June

English, P. R., Smith, W. J. and MacLean, A. (1977a). *The Sow Improving her Efficiency*, p. 107, (Farming Press Ltd.)

English, P. R., Hammond, D., Davidson, F. M., Smith, W. J., Silver, C. L., Dias, M. F. M. and MacPherson, R. M. (1977b). Evaluation of an induced farrowing system using cloprostenol, a synthetic analogue of prostaglandin $F_{2\alpha}$. *Mtg. British Soc. Anim. Prod.* Harrogate, 21–25 March

Envall, R., Einarsson, S., Gustafsson, B. and Larsson, K. (1976). A field study of prostaglandin-induced parturition in the sow. *Proc. 4th Congr. Int. Pig. Vet. Soc.* Iowa, 22–24 June

Envall, R., Einarsson, S., Larsson, K., Hard, C., Segerstad, A. F. and Westerberg, L. (1977). Prostaglandin-induced parturition in swine – a field study on its accuracy after treatment with different amount of $PGF_{2\alpha}$. *Nord. Vet. Med.*, **29**, 376

Esslemont, R. J., Eddy, R. G. and Ellis, P. R. (1977). Planned breeding in autumn-calving dairy herds. *Vet. Rec.*, **100**, 426

Fields, M. J., Schultz, R. H., Bass, J. and Warnick, A. C. (1977). Abortion in beef heifers using cloprostenol (a $PGF_{2\alpha}$ analogue). *Mtg. of So. Div. Am. Soc. Anim. Sci.* Atlanta, Georgia (Abstr.)

First, N. L. (1978). Mechanisms controlling parturition in farm animals. *Beltsville Symposia in Agricultural Research. III. Animal Reproduction.* Beltsville, Maryland

Fonda, E. S., Thrasher, D. M. and Godke, R. A. (1977). Induced farrowing in swine with $PGF_{2\alpha}$ and prostaglandin analogue (ICI 80 996). *69th Ann. Mtg. Amer. Soc. Anim. Sci.* Madison, July

Fulka, J., Motlik, J. and Pavlok, A. (1978). Heat and conception rate after synchronization of oestrus with cloprostenol. *Vet. Rec.*, **103**, 52

Gleeson, A. R. (1974a). Luteal function in the cyclic sow after infusion of prostaglandin $F_{2\alpha}$ through a uterine vein. *J. Reprod. Fertil.*, **36**, 487

Gustafsson, B., Backström, G. and Edqvist, L. E. (1976a). Treatment of bovine pyometra with prostaglandin $F_{2\alpha}$: an evaluation of a field study. *Theriogenology*, **6**, 45

Gustafsson, B., Einarsson, S., Larsson, K. and Edqvist, L. E. (1976b). Sequential changes of estrogens and progesterone at prostaglandin-induced parturition in the sow. *Am. J. Vet. Res.*, **37**, 1017

Guthrie, H. D., Henricks, D. M. and Handlin, D. L. (1972). Plasma oestrogen, progesterone and luteinizing hormone prior to oestrus and during early pregnancy in pigs. *Endocrinology*, **91**, 675

Guthrie, H. D. (1975). Estrous synchronization and fertility in gilts treated with estradiol-benzoate and prostaglandin $F_{2\alpha}$. *Theriogenology*, **4**, 69

Guthrie, H. D. and Polge, C. (1976a). Luteal function and oestrus in gilts treated with a synthetic analogue of prostaglandin $F_{2\alpha}$ (ICI 79 939) at various times during the oestrus cycle. *J. Reprod. Fertil.*, **48**, 423

Guthrie, H. D. and Polge, C. (1976b). Control of oestrus and fertility in gilts with accessory corpora lutea by prostaglandin analogues, ICI 79 939 and ICI 80 996. *J. Reprod. Fertil.*, **48**, 427

Guthrie, H. D. and Polge, C. (1978). Treatment of pregnant gilts with a prostaglandin analogue, cloprostenol, to control oestrus and fertility. *J. Reprod. Fertil.*, **52**, 271

Hafs, H. D. and Manns, J. G. (1975). Onset of oestrus and fertility of dairy heifers and suckled beef cows treated with prostaglandin $F_{2\alpha}$. *Anim. Prod.*, **21**, 13

Hafs, H. D., Manns, J. G. and Drew, B. (1975). Onset of oestrus after prostaglandin $F_{2\alpha}$ in cattle. *Vet. Rec.*, **96**, 134

Hafs, H. D., Manns, J. G. and Wood, P. D. P. (1978). Fertility of heifers and suckled cows inseminated at pre-determined intervals after treatment with prostaglandin $F_{2\alpha}$. *J. Anim. Sci.*, **91**, 479

Hallford, D. M., Wettemann, R. P., Turman, E. J. and Omtvedt, I. T. (1975). Luteal function in gilts after prostaglandin $F_{2\alpha}$. *J. Anim. Sci.*, **41**, 1706

Hallford, D. M., Wettemann, R. P., Turman, E. J., Omtvedt, I. T., Kreider, D. L. and Welty, S. D. (1974). The influence of prostaglandin $F_{2\alpha}$ on oestrus cycle length and the induction of parturition in swine. *Oklahoma Agric. Expt. Stn. Anim. Sci. Res. Rep.*, 187

Hammond, D. and Carlyle, W. W. H. (1976). Controlled farrowing on commercial pig breeding units using cloprostenol – a synthetic analogue of prostaglandin $F_{2\alpha}$. *Proc. 8th Int. Congr. Animal Reproduction and A.I.* Krakow, 12–16 July

Hammond, D. (1978a). Comparative gestation length distribution following the use of cloprostenol to induce farrowing. *5th World Cong. Hyology and Hyoiatrics*. Zagreb, 12–16 June

Hammond, D. (1978b). Management factors related to induced farrowing. *Pig Veterinary Society Meeting*. Bedford, 20–22 November

Hansen, L. H. and Jacobsen, M. J. (1976). Incidence of MMA after prostaglandin-induced parturition. *Nord. Vet. Med.*, **28**, 357

Hansen, L. H. (1978). Reproductive efficiency and incidence of MMA after controlled farrowing using a prostaglandín analogue, cloprostenol. *Institut for Sterilitetsforskning: Annual Report*. Koebenhavn, **21**, 15

Hartl, M. (1974). Inaugural Dissertation, Munich University

Henricks, D. M., Rawlings, N. C., Ellicott, A. R., Dickey, J. F. and Hill, J. R. (1977). Use of prostaglandin $F_{2\alpha}$ to induce parturition in beef heifers. *J. Anim. Sci.*, **44**, 438

Henricks, D. M. and Handlin, D. L. (1974). Induction of parturition in the sow with prostaglandin $F_{2\alpha}$. *Theriogenology*, **1**, 7

Herak, M., Kovacevic, V., Korenic, I., Pivac, J., Dolovcak, Z. and Pavlovic, V. (1977). Sinkronizacija porodjaja u Krma ca Injekcijom prostaglandina. *2nd Yugoslav. Conf. Reprod. Domes. Anim.* Portoroz, October

Herak, M., Kovacevic, V., Culinovic, Z., Pivac, J. and Dolovcak, Z. (1978). Induction of parturition in sows with synthetic prostaglandin (cloprostenol). *5th World Cong. Hyology and Hyoiatrics*. Zagreb, 12–16 June

Hoffman, B., Grunert, E. and Seeger, K. (1975a). Indications for the use of synthetic hypothalamus hormones in animal production and veterinary medicine. *Acta Endocrinol.* (Suppl.), **193**, 166 (Abstr.)

Hoffman, B., Schams, D. and Karg, H. (1975b). Egg transfer in cattle. Cycle synchronization under hormonal control (ICI 80 996). *Agr. Res. Counc.*, **209**

Holness, D. H. and Hurrell, A. D. (1977). Fertility in cows after synchronization of oestrus with prostaglandin $F_{2\alpha}$ and oestradiol benzoate. *S. Afric. J. Anim. Sci.*, **7**, 27

Jackson, P. S. (1977a). Treatment of chronic post-partum endometritis in cattle with cloprostenol. *Vet. Rec.*, **101**, 441

Jackson, P. S. and Cooper, M. J. (1976). The use of cloprostenol (ICI 80 996) in the treatment of infertility in cattle. *Presented at World Ass. for Buiatrics*, 6–9 September, 903

Jackson, P. S. (1977b). The use of cloprostenol for the termination of pregnancy and the expulsion of mummified foetus in cattle. *Vet. Rec.*, **100**, 361

Jeffcot, L. and Rossdale, P. D. (1977). A critical review of current methods for induction of parturition in the mare. *Equine Vet. J.*, **9**, 208

Johnson, C. (1978). Time to onset of oestrus after the injection of heifers with cloprostenol. *Vet. Rec.*, **103**, 204

Joubert, D. M. (1958). Duration of pregnancy and length of the dioestrus cycle in the domestic pig. *S. Afric. J. Sci.*, **54**, 183

Karg, H., Hartl, M., Hoffman, B., Schams, D., Schmidt, W., Gunzler, O., Huber, E. and Muller, S. (1976). Versuche mit einem prostaglandinanalog zur zyklus-synchronization bein rint unter hormonanalytischer und klinischer kontrolle. *Zuchthygienne*, **11**, 7

Kelley, J. S., Morrison, D. G., Loyacano, A. F., Ingraham, R. H. and Godke, R. A. (1978b). Induced calving in beef cattle with a new prostaglandin analogue (cloprostenol). *Proceedings of the 18th Annual Livestock Producers' Day*, Louisiana State University, **18,** 155

Kelley, J. S., Morrison, D. G., Loyacano, A. F., Ingraham, R. H. and Godke, R. A. (1978c).

Induction of parturition in beef cattle with prostaglandin analogue (ICI 80996). *Presented at Amer. Soc. Anim. Sci. Southern Sect.* Houston, Texas, February (49 Abstr. 105)

Kelley, J. S., Longwell, L. C., Ingraham, R. H. and Godke, R. A. (1978a). Attempts to induce abortion during the last trimester of pregnancy in beef cattle with a prostaglandin analogue (ICI 80996). *Presented at 70th Ann. Mtg. Am. Soc. Anim. Sci.* Michigan State University, July (371 Abstr. 389)

Killian, D. B., Garverick, H. A. and Day, B. N. (1973). Peripheral plasma progesterone and corticoid levels at parturition in the sow. *J. Anim. Sci.*, **37**, 1371

King, G. J., Hurnik, J. F. and Robertson, H. A. (1976). Ovarian function and oestrus in dairy cows during early lactation. *J. Anim. Sci.*, **42**, 688

Kupfer, U. (1977). Behandlung von Brunstlosigkeit mit einem Prostaglandin-Analog. *Schweiz. Arch. Tierheijk.*, **119**, 453

Kostov, L., Tomarov, R. and Gruev, A. (1977). Application of prostaglandins in industrial pig breeding. *Vet. Sbirka (Sofia)*, **75**, 25

Kostov, L., Bogdanov, M., Doicheva, M. and Gruev, A. (1978). Synchronization of parturition in pigs using the synthetic analogue of prostaglandin $F_{2\alpha}$–cloprostenol. *5th World Cong. Hyology and Hyoiatrics.* Zagreb, 12–16 June

Kraeling, R. R., Barb, C. R. and Davis, B. J. (1975). Prostaglandin-induced regression of porcine corpora lutea maintained by estrogen. *Prostaglandins*, **9**, 459

Kraeling, R. R. and Rampacek, G. B. (1977). Synchronization of estrus and ovulation in gilts with estradiol and prostaglandin $F_{2\alpha}$. *Theriogenology*, **8**, 103

Krzymowski, T., Kotwica, J., Okrasa, S., Doboszynska, T. and Ziecik, A. (1978). Luteal function in sows after unilateral infusion of $PGF_{2\alpha}$ into the anterior uterine vein on different days of the oestrous cycle. *J. Reprod. Fertil.*, **54**, 21

Lamming, G. E. and Bulman, D. C. (1976). The use of milk progesterone radioimmunoassay in the diagnosis and treatment of subfertility in dairy cows. *Br. Vet. J.*, **132**, 507

Lamond, D. R., Tomlinson, R. V., Drost, M., Henricks, D. M. and Jochle, W. (1973). Studies of prostaglandin $F_{2\alpha}$ in the cow. *Theriogenology*, **4**, 269

Lauderdale, J. W. (1972). Effects of $PGF_{2\alpha}$ on pregnancy and the estrous cycle of cattle. *J. Anim. Sci.*, **35**, 246 (Abstr.)

Lauderdale, J. W. (1978). Beef A.I. and lutalyse. *Proc. 10th World Congr. Buiatrics.* Mexico

Lauderdale, J. W., Seguin, B. E., Stellflug, J. N., Chenault, J. R., Vincent, C. K., Thatcher, W. W. and Loyancano, A. F. (1974). Fertility of cattle following $PGF_{2\alpha}$ injection. *J. Anim. Sci.*, **38** (5), 964

Leaver, J. D., Glencross, R. G. and Pope, G. S. (1975). Fertility of Friesian heifers after luteolysis with a prostaglandin analogue (ICI 80996). *Vet. Rec.*, **96**, 383

Leaver, J. D., Mulvany, P. M., Glencross, R. G. and Pope, G. S. (1976). Synchronization of oestrus in dairy cattle with a prostaglandin analogue (ICI 80996). *Anim. Prod.*, **22**, 145 (Abstr.)

Leidl, W., Bostedt, H., Stolla, R., Schefels, W. and Kuhn, H. (1977). The effect of prostaglandin $F_{2\alpha}$ as seen in the clinical use of the analogue 'Estrumate' especially in the case of non-detected oestrus (silent heat). *Berl. Munch. Tierarztl. Wochenschr.*, **90**, 309

Martinat-Botte, F., Locatelli, A. and Mauleon, P. (1977a). Control of the sexual cycles of nulliparous gilts by means of norethandrolone and prostaglandin analogue (ICI 80996). *Ann. Zootechnie*, **26**, 444

Martinat-Botte, F., Locatelli, A. and Mauleon, P. (1977b). The control of oestrous cycles in gilts using norethandrolone and an analogue of prostaglandin $F_{2\alpha}$ (ICI 80996). *J. Rec. Porcine Fr.*, 23

du Mesnil du Buisson, F. and Dauzier, L. (1957). Influence de l'ovariectomie chez la truie pendant le gestation. *Comptes Rendus Séances Soc. Biol. Filiales*, **151**, 311

Millar, P. G. (1974). Methods of early termination of pregnancy in the cow. *Vet. Rec.*, **94**, 626

Molokwu, E. C. I. and Wagner, W. C. (1973). Endocrine physiology of the puerperal sow. *J. Anim. Sci.*, **36**, 1158

Musson, A. L. (1951). Causes of variation in gestation length in swine. *J. Anim. Sci.* **10**, 1028

Nancarrow, C. D. and Radford, H. M. (1975). Use of oestradiol benzoate to improve synchronization of oestrus in cattle. *J. Reprod. Fertil.*, **43**, 404

Nancarrow, C. D. (1976). Herd fertility following various synchronization techniques. *Proc. of Oestrus Synchronization in Cattle Symposium.* Sydney, 53

Nara, B. S. and First, N. L. (1977). Effect of indomethacin and prostaglandin $F_{2\alpha}$ on porcine parturition. *69th Ann. Mtg. Amer. Soc. Anim. Sci.* Madison, July

Nellor, J. E. and Cole, H. H. (1956). The hormonal control of oestrus and ovulation in the beef heifer. *J. Anim. Sci.*, **15**, 650

Oxender, W. D., Noden, P. A., Louis, T. M. and Hafs, H. D. (1974). A review of prostaglandin $F_{2\alpha}$ for ovulation control in cows and mares. *Am. J. Vet. Res.* **35**, 997

Peters, J. B., Welch, J. A., Lauderdale, J. W. and Inskeep, E. K. (1977). Synchronization of oestrus in beef cattle with $PGF_{2\alpha}$ and estradiol benzoate. *J. Anim. Sci.*, **45**, 230

Rajakoski, E. (1960). The ovarian follicular system in sexually mature heifers with special reference to seasonal, cyclical, and left–right variations. *Data Endocrinol. (Kbh)* (Suppl.), **52**, 1

Refsal, K. R., Seguin, B. E., Mather, E. C. and Gustafsson, B. G. (1976). Estradiol and $PGF_{2\alpha}$ as luteolytic agents and abortifacients in cattle. *Presented at 57th Conf. Research Workers in Anim. Diseases.* Chicago, Illinois

Robertson, H. A., King, G. J. and Elliot, J. I. (1974). Induction of parturition in the pig. *J. Anim. Sci.*, **39**, 994

Robertson, H. A., King, G. J. and Elliot, J. I. (1978). Control of the time of parturition in sows with prostaglandin $F_{2\alpha}$. *Can. J. Comp. Med.*, **42**, 32

Roche, J. F. (1976). Fertility in cows after treatment with a prostaglandin analogue with or without progesterone. *J. Reprod. Fertil.*, **46**, 341

Rowson, L. E. A., Lamming, G. E. and Fry, R. M. (1953). The relationship between ovarian hormones and uterine infection. *Vet. Rec.*, **65**, 335

Russell, C. A. (1978). Prostaglandins in planned breeding. *5th World Cong. Hyology and Hyoiatrics.* Zagreb, 12–16 June

Schultz, R. H. (1978). The use of cloprostenol (ICI 80 996) for the treatment of various infertile states in the bovine. *Proc. 10th World Congr. Buiatrics.* Mexico City, Mexico

Schultz, R. H., Beerwinkle, D. R., Bierschwal, C. J., Fields, M. J., Godke, R. A., Kraemer, D. C., Mawns, J. C., Seguin, B. E. and Vatthauer, R. J. (1977). Synchronizing beef cows with cloprostenol. *Proc. 69th Ann. Mtg. A.S.A.S.* Madison (Abstr. 513)

Schultz, R. H. and Wilson, D. C. (1978). Factors affecting cloprostenol-induced abortion in beef heifers. *Presented at 70th Ann. Mtg. Am. Soc. Anim. Sci.* Michigan, July, 387 (Abstr. 431)

Seguin, B. E., Refsa, L. J. R., Goerke, T. P. and Phatak, A. (1978). Field trial experiences with prostaglandins in Minnesota and Wisconsin beef cattle. *Minnesota Vet.*, **18**, 9

Seguin, B. E., Gustafsson, B. K., Hurtgen, J. P., Mather, E. C., Refsal, K. R., Wescott, R. A. and Whitmore, H. L. (1978). Use of the prostaglandin $F_{2\alpha}$ analogue cloprostenol (ICI 80 996) in dairy cattle with unobserved oestrus. *Theriogenology*, **10**, 55

Short, R. V. (1960). Blood progesterone levels in relation to parturition. *J. Reprod. Fertil.*, **1**, 61

Sugawara, S. (1977). The effect of prostaglandin $F_{2\alpha}$ on induced farrowing in pigs. *Chikusan-No-Kenkyu*, **2**, 31

Sugawara, S., Hashizume, K., Totsukawa, K., Umezu, M., Masaki, J., Watanabe, M., Sato, H., Abe, W., Usami, N., Sata, K. and Yoshida, T. (1976). Induced parturition in swine with prostaglandin $F_{2\alpha}$. *Jap. J. Anim. Reprod.*, **22**, 60

Trimburger, G. W. and Hansel, W. (1955). Conception rate and ovarian function following oestrus control by progesterone injection in dairy cattle. *J. Anim. Sci.*, **14**, 224

Trounson, A. O., Brand, A. and Straver, G. M. (1976). The use of prostaglandins in animal breeding. *Diergeneesk. Memo.*, **23** (5–6), 141

Uwland, J. (1978). Experience of cloprostenol (Estrumate) in dairy cattle. *Tijdschr. Diergeneesk.*, **103**, 480

Walker, N. (1977). The effects of induction of parturition in sows using an analogue of prostaglandin $F_{2\alpha}$. *J. Agri. Sci.*, **89** (part 2), 267

Waters, R. J., and Ball, R. (1978). Commercial ovulation control and fixed time artificial insemination in cattle. *Vet. Rec.*, **103**, 585

Weaver, L. D. and Schultz, R. H. (1977). Synchronization of oestrus and ovulation in lactating dairy cows using cloprostenol. *J. Dairy Sci.*, **60** (Suppl. 1), 81 (Abstr.)

Wenkoff, M. S. (1978). Therapeutic evaluation of the use of prostaglandin analogue ICI 80 996 in cattle. *Can. Vet. J.*, **19**, 277

Wettemann, R. P., Hallford, D. M., Kreider, D. L. and Turman, E. J. (1974). Parturition in swine after prostaglandin $F_{2\alpha}$. *J. Anim. Sci.*, **39**, 228

Wettemann, R. P., Hallford, D. M., Kreider, D. L. and Turman, E. J. (1977). Influence of prostaglandin $F_{2\alpha}$ on endocrine changes at parturition in gilts. *J. Anim. Sci.*, **44**, 106

Wierzchos, E. and Pejsak, Z. (1976). Induction of parturition in sows with prostin $F_{2\alpha}$ in commercial swine farms. *Proc 8th Int. Congr. Animal Reproduction and A.I.* Krakow, 12–16 July

Williamson, N. B., Morris, R. S., Blood, D. C. and Cannon, Christine M. (1972). A study of oestrus behaviour and oestrus detection methods in a large commercial dairy herd. *Vet. Rec.*, **91**, 50

Wilson, D. (1978). The use of cloprostenol (ICI 80 996) for controlled breeding of cattle. *Proc. 10th World Congr. Buiatrics.* Mexico

Youngquist, R. S., Bierschwal, C. J., Elmore, R. G., Jenkins, A. L., Schultz, R. H. and Widmer, J. H. (1977). Induction of abortion in feedlot heifers with cloprostenol (ICI 80 996). *Theriogenology*, **7**, 305

Zemjanis, R., Fahning, M. L. and Schultz, R. H. (1969). Anestrus: The practitioners dilemma. *Scope (Upjohn)*, **XIV**, 14

Zerobin, K., Jochle, W. and Steingruber, C. H. (1973). Termination of pregnancy with prostaglandins F_2 and $F_{2\alpha}$ in cattle. *Prostaglandins*, **4**, 891

Zuber, H. (1978). Practice experiences with the prostaglandin analogue Extrumate in anoestrous cattle. *Dtsch. Tierarztl. Wochenschr.*, **85**, 153

11 Prostaglandins and their Synthesis Inhibitors in Primary Dysmenorrhoea

N. WIQVIST

11.1 INTRODUCTION

Primary dysmenorrhoea may be regarded as a syndrome that includes not only pain in the lower abdomen and back but also a variety of other symptoms. However, pain is the primary complaint, often attributed to uterine cramps, which makes the uterus a focus of attention. Amongst the various factors that may be responsible for this pain, uterine hypercontractility has received particular attention. When it became evident that prostaglandins play a major role in the control of uterine contractility it was logical to try and suppress the synthesis of these substances with prostaglandin synthetase inhibitors (PGSI) and thereby prevent uterine cramps.

This concept seems simple enough and may be true to some extent. The aetiology of primary dysmenorrhoea, however, is complex and there are many other events that are influenced by prostaglandins. In addition other mechanisms not involving prostaglandins may also be responsible for primary dysmenorrhoea. Nevertheless, the use of PGSI represents a new approach in its treatment. The efficacy and side-effects of PGSI have to be balanced against other remedies which range from hot-water bottles, alcohol and psychotherapy to potent analgesics, spasmolytics and oral contraceptives.

That non-steroidal anti-inflammatory drugs inhibit prostaglandin biosynthesis has been recognized only recently and the same applies to their potential in the treatment of primary dysmenorrhoea.

11.2 PATHOPHYSIOLOGY OF DYSMENORRHOEA

Among the various hypotheses on the aetiology of primary dysmenorrhoea that have been discussed over the years, some have gained credence with recent discoveries and experimental findings whereas others seem to have been dismissed. Little importance is now attached to the significance of uterine hypoplasia or the position of the uterus in the aetiology of primary dysmenorrhoea. Psychogenic factors may play a role but there is an impression that these factors have been over-emphasized. Still under discussion are pathophysiological events related to myometrial contractility, uterine blood flow, ovarian steroids, prostaglandins, the uterine innervation and the cervix. There are some arguments in favour of most of these hypotheses and it is now generally recognized that a combination of factors is probably involved in the aetiology of primary dysmenorrhoea.

The present review is aimed at discussing the possible significance of prostaglandins in the aetiology of primary dysmenorrhoea and evaluating the potential of PGSI in the treatment of the disorder. Prostaglandins are present in all mammalian tissues and serve many functions in the body. It is therefore necessary to consider the various factors in conventional order and to try and relate their possible dependence on prostaglandins.

11.2.1 Myometrial contractility

Measurement of uterine activity during the first few days of menstruation in non-dysmenorrhoeic women generally shows a pattern characterized by reasonably regular, low-frequency contractions with a low basal tonus (Figure 11.1). Records of uterine activity from women with primary dysmenorrhoea at the beginning of their menstrual flow exhibit a pattern

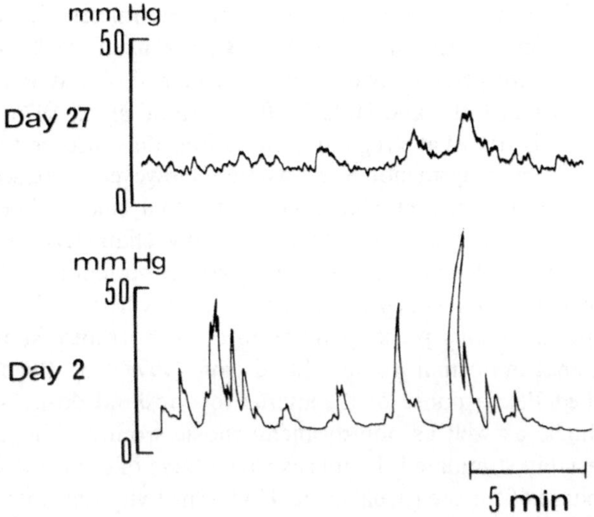

Figure 11.1 Typical uterine contractility pattern on day 27 and day 2 of the cycle in a normal, non-dysmenorrhoeic woman. Note the 'labour-like' pattern and low basal tonus at menstruation. (From the author's material)

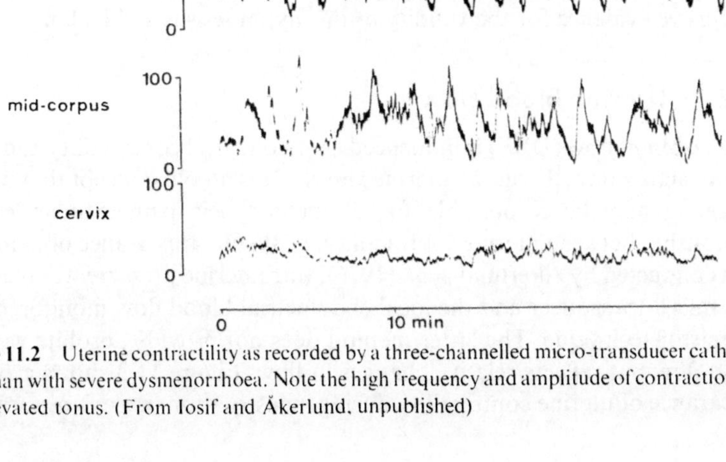

Figure 11.2 Uterine contractility as recorded by a three-channelled micro-transducer catheter in a woman with severe dysmenorrhoea. Note the high frequency and amplitude of contractions and the elevated tonus. (From Iosif and Åkerlund, unpublished)

different from non-dysmenorrhoeic subjects. The typical contractility pattern in women with dysmenorrhoea is characterized by a high tonus, high amplitude and frequent spasmodic contractions (Figure 11.2). Some authors attach more importance to the high amplitude of contractions while others consider high tonus as being the important parameter. However, most investigators seem to recognize that various patterns of markedly increased uterine activity are present (Moir, 1936; Bickers, 1943; Woodbury *et al.*, 1947; Mann, 1963; Filler and Hall, 1970; Åkerlund *et al.*, 1976; Andersson *et al.*, 1978). It is true that irregular contractions may also be found during menstruation in non-dysmenorrhoeic women. However, there seems to be a clear quantitative difference in this respect between dysmenorrhoeic and non-dysmenorrhoeic subjects. The pain is generally characterized by painful intermittent cramps which coincide with uterine contractions.

One problem of relevance in this context is whether the myometrial sensitivity to exogenous prostaglandins in dysmenorrhoeic subjects is different from that in normal women. Lundström (1977) and Bygdeman *et al.* (1979) studied the response of the uterus to threshold doses of $PGF_{2\alpha}$ in dysmenorrhoeic as well as non-dysmenorrhoeic women. They found that $PGF_{2\alpha}$ invariably stimulated the uterus irrespective of the route of administration or phase of the menstrual cycle. High sensitivity was noted in the late secretory phase. The uterine response to PGE_2 was more complex in that intrauterine administration resulted in either stimulation or inhibition of uterine activity. There was some indication that small doses of PGE_2 (2–5 μg) tended to stimulate the uterus whereas high doses (30–40 μg) tended to inhibit the contractility. Bygdeman *et al.* (1979) found that the inhibitory effect was particularly evident during menstruation. These results support Pickles' original hypothesis on the significance of the ratio of $PGF_{2\alpha}$ to PGE_2 in menstrual fluid and disintegrating endometrium (Pickles *et al.*, 1965) and may imply that the reported abnormal contractility pattern during menstruation in dysmenorrhoeic women is due to a dominance of $PGF_{2\alpha}$. It should, however, be emphasized that the experimental findings are not consistent and that conclusive evidence for the validity of this hypothesis is still lacking.

11.2.2 Uterine blood flow

Uterine blood flow (UBF) is influenced by myometrial contractility and other factors acting directly on the uterine vessels. It is an old concept that uterine ischaemia may be responsible for dysmenorrhoeic pain. Studies on the relationship between uterine contractility, UBF and appearance of pain have been conducted by Åkerlund *et al.* (1976). Intrauterine pressure was recorded by a micro-transducer and the local endometrial blood flow monitored by a thermistor technique. The latter method does not provide absolute value of blood flow but reflects relative changes in flow. Figure 11.3 shows a typical appearance of uterine contractility during menstruation in a dysmenorrhoeic woman. Uterine blood flow varied with the individual contractions and pain was generally pronounced when this was low. Intravenous administration of an adrenergic β_2-stimulating drug (0.5 mg terbutaline) caused complete relaxation of the uterus in this individual and a marked increase in UBF. The patient experienced complete pain relief within 1 minute after the injection.

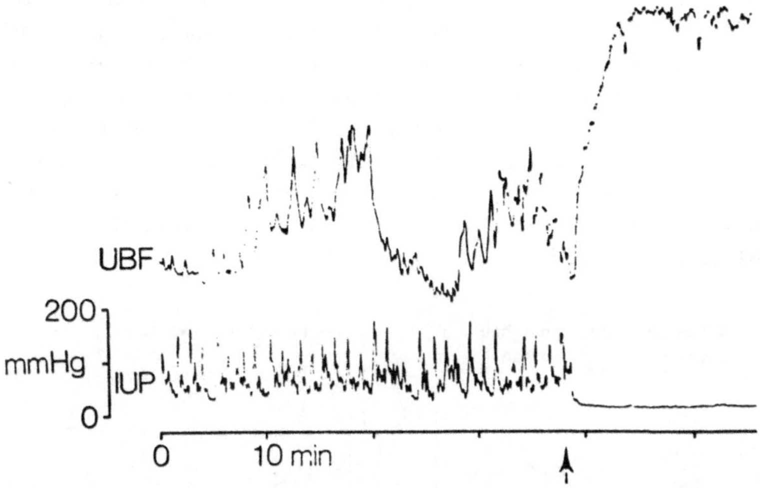

Figure 11.3 Local uterine blood flow, intrauterine pressure, and the effect of terbutaline (0.5 mg intravenously, injection indicated by arrow) on the first day of menstruation in a woman with severe primary dysmenorrhoea. (From Åkerlund *et al.*, 1976, by permission)

The opposite effect, i.e. induction of hypercontractility, a reduction in blood flow and appearance of pain may be obtained by administration of uterine stimulating drugs, such as vasopressin or $PGF_{2\alpha}$. Whatever the exact mechanism of pain may be, there is a strong impression of parallelism between uterine hypercontractility, reduced blood flow and dysmenorrhoeic pain.

11.2.3 Prostaglandin levels in dysmenorrhoea

As early as 1965, Pickles and collaborators suggested that prostaglandins might play a role in the aetiology of dysmenorrhoea. Based on bioassay results they produced evidence of an increased concentration of $PGF_{2\alpha}$ in menstrual fluid of dysmenorrhoeic women. More refined chemical assay methods like radioimmunoassay and gas chromatography–mass spectrometry have subsequently been utilized in the determination of prostaglandin levels in body fluids and tissues. Prostaglandins seem to be produced in most tissues and the rate of formation from essential fatty acid precursors as well as the rate of enzymatic degradation is generally very high.

The levels of PGE_2 and $PGF_{2\alpha}$ in circulation are difficult to determine in view of an artificial formation at sampling. Wilks *et al.* (1973) and Shangold *et al.* (1976) found plasma $PGF_{2\alpha}$ concentrations of the order of 200–400 pg/ml, levels that are probably 100 times higher than can be expected on theoretical considerations. They were not able to confirm any elevated concentrations of $PGF_{2\alpha}$ in dysmenorrhoeic subjects. The major plasma metabolite of $PGF_{2\alpha}$, 15-keto-13,14-dihydro-$PGF_{2\alpha}$, has a longer half-life in circulation and consequently is present in a higher concentration. The metabolite is not formed artificially and the plasma levels are therefore more representative of the true situation. Lundström and Gréen (1978) determined plasma concentration of the metabolite in dysmenorrhoeic and non-dysmenorrhoeic women. They found levels of 25–40 pg/ml before and during menstruation in normal women and around 80 pg/ml on the first day of menstruation in dysmenorrhoeic subjects. Patients treated for dysmenorrhoea with oral contraceptives had normal levels, i.e. around 30–40 pg/ml on the first day of menstruation (Figure 11.4).

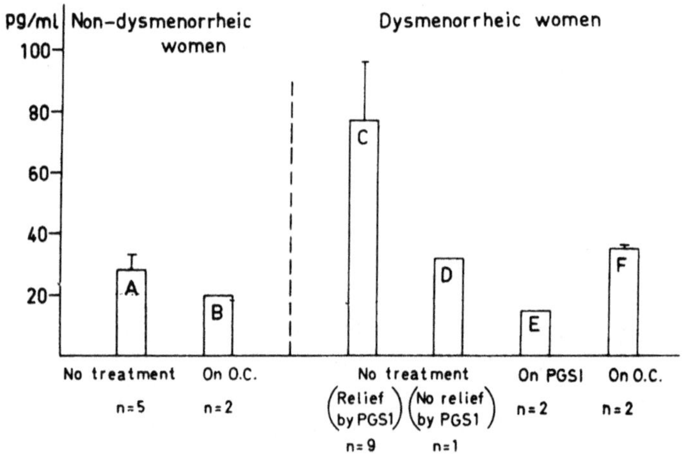

Figure 11.4 Concentrations of 15-keto-13,14-dihydro-$PGF_{2\alpha}$ in plasma on the first day of menstruation. OC = oral contraceptive, PGSI = prostaglandin synthetase inhibitor, n = no. of patients. (From Lundström and Gréen, 1978, by permission)

It is difficult, probably impossible, to get accurate information on tissue concentration of prostaglandins. Even gentle handling or slight mechanical trauma can initiate the biosynthesis of prostaglandins. With these considerations in mind, Lundström and Gréen (1978) estimated the concentration of $PGF_{2\alpha}$ and its metabolites in the endometrium from dysmenorrhoeic and non-dysmenorrhoeic women. The endometrial biopsy specimens were blotted on a filter paper and transferred to a pre-chilled (−60 °C) test tube containing 96% ethanol within 2–3 seconds. Prostaglandins $PGF_{2\alpha}$ and metabolites were measured using a gas chromatography–mass spectrometry method. Their data were not claimed to represent the true concentrations of the above compounds in intact endometrial tissue. However, the results were supposed to reflect the capacity of the tissue to produce the prostaglandins in question with the amounts of precursor acid, cofactors and prostaglandin synthetase available. Figure 11.5 illustrates the mean values obtained premenstrually

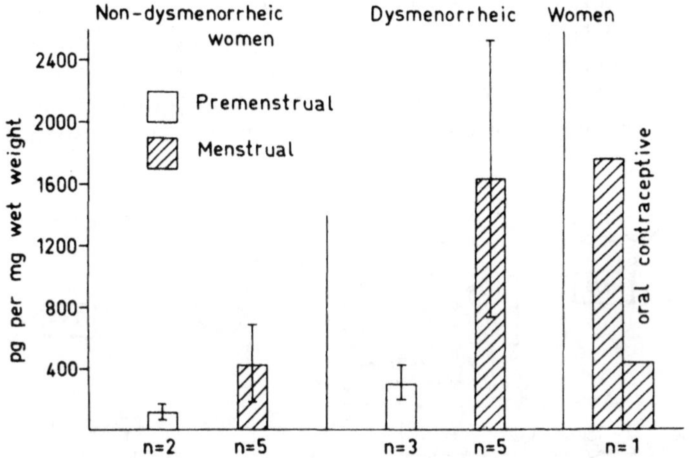

Figure 11.5 Concentrations of $PGF_{2\alpha}$ in the endometrium of normal and dysmenorrhoeic women. (From Lundström and Gréen, 1978, by permission)

and on the first day of menstrual bleeding. There was no significant difference between the premenstrual $PGF_{2\alpha}$ levels in the two groups but the 'concentration' was approximately four times higher in dysmenorrhoeic than in normal women on the first day of menstrual bleeding ($p < 0.05$). The presence of blood in the uterine cavity on the first day of menstruation may lead to an additional formation of prostaglandins. However, this situation is likely to be identical in both groups. Metabolites of $PGF_{2\alpha}$ were generally below the detectable limit of assay which may indicate that catabolic enzymes are not present in the endometrium. In one subject with dysmenorrhoea the endometrial concentration of $PGF_{2\alpha}$ on the first day of bleeding was 1773 pg/ml wet weight and after treatment with oral contraceptives in the next cycle it decreased to 436 pg/ml.

The above data support the concept that the endometrium of dysmenorrhoeic women, at the time when uterine pain is present, has the capacity to synthesize larger amounts of $PGF_{2\alpha}$ than the endometrium of normal subjects. The results also show that the concentration of the major circulating metabolite of $PGF_{2\alpha}$ increases during dysmenorrhoea which may reflect an increased synthesis of $PGF_{2\alpha}$ in the uterus, in the uterine cavity or elsewhere in the body. Oral contraceptives seem to reduce the local and peripheral levels of prostaglandin. This may explain the beneficial effect of oral contraceptives in primary dysmenorrhoea.

11.2.4 Effects of prostaglandin synthetase inhibitors on prostaglandin levels and uterine contractility

Figure 11.6 shows the major pathways of arachidonic acid metabolism (Pace-Asciak, 1977). Most cells and tissues have the capacity to form prostaglandins but the precursor, arachidonic acid, must first be liberated from membrane-bound phospholipids. This process is brought about by the enzyme phospholipase A_2 in response to a variety of specific or non-specific stimuli.

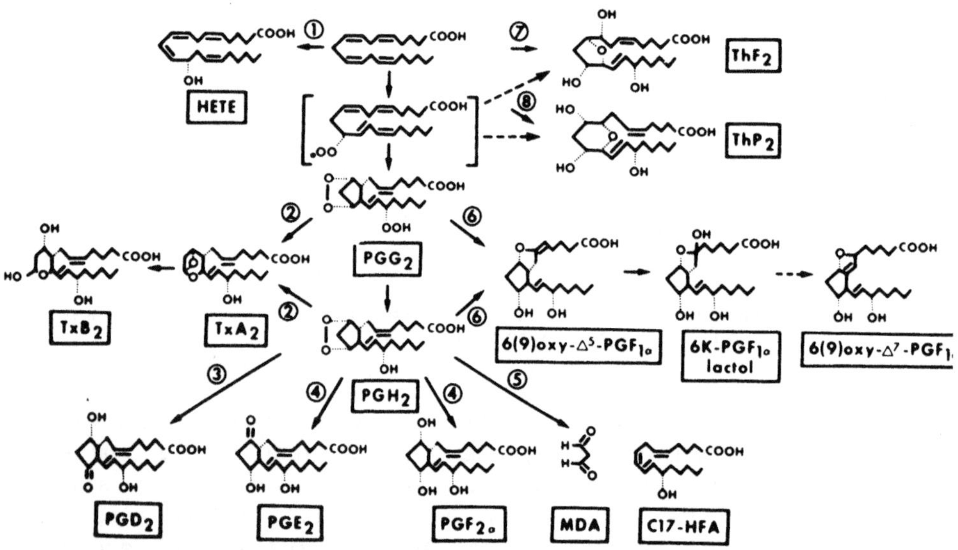

Figure 11.6 Eight established pathways of oxidative biotransformation of arachidonic acid. 6(9)oxy-Δ^5-$PGF_{1\alpha}$ = prostacyclin (PGI_2). TXA_2 = thromboxane A_2. (From Pace-Asciak, 1977, by permission)

Conversion of arachidonic acid into the labile endoperoxides, PGG_2 and PGH_2, is brought about by a reaction catalysed by the enzyme cyclo-oxygenase. The endoperoxides can then be converted into a number of compounds: the classical prostaglandins (PGE_2 and $PGF_{2\alpha}$), the thromboxanes (TXA_2), prostacyclin (PGI_2) and others. All these compounds and possibly also PGG_2 and PGH_2 influence myometrial contractility (Figure 11.7) or vascular smooth muscle. Endoperoxide metabolites (prostacyclin and thromboxane A_2) have a stimulant effect on the human myometrium (Wilhelmsson *et al.*, 1979).

Non-steroidal anti-inflammatory drugs or PGSI, such as aryl carboxylic acids (salicylates, fenamates), aryl alkanoic acids (ibuprofen, naproxen, indomethacin) and enolic acids, inhibit the enzyme cyclo-oxygenase and thereby the formation of endoperoxides (Vane, 1978). This means that PGSI prevent the formation of not only PGE_2 and $PGF_{2\alpha}$ but also other biologically active prostaglandin compounds (Figure 11.8). Administration of these compounds in therapeutic doses causes a marked reduction in uterine contractility both in normal and dysmenorrhoeic subjects. This effect is particularly evident in women with uterine hypercontractility and dysmenorrhoeic pain

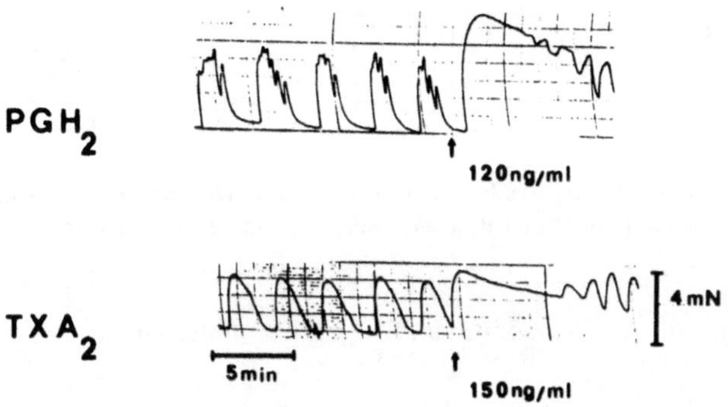

Figure 11.7 The effect of PGH_2 and thromboxane A_2 (TXA_2) on the contractility of human myometrium *in vitro*. (From Wilhelmsson *et al.*, unpublished, by permission)

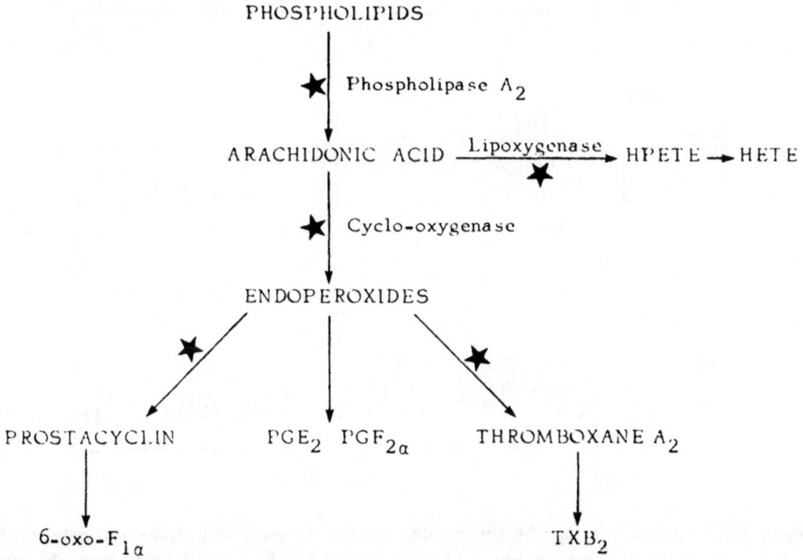

Figure 11.8 Pathways of arachidonic acid metabolism. Pathways marked (★) represent enzymatic stages which can be selectively inhibited under *in vivo* or *in vitro* conditions. (From Whittle, 1979, by permission)

(Lundström *et al.*, 1976; Csapo *et al.*, 1977; Pulkkinen and Kaihola, 1977). The amplitude and frequency of contractions diminish and uterine tonus decreases within 1–2 hours following the first dose. These events are accompanied by a relief from uterine pain (Figure 11.9). If treatment with PGSI is started 2–3 days before the expected onset of bleeding the uterine

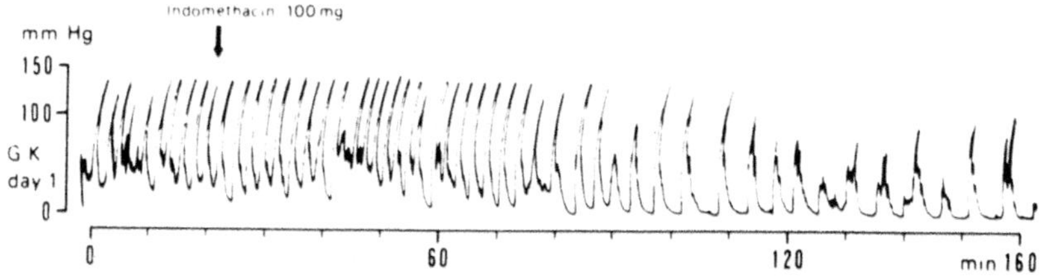

Figure 11.9 The effect of rectal administration of 100 mg indomethacin on uterine contractility during menstruation (day 1) in a dysmenorrhoeic patient. (From Lundström *et al.*, 1976, by permission)

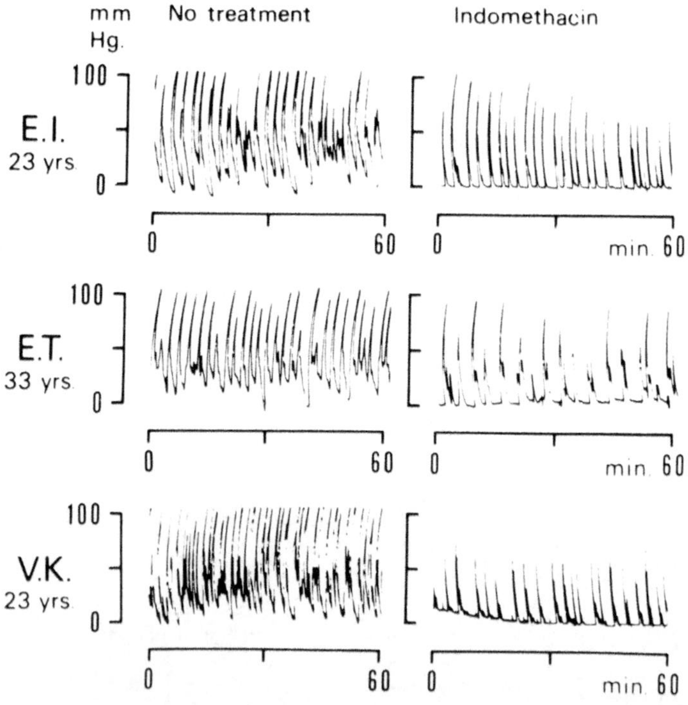

Figure 11.10 Records of uterine contractility in three patients with dysmenorrhoea on the first or second day of menstruation. The tracings to the right were obtained from the same three women during their subsequent cycle following pretreatment with oral indomethacin (25 mg × 3/daily). Note the low uterine tonus after indomethacin treatment. (From Lundström *et al.*, 1976, by permission)

contractility at menstruation is lower than that observed in the same subject in a cycle without treatment (Figure 11.10). However, there seems to be no major difference in effect if PGSI is administered one or more days before the onset of menstrual bleeding or given at the beginning of menstruation. There is rarely complete inhibition of uterine contractility, only a reduction or normalization' of the pattern.

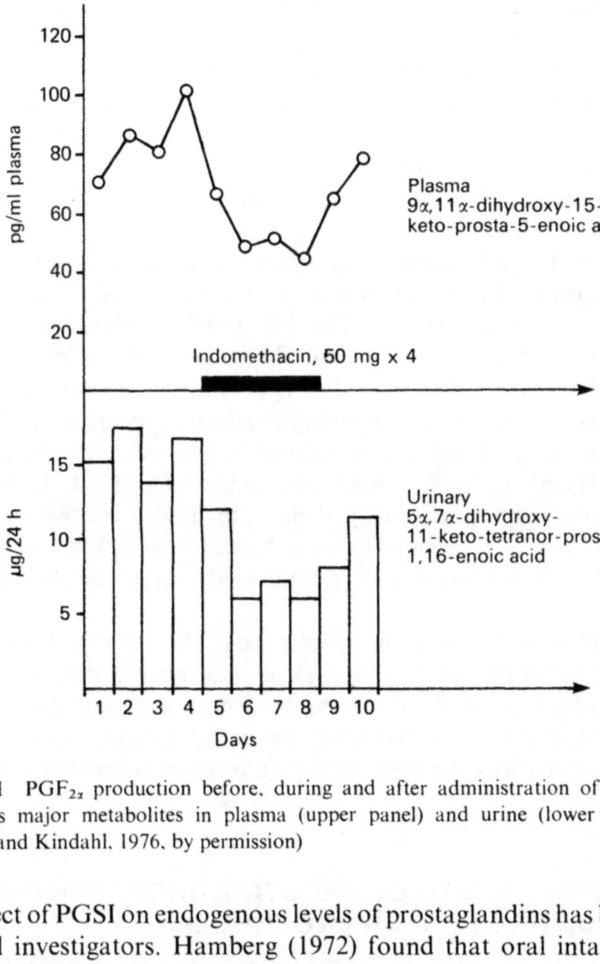

Figure 11.11 $PGF_{2\alpha}$ production before, during and after administration of indomethacin, measured as major metabolites in plasma (upper panel) and urine (lower panel). (From Granström and Kindahl, 1976, by permission)

The effect of PGSI on endogenous levels of prostaglandins has been studied by several investigators. Hamberg (1972) found that oral intake of 50 mg indomethacin four times a day resulted in a 70–80% reduction in the total daily excretion of the major urinary prostaglandin F metabolite as analysed by gas chromatography–mass spectrometry method. Granström and Kindahl (1976) determined the major metabolites of $PGF_{2\alpha}$ in plasma and urine by a specific radioimmunoassay and found a 50–60% decrease in their daily excretion with the same dose of indomethacin (Figure 11.11).

11.2.5 Other pathophysiological factors

The cervix has attracted much attention as a causative factor in the aetiology of primary dysmenorrhoea. The old theory of Hippocrates on the existence of a cervical obstruction and retention of menstrual fluid within the uterus of dysmenorrhoeic women is supported by clinical experience that dysmenorrhoea generally disappears following child-birth and dilatation of the cervix. It is also a fact that dysmenorrhoea tends to disappear temporarily following surgical cervical dilatation. Mann *et al.* (1962) claimed that the leading cause of primary dysmenorrhoea was the failure of the isthmus to relax after the onset of menstruation. Moghissi (1972) suggested that a prolonged presence of menstrual blood containing high concentrations of prostaglandins within the uterus might stimulate uterine contractility and elicit pain. However, Asplund (1952) and Ylikorkala and Dawood (1978) found no evidence of any particularly narrow cervix during the first and second day of menstruation in dysmenorrhoeic women.

The functional significance of uterine nerves (adrenergic and cholinergic) is poorly understood. However, it is well known that presacral nerve resection may cure severe dysmenorrhoea. Thorbert (1979) studied the existence of short adrenergic neurons in the uterus. These nerve structures disappeared almost completely from the uterus during pregnancy and did not regenerate after the end of pregnancy. This may explain the disappearance of dysmenorrhoea after the first pregnancy. The possible importance of cholinergic nerves may be illustrated by the following case report (Åkerlund, 1979). A non-dysmenorrhoeic woman with myasthenia gravis was treated with cholinesterase inhibitors. She developed severe dysmenorrhoea following the onset of treatment. Her dysmenorrhoea disappeared every time she omitted the treatment.

Prostaglandins may have little significance in the context of uterine nerve function and pain. However, it should be remembered that prostaglandin mechanisms are involved in the transmitter process at terminal nerve endings and that prostaglandins can potentiate the pain-producing actions of kinins and hence may sensitize the peripheral pain receptors (Ferreira, 1972; Higgs *et al.*, 1978).

11.3 CLINICAL TRIALS OF PROSTAGLANDIN SYNTHETASE INHIBITORS IN DYSMENORRHOEA

The symptomatology of primary dysmenorrhoea involves a number of widely different complaints. Pain is the dominating symptom but a variety of gastro-intestinal disturbances and symptoms related to the central nervous system also occur. PGSI are also known to produce side-effects some of which resemble certain symptoms within the dysmenorrhoea syndrome. There is a common experience that these generally young patients may have anovulatory cycles, during which the symptoms of dysmenorrhoea are absent. Double blind or double blind crossover trials are difficult to complete in view of the fact that patients with dysmenorrhoea tend to drop out from placebo regimens. Symptom-relieving effects of drugs are generally assessed by a scoring system, sometimes differentiated in three, sometimes in five or more scores, and varying between no relief (or even worse) and complete relief. The scoring systems may be applied to a number of different symptoms. The treatment results may also be evaluated from the patients' general assessment: preference of drugs, absence from work or school, number of additional analgesics, etc.

All these variables, combined with the well-known psychological overlay in some patients, make it difficult to compare results of different clinical trials. Most of the initial reports on the use of PGSI in the treatment of primary dysmenorrhoea were open studies, i.e. no comparison with placebo treatment or with other treatment regimens, and conclusions based on such studies may not be quite accurate. Nevertheless, a few controlled studies have been carried out and the following survey will be mainly concerned with the results from such studies (Table 11.1).

Table 11.1 Double blind crossover studies in the treatment of dysmenorrhoea with prostaglandin synthetase inhibitors

Compound	*Author*	*No. of patients*	*Dose per day*	*Beginning of medication*
Indomethacin Tolfenamic acid Placebo	Kauppila and Ylikorkala, 1977	27	25 mg × 3 133 mg × 3	day −2 day −2
Indomethacin Placebo	Hamann and Laursen, 1977	60	25 mg × 3 + 100 mg	day 1
Flufenamic acid Placebo	Kapadia and Elder, 1978	44	200 mg × 3	day 1
Mefenamic acid Flufenamic acid 'Common analgesic'	Anderson *et al.*, 1978	30	500 mg × 3 200 mg × 3	day 1
Ibuprofen Paracetamol	Layes Molla and Donald, 1974	67	400 mg × 3 1000 mg × 3	day −1
Naproxen-sodium Placebo	Henzl *et al.*, 1977	22	550 mg + 275 mg + 275 mg	day 1
Naproxen-sodium Placebo	Lundström, 1978	26	550 mg + 275 mg + 275 mg	day 1

11.3.1 Pain relief

The characteristic pain sensation experienced by these patients is generally cramp-like, intermittent and with each episode of cramp coinciding with a uterine contraction. The pain is consistently localized in the lower abdominal region, mainly the groin, and nearly always in the lower back region. Occasionally women complain of pain in the legs. Some patients may also have a continuous background ache in the lower abdomen. Most studies on PGSI do not differentiate between these different types of pain.

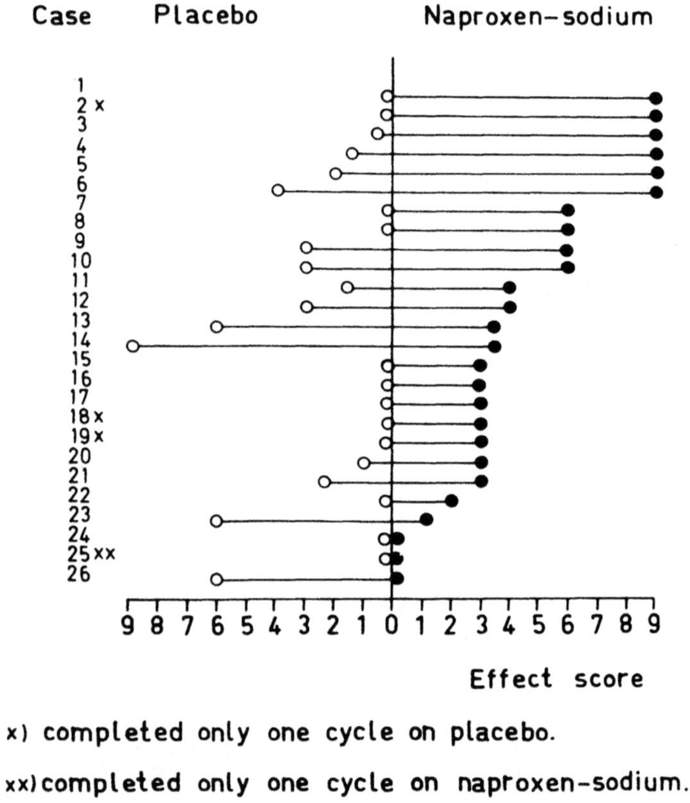

Figure 11.12 Diagram illustrating the results of a double blind crossover study of naproxen-sodium versus placebo in the treatment of dysmenorrhoea. The horizontal bars on each side of the vertical line represent the sum of pain relief scores (see text) during three cycles. (From Lundström, 1978, by permission)

Analysis of results obtained in controlled (placebo) trials shows that a pain-relieving effect was obtained in 65–90% of the patients compared to 10–40% in the placebo group. The typical results of a double blind crossover trial are illustrated in Figure 11.12 (Lundström, 1978). The patients were given naproxen-sodium 550 mg at the beginning of menstruation and thereafter 275 mg every 6th hour (maximum 1100 mg/day) until the pain normally disappeared. This treatment regimen was continued for 3 months followed by placebo treatment for another 3-month period or *vice versa*. Complete pain relief was given a score of 3, marked improvement 2, moderate improvement 1 and no relief 0. The scores for the whole 3-month period were added (score 9 for those who experienced complete pain relief). Score for each patient is separately shown (Table 11.1) irrespective of order of treatment. It is evident that the scores for naproxen-sodium were superior to those of placebo. There were some exceptions. Only four patients considered the placebo treatment as better than the active drug whereas 20 preferred PGSI treatment. Similar results were obtained by Henzl *et al.* (1977) in a double blind trial with naproxen-sodium.

Indomethacin was tested in a study conducted by Hamann and Lauersen (1977). The dose used was 25 mg orally three times a day and additional 100 mg rectally in the evening. Of the 42 who completed the treatment 38 experienced a reduction 'in the duration' of uterine cramps with indomethacin whereas the corresponding number for placebo treatment was four. The need for supplementary analgesics was reduced in 32 of the patients during the indomethacin treatment period but only in two during the placebo period. The significance of these differences is beyond any doubt.

A double blind crossover trial of flufenamic acid (220 mg × 3 per day) and placebo involving 44 patients was carried out by Kapadia and Elder (1978). While on flufenamic acid for 3 months, 82% of the patients experienced significant pain relief. The difference in pain relief between the two regimens, as evaluated by the scoring system applied, was significant at a level of $p < 0.001$. Layes Molla and Donald (1974) published a comparative multicentre study of ibuprofen (400 mg × 3 per day) and paracetamol (1000 mg × 3 per day) in the treatment of dysmenorrhoea. The treatments were found to be of value in reducing the duration and degree of established pain. Although the results appeared to favour ibuprofen, the difference between the two treatments was not of statistical significance. Kauppila and Ylikorkala (1977) compared the effect of indomethacin, tolfenamic acid and placebo in a double blind crossover study. Relief of pelvic pain and lower back pain was obtained by indomethacin in 79% and 91%, by tolfenamic acid in 67% and 77% and by placebo in 34% and 42% respectively. The difference between indomethacin and tolfenamic acid was not statistically significant.

A further comparative trial has recently been published by Anderson *et al.* (1978). The efficacy of mefenamic acid (500 mg), flufenamic acid (200 mg) or a 'common analgesic' (mixture of dextropropoxyphene hydrochloride and paracetamol, 65 mg and 650 mg respectively) all given three times a day, was tested in a double blind crossover study in 26 patients. The results showed that both mefenamic acid and flufenamic acid were more effective in the treatment of primary dysmenorrhoea than the dextropropoxyphene–paracetamol combination. Furthermore, mefenamic acid seemed to be better than flufenamic acid, although the difference was not statistically significant.

11.3.2 Associated symptoms of dysmenorrhoea and side-effects of prostaglandin synthetase inhibitors

In addition to uterine and back pain other symptoms associated with primary dysmenorrhoea include nausea, vomiting, diarrhoea, constipation, headache, sweating, flushes, dizziness, depression, irritability, etc. It is difficult to assess such symptoms with any degree of accuracy. However, many of these occur frequently and may be highly distressing. It would be useful to evaluate the extent to which the associated symptoms are relieved by PGSI.

Treatment with PGSI, on the other hand, is accompanied by certain side-effects such as nausea, headache, mild dyspepsia, dizziness and fatigue. These disturbances are similar to those associated with dysmenorrhoea and it is consequently difficult to separate them from basic symptoms.

Gastro-intestinal complaints are common in women with primary dysmenorrhoea. Nausea and to some extent vomiting occur in approximately 50% of the patients and occasional diarrhoea or loose stool in about 30%. Symptoms related to the central nervous system occur in 40–50% of the patients.

There seems to be a general agreement that PGSI have a beneficial effect on these associated symptoms. Kapadia and Elder (1978) concluded that gastro-intestinal symptoms were relieved by PGSI, although not to the same extent as dysmenorrhoeic pain. Kauppila and Ylikorkala (1977) found that diarrhoea was relieved by indomethacin in 83%, by tolfenamic acid in 55%, and by placebo in 46% of dysmenorrhoea subjects. Indomethacin had a good or moderate effect on nausea and vomiting in 84%, tolfenamic acid in 86% and placebo in 61% of the patients.

The incidence of side-effects of PGSI is even more difficult to assess. Kapadia and Elder (1978) found that 9% of their patients experienced side-effects 'that could have been caused by flufenamic acid'. These were dizziness and mild dyspepsia. Anderson *et al.* (1978) recorded side-effects (dizziness, nausea, headache) in nearly 20% of their cases. One woman developed a deep-vein thrombosis of the leg, late in the first menstrual cycle, 3 weeks after taking mefenamic acid. Lundström (1978) reported data from three separate case materials; two open trials and one double blind crossover study. She found a 23% incidence of side-effects (headache, exanthema, nausea, gastritis) in the first open trial and 8% in the second. However, the corresponding incidence of 'side-effects' in the double blind crossover study was 15% in the naproxen group and 19% in the placebo group, a fact that illustrates the difficulties involved.

Although the incidence of side-effects recorded by different investigators appears relatively high, the nature of these effects is generally mild. Nevertheless, there is no doubt that some of these side-effects are unpleasant and that they represent a limiting factor in the use of these drugs. Whether serious complications like peptic ulcer or thromboembolism do occur following 1 or 2 days of drug administration every month is not known. However, the therapeutic ratio of some of the newly introduced drugs has been claimed to be more acceptable.

11.4 COMMENTS AND CONCLUSION

Even if there are difficulties in the exact evaluation of individual symptoms, there is no doubt that patients in their general assessment give preference to PGSI rather than to placebo or common analgesics. Highly significant differences in favour of PGSI have been documented in current literature when parameters such as absence from work or school, number of 'additional' analgesics taken or days of bed rest have been recorded. The influence of endogenous prostaglandins on menstruation is emphasized by the observation that PGSI tend to reduce the amount and duration of menstrual blood flow (Anderson *et al.*, 1976; Kauppila and Ylikorkala, 1977).

A number of different anti-inflammatory drugs or PGSI have been tested for their efficacy in relieving the symptoms of dysmenorrhoea and the incidence of their side-effects. However, on the basis of available data it is not possible to identify the drug of choice. PGSI in general are potent inhibitors of the enzyme cyclo-oxygenase and hence they interfere with all pathways of arachidonic acid metabolism. Fenamates also inhibit the action of endogenous and exogenous prostaglandins at receptor levels in various tissues. However, there is no clinical evidence that these drugs are superior to other PGSI in relieving symptoms of dysmenorrhoea.

Self medication with 'common' analgesics may provide occasional help in cases of mild, short-lasting, menstrual pain. These common analgesics often contain low potency anti-inflammatory drugs, like salicylates or paracetamol. It seems probable that the alleviation of pain by these remedies is partly due to an inhibition of uterine prostaglandins (and myometrial contractility) and partially to the general analgesic action of PGSI. It is, however, clear that dramatic pain relief in severe cases requires administration of potent PGSI in adequate doses.

Apart from analgesics, conventional treatment of dysmenorrhoea includes dehydro-retro-progesterone and oral contraceptives. Dehydro-retro-progesterone involves daily intake during the major part of the menstrual cycle at a considerable monthly expense. Patients who need a contraceptive and who accept and tolerate the Pill should preferably be recommended oral contraceptives. However, in the remaining cases PGSI treatment may provide a useful alternative. In this context, it should also be mentioned that some women suffer from dysmenorrhoea even when using combined oral contraceptives. These are data indicating that many of these patients may benefit from the use of PGSI and *vice versa* (Lundström, 1978).

One problem of practical significance is whether treatment should be started before the beginning of menstrual bleeding or at the first signs of impending menstruation. Lundström (1978) compared two groups of women treated with indomethacin or naproxen in an open trial. Of the patients who started their medication before the onset of menses 67% experienced pain relief compared with 75% who started at the beginning of menstruation. There is apparently no difference between the two groups and current literature does not provide significant information on this point. However, there is an impression that individual patients may need pretreatment with PGSI for 2 or more days to achieve proper pain relief. In view of the fact that most women are unable to predict the exact day of menstruation and because the duration of medication should be kept to a minimum, treatment should not be given until the first signs of impending menstruation.

A question of great importance is whether or not PGSI should be recommended for general use in the routine treatment of dysmenorrhoea. This would inevitably mean that a significant proportion of women, particularly the young, would be exposed to these drugs. Many practising physicians would undoubtedly hesitate a routine use because anti-inflammatory drugs do produce rare but serious complications. These involve adverse haematological reactions, retinal changes, bronchospasm, ulcerations of the ventricle and gut. Such complications have been reported in connection with long-term use of high doses of the older drugs, e.g. phenylbutazone, oxyphenbutazone, acetyl salicylic acid and indomethacin. There are indications that drugs based on aryl propionic acid, such as ibuprofen and naproxen, may produce fewer serious side-effects. It should, however, be borne in mind that the duration of observation and number of patients treated with these drugs have been limited.

Anyway, it does not seem correct to compare the pattern and incidence of side-effects during long-term treatment of, e.g., rheumatoid arthritis with those observed during short-term therapy of dysmenorrhoea. Most probably the incidence of some side-effects will be lower during short-term treatment.

References

Åkerlund, M. (1978). Pathophysiology of dysmenorrhoea. Symposium on Prostaglandins and Dysmenorrhoea, Helsinki, 1978. *Acta Obstet. Gynec. Scand.* (Suppl.) (In press)

Åkerlund, M., Andersson, K. E. and Ingmarsson, I. (1976). Effects of terbutaline on myometrial activity, endometrial flow and lower abdominal pain in women with primary dysmenorrhoea. *Br. J. Obstet. Gynaecol.*, **83**, 673

Anderson, A. B. M., Guillebaud, J., Haynes, P. J. and Turnbull, A. C. (1976). Reduction of menstrual blood-loss by prostaglandin synthetase inhibitors. *Lancet*, **i**, 774

Anderson, A. B. M., Fraser, I. S., Haynes, P. J. and Turnbull, A. C. (1978). Trial of prostaglandin synthetase inhibitors in primary dysmenorrhoea. *Lancet*, **i**, 345

Andersson, K. E. and Ulmsten, U. (1978). Effects of nifedepin on myometrial activity and lower abdominal pain in women with primary dysmenorrhoea. *Br. J. Obstet. Gynaecol.*, **85**, 142

Asplund, J. (1952). The uterine cervix and isthmus under normal and pathological conditions. *Acta Radiol.* (Suppl.), **91**, 1

Bickers, W. (1943). Primary dysmenorrhoea. *Southern Med. J.*, **36**, 192

Bygdeman, M., Bremme, K., Gillespie, A. and Lundström, V. (1978). Effects of prostaglandins on the uterus. Symposium on Prostaglandins and Dysmenorrhoea, Helsinki, 1978. *Acta Obstet. Gynecol. Scand.* (Suppl.) (In press)

Csapo, A. I., Pulkkinen, M. O. and Henzl, M. R. (1977). The effect of naproxen sodium on the intrauterine pressure and menstrual pain of dysmenorrhoeic patients. *Prostaglandins*, **13**, 193

Ferreira, S. H. (1972). Prostaglandins, aspirin-like drugs and analgesia. *Nature (New Biol.)*, **240**, 200

Filler, W. W. and Hall, W. C. (1970). Dysmenorrhoea and its therapy. A uterine contractility study. *Am. J. Obstet. Gynecol.*, **106**, 104

Granström, E. and Kindahl, H. (1976). Radioimmunoassay for urinary metabolites of prostaglandin $F_{2\alpha}$. *Prostaglandins*, **12**, 759

Hamann, G. O. and Lauersen, B. (1977). Primary dysmenorrhoea treated with indomethacin. *Ugeskr. Laeg.*, **139**, 1899 (In Danish, summary in English)

Hamberg, M. (1972). Inhibition of prostaglandin synthesis in man. *Biochem. Biophys. Res. Commun.*, **49**, 720

Henzl, M., Buttram, V., Segre, E. and Bessler, S. (1977). The treatment of dysmenorrhoea with naproxen sodium. *Am. J. Obstet. Gynecol.*, **127**, 818

Higgs, E. A., Moncada, S. and Vane, J. R. (1978). Inflammatory effects of prostacyclin and 6-oxo-$PGF_{1\alpha}$ in the rat paw. *Prostaglandins*, **16**, 153

Kapadia, L. and Elder, M. G. (1978). Flufenamic acid in treatment of primary spasmodic dysmenorrhoea. *Lancet*, **i**, 348

Kauppila, A. and Ylikorkala, O. (1977). Indomethacin and tolfenamic acid in primary dysmenorrhoea. *Eur. J. Obstet. Gynecol. Reprod. Biol.*, **7/2**, 59

Layes Molla, A. and Donald, J. F. (1974). A comparative study of ibuprofen and paracetamol in primary dysmenorrhoea. *J. Int. Med. Res.*, **2**, 395

Lundström, V. (1977). The myometrial response to intrauterine administration of $PGF_{2\alpha}$ and PGE_2 in dysmenorrhoeic women. *Acta Obstet. Gynecol. Scand.*, **56**, 167

Lundström, V. (1978). Treatment of primary dysmenorrhoea with prostaglandin synthetase inhibitors – a promising therapeutic alternative. *Acta Obstet. Gynecol. Scand.*, **57**, 421

Lundström, V. and Gréen, K. (1978). Endogenous levels of prostaglandin $F_{2\alpha}$ and its main metabolites in plasma and endometrium of normal and dysmenorrhoeic women. *Am. J. Obstet. Gynecol.*, **130**, 640

Lundström, V., Gréen, K. and Wiqvist, N. (1976). Prostaglandins, indomethacin and dysmenorrhoea. *Prostaglandins*, **11**, 893

Mann, E. C. (1963). *Progress in Gynecology*, Vol. IV, p. 123 (New York: Grune and Stratton)

Mann, E. C., Thomas, C. L. and Carmichael, D. E. (1962). Myometrial and isthmic mechanisms in primary dysmenorrhoea. *Gynecol. Obstet.*, **13**, 408

Moghissi, K. S. (1972). Prostaglandins in reproduction. *Obstet. Gynecol. Ann.*, **1**, 297

Moir, C. (1936). Intrinsic dysmenorrhoea. *Proc. R. Soc. Med.*, **29**, 950

Pace-Asciak, C. R. (1977). Minirevue – Oxidative biotransformations of arachidonic acid. *Prostaglandins*, **13**, 811

Pickles, V. R., Hall, W. J., Best, F. A. and Smith, C. N. (1965). Prostaglandins in endometrium and menstrual fluid from normal and dysmenorrhoeic subjects. *J. Obstet. Gynecol. Br. Cmwlth.*, **72**, 185

Pulkkinen, M. O. and Kaihola, H.-L. (1977). Mefenamic acid in dysmenorrhoea. *Acta Obstet. Gynecol. Scand.*, **56**, 75

Shangold, M. M., Aksel, S., Schomberg, D. W. and Hammond, C. B. (1976). Plasma prostaglandin $F_{2\alpha}$ levels in dysmenorrhoeic women. *Fert. Steril.*, **27**, 1171

12
Prostaglandins and their Synthesis Inhibitors in Dysfunctional Uterine Bleeding

M. TOPPOZADA

12.1 INTRODUCTION

Almost half a century ago a factor isolated from menstrual blood was implicated in the mechanism of cyclic endometrial shedding. This substance was referred to as 'The Menstrual Toxin' or 'Menotoxin'. Technical limitations prevented chemical characterization of the active principle (Smith and Smith, 1947). The substance was present in premenstrual endometrium in ovulatory as well as non-ovulatory cycles.

Several decades later, prostaglandins (PG) were shown to be present in the menstrual blood as well as in the endometrium. These compounds share a number of properties attributed to menotoxin (Pickles, 1957; Clitheroe, 1961; Eglington *et al.*, 1963; Pickles and Hall, 1963; Pickles and Ward, 1965). Whether the prostaglandins and menotoxin group of compounds are identical remains a subject of speculation.

A few years ago, pure prostaglandins became available for clinical studies and their administration to non-pregnant women was found to induce uterine bleeding (Wiqvist *et al.*, 1971). This bleeding was believed to result from strong uterine contractions or a vasoconstriction within the uterus. Further evidence for a role of prostaglandins in menstruation has also been presented by investigators who measured levels of different prostaglandins in the peripheral blood, endometrium and menstrual blood (see Karim and Hillier, 1975). The most recent support for a role of prostaglandins in the monthly shedding of the endometrium is derived from observations that menstrual blood loss (MBL) can be significantly reduced by administration of inhibitors of prostaglandin biosynthesis (Anderson *et al.*, 1976; Damarawy and Toppozada, 1976). The factors controlling and regulating MBL are poorly understood. It is obvious that a number of complex interrelated factors are involved in this process with prostaglandins serving as a link in a long chain of events.

In this review an attempt is made to define the role of prostaglandins in the mechanism of uterine bleeding in physiological and pathophysiological conditions. In the latter area, the main emphasis is placed on dysfunctional uterine bleeding. A large section of this chapter is devoted to bleeding associated with intra-uterine contraceptive devices (IUD) despite the fact that this type of bleeding cannot, in the strict sense of the definition, be considered dysfunctional. This inclusion is largely based on the global interest in this type of blood loss and the strong evidence implicating prostaglandins in irregular bleeding associated with IUDs. Finally, the use of inhibitors of prostaglandin synthesis in the control of excessive uterine bleeding will be discussed.

12.2 ROLE OF PROSTAGLANDINS IN NORMAL UTERINE BLEEDING

There is a paucity of information regarding the role of prostaglandins in the mechanism of endometrial bleeding. An understanding of how prostaglandins are involved in MBL or in haemostatic mechanisms that inhibit excessive loss may be helpful in directing future research efforts towards developing therapeutic approaches.

At the local uterine level, four fundamental factors may modify menstrual blood loss. These are: circulating blood, uterine vasculature, myometrial activity and endometrial integrity (Figure 12.1).

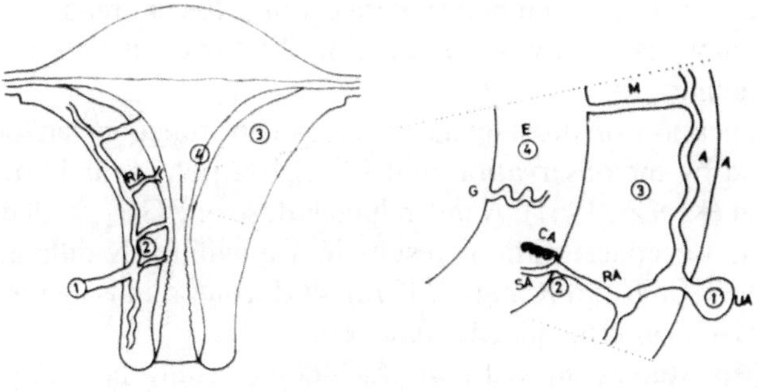

Figure 12.1 Local (uterine) factors involved in the control of uterine bleeding (1) circulating blood, (2) uterine vasculature, (3) myometrial factors, (4) endometrial factors. UA = uterine artery, AA = arcuate artery, RA = radial artery, SA = straight/short artery, CA = coiled or spinal arteriole, M = myometrium, E = endometrium

Each of these factors may be influenced by a large number of secondary factors such as endocrine, nervous and metabolic changes. However, the following section will only deal with the involvement of prostaglandins and the way in which a specific prostaglandin may modify the function of any of these basic uterine factors.

12.2.1 Prostaglandins and blood coagulation

12.2.1.1 *Platelet function*

The function of human platelets in haemostasis is closely linked to prostaglandins. This conclusion is based on the following observations: (1) Some prostaglandins and their intermediates inhibit platelet aggregation or adhesiveness while others stimulate the process. (2) Prostaglandins are released during platelet aggregation. (3) Non-steroidal anti-inflammatory drugs (NSAID) effectively prevent the synthesis of prostaglandins by platelets and inhibit the second phase of platelet aggregation.

As part of the haemostatic mechanism following vessel injury, a platelet plug forms and adhesion of platelets at the injured surface takes place. This is subsequently stabilized by fibrin. The platelet adhesion to the exposed subendothelial collagen (first phase) results in the release of adenosine diphosphate (ADP) (platelet release reaction), which plays a major role in the second phase of platelet aggregation (Gaarder *et al.*, 1961; Hovig, 1963). Other substances are also liberated during this platelet clumping and release reaction. These include serotonin (5-HT), catecholamines, platelet factor 3 and prostaglandins (Smith and Willis, 1970, 1971). The release reaction is blocked by NSAID which also inhibit prostaglandin biosynthesis. This may imply that prostaglandin synthesis is an integral part of the release reaction (Weiss *et al.*, 1968; Zucker and Peterson, 1968). These findings stimulated many investigators to look into the possible application of NSAID in the management of thromboembolic complications. Recent reports also indicate that these substances may prove useful in the treatment of certain types of uterine bleeding.

The implication of prostaglandins in platelet function has been further documented by the observation that PGE_1 is a potent inhibitor of platelet aggregation (Kloeze, 1967). A much higher dose of PGE_2 produces a similar effect but lower concentrations results in a qualitatively different response (Kloeze, 1967; Shio and Ramwell, 1972). PGF compounds on the other hand are ineffective in altering platelet function.

Subsequent studies showed that arachidonic acid (a natural precursor of some prostaglandins) also enhances platelet aggregation and even more potent in this respect are the endoperoxide intermediates PGG_2 and PGH_2. The latter agents were believed to be mediators of platelet clumping effect of arachidonic acid (Vargaftig and Zirinis, 1973; Silver *et al.*, 1973 and Willis *et al.*, 1974). The picture has become more complex by the recent finding that thromboxane A_2 (also formed from arachidonic acid) is a potent aggregator of platelets while PGD_2 and PGI_2 (prostacyclin) have the opposite effect, i.e. they inhibit platelet aggregation. Thus, different products formed from arachidonic acid may result in end products or intermediates with opposite actions on the platelets.

Several platelet aggregating agents (thrombin, collagen, ADP, epinephrine) activate phospholipase enzymes in the platelet membrane and release arachidonic acid which leads to the formation of endoperoxides and thromboxanes (Smith and Silver, 1973; Schoene and Iacono, 1975). The latter compounds may act as a link between the initial stimulus and the release reaction of platelets and aggregation.

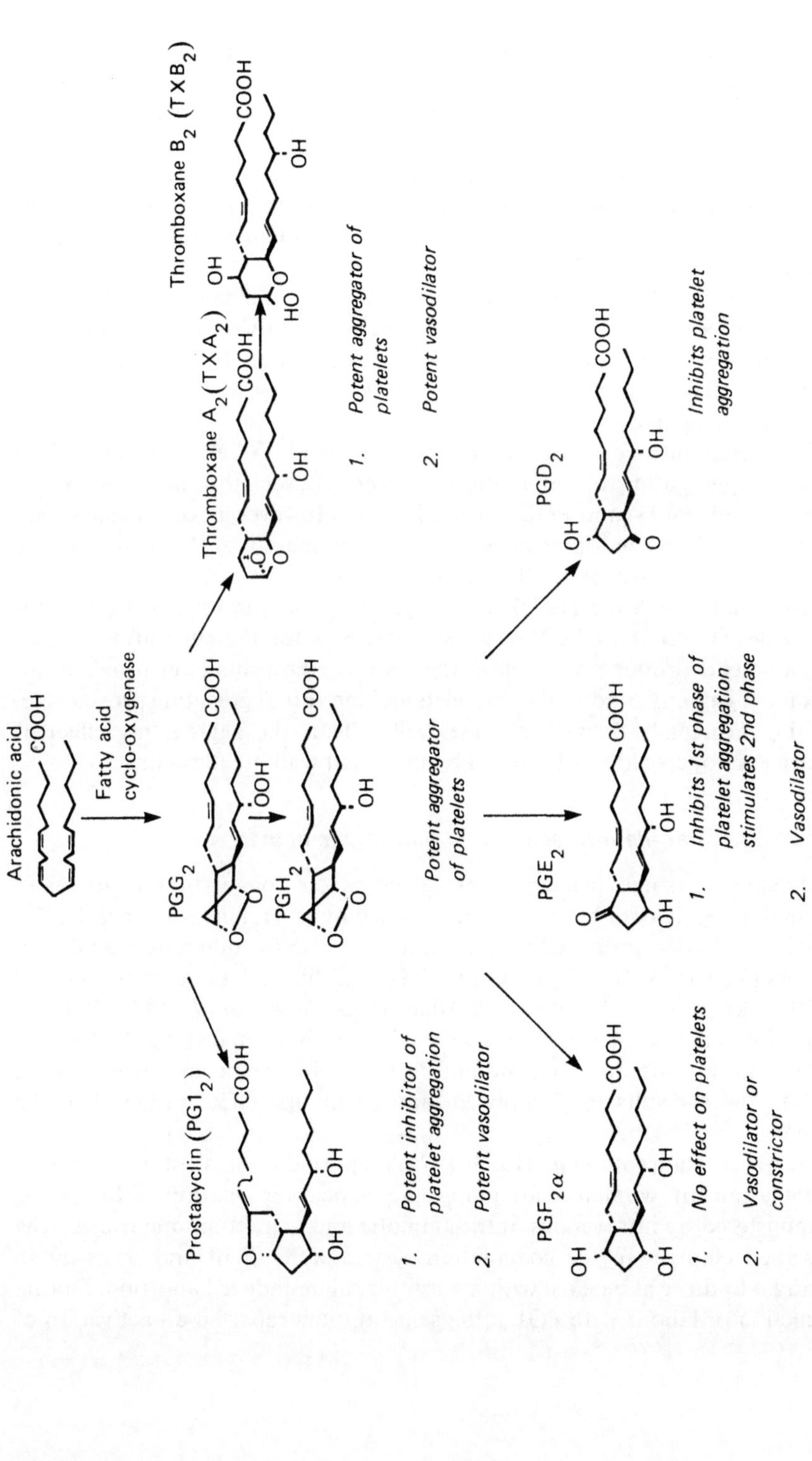

Figure 12.2 Pathways of prostaglandins and thromboxane biosynthesis and their effects on platelets and blood vessels

In summary (Figure 12.2), amongst the primary prostaglandins, PGE_1 is an inhibitor of platelet aggregation and also interferes with clumping induced by different aggregating agents. PGE_2 has an initial weak PGE_1-like inhibitory effect on the first phase of aggregation followed by a stimulatory action on the second phase (ADP induced) of aggregation. $PGF_{2\alpha}$ has no effect on platelet aggregation.

The endoperoxide intermediates (PGG_2 and PGH_2) induce rapid and irreversible aggregation of human platelets. One of the end products of these endoperoxides is thromboxane A_2 which is a potent platelet aggregating agent.

Prostacyclin (PGX or PGI_2) is a potent inhibitor of platelet aggregation. It is 20–30 times more potent than PGE_1 and 10–15 times more potent than PGD_2 in preventing human platelet aggregation induced by arachidonic acid, ADP or collagen. It can also reverse platelet aggregation induced by some aggregating agents.

The mechanism of selective transformation of the endoperoxides into platelet aggregating or inhibiting end products, i.e. thromboxane A_2 or prostacyclin (PGI_2) and PGD_2, is not known. However, at certain sites such as vessel wall, the endoperoxides are converted mainly to PGI_2 while in the platelets, thromboxanes are the major products.

Moncada and Vane (1977) have suggested that the intermediate endoperoxides (PGG_2 and PGH_2) act as substrates for the generation of two unstable end products with opposing actions; the pro-aggregating thromboxane A_2 mainly produced by platelets and the anti-aggregating prostacyclin (PGI_2) principally formed in vessel walls. Thus the aggregating effect of platelet endoperoxides is balanced by the vessel wall prostacyclin.

12.2.1.2 *Coagulation factors and fibrinolytic activity*

The effect of some primary prostaglandins on coagulation factors and fibrinolytic activity of blood has been studied by several investigators. PGE_1, PGE_2 and $PGF_{2\alpha}$ produced insignificant effects on the different coagulation factors (V, VII, VIII, IX, X, XI and XII) and fibrinolytic activity (Kloeze, 1970; Sekhar, 1970; Karim and Filshie, 1972; Howie *et al.*, 1973; Phillips, 1973; Duboff *et al.*, 1974). Increased euglobulin lysis time and antithrombin activity in response to an infusion of PGE_2 has been reported (Howie *et al.*, 1973). These results may imply an antithrombotic effect rather than the reverse.

However, Badraoui *et al.* (1973, 1974a) reported a transient intravascular coagulation in women undergoing pregnancy termination with $PGF_{2\alpha}$ administered by intravenous, intra-amniotic and extra-amniotic routes. The observed changes in the coagulation system were slight and transient in contrast to those associated with hypertonic saline-induced abortion. During induction of labour with PGE_2, the same authors reported an activation of the coagulation system which was more pronounced than the changes noted during spontaneous labour or that induced with oxytocin (Badraoui *et al.*, 1974b). Many of the changes in the coagulation system reported by Badraoui *et al.*(1973, 1974a, 1974b) were attributed (at least in part) to the induced uterine contractions or to the process of foetal expulsion itself.

The findings to date, therefore, suggest that the effects of prostaglandins on blood coagulation and thrombosis are mainly mediated through their influence on platelet function and to a lesser extent by affecting the factors responsible for fibrin formation and fibrinolysis.

12.2.2 Uterine blood vessels

The vascular reactivity to prostaglandins is more complex than initially anticipated. The vascular response depends on the type of prostaglandin and the species. Even in the same animal the effect of a particular prostaglandin may be different on different vascular beds. Sometimes, an alternation in humoral factors may modify vascular reactivity to prostaglandins. The vascular effects of the newly discovered prostaglandins (C_2, D_2, G_2, H_2, I_2) and thromboxanes has made the situation more complex. Moreover, it is not yet fully established whether prostaglandins play a definite physiological role in the vascular system or whether they are only involved in certain pathological situations.

Prostaglandins are locally formed in vessel walls and can thus influence vascular responses at their site of production (Tuvemo and Wide, 1973; Kalsner, 1974; Terragno *et al.*, 1974; Gryglewski and Korbut, 1975). Their action may either be a primary myogenic response or more probably mediated directly or indirectly by other vasoactive agents such as adrenergic neurotransmitters (Greenberg *et al.*, 1974a, 1974b). In most peripheral vascular beds, prostaglandins of the A and E series are potent vasodilators. PGB_2 is a potent vasoconstrictor while $PGF_{2\alpha}$ produces a similar but weaker effect (Greenberg and Sparks, 1969; Kadowitz *et al.*, 1971a, 1971b; Kadowitz, 1972; Greenberg *et al.*, 1974a, 1974b). In this context, recent studies show that PGI_2 (prostacyclin), D_2 and E_1 relax some vascular smooth muscles while the endoperoxide intermediates (PGG_2 and PGH_2) have the opposite effect.

12.2.2.1 *Uterine blood flow*

Very little is known about the effects and role of prostaglandins and thromboxanes in the control of human uterine blood flow. Most of the available information is derived from *in vitro* and animal studies.

The only study in primates on the effect of intrauterine instillation of $PGF_{2\alpha}$ (in approximately physiological doses) showed a dramatic fall in endometrial blood flow (Einer-Jensen, 1973). Whether this effect is due to myometrial contractions or is a result of direct vascular constriction is not clear. Despite the fact that $PGF_{2\alpha}$ produces systemic vasoconstriction, it has little influence on uterine vascular resistance (Brody and Kadowitz, 1974). The E and A series of prostaglandins, on the other hand, cause relaxation of uterine blood vessels and decrease the sensitivity of uterine vascular muscles to adrenergic constrictor stimuli (Clark *et al.*, 1977, 1978). It has been suggested that adrenergic nerve stimulation activates the local release of prostaglandins which produce a local negative feedback effect on uterine vascular smooth muscle. Moreover, inhibitors of prostaglandin synthesis lead to a fall in uterine PGE concentrations with a consequent rise in uterine vascular resistance.

Studies on human endometrial cell cultures indicate that oestrogens are capable of stimulating prostaglandin synthesis whereas progesterone produces an opposite effect (Cane and Villee, 1975). In rodents, prostaglandins have been implicated in oestrogen-induced hyperaemia (Ryan *et al.*, 1974). This assumption was based on the finding that oestrogen-induced increase in blood flow could be blocked by administration of prostaglandin biosynthesis inhibitors. This effect was accompanied by a parallel drop in the uterine levels of E and F prostaglandins.

More information is needed to evaluate the role of prostaglandins in endometrial blood flow. The extent to which different prostaglandins, their intermediates and metabolites, the thromboxanes and other vasoactive substances interact in the endometrium to control its haemodynamics needs to be explored in more detail. The factors which selectively result in the biosynthesis of a specific prostaglandin from its unsaturated fatty acid precursor require further evaluation.

12.2.2.2 *Microcirculation*

Factors other than endometrial blood flow such as increased vascular permeability and minor vascular injury may contribute to the occurrence of uterine bleeding. This is particularly true in certain inflammatory conditions and in the presence of a foreign body within the uterus. The increase in vascular permeability can be achieved by different prostaglandins, histamine, endotoxin, bradykinin, thermal injury, etc.

Both endometrial vascular constriction and dilatation are important components in the production or aggravation of uterine bleeding. It has been known for a long time that menstruation represents a specific and peculiar form of tissue breakdown in which vasoactive changes in the spiral arterioles play an important role. A marked degree of spiral arteriolar spasm has been reported to occur just prior to menstrual bleeding and is sustained throughout menstruation (Markee, 1940, 1950; Salvatore, 1968). The fact that these vessels are end arteries may explain the relation between the observed spasm and onset of uterine bleeding (Bartelmez, 1957). The venous drainage of the endometrium is accomplished via a rich plexus of veins which show some dilatations known as 'venous lakes' (Harris and Ramsay, 1966). The number and degree of dilatation in these veins are increased in endometrial hyperplasia (Beilby *et al.*, 1971).

The actual cause of vascular changes in the endometrium related to menstruation is not completely understood. The role of prostaglandins in this context also remains speculative. Lysosomal stress and release of vasoactive substances such as oxytocin, vasopressin and angiotensin have been suggested as possible contributing factors. However, these substances are also known to induce a release of $PGF_{2\alpha}$ or PGE_2 which are capable of altering arteriolar resistance (Gustavii, 1972; Gimbrone and Alexander, 1975; Roberts *et al.*, 1976; Åkerlund and Andersson, 1976a, 1976b). Infusion of $PGF_{2\alpha}$ for a 48-hour period in the early luteal phase induces uterine bleeding which is associated with local necrosis in the endometrium. This is more likely to be pharmacological than a physiological response (Turksoy and Safaii, 1975). Moreover, a factor capable of inhibiting fatty acid cyclo-oxygenase has been identified in the endometrium. The changes in this factor may be relevant to the marked increase in the capacity of the endometrium in converting arachidonic acid to $PGF_{2\alpha}$ in the late luteal phase (Wlodawer *et al.*, 1976).

Another factor which has to be considered in this context is vascular leakage. This mechanism may contribute to uterine bleeding particularly in relation to abnormal menstrual loss in the presence of an IUD. It is now established that prostaglandins are mediators of inflammation by potentiating or increasing vascular leakage induced by other mediators such as bradykinin or histamine (Williams and Morley, 1973; Lewis *et al.*, 1974; Vane, 1976).

Prostaglandins of the E series are thought to be important in the vascular leakage response (Vane, 1976). $PGF_{2\alpha}$, on the other hand, antagonizes the increased vascular permeability induced by PGE_1 and PGE_2 (Crunkhorn and Willis, 1971).

Microscopic studies of the endometrium in cases of increased vessel permeability showed widened inter-endothelial spaces through which plasma components and red cells could escape into the interstitial spaces (Wilson *et al.*, 1965; Shaw and Moyer, 1978). These changes may prove to be of basic importance in the mechanism of physiological and/or IUD-induced uterine bleeding.

12.2.3 Myometrial factors

The relationship between myometrial function and uterine blood loss has been recognized for a long time. Oxytocic agents are effectively used for the control of abnormal and excessive uterine bleeding particularly in obstetric practice. Because prostaglandins are potent uterine stimulants it is logical to assume that they will be useful in the management of uterine haemorrhages. This has been documented in cases of atonic post-partum haemorrhage where direct intra-uterine injection of 1 mg $PGF_{2\alpha}$ proved to be clinically useful (Takagi *et al.*, 1976). Systemic administration of PGE_1 or $PGF_{2\alpha}$ did not significantly reduce the immediate post-partum blood loss. In one study a slight decrease in blood loss was observed when infusion of $PGF_{2\alpha}$ used for acceleration of labour was continued after delivery (Roth-Brandel *et al.*, 1970b; Persianinov

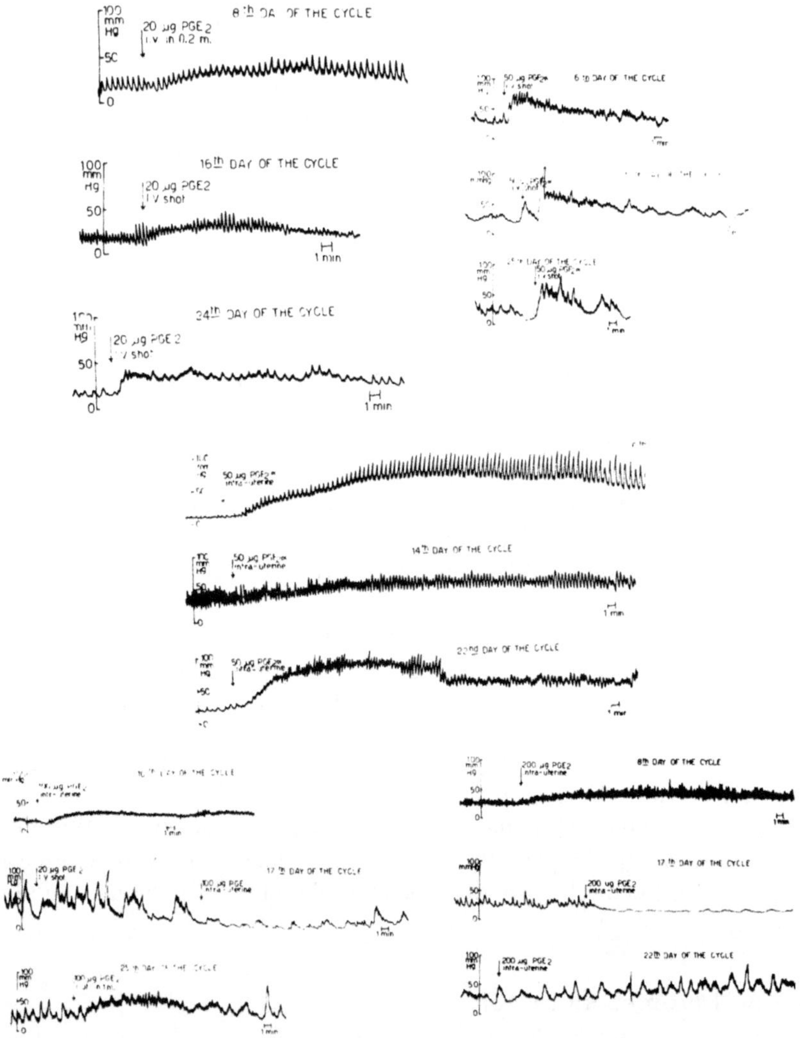

Figure 12.3 Response of the non-pregnant human uterus to intravenous and intra-uterine administration of PGE_2 and $PGF_{2\alpha}$ during different phases of the menstrual cycle. Upper two curves show the stimulatory effect of intravenous injections. Middle section shows uterine stimulation following local instillation of $PGF_{2\alpha}$. The lower two sections illustrate the mid-cycle uterine relaxation in response to intra-uterine administration of PGE_2. The same procedure caused stimulation at other phases of the cycle.

et al., 1973; Takagi *et al.*, 1976). The effectiveness of prostaglandins in the treatment of uterine haemorrhage in non-pregnant state has so far received little attention.

Prostaglandins may control endometrial bleeding by a mechanical effect of the contracting uterus on the blood vessels within the muscular layer. Intra-myometrial injections of $PGF_{2\alpha}$ and 15-methyl-$PGF_{2\alpha}$ at mid-pregnancy result in marked and sustained uterine contractions and extreme blanching due to severe ischaemia of the uterine wall (Morad and Toppozada, 1977).

In *in vitro* studies PGE compounds inhibited the contractility of non-pregnant myometrial strips (Bygdeman, 1964). Magnitude of inhibition was related to the phase of the menstrual cycle. The inhibitory response was initially believed to be mediated via activation of the adrenergic β-receptor system (Lish *et al.*, 1960) but this was later disputed in view of the obvious differences in the character of response to PGE and drugs that act on β-adrenergic receptors.

Embrey (1966) was the first to show a spasmogenic action of pure $PGF_{2\alpha}$ on the human myometrium following intra-uterine instillation in a non-pregnant woman undergoing dilatation and curettage. Subsequently, the uterine response to intra-uterine instillation of $PGF_{2\alpha}$ has been studied in more detail during different phases of the menstrual cycle (Toppozada *et al.*, 1974, 1977a; Shaala *et al.*, 1977). Several other investigators have reported that systemic administration of E and F prostaglandins stimulates the non-pregnant uterus irrespective of the phase of the menstrual cycle (Roth-Brandel *et al.*, 1970b; Karim *et al.*, 1971; Toppozada *et al.*, 1975, 1976; Shaala *et al.*, 1977).

The response of the non-pregnant human uterus to intra-uterine instillation of PGE_2 was first reported by Toppozada *et al.* (1974). Several publications from the same investigators have documented the nature and magnitude of uterine response to local administration of PGE_2 (Toppozada *et al.*, 1975, 1976, 1977b). Intra-uterine administration of PGE_2 in cycling women produced a marked stimulation in the proliferative and luteal phases of the cycle but pronounced inhibition of uterine activity was elicited around the time of ovulation (days 13–18) (Figure 12.3). A similar type of inhibition was also observed in menopausal subjects (Shaala *et al.*, 1974). The authors have suggested that mid-cycle inhibition of uterine activity by local administration of PGE_2 may be of importance in passive sperm transport. Moreover, it was absent in women using combined (oestrogen and progesterone) oral contraceptives and in cases of functional infertility (Toppozada *et al.*, 1976, 1977b). Combined oral contraceptives also suppressed the contractile response of the non-pregnant uterus to systemic and local administration of $PGF_{2\alpha}$ and PGE_2.

In a recent publication the uterotonic effect of small (physiological) doses of PGE_2 and $PGF_{2\alpha}$ in non-pregnant women was evaluated (Martin *et al.*, 1978). The authors reported that the response of the non-pregnant human uterus to locally administered PGE_2 and $PGF_{2\alpha}$ was dependent upon the phase of the menstrual cycle. Stimulation was observed after the cessation of menstruation until 4 days prior to ovulation followed by a phase of relative insensitivity. In the luteal phase the stimulation was characterized by an increase in frequency and amplitude of contractions in contrast to an increase in the tone of the uterus at the beginning of the cycle. A definite suppression of uterine contractility following local instillation of PGE_2 was observed during menstrual bleeding. $PGF_{2\alpha}$ stimulated the uterus during this period.

The available evidence indicated that prostaglandins of the E and F series may be important in the control of uterine activity during the menstrual cycle. The exact physiological significance of these effects is so far not clear. Also, the balance between the E and F prostaglandins and interaction with other humoral substances need to be further explored. The effects of other related substances such as endoperoxides, prostacyclin and thromboxanes on uterine activity in women have not been evaluated.

The effect of uterine activity on endometrial blood flow in non-pregnant women has recently been studied using a microtransducer catheter for recording intra-uterine pressure with simultaneous monitoring of endometrial blood flow with a thermistor probe (Åkerlund *et al.*, 1975; Åkerlund *et al.*, 1976). During the frequent small contractions seen in the proliferative phase and at mid-cycle, the local endometrial blood flow showed only small variations which were not related to individual contractions. However, the blood flow decreased significantly during the well-defined high amplitude and low-frequency contractions recorded at the onset of menstruation (Åkerlund, 1976). The transient decrease in uterine blood flow during strong co-ordinated contractions was attributed to the compression of blood vessels. The authors suggested that in the human non-pregnant uterus, where local and propagated contractions are known to occur (Martinez-Gaudio *et al.*, 1973) there is a redistribution of blood flow from a contracting segment to a non-contracting area.

In view of the above observations one could speculate that there is a correlation between prostaglandins and endometrial blood flow in the human. Since prostaglandins possess potent biological actions both on the myometrium and on the uterine vasculature, they may have important functions in the induction and control of MBL.

12.2.4 Endometrial factors

The bleeding surface at menstruation, the endometrium, is the final target of a large number of factors (systemic or local) involved in the control of cyclic endometrial shedding. However the present section will be restricted to a discussion of whether endometrial prostaglandins play a role in the induction or control of menstrual bleeding. Five major factors warrant consideration in this context:

(1) Endometrial and circulating levels of prostaglandins and their metabolites.
(2) The capacity of endometrial tissue to synthesize prostaglandins.
(3) Prostaglandin receptors in the endometrium and their binding capacity.
(4) Endometrial metabolism of prostaglandins.
(5) Effect of prostaglandin biosynthesis inhibitors.

Several investigators have measured amounts of prostaglandins in the endometrium in an effort to correlate the levels to physiological events. Table 12.1 summarizes the findings of these investigations. Results of most studies

Table 12.1 Relative levels of E and F prostaglandins in the human endometrium during different phases of the menstrual cycle

			Phase of the cycle			
Reference	*Method*	*PG*	*Prolif. (P)*	*Late secretory (S)*	*Menst. (M)*	*PGF: PGE ratio*
Pickles *et al.*, 1965	bioassay	E_2 and $F_{2\alpha}$	low	higher	—	higher at S
Clitheroe, 1973	TLC	$F_{2\alpha}$	low	higher	—	higher at S
Downie *et al.*, 1974	bioassay	E_2 and $F_{2\alpha}$	low	higher	highest	higher at S
Levitt *et al.* 1975	RIA	E_2	low	higher	—	equal at P
		F_2	low	much higher	—	much higher at S
Singh *et al.*, 1975	TD	E_2 and $F_{2\alpha}$	low	higher	highest	much higher at S
Green and Hagenfeldt, 1975	GLC–MS	$F_{2\alpha}$	low	higher	—	—
		15-keto-13,14-dihydro $PGF_{2\alpha}$	low	higher	—	—
Willman *et al.*, 1976	RIA	E_2 and $F_{2\alpha}$	low	higher	highest	low at P ± equal at S and M

TLC = Thin layer chromatography
RIA = Radioimmunoassay
TD = Transmission densitometry
GLC-MS = Gas liquid chromatography and mass spectrometry

indicate a progressive increase in concentrations of $PGF_{2\alpha}$, 15-keto-13,14-dihydro-$PGF_{2\alpha}$ or PGE_2 from the proliferative phase to the secretory phase and reaching peak levels during menstruation (Figure 12.4). In only one study (Levitt *et al.*, 1975) there was an insignificant difference in the endometrial concentration of prostaglandins during proliferative and late secretory phase

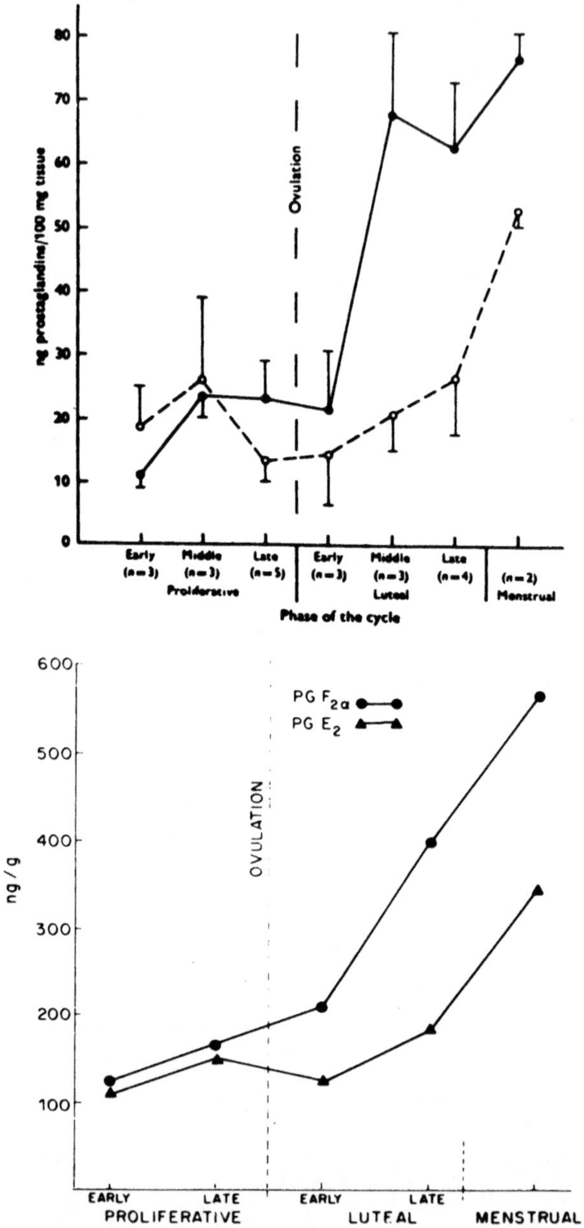

Figure 12.4 Endometrial levels of $PGF_{2\alpha}$ and PGE_2 during different phases of human menstrual cycle. Top: from Downie *et al.* (1974), $PGF_{2\alpha}$ ●–● and ○–○ PGE_2 (by courtesy of *J. Physiol.*). Bottom: from Singh *et al.* (1975) ●–● $PGF_{2\alpha}$ and ▲–▲ PGE_2 (by courtesy of *Am. J. Obstet. Gynecol.*). Both studies show an increase in prostaglandin concentrations in the luteal and menstrual phases of the cycle

of the menstrual cycle. However, when the data were expressed as total endometrial prostaglandins the difference was highly significant. Prostaglandin F levels in endometrial jet washings are also significantly higher in the secretory phase compared to the proliferative phase (Demers *et al.*, 1975).

The ratio of F to E prostaglandins in most of the studies discussed above followed an interesting pattern. This ratio was higher (i.e. relative preponderance of F over E prostaglandins) in the secretory and menstrual phases of the cycle compared to the proliferative phase.

Measurements of tissue levels of prostaglandins pose certain problems and results should be interpreted with caution. These compounds are readily formed and released in response to trauma of sampling and tissue homogenization prior to extraction. The measurement may, therefore, represent 'artificial' formation of prostaglandins by tissues. Most investigators, however, have emphasized that the tissues were handled in a manner that minimized such unphysiological biosynthesis, i.e. snap frozen or homogenized and extracted in the presence of an inhibitor of prostaglandin biosynthesis. Some authors have also expressed a confidence in the significance and interpretation of relative concentrations since samples obtained at different phases of the menstrual cycle were managed in the same way. However, the ability of tissues to synthesize prostaglandins may change significantly under different hormonal conditions and the observed relative changes in levels may simply represent a measurement of the tissues' ability to form prostaglandins.

If the reported levels of prostaglandins in the endometrium are real then it would be important to know the factors controlling the observed changes during the menstrual cycle.

Based on studies in guinea-pigs, Blatchley *et al.* (1972) postulated that oestrogen increases the production of $PGF_{2\alpha}$ by the uterus. Results of experiments in the sheep indicate that the uterus may have to be progesterone primed before the maximum effect of oestrogen is seen (Caldwell *et al.*, 1972). Oxytocin also enhances the release of $PGF_{2\alpha}$ from ovine endometrium *in vitro* in a dose-dependent manner (Roberts *et al.*, 1976). This may involve an interaction between oxytocin and its receptors in the endometrium with steroid hormones.

In the human the situation may be different. Earlier studies indicated a correlation between a rise in progesterone and increased endometrial prostaglandins (Pickles, 1965; Clitheroe, 1973). Downie *et al.* (1974) found maximum levels of $PGF_{2\alpha}$ in the endometrium when oestrogen and progesterone together were at their highest level. The authors suggested that a combination of these two hormones form the physiological stimulus for the production of $PGF_{2\alpha}$ by the human endometrium. In tissue cultures of human endometrium *in vitro* oestradiol stimulates and progesterone inhibits the release of $PGF_{2\alpha}$ (Cane and Villee, 1975). It has been postulated that during the pre-menstrual phase the inhibitory effect of progesterone is removed leading to a marked increase in $PGF_{2\alpha}$ synthesis. However, there is also a concomitant drop in oestrogen levels at this phase of the cycle.

Another factor involved in endometrial production of prostaglandins or occurrence of menstrual bleeding may be related to lysosomal activity. A progressive increase in the number of lysosomes and their enzymes in endometrial cell cytoplasm with advancing luteal phase has been demonstrated (Henzl *et al.*, 1972; Rosada *et al.*, 1977). Oestrogens are known to cause some increase in lysosome numbers and the hydrolase content. Progesterone, on the other hand, may stabilize lysosomal membranes in addition to increasing the number of lysosomes and their enzyme content (Szego, 1972, 1974). A decline in progesterone levels in the late luteal phase probably leads to fragility and breakdown of lysosomal membranes with ultimate leakage of their enzymes. The liberated phospholipase A may act on cell membrane phospholipids to release precursors of prostaglandins. This hypothesis may explain the chain of events leading to an increased production of prostaglandins as menstruation becomes imminent (Gustavii, 1972).

Several investigators have attempted to correlate circulating levels (plasma or serum) of prostaglandins with different phases of the menstrual cycle. Prostaglandin levels in such studies have varied between 5 and 3500 pg/ml which indicate artificially high values in some studies. The short half-life of the measured prostaglandins, their synthesis and metabolism in blood cast doubt on the significance of reported levels. Measurements of stable, circulating metabolites of prostaglandins also suffer from drawbacks, including the presence of a number of metabolites and their daily fluctuations. The levels of 15-keto-13,14-dihydro-$PGF_{2\alpha}$ (a metabolite of $PGF_{2\alpha}$) in serum or plasma did not correlate with any particular event in the menstrual cycle (Levine and Gutierrez-Cernosek, 1973; Kindahl *et al.*, 1976). Measurements of total urinary metabolites in a 24-hour urine sample has its own limitations since these may originate from a number of sites in the body.

High levels of prostaglandins in tissues and biological fluids may be the result rather than a cause of a particular physiological event. The binding of prostaglandins to specific sites at cell membranes could be indicative of a possible physiological role. Two distinct prostaglandin receptor sites have been identified in human uterine tissues. PGE_2 binds with high affinity and capacity with the first site and to a lesser degree with the second site. $PGF_{2\alpha}$ has a high affinity with site two and only at high concentration binds at site one (Schillinger and Prior, 1976).

If prostaglandins are essential in the mechanism of monthly endometrial shedding, then administration of prostaglandin biosynthesis inhibitors would be expected to delay the onset of menstruation. This could not be confirmed in women treated with aspirin or indomethacin (Chaudhury and Elder, 1976; Toppozada *et al.*, 1977a). These findings may imply that prostaglandins do not have an obligatory role in the induction of menstruation. However, in a recent report indomethacin or naproxen administered 1–2 days prior to expected onset of menstruation caused a delay of 4–5 days in the onset of bleeding in some women (Lundström, 1977).

12.3 ROLE OF PROSTAGLANDINS IN DYSFUNCTIONAL BLEEDING AND BLEEDING ASSOCIATED WITH INTRA-UTERINE CONTRACEPTIVE DEVICE (IUD)

The previous section dealt with different aspects of possible involvement of prostaglandins in the mechanism of normal cyclic uterine bleeding. It is clear that a large number of factors may play a role in the control of endometrial bleeding and may influence prostaglandins in a way that ultimately induces tissue breakdown. The primary objective of this section, therefore, is to evaluate whether abnormal production or function of prostaglandins is involved in dysfunctional bleeding or bleeding induced by IUD. Several factors including abnormal hormonal patterns, distorted vascular morphology or physiology, disturbed function of lysosomes, prostaglandins and platelets have been implicated in dysfunctional and IUD-related bleeding. The initial trigger and the exact sequence of events which lead to endometrial bleeding and the precise role of prostaglandins within the complex series of events still remain obscure.

There is a consensus of opinion that dysfunctional, organic and IUD-induced bleeding is associated with overproduction of E and F prostaglandins (Singh *et al.*, 1975; Hillier and Kasonde, 1976; Anderson *et al.*, 1976; Willman *et al.*, 1976; Haynes *et al.*, 1978). Large amounts of PGE_2 and $PGF_{2\alpha}$ are present in endometrial adenocarcinoma (Singh *et al.*, 1975). In patients with dysfunctional uterine bleeding, the concentrations of PGE_2 and $PGF_{2\alpha}$ in endometrial tissue are significantly higher, with minimal cyclical variation, than in normal controls. The increase in PG levels was more marked in women with irregular bleeding than in those with regular but excessive menstrual blood loss (Willman *et al.*, 1976). Recently, $PGF_{2\alpha}$ and PGE_2 were measured by radioimmunoassay in endometrial tissue obtained at different phases of the menstrual cycle from 17 women with dysfunctional menorrhagia and the results were compared with levels in 28 eumenorrhoeic women. Subjects with menorrhagia had significantly higher concentrations of PGE_2 in the pre-menstrual phase compared to women with normal loss (Haynes *et al.*, 1978). The reported alterations in ovarian steroid secretions in dysfunctional uterine bleeding (unopposed oestradiol or elevated levels of oestrogens and progesterones) may influence levels of prostaglandins in the endometrium (Cane and Villee, 1975). However, any correlation between endocrine changes associated with dysfunctional bleeding and increased production of prostaglandins is far from established.

There is considerable evidence from studies in sub-primates to show that the presence of an intra-uterine contraceptive device results in excessive production of prostaglandins. High levels of PGE and PGF have also been reported in endometrial tissue, utero-ovarian vein blood and uterine flushings obtained from rats, rabbits, hamsters, guinea-pigs and sheep bearing IUD (Poyser *et al.*, 1971; Spilman and Duby, 1972; Chaudhury, 1973; Saksena and Harper, 1974; Saksena *et al.*, 1974). These data implicate prostaglandins in the mechanism of action of IUDs. The situation in the human female is not clear. Green and Hagenfeldt (1975) did not find any change in levels of endometrial $PGF_{2\alpha}$ and its 15-keto-13,14-dihydro metabolite in women with IUD. In contrast, Hillier and Kasonde (1976) found a significant increase in concentration of E prostaglandins (but not F) following insertion of inert or copper-bearing IUD. The results of this study has revived the theory put forward by Chaudhury (1971) that the efficacy of IUD is related to a release of prostaglandins within the uterus.

Prostaglandins (especially the E series) produce vascular effects, leukocyte migration and histamine release. Thus prostaglandins may mediate the contraceptive action of IUDs through any of these biological effects. Recently, the macrophages cultured from the surface of extracted IUDs have been implicated as a sourc of excessive prostaglandin production (Myatt, 1975). Moreover, leukocytes are known to have the capability to preferentially release PGE_1 (Zurier, 1976). Overproduction of prostaglandins in the presence of IUDs may be a cause or result of increased leukocytic infiltration.

Apart from mediating the contraceptive effectiveness of IUDs, excessive production of prostaglandins is also thought to be associated with abnormal bleeding, uterine cramps and expulsion of the device. Irregular and excessive bleeding is the most common reason given by women who request removal of IUDs. However, there is a lack of direct evidence showing an overproduction of prostaglandins in IUD users with excessive MBL. Comparative studies on prostaglandin levels in women with IUDs with excessive blood loss and those with normal blood loss have not been reported. Theoretically prostaglandins of the E series and prostacyclin (PGI_2) could be responsible for abnormal bleeding in IUD users because of vascular and platelet effects of these compounds.

The presence of copper or progesterone in IUDs is thought to reduce menstrual blood loss. This effect may be due to an action on prostaglandin synthesizing enzymes. Copper ions have been shown to favour the production of F prostaglandins and inhibit the production of E prostaglandins from arachidonic acid (Maddox, 1973; Lands *et al.*, 1971).

12.4 MANAGEMENT OF DYSFUNCTIONAL UTERINE BLEEDING

Based on theoretical considerations either prostaglandins or their synthesis inhibitors could be employed in the management of dysfunctional uterine bleeding and that associated with IUDs. Such an approach may appear paradoxical. However, by employing a prostaglandin with an antihaemorrhagic prothrombotic action or by inhibiting the formation of prohaemorrhagic antithrombotic prostaglandins (with appropriate prostaglandin synthesis inhibitor), the same end result could be achieved. The situation is far more complex than presented here and the above assumptions cannot be accepted as an established fact.

12.4.1 Use of prostaglandins

Although some of the primary prostaglandins (E and F series) have a potent stimulant action on the non-pregnant human uterus, their clinical application in the control of dysfunctional or IUD-induced bleeding has, to the best of our knowledge, not been attempted. Prostaglandins of the F series would appear to be more suitable compounds in this respect in view of their vascular properties. These compounds may induce haemostatic uterine effects by stimulating uterine contractions and mechanical vascular constriction.

To test the above hypothesis, a pilot investigation has recently been carried out by our group where $PGF_{2\alpha}$ or its 15-methyl analogue were infused at a constant rate for 6 hours in 10 women with dysfunctional haemorrhage (Toppozada *et al.*, 1979). The menstrual blood loss was estimated by a modified alkaline haematin method (Newton *et al.*, 1977) during a 6-hour infusion period and compared to a similar control period prior to treatment. The results are presented in Table 12.2 which shows the drug used, doses,

Table 12.2 Uterine blood loss prior to and during a 6-hour infusion of $PGF_{2\alpha}$ or its 15-methyl analogue in cases of dysfunctional uterine haemorrhage

Prostaglandin	*No. of cases*	*Dose per min* (μg)	*Side-effects* (% cases)			*Mean blood loss in 6 h* (ml)	
			Vomiting	*Diarrhoea*	*Colics*	*Before infusion*	*During infusion*
$PGF_{2\alpha}$	4	50	66%	66%	33%	13.2	6.2
15-methyl $PGF_{2\alpha}$	6	2.5	66%	22%	44%	13.0	8.1

side-effects and amount of blood loss. There was a 40% reduction in the amount of blood loss as a result of prostaglandin infusion in both treatment groups; the decrease being more pronounced in the $PGF_{2\alpha}$ treated group. However, two major drawbacks characterize this therapeutic approach; gastro-intestinal side-effects and a relatively short duration of effect. A longer-acting analogue with fewer side-effects would be a better alternative particularly if it can be administered intramuscularly or vaginally.

12.4.2 Use of inhibitors of prostaglandin biosynthesis

The first report indicating that inhibitors of prostaglandin synthesis may be useful in controlling abnormal bleeding due to IUDs was published in January, 1976 (Damarawy and Toppozada, 1976). The authors based their approach on a theoretical assumption that excessive production of PGEs may be an active factor contributing to excessive blood loss. PGE compounds produce vasodilatation and PGE_1 in addition is an inhibitor of platelet aggregation. At that time, an increased production of PGEs in response to IUD insertion had not been reported (Hillier and Kasonde, 1976). To date, it is not known whether more PGEs are produced in women with IUDs who have an abnormal bleeding pattern than with similar IUDs but normal bleeding.

Soon after the first publication, a second report confirmed the original finding in one subject with a medicated IUD (Cu7). Moreover, the new study introduced the use of prostaglandin biosynthesis inhibitors in the treatment of dysfunctional uterine bleeding (Anderson *et al.*, 1976).

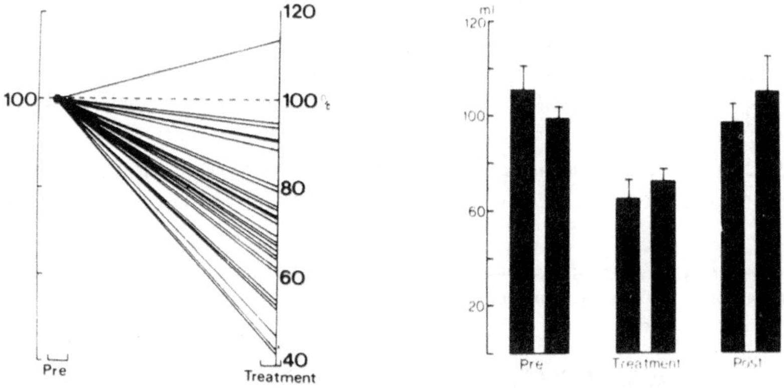

Figure 12.5 Effect of mefenamic acid therapy on mean total menstrual blood loss in women with IUDs. Left: Percentage change (mean of two treatment cycles compared with two pretreatment control periods expressed as 100%). Right: Mean blood loss for six menstrual periods in 15 women with IUD with heavy blood loss (80 ml or more). Treatment resulted in a significant reduction in blood loss. (From Guillebaud *et al.*, 1978, by courtesy of *Br. J. Obstet. Gynaecol.*)

The same group at Oxford recently reported on the use of the same prostaglandin synthetase inhibitor in the control of IUD-induced bleeding with favourable results (Guillebaud *et al.*, 1978). Twenty-five subjects were treated with 500 mg of mefenamic acid every 8 hours during two menstrual periods and the amount of blood loss was compared with that estimated in two pre- and two post-treatment cycles. A highly significant reduction in mean total blood loss was observed regardless of whether the therapy started before or on the first day of menses. The decrease in MBL was more pronounced in women with heavy blood loss (Figure 12.5). These data along with those reported by Damarawy and Toppozada (1976) have established a basis for future research aimed at improving the clinical performance of IUDs.

The effect of treatment with inhibitors of prostaglandin synthesis on the duration of bleeding is less apparent than their effect on the amount of blood loss (Guillebaud *et al.*, 1978). The clinical value of these agents in intermenstrual spotting or bleeding also needs further evaluation (Damarawy and Toppozada, 1976). The best inhibitor of prostaglandin synthesis which produces minimal side-effects and the optimum schedule of administration remains unsettled. However, prolonged local release or systemic therapy throughout the cycle to control excessive blood loss suffers from three major problems. These are a possible interference with the contraceptive action of IUDs, a potential teratogenic effect if pregnancy occurs and the side-effects and complications associated with long-term use of these agents. It has been shown that in rabbits prostaglandin synthesis inhibitors can reverse the anti-implantation action of IUDs (Saksena and Harper, 1974). Accordingly, the use of such drugs in the control of excessive MBL should be restricted to the duration of menstruation. See Table 12.3.

Table 12.3 Effect of treatment with prostaglandin synthesis inhibitors on menstrual blood loss in dysfunctional and IUD-induced bleeding

Ref.	*Drug*	*Cause of bleeding*	*No. of cases*	*Result*
1	Indomethacin	inert IUD	100	90% improvement
2	Mefenamic acid	Cu IUD	1	marked improvement
3	Mefenamic acid	inert and Cu IUDs	25	reduction among heavy losers
2	Mefenamic and flufenamic acid	dysfunctional	6	all improved
4	Mefenamic acid	dysfunctional	20	all improved
5	Indomethacin	dysfunctional	12	all improved

1 Damarawy and Toppozada (1976): By subjective evaluation
2 Anderson *et al.* (1976)
3 Guillebaud *et al.* (1978)
4 Haynes *et al.* (1978)
5 Toppozada *et al.* (1979)
(2–5) By measurement of blood loss

The mechanism of action of prostaglandin synthesis inhibitors in the treatment of dysfunctional and IUD-associated bleeding is not fully understood. It is presumed that these drugs act by interfering with prostaglandin synthetase activity.

If excessive bleeding is related to an overproduction of prostaglandins then one would expect uterine cramps in association with the increased blood loss. This is not always the case. Since the production of E prostaglandins in the endometrium seems to predominate in women with dysfunctional bleeding and those with IUDs (Hillier and Kasonde, 1976; Haynes *et al.*, 1978), heavy uterine bleeding need not necessarily be accompanied with uterine cramps since the uterus relaxes in response to local administration of PGE_2 during menstruation (Martin *et al.*, 1978). It is possible that administration of PGE_2 may in fact prove useful in the treatment of dysmenorrhoea.

Prostaglandins of the E series dilate uterine blood vessels (Clark *et al.*, 1977, 1978), inhibit uterine contractions during the phase of menstrual bleeding (Martin *et al.*, 1978) and interfere with platelet aggregation (Kloeze, 1967). It is therefore reasonable to believe that inhibition of uterine PGE synthesis would alter the balance in favour of other haemostatic mechanisms. In fact, some anti-inflammatory agents selectively inhibit synthesis of PGE compounds without affecting PGF compounds (Maddox, 1973). It is known that the inhibitory activity of some compounds on prostaglandin synthesis can vary from tissue to tissue (Flower and Vane, 1974). Accordingly, the effect of different drugs on prostaglandin synthesis by the endometrium should be evaluated to assist in the selection of the most suitable agent.

12.5 FUTURE DEVELOPMENTS

The role of prostaglandins and thromboxanes in the mechanism of uterine bleeding is still a matter of speculation. A definite evidence for an obligatory role is so far lacking. However, data from few available publications point towards a probable involvement of these substances in the haemostatic as well as haemorrhagic mechanisms related to physiological MBL, IUD-induced haemorrhages and dysfunctional uterine bleeding. There is a need to conduct additional basic and applied clinical studies in this area.

Some suggestions regarding the type of studies that could prove useful towards this end are outlined below.

12.5.1 Basic studies on the role of prostaglandins and thromboxanes in uterine bleeding

(1) Measurement of different prostaglandins, their metabolites, endoperoxides and thromboxanes in the endometrium, uterine jet wash and uterine vein blood in women with normal menstruation, those with IUDs and with dysfunctional bleeding. Comparison of levels of prostaglandins in women with IUDs who bleed excessively with those with similar devices but with normal blood loss.

(2) Effect of endoperoxides, prostaglandins and thromboxanes on uterine activity and vascular reactivity under various physiological and pathological conditions.

(3) Study of the binding capacity of endometrial cells, vascular and myometrial tissue, to prostaglandins, endoperoxides and thromboxanes and the factors controlling this binding.

(4) Study of enzyme activity of the endometrium which favours a specific pathway of prostaglandin biosynthesis. These are different in different tissues and are under the influence of humoral factors.

(5) Histological and cytological changes in the endometrium induced by local instillation of different prostaglandins, endoperoxides and thromboxanes. If any of the changes observed with IUDs or dysfunctional bleeding can be reproduced by intra-uterine administration of these substances then their overproduction may be involved in the pathogenesis of the disorder.

(6) Endometrial blood flow studies. Effect of the newly discovered prostaglandins, e.g. PGD_2, PGG_2, PGH_2, PGI_2 and thromboxanes on endometrial blood flow with concomitant recording of uterine activity may help in the evaluation of whether the observed changes are primary or secondary to myometrial response.

(7) Since PGI_2 is a potent inhibitor of platelet aggregation, a pro-inflammatory substance and a potent dilator of microcirculation, its role in IUD-induced bleeding needs to be evaluated.

12.5.2 Effect of prostaglandin synthesis inhibitors on uterine bleeding

(1) A study of relative potencies of different prostaglandin synthesis inhibitors on the human endometrium and an evaluation of the influence of hormonal status on this inhibition.

(2) The effect of prostaglandin synthesis inhibitors on the prostaglandin binding capacity of the endometrium.

(3) To determine whether any prostaglandin synthesis inhibitors will selectively inhibit the production of a particular prostaglandin. An agent which selectively inhibits the synthesis of PGE_1, PGD_2 and PGI_2 (all inhibitors of platelet aggregation and vasodilators) could prove useful in the control of menstrual blood loss. The role of such agents on fibrinolysis and thrombus formation should also be evaluated.

(4) Histological, electron microscopial and histochemical effects of locally administered prostaglandin synthesis inhibitors on the endometrium in normal and abnormal menstruation.

(5) Based upon the theory that prostaglandins mediate contraceptive effectiveness of IUDs, there is a need to explore whether long-term local or systemic administration of prostaglandin synthesis inhibitors interfere with the contraceptive efficacy of IUDs.

(6) Does the long-term local or systemic administ0ation of prostaglandin synthesis inhibitors throughout the cycle produce a teratogenic effect? This is of particular significance in cases of IUD failures.

(7) Comparative clinical evaluation of different prostaglandin synthesis inhibitors in the control of MBL in order to select the most effective agent with least side-effects and also to determine the best route of drug delivery.

(8) Clinical evaluation of prostaglandin synthesis inhibitors in the control of intermenstrual spotting and bleeding.

References

Åkerlund, M. (1976). Studies on myometrial activity and endometrial blood flow in the non-pregnant human uterus. Thesis presented at the University of Lund, Sweden, p. 20

Åkerlund, M. and Andersson, K. E. (1976a). Effect of terbutaline on human myometrial activity and endometrial blood flow. *Obstet. Gynecol.*, **47**, 529

Åkerlund, M. and Andersson, K. E. (1976b). Vasopressin response and terbutaline inhibition of the uterus. *Obstet. Gynecol.*, **48**, 528

Åkerlund, M., Bengtsson, L. P. and Carter, M. (1975). A technique for monitoring endometrial or decidual blood flow with an intra-uterine thermistor probe. *Acta Obstet. Gynecol. Scand.*, **54**, 469

Åkerlund, M., Bengtsson, L. P. and Ulmsten, U. (1976). Recording of myometrial activity in the non-pregnant human uterus by a microtransducer catheter. *Biophys. Reprod.* (In press)

Anderson, A. B. M., Haynes, P. J., Guillebaud, J. and Turnbull, A. C. (1976). Reduction of menstrual blood loss by prostaglandin synthetase inhibitors. *Lancet*, **i**, 774

Badraoui, M. H. H., Bonnar, J., Hillier, K. and Embrey, M. P. (1973). Coagulation changes during termination of pregnancy by prostaglandins and by vacuum aspiration. *Br. Med. J.*, **1**, 19

Badraoui, M. H. H., Bonnar, J., Hillier, K. and Embrey, M. (1974a). Coagulation changes during induction of labour at 38 weeks by prostaglandin E_2 compared to syntocinon drip. In: M. Toppozada (ed.), *Prostaglandins in Human Reproduction*, p. 45 (Alexandria: Alexandria University Press)

Badraoui, M. H. H., Bonnar, J., Hillier, K. and Embrey, M. (1974b). Blood coagulation changes during induction of abortion by prostaglandin $F_{2\alpha}$ compared to hypertonic saline and vacuum aspiration. In: M. Toppozada (ed.), *Prostaglandins in Human Reproduction*, p. 71 (Alexandria: Alexandria University Press)

Bartelmez, G. W. (1957). The phases of the menstrual cycle and their interpretation in terms of the pregnancy cycle. *Am. J. Obstet. Gynecol.*, **74**, 931

Beilby, J. O. W., Farrer-Brown, G. and Tarbitt, M. H. (1971). The microvasculature of common uterine abnormalities other than fibroids. *J. Obstet. Gynaecol. Br. Cmnwlth.*, **78**, 361

Blatchley, F. R., Donovan, B. T., Horton, E. W. and Poyser, N. L. (1972). The release of prostaglandin and progesterone into the utero-ovarian venous blood of guinea-pigs during the estrous cycle and following estrogen treatment. *J. Physiol.*, **223**, 69

Brody, M. J. and Kadowitz, P. J. (1974). Prostaglandins as modulators of the autonomic nervous system. *Fed. Proc.*, **33**, 46

Bygdeman, M. (1964). The effect of different prostaglandins on human myometrium *in vitro*. *Acta Physiol. Scand.*, **63** (Suppl. 242), 1

Cane, E. M. and Villee, C. A. (1975). The synthesis of prostaglandin F by human endometrium in organ culture. *Prostaglandins*, **9**, 281

Caldwell, B. V., Tillson, S. A., Brock, W. A. and Speroff, L. (1972). The effects of exogenous progesterone and estradiol on prostaglandin F levels in ovariectomized ewes. *Prostaglandins*, **1**, 217

Chaudhury, G. (1971). Intra-uterine device: Possible role of prostaglandins. *Lancet*, **i**, 48

Chaudhury, G. (1973). Release of prostaglandins by the IUCD. *Prostaglandins*, **3**, 773

Chaudhury, G. and Elder, M. G. (1976). Lack of evidence for inhibition of ovulation by aspirin in women. *Prostaglandins*, **11**, 727

Clark, K. E., Farley, D. B., Van Orden, D. E. and Brody, M. J. (1977). Role of endogenous prostaglandins in regulation of uterine blood flow and adrenergic neurotransmission. *Am. J. Obstet. Gynecol.*, **127**, 455

Clark, K. E., Ryan, M. J. and Brody, M. J. (1978). Effect of prostaglandins on vascular resistance and adrenergic vasoconstrictor responses in the canine uterus. *Prostaglandins*, **12**, 71

Clitheroe, H. J. (1961). The separation of three plain muscle stimulants present in the human endometrium. *J. Physiol. (London)*, **155**, 62

Clitheroe, H. J. (1973). Cyclic variations in endometrial prostaglandins during the human menstrual cycle. *Acta Endocrinol. (Kbh.)*, (Suppl.), **177**, 317

Crunkhorn, P. and Willis, A. L. (1971). Interaction between prostaglandin E and F given intradermally in the rat. *Br. J. Pharmacol.*, **41**, 507

Damarawy, H. and Toppozada, M. (1976). Control of bleeding due to IUDs by a prostaglandin biosynthesis inhibitor. *IRCS Med. Sci.*, **4**, 5

Demers, L. M., Halbert, D. R., Jones, D. E. D. and Fontana, J. (1975). Prostaglandin F levels in endometrial jet wash specimens during the normal human menstrual cycle. *Prostaglandins*, **10**, 1057

Downie, J., Poyser, N. L. and Wunderlich (1974). Levels of prostaglandins in human endometrium during the normal menstrual cycle. *J. Physiol.*, **236**, 465

Duboff, G. S., Penner, J. A. and Rohwedder, J. (1974). Effect of prostaglandins E_1, E_2 and $F_{2\alpha}$ on human blood coagulation. *Nature (London)*, **251**, 430

Eglinton, G., Raphael, R. A., Smith, G. N., Hall, W. J. and Pickles, V. R. (1963). The isolation and identification of two smooth muscle stimulants from menstrual fluid. *Nature (London)*, **200**, 960, 993

Einer-Jensen, N. (1973). Decreased endometrial blood flow and plasma progesterone level after instillation of 10 μg $PGF_{2\alpha}$ into the lumen of the uteri of rhesus monkey. *Prostaglandins*, **4**, 517

Embrey, M. P. (1966). Some experiments on the mechanism of action of prostaglandin on the guinea-pig and rat myometrium (quoted by Pickles *et al.*). In: V. R. Pickles and R. J. Fitzpatrick (eds.), *Endogenous Substances Affecting the Myometrium*, Vol. XIV, p. 89 (Cambridge University Press)

Flower, R. J. and Vane, J. R. (1974). Inhibition of prostaglandin biosynthesis. *Biochem. Pharmacol.*, **23**, 1439

Gaarder, A., Jonsen, J., Laland, S., Hellem, A. and Owren, P. A. (1961). Adenosine diphosphate in red cells as a factor in the adhesiveness of blood platelets. *Nature (London)*, **192**, 531

Gimbrone, M. A. and Alexander, R. W. (1975). Angiotensin II stimulation of prostaglandin production in cultured human vascular endothelium. *Science*, **189**, 219

Green, K. and Hagenfeldt, K. (1975). Prostaglandins in the human endometrium. Gas chromatographic mass spectrometric quantitation before and after IUD insertion. *Am. J. Obstet. Gynecol.*, **122**, 611

Greenberg, R. A. and Sparks, H. V. (1969). Prostaglandins and consecutive vascular segments of the canine hind limb. *Am. J. Physiol.*, **216**, 567

Greenberg, S., Howard, L. and Wilson, W. R. (1974a). Comparative effects of prostaglandins A_2 and B_2 on vascular and airway resistances and adrenergic neurotransmission. *Can. J. Physiol. Pharmacol.*, **52**, 699

Greenberg, S., Wilson, W. R. and Howard, L. (1974b). Mechanism of the vasoconstrictor action of prostaglandin B. *J. Pharmacol. Exp. Ther.*, **190**, 59

Gryglewski, R. J. and Korbut, R. (1975). Prostaglandin feedback mechanism limits vasoconstrictor action of norepinephrine in perfused rabbit ear. *Experientia*, **31**, 89

Guillebaud, J., Anderson, A. B. M. and Turnbull, A. C. (1978). Reduction by mefenamic acid of increased menstrual blood associated with intra-uterine contraception. *Br. J. Obstet. Gynaecol.*, **85**, 53

Gustavii, B. (1972). Labour: a delayed menstruation? *Lancet*, **i**, 1149

Harris, J. W. and Ramsay, E. M. (1966). The morphology of human uteroplacental vasculature. *Contrib. Embryol. Carnegie Inst. Wash.*, **38**, 43

Haynes, P. J., Flint, A. P. F., Anderson, A. B. M. and Turnbull, A. C. (1978). Studies on the role of prostaglandins in human menstruation. *Br. J. Obstet. Gynaecol.*, **85**, 78

Henzl, M. R., Smith, R. C., Boost, G. and Tyler, E. T. (1972). Lysosomal concept of menstrual bleeding in humans. *J. Clin. Endocrinol. Metab.*, **34**, 860

Hillier, K. and Kasonde, J. M. (1976). Prostaglandin E and F concentrations in human endometrium after insertion of intra-uterine contraceptive device. *Lancet*, **i**, 15

Hovig, T. (1963). Release of platelet aggregating substance (adenosine diphosphate) from rabbit blood platelets induced by salive 'extract' of tendons. *Thromb. Diath. Haemorrhag.*, **9**, 264

Howie, P. W., Calder, A. A., Forbes, C. D. and Prentice, C. R. M. (1973). Effect of intravenous prostaglandin E_2 on platelet function, coagulation and fibrinolysis. *J. Clin. Pathol.*, **26**, 354

Kadowitz, P. J. (1972). Effect of prostaglandins E_1, E_2 and A_2 on vascular resistance and responses to nor-adrenaline nerve stimulation and angiotensin in the dog hind limb. *Br. J. Pharmacol.*, **46**, 395

Kadowitz, P. J., Sweet, C. S. and Brody, M. J. (1971a). Potentiation of adrenergic venomotor responses by angiotensin, prostaglandin $F_{2\alpha}$ and cocaine. *J. Pharmacol. Exp. Ther.*, **176**, 167

Kadowitz, P. J., Sweet, C. S. and Brody, M. J. (1971b). Blockage of adrenergic vasoconstrictor responses in the dog by prostaglandin E_1 and A_1. *J. Pharmacol. Exp. Ther.*, **179**, 563

Kalsner, S. (1974). Responses to and termination of action of prostaglandins in vascular tissue of the rabbit. *Can. J. Physiol. Pharmacol.*, **52**, 1020

Karim, S. M. M. and Filshie, G. M. (1972). The use of prostaglandin E_2 for therapeutic abortion. *J. Obstet. Gynaecol. Br. Cmnwlth.*, **79**, 1

Karim, S. M. M. and Hillier, K. (1975). Physiological roles and pharmacological actions of prostaglandins in relation to human reproduction. In: S. M. M. Karim (ed.), *Advances in Prostaglandin Research. Prostaglandins and Reproduction*, p. 23 (Lancaster: MTP Press)

Karim, S. M. M., Hillier, K., Somers, K. and Trussell, R. R. (1971). The effects of prostaglandins E_2 and $F_{2\alpha}$ administered by different routes on uterine activity and the cardiovascular system in pregnant and non-pregnant women. *J. Obstet. Gynaecol. Br. Cmnwlth.*, **78**, 172

Kindahl, H., Granstrom, E., Edqvist, L. E. and Eneroth, P. (1976). Prostaglandin levels in peripheral plasma during the reproductive cycle. In: B. Samuelsson and R. Paoletti (eds.), *Advances in Prostaglandin and Thromboxane Research*, Vol. II, p. 667 (New York: Raven Press)

Kloeze, J. (1967). Influence of prostaglandins on platelet adhesiveness and platelet aggregation. In: S. Bergstrom and B. Samuelsson (eds.), *Prostaglandins (Proceedings of Nobel Symposium 2)*, p. 241 (Stockholm: Almqwist and Wiksell)

Kloeze, J. (1970). Influence of prostaglandin E_1 and E_2 on coagulation of rat blood. *Experientia*, **26**, 307

Lands, W., Lee, R. and Smith, W. (1971). Factors regulating the biosynthesis of various prostaglandins. *Ann. N.Y. Acad. Sci.*, **180**, 107

Levine, L. and Gutierrez-Cernosek, R. M. (1973). Levels of 13,14-dihydro-15-keto-PGF$_{2\alpha}$ in biological fluids as measured by radioimmunoassay. *Prostaglandins*, **3**, 785

Levitt, M. J., Tobon, H. and Josimovich, J. B. (1975). Prostaglandin content of human endometrium. *Fertil. Steril.*, **26**, 296

Lewis, A. J., Nelson, D. J. and Sugrue, M. F. (1974). Potentiation by prostaglandin E_1 and arachidonic acid of oedema in the rat paw induced by various phlogogenic agents. *Br. J. Pharmacol.*, **50**, 468P

Lish, P. M., Hillyard, I. W. and Dungan, K. W. (1960). The uterine relaxant properties of isoxuprine. *J. Pharmacol. Exp. Ther.*, **129**, 438

Lundström, V. (1977). The role of prostaglandins in primary dysmenorrhoea. Biochemical, pathophysiological and clinical aspects. Thesis, p. 31, Dept. Obstet. Gynec. Karolinska Hospital, Stockholm, Sweden

Maddox, I. S. (1973). The role of copper in prostaglandin synthesis. *Biochem. Biophys. Acta*, **306**, 74

Markee, J. E. (1940). Menstruation in intra-ocular endometrial transplants in the Rhesus monkey. *Contrib. Embryol.*, **28**, 219

Markee, J. E. (1950). The relation of blood flow to endometrial growth and the inception of menstruation. In: E. T. Engle (ed.), *Menstruation and its Disorders*, p. 165 (Springfield: C. C. Thomas)

Martin, J. N. Jr., Bygdeman, M. and Eneroth, P. (1978). The influence of locally adminitered prostaglandin E_2 and $F_{2\alpha}$ on uterine motility in the intact non-pregnant human uterus. *Acta Obstet. Gynecol. Scand.*, **57**, 141

Martinez-Gaudio, M., Yoshida, T. and Bengtsson, L. P. (1973). Propagated and non-propagated myometrial contractions in normal menstrual cycles. *Am. J. Obstet. Gynecol.*, **115**, 107

Moncada, S. and Vane, J. R. (1977). In: N. Kharasch and J. Fried (eds.), *Biochemical Aspects of Prostaglandins and Thromboxanes*, p. 155 (New York: Academic Press)

Morad, M. and Toppozada, M. (1977). Induction of abortion by intra-uterine administration of prostaglandin via laparoscopy with concurrent sterilization. *Int. J. Gynaecol. Obstet.*, **15**, 256

Myatt, L. (1975). Macrophages on intra-uterine contraceptive devices produce prostaglandins. *Nature (London)*, **257**, 227

Newton, J., Bernard, G. and Collins, W. (1977). A rapid method for measuring menstrual blood loss using automatic extraction. *Contraception*, **16**, 269

Persianinov, L. S., Manuilova, I. A. and Chernukha, E. A. (1973). The results of using prostaglandin $F_{2\alpha}$ for induction and stimulation of labour. *Adv. Biosci.*, **9**, 585

Phillips, L. L. (1973). Effect of prostaglandins on the coagulation mechanism of the pregnant rat. *Am. J. Obstet. Gynecol.*, **115**, 227

Pickles, V. R. (1957). A plain muscle stimulant in the menstrual fluid. *Nature (London)*, 1198

Pickles, V. R. (1965). Prostaglandins in the human endometrium. *Int. J. Fertil.*, **12**, 335

Pickles, V. R. and Hall, W. J. (1963). Some physiological properties of the menstrual stimulant substances A_1 and A_2. *J. Reprod. Fertil.*, **6**, 315

Pickles, V. R. and Ward, P. V. F. (1965). Menstrual stimulants component B and possible prostaglandin precursors in the endometrium. *J. Physiol. (London)*, **178**, 38

Pickles, V. R., Hall, W. J., Best, F. A. and Smith, G. N. (1965). Prostaglandins in endometrium and menstrual fluid from normal and dysmenorrhoeic subjects. *J. Obstet. Gynaecol. Br. Cmnwlth.*, **72**, 185

Poyser, N. L., Horton, E. W., Thompson, C. J. and Los, M. (1971). Identification of $PGF_{2\alpha}$ released by distension of guinea-pig uterus *in vitro*. *Nature (London)*, **230**, 526

Roberts, J. S., McCracken, J. A., Gavagan, J. E. and Soloff, M. S. (1976). Oxytocin stimulated release of prostaglandin $F_{2\alpha}$ from ovine endometrium *in vitro*. Correlation with estrus cycle and oxytocin-receptor binding. *Endocrinology*, **99**, 1107

Rosada, A., Mercado, E., Gallegos, A. J., de Los-Angelees Wens, M. and Aznar, R. (1977). Subcellular distribution of lysosomal enzymes in the human endometrium. I. Normal menstrual cycle. *Contraception*, **16**, 287

Roth-Brandel, V., Bygdeman, M. and Wiqvist, N. (1970a). A comparative study on the influence of prostaglandin E_1, oxytocin and ergometrine on the pregnant human uterus. *Acta Obstet. Gynecol: Scand.*, **49** (Suppl. 5), 1

Roth-Brandel, V., Bygdeman, M. and Wiqvist, N. (1970b). Effect of intravenous administration of prostaglandin E_1 and $F_{2\alpha}$ on the contractility of the non-pregnant human uterus *in vivo*. *Acta Obstet. Gynecol. Scand.*, **49** (Suppl. 5), 19

Ryan, M. J., Clark, K., van Orden, D., Farley, D., Edvisson, L., Sjoberg, N. O., van Orden, L. and Brody, M. J. (1974). Role of prostaglandins in estrogen-induced uterine hyperemia. *Prostaglandins*, **5**, 257

Saksena, S. K. and Harper, M. J. K. (1974). Prostaglandin mediated action of intra-uterine devices: F-prostaglandins in the uterine horns of pregnant rabbits with unilateral intra-uterine devices. *Fertil. Steril.*, **25**, 121

Saksena, S. K., Lau, I. F. and Castracane, V. (1974). Prostaglandin mediated action of IUDs. (II) F-prostaglandins (PGF) in the uterine horn of pregnant rats and hamsters with intrauterine devices. *Prostaglandins*, **5**, 97

Salvatore, C. A. (1968). Arteriole alteration in normal and hyperplastic endometrium. *Am. J. Obstet. Gynecol.*, **102**, 493

Schillinger, E. and Prior, G. (1976). Characteristics of prostaglandin receptor sites in human uterine tissue. In: B. Samuelsson and R. Paoletti (eds.), *Advances in Prostaglandin and Thromboxane Research*, Vol. II, p. 259 (New York: Raven Press)

Schoene, N. W. and Iacono, J. M. (1975). Stimulation of platelet phospholipase A_2 activity by aggregating agents. *Fed. Proc.*, **34**, 257

Sekhar, N. C. (1970). Effect of eight prostaglandins on platelet aggregation. *J. Med. Chem.*, **13**, 39

Shaala, S., Gaafar, A. and Toppozada, M. (1974). Response of the menopausal uterus to prostaglandins. In: M. Toppozada (ed.), *Prostaglandins in Human Reproduction*, p. 95 (Alexandria: Alexandria University Press)

Shaala, S., Khowessah, M., El-Damarawy, H., El-Sahwi, S., Osman, M. and Toppozada, M. (1977). Reduced uterine response to $PGF_{2\alpha}$ under oral contraceptives. *Prostaglandins*, **14**, 523

Shaw, S. T. Jr. and Moyer, D. L. (1978). Uterine bleeding from intra-uterine devices: clinical aspects and pathogenesis. (In press)

Shio, H. and Ramwell, P. (1972). Effect of prostaglandin E_2 and aspirin on the secondary aggregation of human platelets. *Nature (New Biol.)*, **236**, 45

Silver, M. J., Smith, J. B., Ingerman, C. and Kocsis, J. J. (1973). Arachidonic acid-induced human platelet aggregation and prostaglandin formation. *Prostaglandins*, **4**, 863

Singh, E. J., Baccarini, I. and Zuspan, F. (1975). Levels of prostaglandin $F_{2\alpha}$ and E_2 in human endometrium during the menstrual cycle. *Am. J. Obstet. Gynecol.*, April, 1003

Smith, J. B. and Silver, M. J. (1973). Phospholipase A_1 of human blood platelets. *Biochem. J.*, **131**, 615

Smith, O. W. and Smith, G. V. S. (1947). Menstrual toxin. *Am. J. Obstet. Gynecol.*, **54**, 201

Smith, J. B. and Willis, A. L. (1970). Formation and release of prostaglandins by platelets in response to thrombin. *Br. J. Pharmacol.*, **40**, 545

Smith, J. B. and Willis, A. L. (1971). Aspirin selectively inhibits prostaglandin production in human platelets. *Nature (New Biol.)*, **231**, 235

Spilman, C. H. and Duby, R. T. (1972). Prostaglandin mediated luteolytic effect of an intra-uterine device in sheep. *Prostaglandins*, **2**, 159

Szego, C. M. (1972). Lysosomal membrane stabilization and anti-estrogen action in specific hormonal target cells. *Gynecol. Invest.*, **3**, 63

Szego, C. M. (1974). The lysosome as a mediator of hormone action. *Rec. Prog. Horm. Res.*, **30**, 171

Takagi, S., Yoshida, T., Yogo, T., Abe, M., Tochigi, H., Sakata, H. and Takahashi, H. (1976). The effects of uterine intramuscular injection of $PGF_{2\alpha}$ on severe post-partum haemorrhage. In: B. Samuelsson and R. Paoletti (eds.), *Advances in Prostaglandins and Thromboxane Research*, Vol. II, p. 1003 (New York: Raven Press)

Terragno, D. A., Terragno, N. A. and McGiff, J. C. (1974). Bradykinin selectively increases the synthesis of prostaglandin in bovine mesenteric arteries and veins. *Clin. Res.*, **22**, 597A

Toppozada, M., Gaafar, A. and Shaala, S. (1974). *In vivo* inhibition of the human non-pregnant uterus by prostaglandin E_2. *Prostaglandins*, **8**, 401

Toppozada, M., Gaafar, A., Shaala, S. and Osman, M. (1975). The relaxant property of local prostaglandin E_2 on the non-pregnant uterus—a cyclic triphasic response. *Prostaglandins*, **9**, 475

Toppozada, M., Khowessah, M., Shaala, S., Said, S. and Osman, M. (1976). Uterine response to prostaglandin E_2 under oral contraceptives. *Contraception*, **13**, 749

Toppozada, M., Khalil, T. H. and El-Sokkary, H. (1977). The role of prostaglandins in the control of human pituitary ovarian function. *Proc. 6th Asia and Oceania Congress of Endocrinology*, p. 143, January 22–27, Singapore

Toppozada, M., Khowessah, M., Shaala, S., Osman, M. and Rahman, H. A. (1977b). Aberrant uterine response to prostaglandin E_2 as a possible etiologic factor in functional infertility. *Fertil. Steril.*, **28**, 434

Toppozada, M., El-Attar, A. H., El-Ayyat, M. A. and Khamis, Y. (1979). Control of dysfunctional uterine bleeding by PGF infusions. (To be published)

Turksoy, R. N. and Safaii, M. S. (1975). Immediate effect of prostaglandin $F_{2\alpha}$ during the luteal phase of the menstrual cycle. *Fertil. Steril.*, **26**, 634

Tuvemo, T. and Wide, L. (1973). Prostaglandin release from the human umbilical artery *in vitro*. *Prostaglandins*, **4**, 689

Vane, J. R. (1976). Prostaglandins as mediators of inflammation. In: B. Samuelsson and R. Paoletti (eds.), *Advances in Prostaglandin and Thromboxane Research*, Vol. II, p. 791 (New York: Raven Press)

Vargaftig, B. B. and Zirinis, P. (1973). Platelet aggregation induced by arachidonic acid is accompanied by release of potential inflammatory mediators distinct from PGE_2 and $PGF_{2\alpha}$. *Nature (New Biol.)*, **244**, 114

Weiss, H. J., Aledort, L. M. and Kochwa, S. (1968). The effect of salicylates on the haemostatic probe ties of platelets in man. *J. Clin. Invest.*, **47**, 2169

Williams, T. J. and Morley, J. (1973). Prostaglandins as potentiators of increased vascular permeability in inflammation. *Nature (London)*, **246**, 215

Willis, A. L., Vane, F. M., Kuhn, D. C., Scott, C. G. and Petrin, M. (1974). An endoperoxide aggregator (LASS), formed in platelets in response to thrombotic stimuli. *Prostaglandins*, **8**, 453

Willman, E. A., Collins, W. P. and Clayton, S. G. (1976). Studies in the involvement of prostaglandins in uterine symptomatology and pathology. *Br. J. Obstet. Gynaecol.*, **83**, 337

Wilson, J. R., Ledger, W. J. and Andros, G. J. (1965). The effect of an intra-uterine contraceptive device on the histologic pattern of the endometrium. *Am. J. Obstet. Gynecol.*, **93**, 802

Wiqvist, N., Bygdeman, M. and Kirton, K. T. (1971). Non-steroidal antifertility agents in the female. In: E. Diczfalusy and U. Borell (eds.), *Nobel Symposium, 15*, p. 137 (New York: John Wiley)

Wlodawer, P., Kindahl, H. and Hamberg, M. (1976). Biosynthesis of prostaglandin $F_{2\alpha}$ from arachidonic acid and prostaglandin endoperoxides in the uterus. *Biochem. Biophys. Acta*, **431**, 603

Zucker, M. B. and Peterson, J. (1968). Inhibition of adenosine diphosphate-induced secondary aggregation and other platelet functions by acetyl salicylic acid ingestion. *Proc. Soc. Exp. Biol. Med.*, **127**, 547

Zurier, R. B. (1976). Prostaglandin release from human polymorphonuclear leukocytes. In: B. Samuelsson and R. Paoletti (eds.), *Advances in Prostaglandin and Thromboxane Research*, Vol. II, p. 815 (New York: Raven Press)

13 Menstrual Regulation with Prostaglandins

M. BYGDEMAN

13.1 INTRODUCTION

In view of the increasing number of therapeutic abortions, efforts to improve the methods of pregnancy termination in the first trimester are continuing. The operative procedure, vacuum aspiration, is the most effective method available for the termination of first trimester pregnancy. If vacuum aspiration is performed during very early pregnancy it is possible to use a thin flaccid polyethylene catheter which can be introduced into the uterus without cervical dilatation. This procedure is often called menstrual regulation. Initially the term was used only when the uterus was evacuated within 2 weeks following the first missed menstrual period; a period during which it is not always possible to confirm pregnancy. This could be an advantage in countries with restrictive abortion laws.

Today, the term menstrual regulation describes termination of very early pregnancy by surgical as well as medical methods. There is no generally agreed upper limit and menstrual regulation is usually performed during the 3 weeks following a missed menstrual period (49 days amenorrhoea or 7 weeks pregnancy from last menstrual period). For menstrual regulation with drugs, this limit is important since the incidence of incomplete abortion increases significantly if the pregnancy is more advanced.

There are several reasons for exploring the use of prostaglandins for menstrual regulation. If properly developed the drug can be self-administered by the patient or managed by paramedical personnel. Since vacuum aspiration (even when performed during early pregnancy) requires skill and training to achieve high efficacy and a low incidence of complications, a simple pharmacological method would be of great importance in countries with a shortage of trained medical personel. Some women may also prefer a treatment that results in a menstrual-like bleeding instead of surgical evacuation of the uterus.

13.2 VAGINAL ADMINISTRATION

13.2.1 Primary prostaglandins

Karim (1971) originally showed that PGE_2 and $PGF_{2\alpha}$ administered by the vaginal route could terminate early pregnancy. Twelve women with a delay in menstruation of 2–7 days were treated with either 40 mg of PGE_2 or 100 mg of $PGF_{2\alpha}$ administered in two divided doses 4 hours apart. The treatment resulted in menstrual-like bleeding and the pregnancy test was negative in 11 patients 2 weeks later. Side-effects encountered were nausea and/or lower abdominal pain.

The promising preliminary results with this technique resulted in several similar studies to determine the effectiveness and safety of the treatment. From these studies it became obvious that treatment at shorter intervals and for a longer period of time was necessary to achieve acceptable success rate.

Treadway and Mishell (1973) achieved complete abortion in seven patients and incomplete abortion in one following vaginal administration of 50 mg $PGF_{2\alpha}$ to 10 women at intervals of 2–4 h for 24 hours. The total dose ranged from 200 to 600 mg. This high dose resulted in a significant increase in the frequency of side-effects, mainly nausea, vomiting and diarrhoea. Two patients failed to abort. Similar results have been reported (Bolognese and Corson, 1973; Corlett *et al.*, 1972; Pion *et al.*, 1972; Toppozada *et al.*, 1973).

The results with PGE_2 were generally less favourable than in the preliminary study (Cheng *et al.*, 1973). Jones *et al.* (1974) reported that vaginal suppositories containing 20 mg PGE_2 administered every 2 hours until abortion or until a maximum of 120 mg was given, resulted in complete abortion in eight women, incomplete in one and no effect on the pregnancy in one patient. All patients experienced nausea, eight had vomiting and diarrhoea. Temperature elevation over 38 °C was observed in seven of the subjects.

13.2.2 Prostaglandin analogues

The results of vaginal administration of natural PGE_2 and $PGF_{2\alpha}$ for the termination of early pregnancy have generally been discouraging. Treatment with effective doses of these compounds is associated with an unacceptably high frequency of side-effects. During recent years the efficacy of several prostaglandin analogues for menstrual regulation has been explored. Some of these seem to act more selectively on the uterine muscle than natural prostaglandins when administered in therapeutically effective doses by the vaginal route (Table 13.1).

13.2.2.1 *15-methyl-$PGF_{2\alpha}$ methyl ester*

In contrast to many other prostaglandins, 15(S)15-methyl-$PGF_{2\alpha}$ methyl ester is stable in suppository form. Bygdeman *et al.* (1976b, 1976c) treated 75 women with amenorrhoea of 31–49 days with repeated vaginal administration of 15-methyl-$PGF_{2\alpha}$ methyl ester in triglyceride base. Suppositories containing 1.0 or 1.5 mg of the prostaglandin were administered at 3-hourly intervals (maximum 3–4 doses). Sixty-three patients were confirmed pregnant. In these women vaginal bleeding usually started 3–6 hours after the initiation of therapy and continued for 10–14 days. The efficacy of the treatment was judged from clinical course, gynaecological examination and measurement of plasma hCG. There were no failures in the trial but the treatment resulted in incomplete abortion in two cases. In two other patients curettage was performed due to prolonged bleeding but histological examination of the material revealed no remaining signs of pregnancy. Gastro-intestinal side-effects associated with the treatment were within the acceptable range.

Table 13.1 Results of menstrual induction following vaginal administration of prostaglandin analogues in selected studies. No pretreatment sedation was given

Reference	*No. of cases*	*Type of prostaglandin and dose*	*Frequency of complete abortion*	*Side-effects*
Bygdeman *et al.* (1976c)	63	15-methyl-$PGF_{2\alpha}$ methyl ester 0.5–1.5 mg × 3–4	97%	vomiting, diarrhoea 58%; endometritis 0%
Hamberger *et al.* (1978)	42	15-methyl-$PGF_{2\alpha}$ methyl ester 1.0–1.5 mg × 4	93%	vomiting, diarrhoea 50%
Zoremthangi *et al.* (1976)	40	15-methyl-$PGF_{2\alpha}$ methyl ester 1.0–1.5 mg × 4	68%	vomiting 32.5%; diarrhoea 27.5%; endometritis 0%
Karim *et al.* (1977b)	50	16,16-dimethyl-*trans*-Δ^2-PGE_1 methyl ester 1.0 mg × 5	92%	vomiting 4%; diarrhoea 6%; muscular weakness 4%; endometritis 0%
Tagaki *et al.* (1978)	63	16,16-dimethyl-*trans*-Δ^2-PGE_1 methyl ester 0.5 mg × 2 to 1.0 mg × 4	86%	vomiting 1.6%; headache 4.8%; endometritis 0%
Lundström *et al.* (1977)	88	16,16-dimethyl-PGE_2 0.8–1.0 mg × 4	94%	vomiting 12.5%; diarrhoea 13.6%; endometritis 1.1%
Mackenzie *et al.* (1978)	34	16,16-dimethyl-PGE_2 1.0 mg × 2–4	100%	vomiting 26.5%; diarrhoea 35.3%; endometritis 0%
Gréen *et al.* (1979)	38	15-methyl-$PGF_{2\alpha}$ 2.0 mg × 1	76.3%	vomiting 37%; diarrhoea 32%; endometritis 7.9%
Gréen *et al.* (1979)	35	15-methyl-$PGF_{2\alpha}$ 2.5 mg × 1	85.7%	vomiting 32%; diarrhoea 51%; endometritis 0%
Gréen *et al.* (1979)	128	15-methyl-$PGF_{2\alpha}$ 3.0 mg × 1	94.5%	vomiting 54%; diarrhoea 59%; endometritis 0.8%
Mandelin (1978)	104	15-methyl-$PGF_{2\alpha}$ 3.0 mg × 1	91%	vomiting 24%; diarrhoea 37%; endometritis 1.0%

Almost half of the patients suffered no side-effects and in most cases oral or rectal administration of analgesics was sufficient to control the menstrual-like uterine discomfort.

In another group of patients it was shown that a high frequency of complete abortion with prostaglandin could be achieved only if patients with amenorrhoea of more than 49 days are excluded. The incidence of incomplete abortion increased with increasing gestation (Bygdeman *et al.*, 1977).

In a number of other studies (in contrast to those of Bygdeman *et al.*, 1976b,

1976c) a fixed dose schedule was used. Four suppositories, each containing 1.0 or 1.5 mg 15-methyl-$PGF_{2\alpha}$ methyl ester were administered at 3-hourly intervals. With this treatment Hamberger *et al.* (1978) reported that all 42 patients started to bleed within 1–12 h after the initiation of therapy. The bleeding lasted for 11 days (range 5–25 days). Pregnancy was terminated in all and abortion without further intervention was accomplished in 93% of the patients. Side-effects (pain, diarrhoea and/or vomiting) occurred in approximately half of the patients with a higher incidence in the 1.5 mg group. These side-effects were not severe.

Satisfactory results following repeated vaginal administration of 15-methyl-$PGF_{2\alpha}$ methyl ester have also been reported by Fylling and Jerve (1977). In their study of 30 patients all but one aborted completely. Ylikorkala *et al.* (1976) treated 40 women and pregnancy was terminated in all but curettage (due to incomplete expulsion of the conceptus) was necessary in seven women. Zoremthangi *et al.* (1976) and Puri *et al.* (1977) failed to terminate pregnancy in eight out of 40 patients (20%) treated with 15-methyl-$PGF_{2\alpha}$ methyl ester. The incidence of incomplete abortion was also high (12.5%).

Attempts to develop devices or suppositories which would give a slow release of prostaglandins for a longer duration have also been made in order to overcome the disadvantages associated with repeated vaginal administration. Spilman *et al.* (1976) developed a polysiloxane device containing 15-methyl-$PGF_{2\alpha}$ methyl ester for insertion into the vagina. Treatment with such a device (3–5 mg) was generally associated with an unacceptable incidence of side-effects (Brenner *et al.*, 1977; Corson and Bolognese, 1977; Duenhoelter *et al.*, 1978; Robins, 1977). Measurements of the plasma concentrations of the free acid and methyl ester forms of 15-methyl-$PGF_{2\alpha}$ after vaginal insertion of the polysiloxane device indicated variable release rate. The frequency of side-effects was significantly higher than encountered with repeated vaginal (pessary) administration of the compound (Bygdeman *et al.*, 1976a).

Slow and gradual absorption from the vagina was obtained with specially formulated suppository. The efficacy and safety of a single suppository containing 2.0, 2.5, or 3.0 mg 15-methyl-$PGF_{2\alpha}$ methyl ester for termination of early pregnancy was recently evaluated in 201 women (Gréen *et al.*, 1979). All patients but one aborted following treatment. The frequency of complete abortion increased from 76.3% with the 2.0 mg to 94.5% with the 3.0 mg suppository. Bleeding generally started 4–6 hours after the start of treatment and lasted for 10–14 days. Gastro-intestinal side-effects were related to the dose and were in most patients limited to one or two episodes. Out of the 128 women treated with a 3.0 mg suppository, only one patient developed endometritis.

Mandelin (1978) reported somewhat less positive results. Out of a total of 104 women, pregnancy was terminated in 95 (91.3%) following vaginal administration of a slow release suppository containing 3.0 mg 15-methyl-$PGF_{2\alpha}$ methyl ester. One of the nine patients with failed treatment experienced neither bleeding nor uterine contractions and early expulsion of the suppository from the vagina may have taken place. In two patients clinical findings indicated a missed abortion but in the remaining six the uterine growth was obvious.

Bleeding after prostaglandin treatment was considered by most patients to be heavier than during normal menstruation and the mean duration was 12.7 days. About 53% of the patients had no gastro-intestinal side-effects and 30% required one or more injections of meperidine hydrochloride to alleviate the pain due to uterine contractions.

13.2.2.2 *Other analogues*

Experience with other analogues is more limited. Mocsary (1977) and Csapo and Mocsary (1976b) have reported on vaginal infusion or vaginal application of a $PGF_{2\alpha}$ analogue ICI 81008. The side-effects, mostly vomiting and increased blood pressure, were transient and subjectively and medically acceptable. In most patients bleeding was induced with prostaglandin treatment but pregnancy test 2 weeks after therapy remained positive in 20% necessitating a curettage.

Preliminary results with two analogues of PGE appear more promising. Vaginal administration of 1.0 mg 16,16-dimethyl-*trans*-Δ^2-PGE_2 methyl ester in triglyceride base five times at 4-hourly intervals resulted in complete abortion in 46 out of 50 women with a delay in menstruation of up to 14 days. The mean duration of bleeding was 6.8 days. Uterine cramps were experienced by most patients but these were mild and only seven resorted to mild analgesics for pain relief. Gastro-intestinal side-effects were very infrequent (Karim *et al.*, 1977b). Takagi *et al.* (1978) also found a very low frequency of gastro-intestinal side-effects following repeated vaginal administration of this analogue. The frequency of incomplete abortion was, however, higher (14%; nine out of 63 patients).

According to Lundström *et al.* (1977) and more recently Mackenzie *et al.* (1978), the analogue 16,16-dimethyl-PGE_2 is effective in inducing an abortion during early pregnancy following vaginal administration. The treatment is associated with a significantly lower frequency of gastro-intestinal side-effects than encountered with 15-methyl-$PGF_{2\alpha}$ methyl ester. Vaginal administration of suppositories containing 0.8–1.0 mg four times at 3-hourly intervals resulted in complete abortion in approximately 95% of the patients. The *p*-benzaldehyde semicarbazone ester of 16,16-dimethyl-PGE_2 seems equally effective in the termination of early pregnancy (Karim, 1976).

13.3 INTRAUTERINE ADMINISTRATION

The efficacy and safety of intrauterine administration of prostaglandins for termination of early pregnancy has been evaluated by several investigators.

Both primary prostaglandins and synthetic analogues have been used (Tables 13.2 and 13.3).

Table 13.2 Results of menstrual induction following intrauterine administration of primary prostaglandins in selected studies

Reference	*No. of cases*	*Type of prostaglandin and dose*	*Frequency of complete abortion*	*Side-effects*
Mocsary and Csapo (1975)	114	PGE_2, 1.5 mg	93.8%	vomiting 8.7%* diarrhoea 4.3% BP change 5.2% pyrexia 14.9% endometritis 10.4%
Mackenzie *et al.* (1976)	12 26	PGE_2, 0.1 mg PGE_2, 0.5 mg	58% 85%	0%† 0%†
Karim (1973)	12 4	PGE_2, 1.0 mg $PGF_{2\alpha}$, 4 mg	100% 100% }	vomiting 37%† endometritis 0%
Mocsary and Csapo (1975)	428	$PGF_{2\alpha}$, 5 mg	95.3%	vomiting 15.1%* diarrhoea 1.1% BP change 3.2% pyrexia 2.1% endometritis 9.3%
Ragab and Edelmann (1976)	100	$PGF_{2\alpha}$, 5 mg	100%	nausea 3%* vomiting 30% endometritis 0%
Lichtman *et al.* (1974)	20	$PGF_{2\alpha}$, 5 mg	65%	BP change 100%* vomiting 80% endometritis 15%
Ylikorkala *et al.* (1974)	12	$PGF_{2\alpha}$, 1.0 mg	83%	nausea 83%† vomiting 58% diarrhoea 0%
Ylikorkala *et al.* (1974)	22	$PGF_{2\alpha}$, 2 or 4 mg	100%	nausea 88% vomiting 50% diarrhoea 6% endometritis 3%

* Strong sedation prior to therapy
† Mild or no pretreatment

13.3.1 Primary prostaglandins

The first recorded study utilizing the intrauterine route for menstrual induction was reported by Bygdeman *et al.* (1972). Four women with a delay in menstruation of up to 14 days were given a single intrauterine dose of 500 μg of $PGF_{2\alpha}$. The treatment was successful in two. Csapo and co-workers have treated a total of 542 patients with 5.0 mg $PGF_{2\alpha}$ or 1.5 mg PGE_2 by the intrauterine route (Csapo *et al.*, 1973; Csapo, 1974; Mocsary and Csapo, 1975). The prostaglandin was delivered transcervically in the fundus region of the uterine cavity through a semistiff catheter. The amount of solvent was normally 1 ml. Prior to the administration of prostaglandin the patients were sedated with 50 mg pethidine, 20 mg diazepam and 0.4 mg atropine. Treatment with 5.0 mg $PGF_{2\alpha}$ or 1.5 mg PGE_2 was equally effective. 95% of the gravidas had complete evacuation of the uterus with bleeding lasting for approximately 10 days following the treatment. Spontaneous menstruation resumed after an average of 34 days following prostaglandin administration.

Table 13.3 Results of menstrual induction following intrauterine administration of prostaglandin analogues in selected studies. No pretreatment was given prior to therapy

Reference	*No. of cases*	*Type of prostaglandin and dose*	*Frequency of complete abortion*	*Side-effects*
Karim (1976) Karim and Ratnam (1976)	142	15-methyl-PGE_2 methyl ester 10 μg 15-methyl-$PGF_{2\alpha}$ methyl ester 100 μg	96%	vomiting 11.3% diarrhoea 7% endometritis 1.4%
Ylikorkala *et al.* (1975)	10	15-methyl-$PGF_{2\alpha}$, 125 μg	90%	nausea 40% vomiting 20% diarrhoea 40%
Ylikorkala *et al.* (1975)	10	15-methyl-$PGF_{2\alpha}$ 200 μg	70%	nausea 30% vomiting 30% diarrhoea 30%
Ylikorkala *et al.* (1975)	10	15-methyl-$PGF_{2\alpha}$ 300 μg	100%	nausea 39% vomiting 30% diarrhoea 20% endometritis 0%
Karim *et al.* (1977a)	240	16-phenoxy-ω-tetranor-PGE_2 methylsulphonylamide 50 μg	95%	vomiting 5.4% headache 3.8% endometritis 0.8% diarrhoea 0%
Tagaki *et al.* (1977)	45	16,16-dimethyl-*trans*-Δ^2-PGE_1 methyl ester 20–80 μg	93%	nausea 20% vomiting 16% endometritis 0% diarrhoea 0%

Vomiting occurred more frequently in $PGF_{2\alpha}$ treated group (15.1%) than in PGE_2 group (8.7%). The opposite was true for diarrhoea and transient pyrexia. The frequency of endometritis was similar in the two treatment groups (8%). Adnexitis was encountered in 1.5% of the patients (Table 13.2).

That intrauterine instillation of $PGF_{2\alpha}$ is a safe and effective procedure for terminating early pregnancy has also been shown by Ragab and Edelmann (1976). One hundred patients were successfully treated with 5.0 mg $PGF_{2\alpha}$ after premedication suggested by Csapo. Vomiting occurred in 30% of the patients.

In two other studies, however, the results with intrauterine administration of 5.0 mg $PGF_{2\alpha}$ were less satisfactory. Lichtman *et al.* (1974) reported that out of 20 patients treated with a single intrauterine dose of $PGF_{2\alpha}$ (5 mg) seven failed to abort. Seven patients had severe adverse reactions including fever, haemorrhage and hypertension. Three women developed septic incomplete abortion. Jones *et al.* (1975) reported complete abortion in only 11 patients out of 14 treated with $PGF_{2\alpha}$. The incidence of infection was high and six patients underwent a dilatation and curettage because of persistent bleeding.

Karim (1973) reported that if the dose of $PGF_{2\alpha}$ was increased to 8.0 mg and that of PGE_2 to 2.0 mg all patients experienced severe uterine cramps and vomiting. If the dose was reduced to 4.0 mg $PGF_{2\alpha}$ or 1.0 mg PGE_2, the efficacy was still high but the frequency of side-effects significantly lower.

Ylikorkala *et al.* (1974) administered a single intrauterine dose of 1.0 mg, 2.0 mg or 4.0 mg $PGF_{2\alpha}$ in 34 women during very early pregnancy. After 3 weeks' observation period all patients but one, treated with 1.0 mg, had aborted. The abortion was complete in 83% of the patients induced with 1.0 mg and in 100% of the patients induced with either 2.0 mg or 4.0 mg $PGF_{2\alpha}$. All patients experienced uterine pain. With 2.0 mg dose, nine out of 18 patients had vomiting and one had diarrhoea. In the latter case a fall in blood pressure was also observed.

A further reduction in the dose of PGE_2 to 0.5 mg or 0.1 mg significantly reduced the frequency of side-effects but this was associated with a reduction in efficacy of the treatment to 84.6% and 58.3% respectively (Mackenzie *et al.*, 1976, 1978).

13.3.2 Prostaglandin analogues

Intrauterine administration of PGE_2 or $PGF_{2\alpha}$ as described above is an effective therapy for the termination of early pregnancy, but because of the associated side-effects the procedure would have limited application. Efforts with drug formulation and the use of synthetic analogues indicated that side-effects could be reduced (Toppozada *et al.*, 1973).

Karim and collaborators have shown that with the use of several prostaglandin analogues there is a significant reduction in the frequency of side-effects while the efficacy remains high. Intrauterine administration of a mixture of 10 μg 15-methyl-PGE_2 methyl ester and 100 μg 15-methyl-$PGF_{2\alpha}$ methyl ester dissolved in 2 ml water was given to 142 pregnant women. Only patients up to 6 weeks gestation and showing a positive pregnancy test were included (Karim and Ratnam, 1976; Karim, 1976). Uterine bleeding followed by a negative pregnancy test within 2 weeks of prostaglandin treatment was the criterion for successful treatment and was achieved in 132 patients (96%). Vaginal bleeding started within 2–8 hours after prostaglandin administration and lasted for 3–12 days. Two patients were admitted to the hospital with suspected infection and were successfully treated with antibiotics. Side-effects consisted of vomiting in 16 patients (1–3 episodes) and diarrhoea in 10 (1–2 episodes). Most patients experienced uterine cramps but only 27 required analgesics.

Equally effective was another analogue, 16-phenoxy-ω-tetranor-PGE_2 methyl sulphonylamide (Karim *et al.*, 1977a). A single dose of 50 μg of this compound into the uterine cavity resulted in successful termination of the pregnancy in 228 out of 240 women with a delay in menstruation of 6–14 days. The prostaglandin analogue was instilled into the uterine cavity via a 6 mm catheter introduced through the cervix. The patients were asked to stay on their backs for 1 hour. Initially they were observed for 6 hours but subsequently the patients were allowed to go home 60 minutes after prostaglandin administration. Only four patients (1.7%) needed intramuscular injection of pentazocine to relieve the pain caused by uterine cramps. Side-effects included vomiting in 13 patients and headache in nine. Two patients developed signs of pelvic infection. The uterus was evacuated for failed treatment (12 patients) prolonged bleeding (three patients) or heavy bleeding (two patients).

More limited data are available for other analogues. Promising results have been reported for 16,16-dimethyl-*trans*-Δ^2-PGE_1 methyl ester (Tagaki *et al.*, 1977). Intrauterine administration of 15-methyl-$PGF_{2\alpha}$ was also effective and associated with fewer side-effects than $PGF_{2\alpha}$ (Ylikorkala *et al.*, 1975). At the doses used, the efficacy of $PGF_{2\alpha}$ analogues ICI 74205 (Embrey *et al.*, 1973) and ICI 81008 (Csapo and Mocsary, 1976a, 1976b) was not satisfactory.

13.4 COMPARISON OF CLINICAL EVENTS FOLLOWING VAGINAL OR INTRAUTERINE ADMINISTRATION OF PROSTAGLANDINS

13.4.1 The intrauterine versus the vaginal route

The advantages of intrauterine administration of prostaglandins compared to vaginal treatment for menstrual regulation are (1) the effective dose is lower, (2) the absorption of the drug is less variable, and (3) the effect on the myometrium is more predictable. The disadvantages include the skill necessary to introduce a catheter into the uterine cavity and an increased risk of endometritis. The most important advantage of the vaginal route is the simplicity of the treatment which allows for self-administration of the drug.

A self-administered pharmacological method of menstrual regulation is often regarded as an ideal complement to conventional contraceptive methods. Self-administration, however, could lead to a misuse of the drug. In certain situations intrauterine administration may be preferable since the treatment is in the hands of trained personnel.

13.4.1.1 *Bleeding*

When effective doses of prostaglandins are administered by the vaginal or intrauterine route for menstrual regulation, the time intervals before the onset of bleeding and the duration of bleeding are very similar. Bleeding generally starts 3–6 hours after initiation of therapy and lasts for 1–2 weeks. The amount of bleeding is described by most patients as heavier than their normal menstrual periods but does not generally affect the haemoglobin values. Heavy bleeding seems to occur in less than 2% of the patients (Gréen *et al.*, 1979; Karim, 1976; Karim *et al.*, 1977a, 1977b; Lundström *et al.*, 1977; Mocsary and Csapo, 1975).

The only study reporting on quantitative determination of blood loss is that of Hamberger *et al.* (1978). Abortion was induced by repeated vaginal administration of 15-methyl-$PGF_{2\alpha}$ methyl ester. Vaginal bleeding started 3.3 hours (mean) after insertion of the first suppository and lasted for 11 days (range 5–25 days). The average blood loss during the first 24 hours was 37 ml. Thirty-five of the 42 patients had a blood loss less than 100 ml. During the remaining period of bleeding the additional blood loss was 94 ml. All but three patients experienced a total blood loss of less than 225 ml. The mean total blood loss, 131 ml corresponds to that of a heavy menstruation and is greater than that generally reported for menstrual regulation by vacuum aspiration.

13.4.1.2 *Efficacy of treatment*

When prostaglandins are used for menstrual induction, it is difficult to assess whether the conceptus is expelled and whether abortion is complete. Similarly in the rate of decrease in plasma hCG following vacuum aspiration and menstrual induction with vaginal administration of 16,16-dimethyl-PGE_2 in a randomized study (Lundström *et al.*, 1977) indicate that most patients abort during the 24 hours following prostaglandin treatment. Minor products of conception may be retained in the uterine cavity even after the first menstruation but these are not of any clinical importance (Mandelin, 1978).

Estimation of plasma hCG seems to be a very useful parameter for predicting the efficacy of prostaglandin therapy. In uncomplicated cases plasma hCG levels drop significantly faster than in patients with failed treatment, incomplete abortion or prolonged bleeding (Corson and Bolognese, 1977; Duenhoelter *et al.*, 1978; Gréen *et al.*, 1979; Hamberger *et al.*, 1978; Mandelin, 1978). The same is true for plasma progesterone (Csapo, 1976).

Mandelin (1978) found that hCG levels in uncomplicated cases had dropped below 1000 U/l within 1 week of therapy in 96%, within 2 weeks in 97.5% and within 4 weeks in 100% of the patients. Gréen *et al.* (1979) reported that all patients (21 out of 201) in whom curettage was eventually performed, had hCG values of over 2000 U/l, 2 weeks after treatment. This is also a border line for conventional pregnancy tests. A negative urine pregnancy test 2 weeks after treatment is thus a very good indicator of successful therapy and in such cases complications due to an incomplete abortion are unlikely.

13.4.1.3 *Side-effects*

The most frequently encountered side-effects associated with prostaglandin therapy are due to stimulation of the gastro-intestinal tract. Vomiting and diarrhoea occur more frequently with PGF compounds than with PGE compounds. The opposite is true for pyrexia.

Intrauterine administration of primary prostaglandins is associated with a very high frequency of side-effects which can be reduced to acceptable limits only by premedication of the patients with a combination of analgesics, sedatives, anti-emetics and antidiarrhoeals. The incidence of side-effects with some prostaglandin analogues is very low. Extensive clinical trials with such analogues are therefore justified (Tables 13.2 and 13.3).

A similar progress has also been achieved with some analogues administered vaginally (Table 13.1). The main problem at present is that the analogues which give a high efficacy and a low incidence of side-effects are chemically unstable in suppository form. Large-scale clinical trials with vaginal administration of prostaglandin will therefore have to await a new analogue which combines a high therapeutic efficacy and chemical stability.

13.4.1.4 *Comparison with vacuum aspiration*

In only two studies has treatment with prostaglandins been compared with surgical procedure for menstrual regulation. In one study intrauterine administration of a single dose of 5.0 mg $PGF_{2\alpha}$ was compared with vacuum aspiration in patients with amenorrhoea of up to 56 days. The second study involved a comparison between repeated vaginal administration of 16,16-dimethyl-PGE_2 with the operative procedure (Ragab and Edelmann, 1976; Lundström *et al.*, 1977). It was concluded from these two studies that administration of a suitable prostaglandin by the intrauterine or vaginal route is as effective as vacuum aspiration for termination of early pregnancy. Both the surgical and non-surgical methods were considered suitable for outpatient treatment. Vacuum aspiration required less hospital time, caused fewer gastro-intestinal side-effects and resulted in a shorter period of bleeding than either intrauterine or vaginal administration of prostaglandins. The acceptability of vaginal treatment and vacuum aspiration has also been evaluated (Rosén *et al.*, 1979). Patients' attitude and preferences were assessed by an interview and rating scales before assignment to abortion procedure, immediately after treatment and 2 weeks later. Both methods were positively evaluated. Preference for a method that could be used by the patient herself increased in both groups. The proportion of patients that had a positive attitude to a method that lends itself to self-administration increased significantly in the group that received prostaglandin by the vaginal route.

13.5 CONCLUSION

Many compounds have an abortifacient activity in animals but very few have been found useful for regulating human fertility. When administered after implantation, they have either been ineffective or too toxic. The recent findings that prostaglandins are effective abortifacients without producing severe complications during very early pregnancy is therefore a significant breakthrough.

The clinical importance of the findings is, however, dependent on the possibility of prostaglandin treatment being equally effective and safe as surgical procedures used to terminate pregnancy during the first few weeks following the first missed menstrual period.

During the initial stages of development the superiority of vacuum aspiration for menstrual regulation was obvious. However, today intrauterine administration of prostaglandin analogues may be regarded as an acceptable alternative to the surgical procedure. Attempts to reduce gastro-intestinal side-effects and duration of bleeding following vaginal treatment are continuing. The simplicity of vaginal administration, its potential for self-administration and anonymity of the treatment should make this method the most attractive alternative to surgical menstrual regulation.

Acknowledgements

Part of this work was supported by research grants from the Special Programme of Research, Development and Research Training in Human Reproduction of the World Health Organization.

References

Bergström, S., Gréen, K. and Bygdeman, M. (1976). Metabolism and pharmaco-kinetics of 15-methyl-PGF$_{2\alpha}$ and its ester after administration via various routes. *Prostaglandins*, **12** (Suppl.), 17

Bolognese, R. and Corson, S. (1973). Abortion of early pregnancy by the intravaginal administration of prostaglandin F$_{2\alpha}$. *Am. J. Obstet. Gynecol.*, **117**, 246

Brenner, P., Ballard, C. and Mishell, D. R. Jr. (1977). Termination of early gestation with a vaginal polysiloxane device impregnated with 15(S)15-methyl prostaglandin F$_{2\alpha}$ methyl ester. *Prostaglandins*, **14**, 771

Bygdeman, M., Beguin, F., Toppozada, M., Wide, L. and Wiqvist, N. (1972). Postconceptional fertility control by prostaglandin F$_{2\alpha}$. In: S. Bergström, K. Gréen and B. Samuelsson (eds.), *Prostaglandin in Fertility Control*, WHO Res. Training Centre on Human Reprod, **2**, 175

Bygdeman, M., Gréen, K. and Lundström, V. (1977). Interruption of first trimester pregnancy by prostaglandins. *Int. J. Gynaecol. Obstet.*, **15**, 69

Bygdeman, M., Gréen, K., Lundström, V., Ramadan, M., Fotiou, S. and Bergström, S. (1976a). Induction of abortion by vaginal administration of 15(S)15-methyl prostaglandin F$_{2\alpha}$ methyl ester. A comparison of two delivery systems. *Prostaglandins*, **12** (Suppl.), 27

Bygdeman, M., Martin, J. N. Jr., Eneroth, P., Leader, A. and Lundström, V. (1976b). Outpatient postconceptional fertility control with vaginally administered 15(S)15-methyl-PGF$_{2\alpha}$ methyl ester. *Am. J. Obstet. Gynecol.*, **124**, 495

Bygdeman, M., Martin, J. N. Jr., Leader, A., Lundström, V., Ramadan, M., Eneroth, P. and Gréen, K. (1976c). Early pregnancy interruption by 15(S)15-methyl-PGF$_{2\alpha}$ methyl ester. *Obstet. Gynecol.*, **48**, 221

Cheng, M. C. E., Tan, P. M. and Ratnam, S. S. (1973). Prostaglandin vaginal pessary as a fertility regulating agent. *Proc. 8th Singapore–Malaysia Congress of Medicine*, **8**, 111

Cortlett, R. C., Sribyatta, B., Mishell, D. R. Jr., Ballard, C., Nakamura, R. and Thorneycroft, I. H. (1972). Termination of early gestation with vaginal prostaglandin F$_{2\alpha}$ tablets. *Prostaglandins*, **2**, 453

Corson, S. and Bolognese, R. (1977). Abortion of early pregnancy on an outpatient basis using silastic 15(S)15-methyl-prostaglandin F$_{2\alpha}$ vaginal devices. *Fertil. Steril.*, **28**, 1056

Csapo, A. J. (1974). 'Prostaglandin impact' for menstrual induction. *Popul. Report*, Ser. G, No. 4, p. 33

Csapo, A. J. (1976). Prostaglandin impact. In: B. Samuelsson and R. Paoletti (eds.), *Advances in Prostaglandin and Thromboxane Research*, p. 705 (New York: Raven Press)

Csapo, A. I. and Mocsary, P. (1976a). Menstrual induction with the PGF$_{2\alpha}$ analogue ICI 81008. *Prostaglandins*, **11**, 155

Csapo, A. I. and Mocsary, P. (1976b). Menstrual induction by the vaginal administration of ICI 81008 gel. *Prostaglandins*, **12**, 455

Csapo, A. I., Mocsary, P., Nagy, T. and Kaikola, H. L. (1973). The efficacy and acceptability of the 'Prostaglandin Impact' in inducing complete abortion during the second week after the missed menstrual period. *Prostaglandins*, **3**, 125

Duenhoelter, J. H., Santos Ramos, R., Milewich, L. and MacDonald, P. C. (1978). Interruption of early pregnancy with a silastic device containing 15(S)15-methyl prostaglandin F$_{2\alpha}$ methyl ester. Efficacy and mode of action. *Contraception*, **17**, 51

Embrey, M. P., Hillier, K. and Calder, A. A. (1973). Early abortion induced with prostaglandin F$_{2\alpha}$ and a prostaglandin analogue ICI 74205. *Lancet*, **ii**, 1100

Fylling, P. and Jerve, F. (1977). 15(S)15-methyl-prostaglandin F$_{2\alpha}$ for termination of very early pregnancy. A comparative study of a single intramuscular injection and vaginal suppositories. *Prostaglandins*, **14**, 785

Gréen, K., Bygdeman, M. and Bremme, K. (1979). Interruption of early first trimester pregnancy by single vaginal administration of 15-methyl-PGF$_{2\alpha}$ methyl ester. *Contraception*. (In press)

Hamberger, L., Nilsson, L., Björn-Rasmussen, E., Atterfelt, P. and Wiqvist, N. (1978). Early abortion by vaginal prostaglandin suppositories. *Contraception*, **17**, 183

Jones, J. R., Gentile, G. P., Kemmann, E. K. and Soriero, A. A. (1975). Intrauterine instillation of prostaglandin F$_{2\alpha}$ in early pregnancy. *Prostaglandins*, **9**, 881

Jones, J. R., Perez, R. J. and Bienart, W. (1974). Intravaginal PGE$_2$ in early abortion. *Prostaglandins*, **7**, 149

Karim, S. M. M. (1971). Once a month vaginal administration of prostaglandins E$_2$ and F$_{2\alpha}$ for fertility control. *Contraception*, **3**, 173

Karim, S. M. M. (1973). Intrauterine prostaglandins for outpatient termination of very early pregnancy. *Lancet*, **ii**, 794

Karim, S. M. M. (1976). Singapore experience with prostaglandins. Routine use and recent advances. In: S. M. M. Karim (ed.), *Obstetric and Gynecological Uses of Prostaglandins*, p. 127 (Lancaster: MTP Press)

Karim, S. M. M., Rao, B., Ratnam, S. S., Prasad, R. N. V., Wong, Y. M. and Ilancheran, A. (1977a). Termination of early pregnancy (menstrual induction) with 15-phenoxy-ω-tetranor PGE$_2$ methylsulphonylamide. *Contraception*, **16**, 377

Karim, S. M. M. and Ratnam, S. S. (1976). Termination of pregnancy with prostaglandin analogues. In: B. Samuelsson and R. Paoletti (eds.), *Advances in Prostaglandin and Thromboxane Research*, Vol. II, p. 727 (New York: Raven Press)

Karim, S. M. M., Ratnam, S. S. and Ilancheran, A. (1977b). Menstrual induction with vaginal administration of 16,16-dimethyl-*trans*-Δ^2-PGE_1 methyl ester (ONO-802). *Prostaglandins*, **14**, 615

Lichtman, A. S., Brenner, P. and Mishell, D. R. Jr. (1974). Intrauterine administration of prostaglandin $F_{2\alpha}$ as an outpatient procedure for termination of early pregnancy. *Contraception*, **9**, 403

Lundström, V., Bygdeman, M., Fotiou, S., Gréen, K. and Kinoshita, K. (1977). Abortion in early pregnancy by vaginal administration of 16,16-dimethyl PGE_2 in comparison with vacuum aspiration. *Contraception*, **16**, 167

Mackenzie, I. Z., Embrey, M. P., Davies, A. J. and Guillebaud, J. (1978). Very early abortion by prostaglandins. *Lancet*, **i**, 1223

Mackenzie, I. Z., Hillier, K. and Embrey, M. P. (1976). Intrauterine prostaglandin $E_{2\alpha}$ as an early postconceptional abortifacient. In: B. Samuelsson and R. Paoletti (eds.), *Advances in Prostaglandins and Thromboxane Research*, Vol. II, p. 687 (New York: Raven Press)

Mandelin, M. (1978). Termination of early pregnancy by a single dose 3 mg 15-methyl $PGF_{2\alpha}$ methyl ester vaginal suppository. *Prostaglandins*, **16**, 143

Mocsary, P. (1977). Menstrual induction with vaginal infusion of the $PGF_{2\alpha}$ analogue ICI 81008. *Prostaglandins*, **13**, 807

Mocsary, P. and Csapo, A. I. (1975). Menstrual induction with $PGF_{2\alpha}$ and PGE_2. *Prostaglandins*, **10**, 545

Pion, R. J., Hale, R. W. and Reich, L. (1972). Vaginal administration of prostaglandins and early abortion. In: E. M. Southern (ed.), *The Prostaglandins*, p. 367 (New York: Futura Publishing Company)

Puri, C. P., Laumas, V., Agarwal, N., Zoremthangi, B., Hingorani, V. and Laumas, K. R. (1977). Effect of 15(S)15-methyl-$PGF_{2\alpha}$ methyl ester vaginal suppositories on circulating hormone levels in early pregnancy. *Prostaglandins*, **13**, 363

Ragab, M. I. and Edelmann, D. A. (1976). Early termination of pregnancy. A comparative study of intrauterine prostaglandin $F_{2\alpha}$ and vacuum aspiration. *Prostaglandins*, **11**, 275

Robins, J. (1977). Early first trimester abortion induction by silastic vaginal devices for continuous release of 15(S)15-methyl prostaglandin $F_{2\alpha}$ methyl ester. *Fertil. Steril.*, **28**, 1048

Rosén, A.-S., Nystedt, L., Bygdeman, M. and Lundström, V. (1979). Acceptability of a non-surgical method to terminate very early pregnancy in comparison to vacuum aspiration. *Contraception*. (In press)

Spilman, C. H., Beuving, D. C., Forbes, A. D., Roseman, T. J. and Larion, L. J. (1976). Evaluation of vaginal delivery systems containing 15(S)15-methyl $PGF_{2\alpha}$ methyl ester. *Prostaglandins*, **12** (Suppl.), 1

Tagaki, S., Sakata, H., Yoshida, T., Den, K., Fujii, T. K., Ameniya, H. and Tomita, M. (1978). Termination of early pregnancy by Ono-802 suppositories (16,16-dimethyl-*trans*-Δ^2-PGE_1 methyl ester). *Prostaglandins*, **15**, 913

Tagaki, S., Sakata, H., Yoshida, T., Nakazawa, S., Fujii, T. K., Tominaga, Y., Iwasa, Y., Ninagawa, T., Hiroshima, T., Tomida, Y., Itoh, K. and Matsukawa, R. (1977). Termination of very early pregnancy by Ono-802 16,16-dimethyl-*trans*-Δ^2-PGE_1 methyl ester. *Prostaglandins*, **14**, 791

Toppozada, M., Beguin, F., Bygdeman, M., Wide, L. and wiqvist, N. (1973). Postconceptional fertility control by prostaglandins. In: S. Bergström, (ed.), *Advances in the Biosciences*, Vol. IX, p. 567

Treadway, D. and Mishell, D. R. Jr. (1973). Therapeutic abortion of early human gestation with vaginal suppositories of prostaglandin $F_{2\alpha}$. *Am. J. Obstet. Gynecol.*, **116**, 795

Ylikorkala, O., Jouppila, P., Ylöstalo, R. and Järvinen, P. A. (1974). Intrauterine injection of prostaglandin $F_{2\alpha}$ for termination of early pregnancy. *Prostaglandins*, **7**, 57

Ylikorkala, O., Järvinen, P. A., Puukka, M. and Vinikka, L. (1976). Abortifacient efficiency of 15(S)15-methyl-prostaglandin $F_{2\alpha}$ methyl ester administered vaginally during early pregnancy. *Prostaglandins*, **12**, 609

Ylikorkala, O., Kirkinen, P., Jouppila, P. and Järvinen, P. A. (1975). Intrauterine injection of 15(S)15-methyl-prostaglandin $F_{2\alpha}$ for termination of early pregnancy in out-patient. *Prostaglandins*, **10**, 333

Zoremthangi, B., Agarwal, N., Puri, C. P., Laumas, K. R. and Hingorani, V. (1976). Evaluation of 15(S)15-methyl $PGF_{2\alpha}$ methyl ester suppositories with a two-dose schedule for termination of early pregnancy. *Contraception*, **14**, 519

14
Preoperative Cervical Dilatation with Prostaglandins

S. M. M. KARIM and R. N. V. PRASAD

14.1 INTRODUCTION

Prostaglandins in appropriate doses can be used to terminate a pregnancy at any stage of gestation. However, in the first trimester of pregnancy, the abortion process takes several hours and the doses required to terminate such a pregnancy produce some gastro-intestinal side-effects. When prostaglandins are used to terminate pregnancies between 7 and 12 weeks the incidence of incomplete abortion is high necessitating surgical intervention to achieve complete evacuation of the uterus. Hence, termination of first trimester pregnancies (particularly between 7 and 12 weeks gestation) is carried out by dilatation of the cervix followed by vacuum aspiration or curettage. Before the introduction of prostaglandins, dilatation of the cervix prior to uterine evacuation was achieved by mechanical means. In a proportion of patients because of a tightly closed cervix, mechanical dilatation may result in damage to the cervix or the uterus. Cheng *et al.* (1975) encountered a high incidence of immediate complication resulting from manual dilatation of the cervix. The incidence of damage to the cervix during manual dilatation has been estimated to be between 0.4 and 4.0% (Hillier and Mackenzie, 1976). Several authors have expressed a concern over the possible long-term sequela of forceful dilatation of the cervix prior to curettage in the first trimester of pregnancy. These include cervical incompetence leading to a higher incidence of spontaneous abortion and premature labour in subsequent pregnancies (Klinger, 1970; Pantelakis *et al.*, 1973; Wright *et al.*, 1972; Moriyama and Hirokawa, 1966). Beric *et al.* (1973) however, did not find any change in prematurity rate in Yugoslavia over a period of 10 years.

In view of the potential hazards of mechanical dilatation, any drug that would soften and dilate the cervix gradually would be expected to reduce the trauma to the cervix during termination of pregnancy. Several prostaglandins have been shown to possess this property. A review of world literature on the subject is presented in this chapter.

14.2 ACTION OF PROSTAGLANDINS ON THE CERVIX

14.2.1 *In vitro* studies

Although the cervix was initially thought to be mainly composed of fibrous tissue exhibiting little spontaneous contractile activity, it has now been recognized that this is not so (Rorie and Newton, 1967; Hawkins, 1961, 1964; Hughesden, 1952; Schild *et al.*, 1951). It has been shown that the human cervix *in vitro* exhibits spontaneous activity which can be modified by drugs (Najak *et al.*, 1970; Hillier and Karim, 1970). The effects of the natural prostaglandins E_1, E_2 and $F_{2\alpha}$ on the isolated pregnant human cervix *in vitro* are variable and may be dose related (see Hillier, 1976 for references). Conrad and Ueland

(1976) in a study on the stretch modulus of the human cervix found that PGE_2 effectively reduced cervical stiffness.

14.2.2 *In vivo* studies

There is ample clinical evidence to suggest that prostaglandins have an effect on the human cervix. In failed cases of prostaglandin-induced mid-trimester abortions, the cervix has softened and at times dilated (Wentz *et al.*, 1973; Igel *et al.*, 1973; Pion *et al.*, 1972; Naftolin *et al.*, 1972; Pitkanen and Rauramo, 1974). Objective proof was obtained when Dingfelder and associates (1975) using electronic force monitors showed that PGE_2 and $PGF_{2\alpha}$ lowered the cervical resistance to mechanical dilatation in 60 nulliparae at 6–12 weeks of gestation. In a double-blind clinical study in 50 nulliparous women in the first trimester of pregnancy the efficacy of prostaglandin analogue, 15(S)15-methyl-PGE_2 was compared with a control group of similar patients given 2 ml of vehicle 20 hours before vacuum aspiration (Cheng *et al.*, 1975). The authors found that the prostaglandin analogue was very effective in softening and dilating the cervix in all cases; in the control group there was no effect on the cervix.

14.2.3 Mode of action

The mechanism by which prostaglandins soften and dilate the cervix is unknown. Since the use of prostaglandins for preoperative cervical dilatation is associated with uterine cramps, it is likely that the effect on the cervix is a result of uterine stimulation. However, a direct effect on the cervix cannot be ruled out. It is possible that prostaglandins evoke some change in the collagen material of the cervix (e.g. breakdown of the collagen by enzymes or alterations in the arrangements of collagen fibres due to changes in the composition of the ground substance) to cause cervical softening (see Danforth, 1947, 1954, 1964; Danforth *et al.*, 1974; Liggins, 1978; Hillier, 1976, for detailed account of the subject).

14.3 CLINICAL EXPERIENCE WITH PROSTAGLANDINS FOR PREOPERATIVE CERVICAL DILATATION

14.3.1 PGE_2 and $PGF_{2\alpha}$

PGE_2 and $PGF_{2\alpha}$ given by the vaginal and extra-amniotic routes have been used by several investigators to produce cervical softening and dilatation prior to vacuum aspiration or curettage in the first trimester of pregnancy. Their use, however, has generally proved to be disappointing because of a high incidence of side-effects. These include nausea, vomiting, diarrhoea, pyrexia and uterine cramps requiring analgesics. In addition, the time interval between prostaglandin administration and adequate cervical dilatation was such that overnight hospitalization of the patients was necessary.

14.3.1.1 *Extra-amniotic route*

Wiqvist *et al.* (1972) first reported on the extra-amniotic route of prostaglandin administration for preoperative cervical dilatation. They used 175–220 μg PGE_2 (5–10 doses) or 1.0–3.5 mg $PGF_{2\alpha}$ (3–5 doses) in 10 patients and found that the cervix had dilated sufficiently in all to allow easy insertion of the curette into the uterine cavity within 1½ to 8 hours. Side-effects included uterine cramps and three episodes of vomiting in each of three patients. Haspels and Neth (1973) used a single extra-amniotic dose of 0.5 mg $PGF_{2\alpha}$ in 11 first trimester patients and found varying degree of cervical dilatation in most patients 4½ to 20 hours after prostaglandin instillation. Side-effects included nausea, vomiting and uterine cramps.

More recently, Andriesse *et al.* (1976) administered a single extra-amniotic dose of 0.5 mg $PGF_{2\alpha}$ in each of 50 first trimester patients at 7–14 weeks gestation. After an interval of 18–20 hours, 16% of the patients had aborted and in an additional 36% the cervix had dilated to 9 mm or more. There was no relationship between the length of gestation and the degree of cervical dilatation. No information on the incidence of side-effects was given (see Table 14.1 for detailed results).

14.3.1.2 *Vaginal route*

Brenner *et al.* (1973) and Craft (1973) have evaluated the efficacy of natural prostaglandins given by the vaginal route for preoperative cervical dilatation in the first trimester of pregnancy. In a controlled study Brenner *et al.* (1973) compared the efficacy of a single dose 50 mg $PGF_{2\alpha}$ in 20 first trimester nulliparae with a similar control group of 20 patients without treatment. Three hours after prostaglandin administration the cervix had dilated adequately in 55% of the patients to enable evacuation of the uterus without mechanical dilatation. In the control group only 5% of the patients did not require mechanical dilatation. The patients in the prostaglandin group experienced vomiting and diarrhoea (43%), and severe uterine cramps requiring analgesics (13%). The incidence of cervical trauma in the control group was 15% whereas in the prostaglandin group it was 3%.

Craft (1973) administered 200 mg $PGF_{2\alpha}$ vaginally in two divided doses over a period of 24 hours in 10 first trimester patients. In only two patients was there adequate cervical dilatation. Side-effects included headache (10%), pyrexia (50%), chest pain (10%) and uterine cramps (10%). Detailed results are given in Table 14.1.

Table 14.1 **The use of natural prostaglandins (PGE_2 and $PGF_{2\alpha}$) for cervical dilatation prior to vacuum aspiration or uterine curettage**

References	*No. of cases*	*Gestation (weeks)*	*Parity*	*Prostaglandin, dose, route*	*Prostaglandin-evacuation interval (hours)*	*Success* rate (percentage)*	*Side-effects*
Wiqvist *et al.* (1972)	10	12	0–4	PGE_2, 175–200 μg 5–10 doses, E/A $PGF_{2\alpha}$, 1.0–3.5 mg 3–5 doses, E/A	$1\frac{1}{2}$–8	100	vomiting (3) uterine cramps
Brenner *et al.* (1973)	20	5–12	0	$PGF_{2\alpha}$, 50 mg vaginal solution single dose	3	55	vomiting and diarrhoea (17) uterine cramps
Craft (1973)	10	9–12	0–9	$PGF_{2\alpha}$, 2 × 100 mg vaginal pessaries over 24 hours	24	20	headache (1) pyrexia (5) diarrhoea (5) chest pain (1) uterine cramps
Haspels and Neth (1973)	11	7–13	0–5	$PGF_{2\alpha}$, 0.5 mg single dose, E/A	$4\frac{1}{2}$–20	varying degree of dilatation in most patients	nausea (2) vomiting (3) hypotension (1) uterine cramps
Ostergard (1973)	5	non-pregnant	—	PGE_2, 20 mg vaginal solution single dose	12	0	rigor (5) nausea (4) pyrexia (4) vomiting (3) diarrhoea (2) hypertension (1) uterine cramps
Andriesse *et al.* (1976)	50	7–14	0–7	$PGF_{2\alpha}$, 0.5 mg single dose	18–20	abortion 16% cervical dilatation 9 mm 36%	not stated

E/A = Extra-amniotic

*Criteria for success: Adequate cervical dilatation to enable evacuation of the uterus without mechanical dilatation

Table 14.2 Extra-amniotic administration of prostaglandin analogues for cervical dilatation prior to evacuation of the uterus in the first trimester of pregnancy

References	*No. of cases*	*Gestation (weeks)*	*Parity*	*Prostaglandin, dose*	*Prostaglandin-evacuation interval (hours)*	*Success* rate (percentage)*	*Side-effects*
Choo *et al.* (1973)	425	7–16	0–4	15(S)15-methyl-PGE_2 methyl ester, 25 μg single dose	12–14	95	vomiting (17) diarrhoea (31) pyrexia (13)
Toppozada *et al.* (1973)	45	9–13	0–4	15(S)15-methyl-$PGF_{2\alpha}$, 200–500 μg single dose	17½ (mean)	84	vomiting (15) diarrhoea (2)
Karim *et al.* (1935)	25	8–13	0	15(S)15-methyl-PGE_2, 25 μg single dose	12–14	92	vomiting (7) diarrhoea (12) pyrexia (11) shivering (8)
Karim *et al.* (1975)	25	8–13	0	15(S)15-methyl-PGE_2 methyl ester, 25 μg single dose	12–14	88	
Karim *et al.* (1975)	25	8–13	0	15(S)15-methyl-$PGF_{2\alpha}$, 250 μg single dose	12–14	84	vomiting (21) diarrhoea (5) pyrexia (2)
Karim *et al.* (1975)	25	8–13	0	15(S)15-methyl-$PGF_{2\alpha}$ methyl ester, 250 μg single dose	12–14	84	

Table 14.2 *continued*

Karim *et al.* (1975)	25	8–13	0	15(S)15-methyl-PGE_2 methyl ester, 12.5 μg + 15(S)15-methyl-$PGF_{2\alpha}$, 125 μg	12–14	96	vomiting (4) diarrhoea (4)
Cheng *et al.* (1975)	25	7–14	0	15(S)15-methyl-PGE_2 methyl ester, 25 μg single dose	20	88	vomiting (6) diarrhoea (3) rigor (1)
Cheng *et al.* (1976)	75	7–13	0	15(S)15-methyl-PGE_2 methyl ester, 25 μg single dose	3	48	vomiting (9)
Choo *et al.* (1976)	1785	7–14	0–5	15(S)15-methyl-PGE_2 methyl ester, 25 μg single dose	12–14	96	vomiting (68) diarrhoea (134) pyrexia (72) chills and rigors (74)

* Criteria for success: adequate cervical dilatation to enable evacuation of the uterus without mechanical dilatation of the cervix

Table 14.3 Intramuscular, intracervical and oral administration of prostaglandin analogues for pre-evacuation cervical dilatation in the first trimester of pregnancy

References	*No. of cases*	*Gestation (weeks)*	*Parity*	*Prostaglandin, dose, route*	*Prostaglandin-evacuation interval (hours)*	*Success* rate (percentage)*	*Side-effects*
Toppozada *et al.* (1973)	22	9–13	0–4	15-methyl-$PGF_{2\alpha}$ 300–800 μg 3 doses 6 hourly I/M	$17\frac{1}{2}$ (mean)	73	high incidence of vomiting and diarrhoea, uterine cramps
Karim *et al.* (1978)	80	7–12	0	16-phenoxy-ω-17,18,19, 20-tetranor-PGE_2 methyl sulphonylamide, 0.5 mg single dose, I/M	3	75	vomiting (4) pyrexia (2) severe uterine cramps requiring analgesics (3)
Karim and Ratnam (1977)	55	7–12	0	16,16-dimethyl-PGE_2 *p*-benzaldehyde semi-carbazone ester, 300 μg single dose I/M	5	85.5	vomiting (3) diarrhoea (9) pyrexia (8)
Karim *et al.* (1977a)	180	6–13	0	16,16-dimethyl-PGE_2 *p*-benzaldehyde semi-carbazone ester, 200 μg single dose, intracervical	3	80	vomiting (20) diarrhoea (12) pyrexia (12) severe uterine cramps requiring analgesics (6)
Karim (1976)	12	8–13	0	16,16-dimethyl-PGE_2 methyl ester, 100 μg 3 doses, 3 hourly, oral	9	66	vomiting (1)
Karim (1976)	16	8–13	0	16,16-dimethyl-PGE_2 *p*-benzaldehyde semi-carbazone ester, 300 μg 3 doses, 3 hourly, oral	9	100	vomiting (3)

I/M = Intramuscular

* Criteria for success: adequate cervical dilatation to enable evacuation of the uterus without mechanical dilatation

14.3.2 Synthetic analogues

The search for an effective drug that would produce cervical dilatation within a short time without producing systemic side-effects, has led to clinical evaluation of several prostaglandin analogues. The results are summarized in Tables 14.2, 14.3 and 14.4. The prostaglandins have been given by several different routes.

14.3.2.1 *Extra-amniotic route*

This route of prostaglandin administration for preoperative cervical dilatation has been used by several investigators. Toppozada *et al.* (1973) studied the effect of a single extra-amniotic dose of 200–500 μg 15(S)15-methyl-$PGF_{2\alpha}$ on cervical dilatation in 45 subjects. These patients were between 9 to 13 weeks pregnant and 60% of them were nulliparae. They were assessed 17½ hours after drug administration (mean time). Of the patients 47% had aborted before the scheduled time of evacuation and the cervix had dilated to 10 mm or more in 34 of the patients (84%). Many of the patients had side-effects. Vomiting (a total of 45 episodes) occurred in 15 patients and diarrhoea in two. All patients had to be given analgesic injections because of painful uterine cramps. Eleven patients bled 100–500 ml at the time of surgical evacuation, and in two, there was more than 500 ml blood loss at operation (Table 14.2).

Choo *et al.* (1973) conducted a study in which they instilled 25 μg of 15(S)15-methyl-PGE_2 methyl ester as a single extra-amniotic dose in 425 women. Twelve to 14 hours after drug instillation, the cervix had softened and dilated sufficiently (8 mm or more) in 95% of the subjects and vacuum aspiration could be performed without further mechanical dilatation. Operative blood loss was less than 30 ml in 420 patients, 100 ml in three, 300 ml in one and 500 ml in one. Most of the patients experienced mild uterine cramps. Other side-effects included vomiting (17), diarrhoea (31) and pyrexia of 1 °C (18 women).

Karim *et al.* (1975) have studied the effect of several prostaglandin analogues given by the extra-amniotic route for preoperative cervical dilatation in 125 nulliparous women in the first trimester of pregnancy. Details of the analogues and doses instilled are given (Table 14.2). Evacuation of the uterus without mechanical dilatation of the cervix was possible in 111 (90%) of the patients. In another 10 patients, the cervix had softened enough to allow easy dilatation to the required size. The results showed that highest efficacy with lowest incidence of side-effects was achieved in the group of patients treated with a mixture of 15-methyl analogues of PGE_2 and $PGF_{2\alpha}$.

Choo *et al.* (1976) used prostaglandin in 1785 women of mixed parity with unwanted first trimester pregnancy. They were given 25 μg 15(S)15-methyl-PGE_2 methyl ester as a single extra-amniotic dose. Adequate preoperative cervical dilatation (8 mm and more) was achieved in 96% of the patients 12–14 hours after prostaglandin administration. In 157 of these patients (8%), the foetus was expelled before the scheduled time of operation. In a further 559 patients (32%), the foetus was found at the dilated cervical os. Vomiting was seen in 4% of the patients and diarrhoea in 7.5%. Transient pyrexia (<1 °C) was recorded in 72 patients (4%). The pyrexia usually appeared 2 hours after prostaglandin administration and lasted for 2–3 hours. Chills and rigors were noted in 4% of the subjects and lasted for 5–15 min. Uterine pain was experienced by most patients, 82 of them needed analgesics. Blood loss was less than 30 ml in 90% of the patients. Uterine perforation and cervical laceration requiring repair occurred during evacuation in one patient each. Cheng *et al.* (1975) explored the efficacy of a single extra-amniotic dose of 25 μg 15(S)15-methyl-PGE_2 methyl ester in dilating the cervix within 3 hours in a group of 75 first trimester nulliparous women. The uterine size ranged between 7 and 13 weeks. None of the patients aborted during the interval between prostaglandin administration and scheduled time of evacuation (3 hours) although 30 had slight bleeding. Cervical dilatation of 8–12 mm was achieved in 37 patients and the uterus in these could be evacuated without further mechanical dilatation. In the remainder 38 patients the degree of cervical dilatation ranged between 5 and 7 mm. In 34 of these patients additional mechanical dilatation could be performed with ease. In the remaining four, some difficulty was encountered in dilating the cervix due to a tight internal os in three patients and an acutely retroverted uterus in one. There was no injury to the cervix in any of the patients and no complications were encountered during the operative procedure.

Vomiting occurred in nine patients (one episode each) after prostaglandin and pethidine administration and diarrhoea in two. One patient had rigor lasting 10 minutes shortly after prostaglandin administration (Table 14.2).

14.3.2.2 *Oral route*

In only one study the oral route of prostaglandin administration for preoperative cervical dilatation has been explored. Twelve nulliparae in the first trimester of pregnancy were given three 100 μg doses of 16,16-dimethyl-PGE_2 at 3-hourly intervals. The uterus was evacuated 9 hours after the first dose of prostaglandins. The degree of cervical dilatation in eight patients ranged between 9 and 10 mm and the uterus was evacuated without further mechanical dilatation. In the remaining four patients the cervix was 7–8 mm dilated at the end of 9 hours and additional mechanical dilatation to 9 or 10 mm was easily performed prior to evacuation of the uterus. Three patients had one episode each of vomiting (Karim, 1976; see Table 14.3).

Another group of 16 first trimester nulliparae were given three 300 μg doses of 16,16-dimethyl-PGE_2 *p*-benzaldehyde semicarbazone ester at 3-hourly intervals. Nine hours after the first dose the cervix had dilated to 9 or 10 mm in all patients and the uterus was evacuated without further dilatation of the cervix. One patient expelled the foetus before the scheduled time of evacuation. Three patients had vomiting.

All patients in the above study received loperamide (4 mg) orally 15 minutes before and 5 hours after the first dose of prostaglandin to prevent diarrhoea (Table 14.3).

14.3.2.3 *Intramuscular route*

Toppozada *et al.* (1973) administered 300–800 μg 15(S)15-methyl-$PGF_{2\alpha}$ by the intramuscular route every 6th hour in 22 first trimester patients (para 9–13) for preoperative dilatation of the cervix. In 16 patients the cervix dilated to 10 mm or more after a mean time of 17½ hours from the first dose. The treatment was associated with a high incidence of vomiting, diarrhoea and strong uterine cramps. Karim and Choo (unpublished) also encountered a high incidence of side-effects with intramuscular administration of 25 μg 15(S)15-methyl-PGE_2 methyl ester in a group of first trimester nulliparae. Adequate cervical dilatation (to enable evacuation of the uterus without mechanical dilatation) was achieved in 70% of the patients.

Lower incidence of side-effects was reported with the use of 16,16-dimethyl-PGE_2 *p*-benzaldehyde semicarbazone ester given intramuscularly. Five hours after a single intramuscular dose of 300 μg of this analogue the cervix had dilated to 8 mm or more in 47 out of 55 (85.5%) first trimester nulliparae. In the remaining eight the cervical dilatation ranged between 5 and 7 mm. Side-effects included vomiting (5.5%), diarrhoea (16.3%) and pyrexia of 1–1.5 °C (14.5%) (Karim and Ratnam, 1977; see Table 14.3).

Similar results were obtained in a recent study reported by Karim *et al.* (1978) with another prostaglandin analogue. Eighty nulliparous women (7–12 weeks gestation) were given a single intramuscular injection of 500 μg 16-phenoxy-ω-17,18,19,20-tetranor-PGE_2 methyl sulphonylamide and the uterus evacuated by vacuum aspiration 3 hours later. Success (i.e. cervical dilatation of 8 mm or more) was achieved in 80% of the patients, and in the remainder mechanical dilatation was achieved easily. Side-effects consisted of vomiting (4 women), transient pyrexia (2 women) and uterine cramps requiring analgesics (3 women) (Table 14.3).

14.3.2.4 *Intracervical route*

Karim *et al.* (1977a) injected 200 μg 16,16-dimethyl-PGE_2 *p*-benzaldehyde semicarbazone ester into the ectocervical tissue in 180 first trimester nulliparae. Three hours after prostaglandin injection the cervix had dilated 8 mm or more in 80% of the patients. Side-effects included vomiting (20 patients), diarrhoea (12 patients) and transient pyrexia (12 patients). Six patients experienced severe uterine cramps and required analgesics. It was suggested that injection of prostaglandin into the cervix may produce a direct local effect resulting in cervical softening and dilatation. However, in recent studies it was found that intramuscular injection of this prostaglandin analogue (into the gluteal muscle) has a similar effect on the cervix in first trimester nulliparae (Karim and Ratnam, 1977).

14.3.2.5 *Vaginal route*

Several investigators have studied the efficacy of prostaglandin analogues given by the vaginal route for preoperative cervical dilatation in the first trimester of pregnancy. Leader *et al.* (1975) administered vaginal pessaries containing 400 μg 16,16-dimethyl-PGE_2 at 3-hourly intervals in a group of 21 patients at 10–12 weeks gestation. Of the patients 60% were multiparous. Twelve hours after the start of treatment the cervix had dilated to 10 mm or more in 90.5% of the patients. Gastro-intestinal side-effects were mild.

Karim *et al.* (1977b) evaluated the efficacy of 16,16-dimethyl-PGE_2 *p*-benzaldehyde semicarbazone ester for pre-evacuation cervical dilatation in 124 first trimester nulliparae. A single pessary containing 0.5 mg of the analogue inserted into the posterior fornix 5 hours before evacuation of the uterus produced a cervical dilatation of 8 mm or more in 70% of the patients. In the remainder the cervix was soft and dilated up to 7 mm and additional mechanical dilatation to 8 mm or more could be performed with ease. Side-effects were trivial and included vomiting (two patients), diarrhoea (one patient) and transient pyrexia (two patients). The same group of investigators (see Prasad *et al.*, 1978) achieved a success rate of 80% (cervical dilatation of 8 mm or more) in a group of 90 first trimester nulliparae 3 hours after vaginal administration of a single pessary containing 1 mg 16,16-dimethyl-*trans*-Δ^2-PGE_1 methyl ester. Side-effects were negligible (Table 14.4).

Borell *et al.* (1976) used vaginal pessaries containing 15(S)15-methyl-$PGF_{2\alpha}$ methyl ester for termination of first trimester pregnancy in 58 women (gestation 8–13 weeks; parity 0–4). A total of 4 or 6 mg of the compound was given over a 12-hour period and vacuum aspiration was performed 18 hours after the start of therapy. All patients aborted prior to vacuum aspiration and cervical dilatation was sufficient to perform easy curettage. All patients were given oral Retardin (5 mg diphenoxylate chloride and 50 μg atropine sulphate) with each of the first two doses of prostaglandin. Vomiting occurred in four patients and some patients experienced moderate uterine cramps.

Ganguli *et al.* (1977) also used vaginal pessaries containing 15(S)15-methyl-$PGF_{2\alpha}$ methyl ester for preoperative cervical dilatation in two groups of patients in the first trimester of pregnancy. In the first group the cervix was assessed 6 hours after vaginal administration of a single pessary containing 2.0 mg of the analogue. Adequate cervical dilatation was achieved in 75% of the patients. With an increase in dose to 2.5 mg in the second group of patients the success rate increased to 100% 12 hours after administration. The incidence of side-effects and painful uterine cramps increased with the higher dose.

Table 14.4 Vaginal administration of prostaglandin analogues for pre-evacuation cervical dilatation in the first trimester of pregnancy

References	*No. of cases*	*Gestation (weeks)*	*Parity*	*Prostaglandin, dose, route*	*Prostaglandin-evacuation interval (hours)*	*Success* rate (percentage)*	*Side-effects*
Leader *et al.* (1975)	21	10–12	0–60% nullips.	16,16-dimethyl-PGE_2, 400 μg vaginal pessary 4 doses	18	90.5	mild and variable gastro-intestinal symptoms, uterine cramps
Borell *et al.* (1976)	58	8–13	0–4	15(S)15-methyl-$PGF_{2\alpha}$ methyl ester, 4–6 mg vaginal pessaries over 12 hours	18	100	vomiting (4)
Ganguli *et al.* (1977)	20	10–12	0–1	15(S)15-methyl-$PGF_{2\alpha}$ methyl ester, single vaginal pessary, 2.0 mg	6	75	occasional gastro-intestinal symptoms
Ganguli *et al.* (1977)	20	10–12	0–1	15(S)15-methyl-$PGF_{2\alpha}$ methyl ester, 2.5 mg single dose	12	100	painful uterine cramps
Karim *et al.* (1977b)	124	0	7–12	16,16-dimethyl-PGE_2 *p*-benz-aldehyde semi-carbazone ester, 0.5 mg single vaginal pessary	5	70	vomiting (2) diarrhoea (1) pyrexia (2)
Prasad *et al.* (1978)	90	8–12	0	16,16-dimethyl-*trans*-Δ^2-PGE_1 methyl ester, 1 mg single vaginal pessary	3	80	nil

* Criteria for success: adequate cervical dilatation to enable evacuation of the uterus without mechanical dilatation

14.4 CERVICAL DILATATION WITH PROSTAGLANDIN IN NON-PREGNANT WOMEN

The use of prostaglandins for dilatation of the non-pregnant cervix is virtually unexplored. The comments pertaining to the late sequelae of forceful cervical dilatation may also apply to the non-pregnant cervix. In addition, it would be an advantage if prostaglandins can be used to soften a non-pregnant cervix which is firm and difficult to dilate.

In the only study reported so far, Ostergard (1973) measured cervical dilatation before and 12 hours after vaginal administration of 20 mg PGE_2 in five women in the mid-luteal phase of the menstrual cycle. The treatment was without effect in four patients and in the fifth it dilated the cervix by only 1 mm. All patients experienced severe side-effects (Table 14.1).

In contrast Sivasamboo and Karim (unpublished) achieved a cervical dilatation of 3–6 mm in a group of patients with a single intracervical injection of 25 μg 15(S)15-methyl-PGE_2 or a single intramuscular dose of 300 μg 16,16-dimethyl-PGE_2 *p*-benzaldehyde semicarbazone ester.

14.5 CONCLUSION AND COMMENTS

Although the use of prostaglandins for cervical dilatation prior to evacuation of the uterus in the first trimester of pregnancy has become established in many centres, there are some who feel that such preliminary cervical dilatation prior to vacuum aspiration is not necessary. They consider that a great majority of first trimester pregnancies can be terminated with Karman cannulae without mechanical dilatation of the cervix (Amy, 1974; Lewis *et al.*, 1971). Others however, find a need to dilate the cervix, even when using Karman cannulae, particularly in nulliparae and during the late first trimester of pregnancy (Cheng *et al.*, 1975; Choo *et al.*, 1976; Toppozada, 1974; Liu and Hudson, 1974). The controversy can be resolved by carrying out comparative studies, i.e. vacuum aspiration using Karman cannula with and without prior treatment with prostaglandin analogues. Factors such as cervical laceration, total blood loss, completeness of evacuation and cervical incompetence will have to be evaluated.

Results of studies with natural prostaglandins clearly indicate that these substances are not suitable for preoperative cervical dilatation for several reasons. These include a high incidence of gastro-intestinal side-effects, a need for repeated dosage, need to administer the drug by extra-amniotic route and the long time interval between prostaglandin administration and adequate cervical dilatation.

The efficacy of several analogues, 15-methyl-$PGF_{2\alpha}$, 16,16-dimethyl-PGE_2 (acid and esters), 16-phenoxy-ω-17,18,19,20-tetranor-PGE_2 methyl sulphonylamide, 16,16-dimethyl-*trans*-Δ^2-PGE_1 methyl esters, given by the intramuscular or vaginal routes has been confirmed in many studies. With the exception of 15-methyl-$PGF_{2\alpha}$ the incidence of side-effects with most analogues is low and cervical dilatation necessary to evacuate the uterus without mechanical dilatation can be achieved within 3–6 hours thus enabling termination of first trimester pregnancy in an outpatient clinic.

Although it is assumed that prostaglandin-induced dilatation is less traumatic to the cervix than mechanical dilatation, there is no concrete evidence for such an assumption. Long-term follow-up of patients treated with prostaglandins is necessary to confirm this.

References

Amy, J. J. (1974). Letter to the editor. On the administration of prostaglandins as a preoperative means of cervical dilatation. *Prostaglandins*, **5**, 302

Andriesse, R., Hart, H. and Haspels, A. A. (1976). Preoperative cervical dilatation by small doses of prostaglandin $F_{2\alpha}$. *Contraception*, **14**, 93

Beric, B., Kupersanin, M. and Kapor Stanulovic, N. (1973). Accidents and sequalae of medical abortions. *Am. J. Obstet. Gynecol.*, **116**, 813

Borell, U., Bygdeman, M., Leader, A., Lundström, V. and Martin, J. N. Jr. (1976). Successful first trimester abortion with 15(S)15-methyl prostaglandin $F_{2\alpha}$ methyl ester vaginal suppositories. *Contraception*, **13**, 87

Brenner, W. E., Dingfelder, J. R., Staurovsky, L. G. and Hendricks, C. H. (1973). Vaginally administered $PGF_{2\alpha}$ for cervical dilatation in nulliparas prior to suction curettage. *Prostaglandins*, **4**, 819

Cheng, M. C. E., Karim, S. M. M. and Ratnam, S. S. (1975). Preoperative cervical dilatation with 15(S)15-methyl prostaglandin E_2 methyl ester in first trimester nulliparae – A double-blind study. *Contraception*, **12**, 59

Cheng, M. C. E., Ahmed, R., Selvadurai, V. and Ratnam, S. S. (1976). The use of prostaglandins for preoperative cervical dilatation in first trimester nulliparous pregnancy. In: S. M. M. Karim (ed.), *Proceedings of Asian Federation of Obstetrics and Gynaecology, First Intercongress, April, 1976. Obstetrical and Gynaecological uses of Prostaglandins*, p. 187 (Lancaster: MTP Press)

Choo, H. T., Karim, S. M. M. and Cheng, P. (1973). Extra-amniotic administration of single dose of 15(S)15-methyl prostaglandin E_2 methyl ester for preoperative cervical dilatation. *J. Asian Fed. Obstet. Gynecol.*, **4**, 71

Choo, H. T., Cheng, P., Yam, K. L. and Karim, S. M. M. (1976). Cervical dilatation with prostaglandin analogue prior to evacuation of the first trimester pregnant uterus. In: S. M. M. Karim (ed.), *Proceedings of the Asian Federation of Obstetrics and Gynaecology, First Intercongress, April, 1976. Obstetric and Gynaecological Uses of Prostaglandins*, p. 191 (Lancaster: MTP Press)

Conrad, J. T. and Ueland, K. (1976). Reduction of the stretch modulus of human cervical tissue by PGE_2. *Am. J. Obstet. Gynecol.*, **126**, 218

Craft, I. (1973). The use of prostaglandin pessaries prior to vaginal termination. *Prostaglandins*, **3**, 377

Danforth, D. N. (1947). The fibrous nature of the cervix and its relation to the isthmic segment in gravid and non gravid uteri. *Am. J. Obstet. Gynecol.*, **53**, 541

Danforth, D. N. (1954). The distribution and functional activity of the cervical musculature. *Am. J. Obstet. Gynecol.*, **68**, 1261

Danforth, D. N. (1964). Connective tissue mechanisms and their relation to pregnancy. *Obstet. Gynecol. Survey.*, **19**, 715

Danforth, D. N., Veis, A., Breen, M., Weinstein, H., Buckingham, J. and Manalo, P. (1974). The effect of pregnancy and labour on the human cervix: changes in collagen, glycoproteins and glycosaminoglycans. *Am. J. Obstet. Gynecol.*, **120**, 641

Dingfelder, J. R., Brenner, W. D., Hendricks, C. H. and Staurovksy, L. G. (1975). Reduction of cervical resistance by prostaglandin suppositories prior to dilatation for induced abortion. *Am. J. Obstet. Gynecol.*, **122**, 25

Ganguli, A. C., Gréen, K. and Bygdeman, M. (1977). Preoperative dilatation of the cervix by single vaginal administration of 15-methyl-$PGF_{2\alpha}$ methyl ester. *Prostaglandins*, **14**, 779

Haspels, A. A. and Neth, F. (1973). Induction of abortion (1) by intravenous and (2) by intrauterine administration of $PGF_{2\alpha}$ (extra- and intra-amniotic). *Adv. Biosci.*, **9**, 515

Hawkins, D. F. (1961). In discussion. *Proc. R. Soc. Med.*, **54**, 719

Hawkins, D. F. (1964). In: D. R. Lawrence and A. L. Bacharach (eds.), *Evaluation of Drug Activities, Pharmacometric*, Vol. II, p. 665 (London: Academic Press)

Hillier, K. (1976). The effect of prostaglandins. In: J. A. Jordan and A. Singer (eds.), *The Cervix*, p. 236 (Saunders)

Hillier, K. and Karim, S. M. M. (1970). The human isolated cervix: A study of its spontaneous motility and responsiveness to drugs. *Br. J. Pharmacol.*, **40**, 576

Hillier, K. and Mackenzie, I. Z. (1976). Experiences and advances in the use of prostaglandins in obstetrics and gynaecology in the United Kingdom. In: S. M. M. Karim (ed.), *Proceedings of the Asian Federation of Obstetrics and Gynaecology, First Intercongress, April, 1976. Obstetric and Gynaecological Uses of Prostaglandins*, p. 83 (Lancaster: MTP Press)

Hughesden, P. E. (1952). The fibromuscular structure of the cervix and its changes during pregnancy and labour. *J. Obstet. Gynaecol. Br. Emp.*, **59**, 763

Igel, H., Lau, Hu. Hengst, P. and Halle, It. (1973). Erste Erfahrungen mit dem Prostaglandin $F_{2\alpha}$ bei der kiinstlichen Abortusaushosiing. *Zentral Gynakol.*, **95**, 353

Karim, S. M. M. (1976). Singapore experience with prostaglandins – routine use and recent advances. In: S. M. M. Karim (ed.), *Proceedings of the Asian Federation of Obstetrics and Gynaecology, First Intercongress, April, 1976. Obstetric and Gynaecological Uses of Prostaglandins*, p. 127 (Lancaster: MTP Press)

Karim, S. M. M., Choo, H. T. and Cheng, P. (1975). Cervical dilatation with prostaglandin analogues prior to vaginal termination of first trimester pregnancy in nulliparous patients. *Prostaglandins*, **9**, 631

Karim, S. M. M., Ilancheran, A., Winnie Wun, Ho, T. H. and Ratnam, S. S. (1978). Intramuscular administration of 16-phenoxy-ω-17,18,19,20-tetranor-PGE_2 methyl sulphonylamide for preoperative cervical dilatation in first trimester nulliparae. *Prostagland. Med.*, **1**, 71

Karim, S. M. M. and Ratnam, S. S. (1977). Newer aspects of practical applications of prostaglandin in obstetrics and gynaecology. In: N. Kharasch and J. Fried (eds.), *Biochemical Aspects of Prostaglandins and Thromboxanes*, p. 115 (New York: Academic Press)

Karim, S. M. M., Ratnam, S. S., Selvadurai, V., Wun, W. and Prasad, R. N. V. (1977a). Cervical dilatation with 16,16-dimethyl-PGE_2 *p*-benzaldehyde semicarbazone ester prior to vacuum aspiration in first trimester nulliparae. *Prostaglandins*, **13**, 333

Karim, S. M. M., Ratnam, S. S., Prasad, R. N. V. and Wong, Y. M. (1977b). Vaginal administration of a single dose of 16,16-dimethyl prostaglandin E_2 *p*-benzaldehyde semicarbazone ester for preoperative cervical dilatation in first trimester nulliparae. *Br. J. Obstet. Gynaecol.*, **84**, 269

Klinger, A. (1970). Demographic consequences of the legalization of induced abortion in Eastern Europe. *Int. J. Gynaecol. Obstet.*, **8**, 680

Leader, A., Bygdeman, M., Gréen, K., Martin, J. N. Jr. and Wiqvist, N. (1975). Vaginally administered 16,16-dimethyl-PGE_2 as an agent for preoperative cervical dilatation. *Prostaglandins*, **10**, 357

Lewis, S. C., Lal, S., Branch, B. and Beard, R. W. (1971). Outpatient termination of pregnancy. *Br. Med. J.*, **4**, 606

Liggins, G. C. (1978). Ripening of the cervix. In: T. K. Oliver and T. H. Kirschbaum (eds.), *Seminars in Perinatology*, Vol. II, No. 3, p. 261 (New York: Grune and Stratton)

Liu, D. T. Y. and Hudson, I. (1974). Karman cannula and first trimester termination of pregnancy. *Am. J. Obstet. Gynecol.*, **118**, 906

Moriyama, Y. and Hirokawa, O. (1966). The relationship between artificial termination of pregnancy and abortion and premature birth. In: *Harmful Effects of Induced Abortions*, p. 64 (Family Planning Federation of Japan)

Naftolin, F., Kirshen, E. J. and Ryan, K. J. (1972). Therapeutic abortion utilizing local application of prostaglandin $F_{2\alpha}$. In: E. M. Southern (ed.), *The Prostaglandins – Clinical Applications in Human Applications*, p. 423 (Mount Kisco, New York: Futura)

Najak, Z., Hillier, K. and Karim, S. M. M. (1970). The action of prostaglandins on the human isolated non-pregnant cervix. *J. Obstet. Gynaecol. Br. Cmnwlth.*, **77**, 701

Ostergard, D. R. (1973). The cervical relaxant properties of prostaglandin E_2 in non-pregnant subjects. *Prostaglandins*, **4**, 701

Pantelakis, S. N., Papadimitriou, G. C. and Doxiadis, S. A. (1973). Influence of induced and spontaneous abortions on the outcome of subsequent pregnancies. *Am. J. Obstet. Gynecol.*, **116**, 799

Pion, R. J., Hale, R. W. and Reich, L. (1972). Vaginal administration of prostaglandins and early abortion. *J. Reprod. Med.*, **9**, 413

Pitkanen, Y. and Rauramo, L. (1974). The efficacy of the extravular prostaglandin – impact in provoking first trimester abortion. *Prostaglandins*, **5**, 269

Prasad, R. N. V., Charles, Lim, Wong, Y. C., Karim, S. M. M. and Ratnam, S. S. (1978). Vaginal administration of 16,16-dimethyl-*trans*-Δ^2-PGE_1 methyl ester (ONO 802) for preoperative cervical dilatation in first trimester nulliparous pregnancy. *Singapore J. Obstet. Gynecol.*, **9**, 69

Rorie, D. K. and Newton, M. (1967). Histological and chemical studies of the smooth muscle in the human cervix and corpus uterus. *Am. J. Obstet. Gynecol.*, **99**, 466

Schild, H. O., Fitzpatrick, R. J. and Nixon, W. C. W. (1951). Activity of the human cervix and corpus uteri. Their responses to drugs in early pregnancy. *Lancet*, **i**, 250

Toppozada, M. (1974). In author's reply. *Prostaglandins*, **5**, 303

Toppozada, M., Bygdeman, M., Papageorgiou, C. and Wiqvist, N. (1973). Administration of 15-methyl prostaglandin $F_{2\alpha}$ as a preoperative means of cervical dilatation. *Prostaglandins*, **4**, 371

Wentz, A. C., Burnett, L. S., Atienza, M. F. and King, T. M. (1973). Experience with intra-amniotic $PGF_{2\alpha}$ for abortion. *Am. J. Obstet. Gynecol.*, **117**, 513

Wiqvist, N., Beguin, F., Bygdeman, M., Fernstrom, I. and Toppozada, M. (1972). Induction of abortion by extra-amniotic prostaglandin administration. *Prostaglandins*, **1**, 37

Wright, C., Campbell, S. and Beazley, J. (1972). Second trimester abortion after vaginal termination of pregnancy. *Lancet*, **i**, 1278

15
Prostaglandins for Pre-induction Cervical Ripening

A. A. CALDER

15.1 INTRODUCTION

This chapter deals with the use of prostaglandins in the management of pregnancies in which induction of labour is indicated but the uterine cervix is found to be unripe. There are two main types of clinical situation in which this may arise:

(1) In pre-term gestations: the cervix may be unripe because the normal process of ripening is not sufficiently advanced.

(2) In term or post-term gestations: the cervix is unripe because the normal ripening process has failed to occur. This is the more common clinical problem.

Before discussing the role of prostaglandins in cervical ripening it is necessary to consider briefly the normal pattern of ripening and the clinical problems associated with an unripe cervix. It is important to stress here that in both these respects there are important differences between primigravida and multigravida subjects. Primigravidae represent the more common and difficult clinical problem and so more attention will be paid to them.

15.2 NORMAL PATTERN OF CERVICAL RIPENING

Every obstetrician is aware of the striking physical differences between the cervix in early and late pregnancy. During this time a long, firm, closed, fibrous tube is usually transformed into a soft, compliant structure that is already effaced and partially dilated.

These changes, which are especially obvious in the primigravida, would seem to be an essential prelude to normal labour. Whereas in other species such as the sheep, cervical ripening appears to occur rapidly just before the onset of labour, the process is much more gradual in the human. Anderson and Turnbull (1969) and Hendricks, Brenner and Kraus (1970) have studied the development of these changes by recording the findings at serial vaginal examinations through the course of large numbers of human pregnancies. Both studies confirm the gradual nature of the process and show that it occurs at an increasing rate throughout the third trimester of pregnancy. Bishop (1964) has shown a clear temporal relationship between the development of ripening and the onset of labour.

Thus, during the few days preceding spontaneous labour it is usual to find a cervix that is soft, distensible and already 3 or 4 cm dilated. In the primigravida it is usually also well effaced and thin; in the multigravida this is more variable.

Ripening may thus be considered to consist of two identifiable physical changes in the cervix:

(1) The shape change – effacement and dilatation (these are the changes which continue much more rapidly during parturition).

(2) The physical change in the nature of the cervical tissue which makes it softer and more compliant.

Ripening was thought to be a result of increasing uterine contractility in late pregnancy (the so-called Braxton–Hicks contractions). Whereas these are probably partly responsible for the shape change in the cervix during ripening, it is now clear that this could not come about without fundamental changes in the biomechanics of the cervical tissue. Considering the importance of cervical biomechanics in human labour, it is perhaps surprising that more attention has not been focused on this. Over the years, Danforth (Danforth, 1947, 1954; Danforth and Buckingham, 1964, 1973; Danforth *et al.*, 1960, 1974) has been the outstanding contributor to our knowledge of the nature and behaviour of the cervix. He has repeatedly emphasized the importance of collagen rather than muscle in the cervix. The former is not only much more abundant but would appear to have a more important role in the ripening process. From these and other workers the following picture of the collagen changes during ripening has emerged:

(1) Breakdown of collagen by collagenase and other proteases.

(2) Alterations in the spatial arrangements of collagen fibres due to changes in the composition of the ground substance (in particular glycosaminoglycans and proteoglycans) causing reduction in the tensile strength of the tissue. These changes, which all appear to be under the control of fibroblasts, have been elegantly reviewed by Liggins (1978) but our understanding of them is far from complete.

15.3 MEASUREMENT OF CERVICAL RIPENESS

An accurate method of assessing the ripeness of the cervix is an essential requirement for identifying patients in need of ripening therapy and also to allow for valid comparisons between patients and between different methods of treatment. Clinicians may give quite different views if they rely on the vague impression gained from a vaginal examination. Greater objectivity has been

Table 15.1 Pelvic scoring system devised by Bishop (1964)

Characteristic	*Pelvic score*			
	0	*1*	*2*	*3*
Dilatation (cm)	0 __	1–2 __	3–4 __	5–6 __
Effacement (%)	0–30 __	40–50 __	60–70 __	80 __
Consistency	firm __	average __	soft __	______
Position	posterior __	mid __	anterior __	______
Level	0–3 __	0–2 __	0–1; 0 __	+ __
				Total score __

(Bishop, 1964)

achieved by the use of a scoring system and among a number that have been described, that of Bishop (1964) or a modification of this has been most widely applied (Table 15.1). For ease of use we have employed a slight modification of the Bishop system (Table 15.2, Calder *et al.*, 1974).

Table 15.2 Modification of the Bishop system used to assess cervical ripeness

Characteristic	*Cervical score*			
	0	*1*	*2*	*3*
Dilatation (cm)	less than 1 __	1–2 __	2–4 __	more than 4 __
Length (cm)	more than 4 __	2–4 __	1–2 __	less than 1 __
Consistency	firm __	average __	soft __	______
Position	posterior __	mid-anterior __	______	______
Level	0–2 __	0–1 : 0 __		+ __
				Total score __

(Calder, Embrey and Hillier, 1974)

15.4 PROBLEMS ASSOCIATED WITH FAILURE OF THE CERVIX TO RIPEN

Acceptance that cervical ripening is a necessary prelude to spontaneous parturition implies that if the cervix is unripe we may expect labour to be delayed. This is borne out in clinical practice where the patient with an unripe cervix at term faces prolongation of pregnancy and its associated dangers. The greatest fear is placental failure leading to foetal hypoxia in labour and birth asphyxia or even intrauterine death of the foetus before labour. These dangers increase the longer pregnancy continues beyond term (Walker, 1954). Furthermore, when labour eventually does occur it is likely to be incoordinate and prolonged (Clayton, 1941). It may be that pregnancy and labour are both prolonged because of the failure of cervical ripening but a more attractive explanation is that the cervix remains unripe and labour is delayed as a result of an endocrine abnormality which affects both the cervix and the myometrium. Indeed it appears that similar endocrine mechanisms may control both cervical ripening and myometrial contractility (Liggins, 1978).

To avoid the problems associated with prolonged pregnancy, obstetricians are tempted to intervene at 41 or 42 weeks gestation but have often in the past had a cause to regret attempted induction of labour in the presence of an unripe cervix. The most reliable method of labour induction was amniotomy and intravenous oxytocin infusion but several authors (Garett, 1960; Embrey and Anselmo, 1962; Bishop, 1964; Turnbull and Anderson, 1968) showed that its success was closely related to the state of the cervix. 'Failed induction' in such cases meant resort to caesarean section when effective uterine contractility had not been achieved 36 or 48 hours after amniotomy. With the more aggressive doses of oxytocin used during the past decade, it is almost always possible to produce strong uterine contractions and while this may have altered the pattern of the outcome it has not overcome the problems of the unripe cervix. Calder (1978) has shown that when the cervix is unripe, this form of induction is associated with unacceptable rates of maternal and foetal morbidity in the form of pyrexia in labour, caesarean section and birth asphyxia. In contrast, the rates of these complications are very low if the cervix is ripe at the outset (Table 15.3). These observations point to the desirability of patients coming to term in a 'labour ready' condition as indicated by a ripe cervix and of the need to produce this condition where it is found wanting.

Table 15.3 Influence of cervical score on the outcome of labour induced by amniotomy and intravenous oxytocin infusion

	Cervical score	
	0–3	*4–11*
Number of patients	31	94
Induction–delivery interval	14.9	8.2
(hours; mean ± SD)	± 5.5	± 2.9
Caesarean section	10	3
(%)	(32%)	(3.2%)
Maternal pyrexia	10	2
(%)	(32%)	(2.1%)
Birth asphyxia	7	4
(%)	(23%)	(4.3%)

Maternal pyrexia is defined as a temperature greater than 38 °C occurring during labour, and birth asphyxia as a 1 minute Apgar score of 4 or less (Calder, 1978)

15.5 EVIDENCE FOR A PHYSIOLOGICAL ROLE OF PROSTAGLANDINS IN CERVICAL RIPENING

15.5.1 Studies in sheep

The pattern of cervical ripening in the pregnant ewe differs from that in the human mother. In contrast to the gradual nature of the process in the human (see p. 302), the cervix of the ewe remains long and firm for almost the entire period of gestation and ripens very suddenly and predictably during the 12 hours or so preceding the onset of labour (Liggins, 1978). By employing an elegant surgical technique of isolating the cervix from the mechanical influence of the uterus, Stys *et al.* (1978) have shown that the dramatic increase in compliance of the cervix at this time is independent of uterine contractility. Fitzpatrick (1977) has studied changes in cervical compliance in the sheep *in vivo* around the time of parturition and correlated these with endocrine changes in the peripheral blood. He found that the sudden increase in compliance was first detectable after the levels of oestradiol-17β began to rise but before there was any detectable rise in $PGF_{2\alpha}$. However, Liggins *et al.* (1977) have been able to produce softening, shortening and dilatation of the sheep cervix as early as 25 days before term by infusing $PGF_{2\alpha}$ into the uterine artery. These changes appear to occur with little or no uterine contractility.

Of crucial importance to the concept of a physiological role of prostaglandins in cervical ripening is their source. In this context a recent report from Elwood *et al.* (1978) is of special interest. These workers have studied cervical tissue *in vitro* using a continuous superfusion system and have shown that such tissue is capable of synthesizing PGE and that the production rate is greater in cervical tissue taken at the time of delivery than during late pregnancy.

15.5.2 Human studies

There is good circumstantial evidence that prostaglandins play a physiological role in human cervical ripening although this is by no means conclusive. The most obvious pointer is the already established clinical value of the prostaglandins for pre-operative cervical dilatation (see Chapter 14) and for pre-induction cervical ripening (see following section). In the second trimester of pregnancy it is possible to stimulate uterine contractions with oxytocin, albeit in large doses, but this rarely induces an abortion. The much

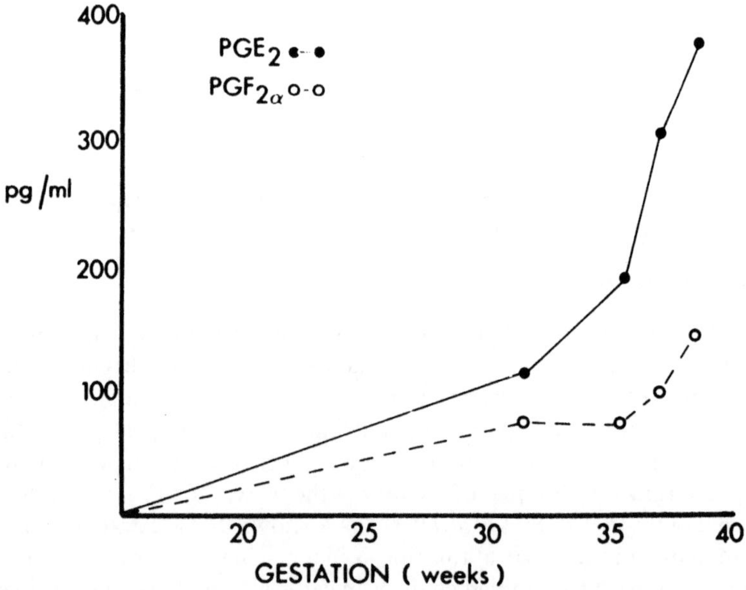

Figure 15.1 Levels of PGE_2 and $PGF_{2\alpha}$ in amniotic fluid samples obtained by amniocentesis during the third trimester of human pregnancy (data from Dray and Frydman, 1975)

greater effectiveness of prostaglandins for this purpose may be largely due to their ability to alter cervical resistance.

Conrad and Euland (1976) have studied the stretch modulus of strips of human cervix obtained immediately post-partum and showed that this was

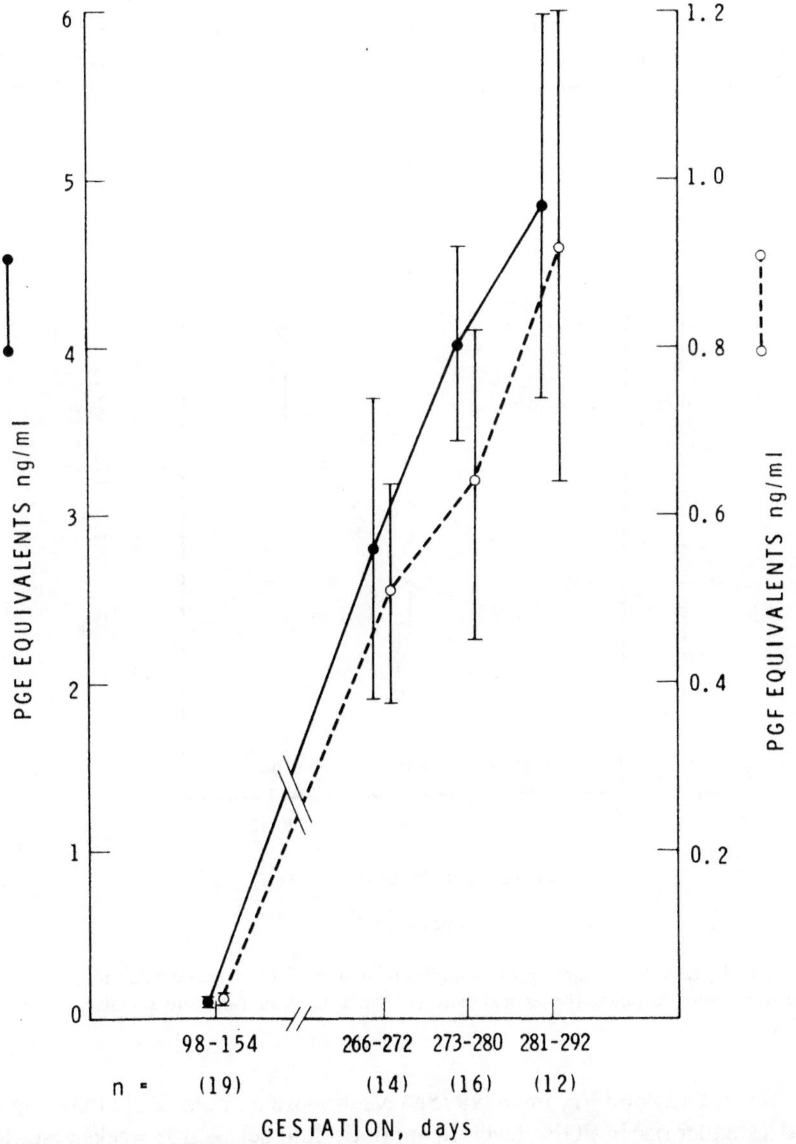

Figure 15.2 Levels of E and F prostaglandins in amniotic fluid in early and late human gestation, measured by radioimmunoassay. (Unpublished data from Calder, Dilley, Hillier, and MacKenzie, 1975)

greater in women whose labours had been induced with PGE_2 than in those who had laboured spontaneously. They further demonstrated that for both types of tissue addition of PGE_2 to the bathing medium caused a further increase in tissue compliance.

There has been no convincing demonstration of a rise in circulating levels of primary prostaglandins before the onset of labour. This is hardly surprising in view of their rate of metabolic breakdown but neither has an increase in the major metabolites been noted before labour is established (Gréen *et al.*, 1974).

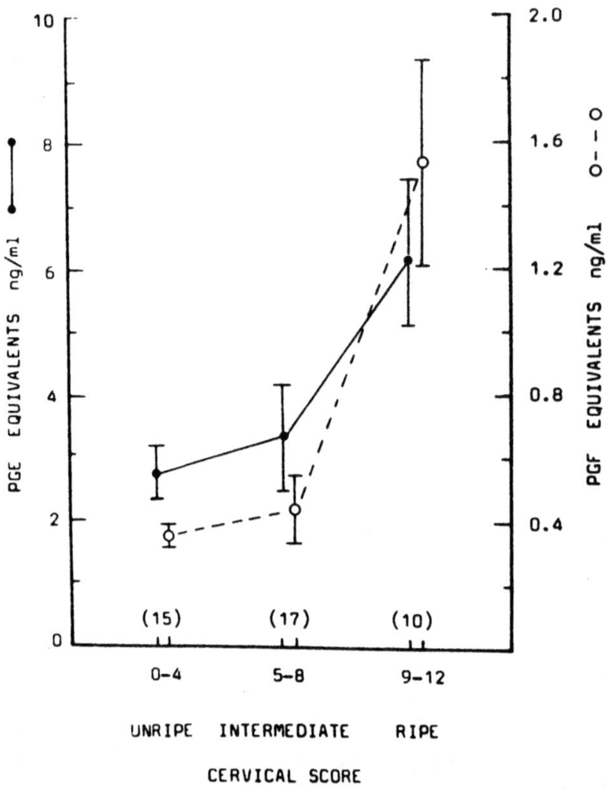

Figure 15.3 Levels of E and F prostaglandins in amniotic fluid obtained by amniotomy in late human gestation related to the cervical score. (Unpublished data from Calder, Dilley, and Hillier, 1975)

However, Dray and Frydman (1975) have shown a marked rise in PGE_2 levels and a smaller rise in $PGF_{2\alpha}$ levels in amniotic fluid between 33 weeks gestation and term (Figure 15.1) i.e. during the most rapid period of cervical ripening. This observation is supported by our own data (Calder *et al.*, 1975; unpublished observations, Figure 15.2). Moreover, the levels of both E and F prostaglandins found in samples from 42 primigravidae around term show a correlation with the degree of cervical ripeness (Figure 15.3). Tambyraja *et al.* (1977) have found a similar correlation in postmature pregnancies for $PGF_{2\alpha}$ but not for PGE_2.

While not firmly established, an important role of prostaglandins in cervical ripening seems highly probable. Their mode of action, however, is not clear. Hillier and Karim (1970) and Najak *et al.* (1970) have shown that prostaglandins can modify the motility of the cervix *in vitro* but the muscle is sparse in the cervix and its importance to the process or ripening is at best uncertain. An influence on cervical collagen or ground substance seems a more likely mechanism and evidence has recently been advanced that prostaglandins, especially $PGF_{2\alpha}$, may cause an increased production of glycosaminoglycans from fibroblasts in culture (Chang *et al.*, 1977). As pointed out earlier (p. 303) these substances appear to determine the binding forces between collagen bundles in the cervix and thereby the tensile strength of the tissue.

15.6 PROSTAGLANDIN THERAPY FOR PRE-INDUCTION CERVICAL RIPENING

Prostaglandins have been employed in a variety of different forms in an effort to ripen the unripe cervix and these will be reviewed according to the route of administration. In common with many attempts to review literature related to clinical research, the task is complicated not only by differences in methods of assessing the value of treatment but by basic differences in the type of patients selected for ripening therapy, especially with regard to parity, gestational age and cervical state. The objective of ripening therapy is a reduction or even elimination of foetal and maternal morbidity so that on the face of it a low incidence of caesarean sections and birth asphyxia in the treatment group should indicate successful treatment. This only holds true if the study group was indeed facing a high morbidity rate. Multiparous patients, for instance, seem less at risk than nulliparae and there are varying degrees of unripeness within any unripe group. Perhaps the best yardstick is the cervical score but this is subject to observer error. It also shows a tendency to increase with the passage of time, and as a result of interference by vaginal examination or catheter insertion, all of which probably release endogenous prostaglandins locally (Mitchell *et al.*, 1977).

These difficulties highlight the virtues of randomized controlled trials. Unfortunately there are very few studies that conform to this requirement. In some the number of patients involved is small or the studies are not restricted to patients with highly unripe cervices. Nevertheless, the literature now contains a dozen or more reports on the use of prostaglandins for cervical ripening and from these a picture of the most effective form of therapy is emerging.

15.6.1 Oral

Friedman and Sachtleben (1975) conducted a randomized double-blind study in 30 patients with a Bishop score less than six. The treatment and control groups each consisted of 15 patients of whom seven were multiparous. The former group received tablets containing 1 mg PGE_2 on three occasions at 3-hourly intervals while the latter received placebo tablets. Success of treatment was assessed from changes in the Bishop score and the response to a standard regime of intravenous oxytocin (without amniotomy) commenced 8–12 h after the last tablets. The results in the two groups were as follows:

Treatment group: improvement in Bishop score 1.4, spontaneous labour before oxytocin (3 patients), failed induction (3 patients).

Control group: improvement in Bishop score 1.5, spontaneous labour before oxytocin (3 patients), failed induction (4 patients).

The authors concluded that oral PGE_2 in this form was of no value for pre-induction cervical ripening. The study highlights a number of points. The control group showed an increase in the Bishop score of 1.5 at the end of 6 hours of placebo 'therapy'. This probably reflects the influence of mechanical interference in the form of sequential vaginal examinations. A surprisingly large number (one in five) of patients in this group went into labour without oxytocin stimulation suggesting that they were not in need of ripening therapy. In contrast labour induction was considered to have failed in 23% of all the patients studied which serves to emphasize the inefficiency of oxytocin when not combined with amniotomy.

Weiss *et al.* (1975) reported positive results in an almost identical study although none of their 56 patients was primigravida. They found a rise of more than 2 points in the Bishop score in two-thirds of their patients treated with PGE_2 against only one in eight in the placebo group. No difference was seen between groups in their response to oxytocin but nine out of the 32 control patients (28%) delivered during the priming period as did one from the control group. The mean Bishop score before priming was 4.7 in the treatment group and 5.0 in the controls; this hardly suggests that the cervices were very unripe and it is doubtful whether similar improvements in Bishop score would have been achieved among primigravida patients with lower starting scores.

Valentine (1977) studied 60 patients of whom 48 were primigravida and all had Bishop scores of 4 or less. Two study groups received either 0.5 mg or 1.0 mg PGE_2 every hour for 10 hours the day before induction and these were compared with two control groups one of which received no treatment and the other 30 units of oxytocin intravenously over the course of 10 hours. The mean improvement in Bishop score in the four groups was as follows: No treatment – no change; intravenous oxytocin – 2 points increase; 0.5 mg PGE_2 group – 4 points increase; 1.0 mg PGE_2 – almost a 6 point increase.

Unfortunately, in spite of these impressive changes in the cervical score the rate of caesarean section in each of the four groups was very high, and accounted for 23% of all prostaglandin treated subjects. No mention is made of any maternal side-effects with the fairly high dose of PGE_2 used but the author concluded that the method was efficient and safe.

15.6.2 Intravenous

In spite of several reports which testify to the value of intravenous prostaglandins for induction of labour when the cervix is unripe (Anderson *et al.*, 1971; Friedman and Sachtleben, 1974; Karim *et al.*, 1970; Calder and Embrey, 1975; Thiery and Amy, 1975) there are no detailed reports of their use by this route for pre-induction cervical ripening. Liggins, however, has recently described some hitherto unpublished observations made by Hutton and himself (Liggins, 1978) which are of considerable interest. They infused $PGF_{2\alpha}$ intravenously in 23 gravidae in increasing doses until the oxytocic threshold for each patient was determined. The dose was then decreased by 50% and continued for 24 hours. This produced an increase in the Bishop score of 3 or more in 18 of the patients, including three patients who did not have detectable uterine contractions.

Intravenous prostaglandin therapy has been largely superseded in obstetric practice by local routes of administration which are more reliable and are associated with fewer side-effects. It is worth remembering, however, that local prostaglandin therapy may occasionally be contraindicated, e.g. in haemorrhage, infection or ruptured membranes. In these situations, intravenous prostaglandin therapy may be considered to ripen the cervix.

15.6.3 Extra-amniotic

The extra-amniotic (or 'extra-ovular') route of prostaglandin administration for therapeutic abortion was independently developed by Wiqvist and Bygdeman (1970) and Embrey and Hillier (1971) in order to overcome the troublesome side-effects associated with systemic routes. It quickly became an established method for this purpose and was extended to the management of abnormal intrauterine pregnancies including anencephaly, hydatidiform mole and foetal death *in utero* (Embrey *et al.*, 1974). From there it was a short step to demonstrate its effectiveness for induction of labour in normal pregnancies (Calder *et al.*, 1974). With wider experience, it quickly became apparent that this approach was particularly valuable for potentially difficult cases of induction with an unripe cervix (Calder and Embrey, 1973; Miller and Mack, 1974; Neuberg, 1975).

The technique consists of passing a catheter (usually a Foley catheter with a small self-retaining balloon) through the cervix to lie in the space between the intact foetal membranes and the wall of the lower uterine segment. Through this a dilute solution of prostaglandins is administered as a continuous infusion. This is the most effective and reliable method of inducing human labour while preserving the integrity of the foetal membranes. Further modification of this technique has allowed the use of prostaglandins on a wider scale for pre-induction cervical ripening.

Calder *et al.* (1975) described a technique of single-shot extra-amniotic PGE_2 therapy which employed a viscous gel for sustained prostaglandin release to ripen the cervix as a prelude to induction of labour. A single application of 5 ml 5% Tylose gel (methyl-hydroxyethyl cellulose, Hoechst) containing 400 μg PGE_2 is given via a Foley catheter with a 20 ml balloon the day before induction of labour is contemplated. Some low-grade uterine contractility is usually experienced during the ensuing 4–6 h before the Foley catheter is extruded from the cervix which is then usually about 3 cm dilated but may not yet be fully effaced. Effacement may continue during the next 12 hours but most patients are able to sleep overnight. A proportion of patients so treated become established in labour and this appears to depend mainly on the initial state of the cervix.

Calder *et al.* (1977) employed this technique in 121 primigravida patients around term with cervical scores of 0–3 (mean 2.3). Twenty-four patients were in established labour before the following morning. The remaining 97 had a mean cervical score of 6.3 and labour was induced by amniotomy and intravenous oxytocin infusion. The overall rate of maternal pyrexia in labour was 4% and that of birth asphyxia 7%. Seventeen mothers (14%) required delivery by caesarean section including seven (from 15 mothers) who were either small in stature (less than 5 feet) or had breech presentation of the foetus. The section rate among the remaining 106 mothers was 9.4% compared with 32% among 31 matched control primigravidae who had no ripening therapy. Birth asphyxia and maternal pyrexia were also at least three times higher among the untreated controls. There were no serious foetal or maternal side-effects from the prostaglandin gel therapy.

Thiery *et al.* (1977) used a similar technique in 92 patients (68 primigravida and 24 multigravida) with Bishop scores 0–4. The same gel was employed and a dose of either 250 μg or 500 μg PGE_2 was given at around midnight. Amniotomy was performed 7–8 h later if the cervix had ripened sufficiently (Bishop score >6); if not a second dose of prostaglandin gel was given (this applied to only three patients). A mean increase in Bishop score of 3.7 was achieved in primigravidae and 4.1 in multigravidae. Eighty-seven mothers were delivered vaginally. In the remaining five caesarean section was carried out because of cephalopelvic disproportion.

In a second study, Thiery *et al.* (1978a) carried out detailed investigation of the foetal and neonatal condition during ripening therapy and labour, and after delivery. This consisted of continuous foetal heart monitoring together with foetal blood sampling at the time of amniotomy and again during the second stage of labour. The acid–base and lactate–pyruvate status was measured in these samples and also in cord blood samples and the Apgar score of the neonate was recorded. These careful investigations revealed no deleterious effects of PGE_2 gel on the foetus. This group of workers (Thiery, *et al.*, 1978b) has recently completed a small study of 22 patients (13 nulliparas and 9 multiparas) treated with 5 mg $PGF_{2\alpha}$ in 8 ml 5% Tylose. The initial Bishop scores of the group were not so low as in the previous studies (mean about 3.5) but this increased by a mean of 4 points and vaginal deliveries were achieved in all cases.

The role of the Foley catheter in these studies has often been the subject of debate especially in view of its known cervical ripening effect (Embrey and Mollison, 1967). The influence of the gel has also been questioned. Shepherd *et al.* (1976) provided at least partial answers to these questions in an elegant study which compared the effect of a single extra-amniotic dose of 250 µg PGE_2 in 10 ml 6% Tylose with that of the same volume of Tylose without prostaglandin. In both groups the catheter was immediately withdrawn. There was a modest increase in Bishop score (from 2.7 to 3.5) in the control group probably due to a local mechanical stimulus releasing endogenous prostaglandins. The increase in Bishop score in the PGE_2 treated group was much greater (from 2.1 to 7.0). This study suggests that whereas the Foley's catheter and the volume of gel may play contributory roles, the major influence on cervical ripening is due to the administered prostaglandin.

15.6.4 Vaginal

MacKenzie and Embrey (1977) have described a simplified technique of cervical ripening in which a single dose of PGE_2 in viscous gel is placed high in the vagina on the day prior to induction of labour. They report a series of 168 primigravida patients with cervical scores 0–3 who received either 2 mg or 5 mg PGE_2 in 2% or 4% sodium carboxymethyl cellulose. A pilot double-blind study was first conducted which compared the effect of gel containing 2 mg PGE_2 with that of gel containing no PGE_2 in two groups of 12 patients. The mean cervical score in the treatment group rose from 2.4 to 7.6 and that in the control group from 2.5 to 3.6. Patients in the treatment group had significantly shorter labour with oxytocin and the babies had better Apgar scores than those in the control group.

In the main study 102 patients received 2 mg PGE_2. The mean cervical score improved from 2.4 to 5.6 and 24 became established in labour before the planned oxytocin induction. A further 66 patients received 5 mg PGE_2. The mean cervical score rose from 2.5 to 6.1 and about half the patients (32) were established in labour before the scheduled induction with oxytocin. Out of the total of 168 patients, 21 (12.5%) were delivered by caesarean section and 15 (9%) showed evidence of birth asphyxia (one minute Apgar score of 4 or less). The caesarean section rate was slightly lower in the group receiving 5 mg PGE_2. No adverse foetal effects were seen and maternal side-effects were rare.

The rate of maternal pyrexia in labour was remarkably low at only 2% and there were no episodes of nausea, vomiting or diarrhoea following prostaglandin therapy.

This latter finding is especially gratifying in the light of the large doses of PGE_2 used and previous experience with vaginal administration of prostaglandins. The explanation for this presumably lies in the property of the gel used which may have given a more sustained and uniform release of prostaglandin than Tylose since some observers using similar doses of PGE_2 in Tylose have encountered troublesome side-effects (A. D. Boyle; personal communication). The results of this study compare very favourably with those achieved by the extra-amniotic route. The vaginal route has advantages of convenience and safety and if equally effective, it should supplant the extra-amniotic technique.

Wilson (1978) has shown that PGE_2 tablets placed high in the vagina may also be effective for ripening the cervix. This paper will be discussed in detail in the next section.

A recent report from MacLennan and Green (1979) suggests that $PGF_{2\alpha}$ may also be effective for cervical ripening. The authors administered 50 mg $PGF_{2\alpha}$ in 10 ml 8% methyl cellulose gel or sterile water in the same volume of gel in a randomized double-blind study of 80 patients. Multiparous patients were included in the study and the mean starting cervical score was rather high at 4.7. The technique produced an average rise in the cervical score of 5.1 in the treatment group against 1.6 among the controls. Of the treated patients 50% went into labour against only 8% of the controls. The caesarean section rate was the same in both groups at approximately 8%.

It is perhaps unfortunate that this study did not concentrate on patients with unripe cervices (the majority of patients presumably had cervical scores greater than 4). Nevertheless, it does suggest that $PGF_{2\alpha}$ given by the vaginal route may be valuable in the management of the unripe cervix.

The effectiveness of the vaginal route of prostaglandin therapy for cervical ripening raises the intriguing possibility that prostaglandins may be absorbed directly into the cervix from the upper vagina. It used to be thought that vaginally administered prostaglandins depended on systemic absorption for their effect on the uterus (Embrey, 1975) but the superiority of the results of these studies over those which employed oral PGE_2 in equivalent or even higher dosage points to the likelihood of direct cervical absorption. More work, however, requires to be done to answer this question.

15.6.5 Comparative studies

It will be seen from the foregoing studies that PGE_2 and $PGF_{2\alpha}$ given by a variety of routes may be effective in ripening the cervix. Even with the help of literature, the clinician may find it difficult to choose the best method. Differences in study populations and criteria for success used by different investigators do not allow for strictly valid comparisons. Studies in which different methods are compared on a randomized basis are required.

The first such study has been reported by Wilson (1978). Sixty primigravidae with cervical scores of 0–4 were randomly allocated to four groups of 15 patients. One group received intravenous oxytocin in a dose range of 1–128 milliunits per minute which was increased until regular contractions were occurring every 2–3 min and continued for a total of 8 h. Another group received oral PGE_2 tablets (1 mg every hour) for 10 h. A third received 400 μg PGE_2 in 5% Tylose extra-amniotically and the last group received 2 mg PGE_2 in tablet form placed high in the posterior vaginal fornix.

The results in all three prostaglandin treated groups were superior to those in the oxytocin treated group and the best results were seen in the extra-amniotic PGE_2 group. In the oxytocin group the mean Bishop score rose by only 1.1 and five patients required caesarean section. The score in the oral PGE_2 group increased by a mean of 1.6 and four patients required caesarean section. In the vaginal PGE_2 group the score rose by 2.5 and three required caesarean section and in the extra-amniotic PGE_2 group the score increased by 4.5 and there was only one caesarean section; this group also had the shortest labour.

Although the study was relatively small it demonstrated the superiority of locally administered PGE_2 over both intravenous oxytocin infusion and oral PGE_2 therapy. The oral PGE_2 tablet regime employed corresponded to the highest dose in any of the published studies (Valentine, 1977) but the results were disappointing. The comparison between the extra-amniotic and the vaginal route may be less fair in that the 2 mg dose used corresponds to the lower dose of the MacKenzie and Embrey (1977) study and the vaginal administration of tablets rather than a gel formulation was a hitherto unexplored method for this purpose. The simplicity of this approach and the results commend it for further investigation.

The results of such comparative studies are bound to be governed to some degree by the doses employed but more studies of this sort are necessary to establish the best method of cervical ripening. Better methods of cervical ripening will surely emerge as the physiological control of the process becomes fully understood. The objectives must be to improve the efficacy, increase the safety and simplify the patient management. To date there are no reports of the use of longer-acting synthetic analogues of prostaglandins for cervical ripening.

15.7 CONCLUSIONS

Cervical ripening is a necessary prerequisite to normal parturition. It usually occurs gradually during the latter weeks of pregnancy in the form of a change in the shape and consistency of the cervix so that it can be rapidly dilated in labour. Failure of the cervix to ripen is a serious clinical problem especially in primigravidae. It is associated with prolongation of pregnancy, long and difficult labour, a poor response to conventional labour induction and high rates of caesarean section and birth asphyxia. There is good circumstantial evidence for a physiological role of prostaglandins of the E and F series in the ripening process and these compounds have been successfully employed in improving the clinical outcome in patients with unfavourable cervices.

PGE_2 has been the more widely used agent. In common with the experience in the use of prostaglandins for other indications in obstetrics and gynaecology, systemic routes (oral and intravenous) have been relatively less effective than local routes of administration probably because of the rapid metabolic breakdown in the systemic circulation. The most widely used and successful route has been the extra-amniotic using a viscous gel for sustained release but the much simpler technique of vaginal administration may prove equally effective. It has the added advantage of being potentially safer.

PGE_2 is probably more effective than $PGF_{2\alpha}$ although experience with the latter is limited. As yet there are no reports of the use of prostaglandin analogues for cervical ripening although such compounds might be well suited to the purpose. We should look to the future for the development of analogues with highly specific cervical ripening properties and little or no stimulant effects on the uterus. Such a compound, capable of ensuring that all labours start with a fully ripe cervix, would represent a considerable boon to the practising obstetrician and his patients.

References

Anderson, A. B. M. and Turnbull, A. C. (1969). Relationship between length of gestation and cervical dilatation, uterine contracility and other factors during pregnancy. *Am. J. Obstet. Gynecol.*, **105**, 1207

Anderson, G., Hobbins, J., Cordero, L. and Speroff, L. (1971). Clinical use of prostaglandins as oxytocin substances. *Ann. N.Y. Acad. Sci.*, **180**, 499

Bishop, E. H. (1964). Pelvic scoring for elective induction. *Obstet. Gynecol.*, **24**, 266

Calder, A. A. (1978). *The Unripe Cervix* (M.D. Thesis, University of Glasgow)

Calder, A. A. and Embrey, M. P. (1973). Prostaglandins and the unfavourable cervix. *Lancet*, **ii**, 1322

Calder, A. A. and Embrey, M. P. (1975). Comparison of intravenous oxytocin and prostaglandin E_2 for induction of labour using automatic and non-automatic techniques. *Br. J. Obstet. Gynaecol.*, **82**, 728

Calder, A. A., Embrey, M. P. and Hillier, K. (1974). Extra-amniotic prostaglandin E_2 for the induction of labour at term. *J. Obstet. Gynaecol. Br. Cmnwlth.*, **81**, 39

Calder, A. A., Embrey, M. P. and Tait, T. (1977). Ripening of the cervix with extra-amniotic prostaglandin E_2 in viscous gel before induction of labour. *Br. J. Obstet. Gynaecol.*, **84**, 264

Calder, A. A., Hillier, K. and Embrey, M. P. (1975). Prostaglandin therapy for cervical ripening prior to induction of labour. In: B. Samuelsson and R. Paoletti (eds.), *Advances in Prostaglandin and Thromboxane Research*, Vol. II, p. 993 (New York: Raven Press)

Chang, W. C., Abe, M. and Murota, S. (1977). Stimulation by prostaglandin $F_{2\alpha}$ of acid glycosaminoglycan production in cultured fibroblasts. *Prostaglandins*, **13**, 711

Clayton, S. G. (1941). Foetal mortality in postmaturity. *J. Obstet. Gynaecol. Br. Emp.*, **48**, 450

Conrad, J. T. and Euland, K. (1976). Reduction of the stretch modulus of human cervical tissue by prostaglandin E_2. *Am. J. Obstet. Gynecol.*, **126**, 218

Danforth, D. N. (1947). The fibrous nature of the cervix and its relation to the isthmic segment in gravid and non-gravid uteri. *Am. J. Obstet. Gynecol.*, **53**, 541

Danforth, D. N. (1954). The distribution and functional activity of the cervical musculature. *Am. J. Obstet. Gynecol.*, **68**, 1261

Danforth, D. N. and Buckingham, J. C. (1964). Connective tissue changes and their relation to pregnancy. *Obstet. Gynecol. Surv.*, **19**, 715

Danforth, D. N. and Buckingham, J. C. (1973). The effects of pregnancy and labour on the amino acid composition of the human cervix. In: R. J. Blandau and K. Moghissi (eds.), *The Biology of the Cervix*, p. 351 (Chicago: University of Chicago Press)

Danforth, D. N., Buckingham, J. C. and Roddick, J. W. (1960). Connective tissue changes incident to cervical effacement. *Am. J. Obstet. Gynecol.*, **80**, 939

Danforth, D. N., Veis, A., Breen, M., Weinstein, H. G., Buckingham, J. and Manalo, P. (1974). The effect of pregnancy and labour on the human cervix: Changes in collagen, glycoproteins and glycosaminoglycans. *Am. J. Obstet. Gynecol.*, **120**, 641

Dray, F. and Frydman, R. (1975). Primary prostaglandins in amniotic fluid of normal pregnancy. In: B. Samuelsson and R. Paoletti (eds.), *Advances in Prostaglandin and Thromboxane Research*, Vol. II (New York: Raven Press)

Elwood, D. A., Mitchell, M. D., Anderson, A. B. M. and Turnbull, A. C. (1978). A significant increase in the *in vitro* production of prostaglandin E by ovine cervical tissue at delivery. Paper presented at the Society for Endocrinology, London, November 1978

Embrey, M. P. (1975). *The Prostaglandins in Human Reproduction*, p. 57 (Edinburgh: Churchill Livingstone)

Embrey, M. P. and Anselmo, J. F. (1962). The effects of intravenous oxytocin on uterine contractility. *J. Obstet. Gynaecol. Br. Cmnwlth.*, **69**, 918

Embrey, M. P., Calder, A. A. and Hillier, K. (1974). Extra-amniotic prostaglandins in the management of intra-uterine foetal death, anencephaly and hydatidiform mole. *J. Obstet. Gynaecol. Br. Cmnwlth.*, **81**, 47

Embrey, M. P. and Hillier, K. (1971). Therapeutic abortion by intrauterine instillation of prostaglandins. *Br. Med. J.*, **1**, 588

Embrey, M. P. and Mollison, B. G. (1967). The unfavourable cervix and induction of labour using a cervical balloon. *J. Obstet. Gynaecol. Br. Cmnwlth.*, **74**, 44

Fitzpatrick, R. J. (1977). Changes in cervical function at parturition. *Ann. Rech. Vet.*, **8**, 438

Friedman, E. A. and Sachtleben, M. R. (1974). Oral prostaglandin E_2 for induction of labour at term. *Obstet. Gynecol.*, **43**, 178

Friedman, E. A. and Sachtleben, M. R. (1975). Pre-induction priming with oral prostaglandin E_2. *Am. J. Obstet. Gynecol.*, **121**, 521

Garrett, W. J. (1960). Prognostic signs in surgical induction of labour. *Med. J. Aust.*, **1**, 929

Green, K., Bygdeman, M., Toppozada, M. and Wiqvist, N. (1974). The role of prostaglandin $F_{2\alpha}$ in human parturition. *Am. J. Obstet. Gynecol.*, **120**, 25

Hendricks, C. H., Brenner, W. E. and Kraus, G. (1970). Normal cervical dilatation pattern in late pregnancy and labor. *Am. J. Obstet. Gynecol.*, **106**, 1065

Hillier, K. and Karim, S. M. M. (1970). The human isolated cervix: a study of its spontaneous motility and responsiveness to drugs. *Br. J. Pharmacol.*, **40**, 576

Karim, S. M. M., Hillier, K., Trussell, R. R., Patel, R. C. and Tamusange, S. (1970). Induction of labour with prostaglandin E_2. *J. Obstet. Gynaecol. Br. Cmnwlth.*, **77**, 200

Liggins, G. C. (1978). Ripening of the cervix. In: T. K. Oliver and T. H. Kirschbaum (eds.), *Seminars in Perinatology*, Vol. II, No. 3, p. 261 (New York: Grune and Stratton)

Liggins, G. C., Fairclough, R. J., Grieves, S. A., Foster, C. and Knox, B. S. (1977). Parturition in the sheep. *Ciba Found. Symp.*, **47**, 31

Mackenzie, I. Z. and Embrey, M. P. (1977). Cervical ripening with intravaginal PGE_2 gel. *Br. Med. J.*, **2**, 1369

MacLennan, A. H. and Green, R. C. (1979). Cervical ripening and induction of labour with intravaginal prostaglandin $F_{2\alpha}$. *Lancet*, **i**, 117

Miller, A. W. F. and Mack, D. S. (1974). Induction of labour by extra-amniotic prostaglandins. *J. Obstet. Gynaecol. Br. Cmnwlth.*, **81**, 706

Mitchell, M. D., Flint, A. P. F., Bibby, J., Brunt, J., Arnold, J. M., Anderson, A. B. M. and Turnbull, A. C. (1977). Rapid increases in plasma prostaglandin concentrations after vaginal examination and amniotomy. *Br. Med. J.*, **2**, 1183

Najak, Z., Hillier, K. and Karim, S. M. M. (1970). The action of prostaglandins on the human isolated non-pregnant cervix. *J. Obstet. Gynaecol. Br. Cmnwlth.*, **77**, 701

Neuberg, R. (1975). The 'uninducible' cervix: induction of labour using extra-amniotic prostaglandin E_2. *Int. J. Gynaecol. Obstet.*, **13**, 171

Shepherd, J., Sims, C. and Craft, I. (1976). Extra-amniotic prostaglandin E_2 and the unfavourable cervix. *Lancet*, **ii**, 709

Stys, S. J., Clewell, W. H., Beschia, G. (1978). Changes in cervical compliance at parturition independent of uterine activity. *Am. J. Obstet. Gynecol.*, **130**, 414

Tambyraja, R. L., Karim, S. M. M., Salmon, J. A. and Ratnam, S. S. (1977). Prostaglandins and postmaturity. *Aust. N.Z. J. Obstet. Gynaecol.*, **17**, 89

Thiery, M. and Amy, J. J. (1975). Induction of labour with prostaglandins. In: S. M. M. Karim (ed.), *Advances in Prostaglandin Research. Prostaglandins and Reproduction*, pp. 149–228 (Lancaster: MTP Press)

Thiery, M., Defoort, P., Benijts, G., Van Eyck, J., Hennay, T., Van Kets, H. and Martens, G. (1977). Effectiveness of extra-ovular injection of prostaglandin E_2 in Tylose gel to ripen the cervix prior to elective induction of labour. *Prostaglandins*, **14**, 381

Thiery, M., Defoort, P., Benijts, G., Derom, R., Martens, G., Amy, J. J., Van Kets, H. and Deschrijver, D. (1978a). Fetal effects of cervical ripening with extra-amniotic prostaglandin E_2 gel. *Prostaglandins*, **15**, 175

Thiery, M., Parewyck, W., De Gezelle, H., Van Kefs, H., Derom, R. and Martens, G. (1978b). Extra-amniotic prostaglandin $F_{2\alpha}$ in gel for prelabor cervical ripening. *Z. Gebrutsh Perinat.*, **182**, 299

Turnbull, A. C. and Anderson, A. B. M. (1968). Induction of labour. Part II: Intravenous oxytocin infusion. *J. Obstet. Gynaecol. Br. Cmnwlth.*, **75**, 24

Valentine, B. H. (1977). Intravenous oxytocin and oral prostaglandin E_2 for ripening of the unfavourable cervix. *Br. J. Obstet. Gynaecol.*, **84**, 846

Walker, J. (1954). Foetal anoxia. *J. Obstet. Gynaecol. Br. Emp.*, **61**, 162

Weiss, R. R., Tejani, N., Israeli, I., Evans, M. I., Bhakthavathsalan, A. and Mann, L. I. (1975). Priming of the uterine cervix with oral prostaglandin E_2 in term multigravidae. *Obstet. Gynaecol.*, **46**, 181

Wilson, P. D. (1978). A comparison of four methods of ripening the unfavourable cervix. *J. Obstet. Gynaecol. Br. Cmnwlth.*, **85**, 941

Wiqvist, N. and Bygdeman, M. (1970). Therapeutic abortion by local administration of prostaglandin. *Lancet*, **ii**, 716

16
Termination of Abnormal Intrauterine Pregnancy with Prostaglandins

S. M. M. KARIM, S. C. NG and S. S. RATNAM

16.1 INTRODUCTION

Abnormal intrauterine pregnancy constitutes abnormal products of conception and deviation from the normal course of pregnancy. The former includes molar pregnancy and gross congenital abnormality of the foetus. The latter comprises threatened, inevitable, incomplete and missed abortion and intrauterine foetal death. Threatened premature labour is not relevant to the present discussion since prostaglandins are not used in its management.

The use of prostaglandins in the termination of abnormal intrauterine pregnancy is a recent development. Karim (1970) first reported successful termination of pregnancies with PGE_2 in cases of missed abortion, intrauterine foetal death and hydatidiform mole. Since then, several prostaglandins given by different routes have been used in the termination of such and other types of abnormal intrauterine pregnancies. The subject was briefly reviewed by Thiery and Amy (1975) and Karim and Amy (1975). In this chapter the current status of the use of prostaglandins in the management of different types of abnormal intrauterine pregnancies will be discussed.

16.2 INTRAUTERINE FOETAL DEATH AND MISSED ABORTION

Intrauterine foetal death is defined as the demise of a foetus *in utero* after 28 weeks of gestation. If the death occurs before the 28th week of pregnancy the condition is described as a missed abortion. Most investigators have adopted an identical management in the termination of pregnancy with prostaglandins in cases of missed abortion and intrauterine foetal death. Published reports often give combined results of treatment with prostaglandins in the two situations. In this section, therefore, the use of prostaglandins in the management of missed abortion and intrauterine foetal death will be reviewed together and the term death *in utero* will be used to describe the two conditions.

A large number of unsuccessful pregnancies end in spontaneous expulsion of the products of conception within a few weeks of death *in utero* (Tricomi and Kohl, 1957). Retention of the dead foetus for a few weeks or even months, however, is not uncommon. The longest recorded duration of a retained dead foetus *in utero* is 2½ years (El-Sherbini, 1963).

Retention of the dead foetus *in utero* is associated with increased risk of infection, disturbance in coagulation mechanism and psychological distress (see Karim, 1970; Lewis, 1976). The recognition of coagulation disorder (Hodgkinson *et al.*, 1954; Pritchard and Ratnoff, 1955; Quinn and Harper, 1955; Corbett, 1958) had led to a more active management of death *in utero*. It is estimated that retention of a foetus *in utero* for 1 month after death results in coagulation disorder in one out of three women (Hardisty and Ingram, 1965). Intravascular coagulation is thought to occur as a result of thromboplastin release from the dead foetus and placenta resulting in depletion of plasma fibrinogen. It is therefore logical that pregnancy should be terminated at the earliest possible moment after confirmation of intrauterine death.

In the first trimester, the termination of pregnancy in cases of death *in utero* poses few problems and is effected by a simple dilatation and vacuum aspiration or curettage. Although in the second trimester of pregnancy the products of conception can be evacuated *per vaginum*, there is an increased morbidity mainly due to a difficulty in evacuating foetal bones and skull. Termination of pregnancies in cases of death *in utero* in the last two trimesters is therefore preferably carried out by medical methods.

Before the advent of prostaglandins, methods for the management of deaths *in utero* were either not effective or were not safe. Many hormones and drugs have been used to stimulate uterine contractility in such cases. Of these, oestrogen treatment has in the past enjoyed the widest popularity since its introduction by Robinson *et al.* in 1935 (see also Jeffcoate, 1940). In a critical assessment of the efficacy of oestrogen therapy, however, Martin and Menzies (1955) showed that it has no merit when used in the treatment of missed abortion and intrauterine foetal death and that where such a therapy was successful, the time required for expulsion of uterine contents was on an average longer than 1 week.

Intravenous oxytocin, given alone, is often not successful in expelling a dead foetus. In addition the high doses required may result in water intoxication and convulsion (Liggins, 1962). A combination of amniotomy and oxytocin infusion increases the success rate and shortens the induction–delivery interval (Ursell, 1972) but carried with it the risk of amnionitis and amniotic fluid embolism (Peterson and Taylor, 1970). Failure to initiate uterine activity by amniotomy leaves one with no choice but to resort to hysterotomy and in the presence of severe infection to hysterectomy. The use of intra-amniotic hypertonic saline occasionally results in hypernatraemia and brain damage (Wagatsuma, 1965; Cameron and Dayan, 1966) while intra-amniotic hypertonic glucose carries an increased risk of intrauterine infection. Hysterotomy and caesarean section in the presence of a dead foetus are undesirable but may be the only alternative in an unsuccessful attempt at medical termination of such pregnancies.

Prostaglandins given by various routes have proved very effective in the management of death *in utero*. The incidence of serious complications has so far been low. It has been observed in many studies that there are no significant alterations in either the coagulation or fibrinolytic systems attributable to the use of prostaglandins. This is an important consideration in the management of death *in utero* since the patient with a prolonged retention of a dead foetus is at risk from a chronic consumptive coagulopathy (Kent, 1977). Briel *et al.* (1976) have demonstrated that in missed abortions and intrauterine foetal deaths, intravenous infusion of $PGF_{2\alpha}$ resulted in a significant decrease in maximal platelet aggregation and speed of platelet aggregation. There was also a significant increase in maximal disaggregation and speed of disaggregation. The authors postulate that prostaglandins may have 'a protective effect on the beginning consumptive coagulability' because the inhibition of platelet aggregation reduces the development of disseminated intravascular coagulation.

16.2.1 Intravenous route

Three naturally occurring prostaglandins (E_1, E_2 and $F_{2\alpha}$) and one synthetic analogue (sulprostone) given by intravenous infusions have been used in the management of death *in utero* in the second and third trimesters of pregnancy.

16.2.1.1 *PGE_2*

This was the first prostaglandin used for the termination of pregnancy in cases of death *in utero* in the last two trimesters (Karim, 1970). PGE_2 was infused at a rate of 5 μg/min in six patients with a missed abortion and at 0.5 to 2.0 μg/min in 15 patients with intrauterine foetal death. All six patients with a missed abortion aborted in a mean time of 8 h. Fourteen out of 15 patients with an intrauterine foetal death delivered in a mean time of 12 h 10 min. One patient who received PGE_2 infusion for 14 h failed to deliver despite good uterine stimulation during the duration of infusion and for at least 12 h after stopping the infusion. Pregnancy in this patient was terminated by caesarean section (Karim, 1970). The efficacy of intravenously administered PGE_2 in the management of missed abortion and intrauterine foetal death has since been confirmed by many investigators. A summary of results from 11 published papers covering a total of 269 patients is shown in Table 16.1. The duration of death *in utero* has ranged from 1 day to 112 days. Patients with a prolonged retention of the dead foetus *in utero* generally required PGE_2 infusion for a longer duration (Karim and Trussell, 1971). The rate of infusion of PGE_2 used by different investigators ranged between 0.25 and 6 μg/min although in one study (Naismith and Barr, 1974) a maximum infusion rate of 12 μg/min was employed. The total dose of PGE_2 varied between 0.1 mg and 7.3 mg in different studies.

The uterus usually responded to intravenous PGE_2 15–45 min after the start of infusion (Karim, 1970; Filshie, 1971; Ring, 1972; Ruppen *et al.*, 1972).

Out of a total of 269 cases of death *in utero* treated with intravenous infusion of PGE_2, the treatment was successful in 255 (94.8%). The average interval between the start of infusion and the expulsion of the foetus ranged between 7 h 42 min and 14 h in different studies. Some patients who failed to deliver with one infusion and were successfully treated with a repeat infusion the following day were classified as failures (Gordon and Pipe, 1975; Murray and Clinch, 1975).

In most studies amniotomy was not performed because of the risk of intrauterine infection (see Thiery and Amy, 1975). Roberts (1974), however, performed amniotomy to reduce the risk of amniotic fluid embolism once adequate uterine activity had been established.

Details of some selected studies are given below:

Filshie (1971) successfully treated five patients with a missed abortion and seven cases of intrauterine foetal death with intravenous infusion of 0.5–5.0 μg/min PGE_2. The mean interval between the start of infusion and expulsion of the foetus was 11 h 36 min and 8 h 30 min respectively. Similar results were obtained by Miller (1973) in a group of 17 patients with death *in utero* treated with 2.5 to 5.0 μg/min infusion of PGE_2.

Roberts (1974) used PGE_2 in five patients with a missed abortion and three

Table 16.1 Termination of pregnancy in cases of intrauterine foetal death and missed abortion with intravenous infusion of PGE_2

No. of cases	*No. successfully treated*	*Gestation (weeks)*	*Duration of death (days)*	*Infusion rate* (μg/min)	*Mean total dose* (mg)	*Mean ind.-del. interval* (h:min)	*Side-effects*	*References*
6	6	14–22	28–84	5.0	2.40	8:00	V	Karim (1970)
15	14	30–40	28–84	0.5–2.0	0.58	10:10	0	
12	12	<28	28–84	5.0	—	8:30	V	Karim and Trussell (1971)
33	31	>28	28–84	0.5–2.0	—	11:30	V	
8	5	—	—	0.21–6.70	—	—	—	Beazley and Gillespie (1971)
5	5	14–26	7–49	0.5–5.0	1.90	11:30	0	Filshie (1971)
7	7	29–40	1–21	0.5–2.5	0.76	8:30	0	
10	10*	14–30	2–112	2.5–5.0	3.40	12:30	P. N. V. D	Miller (1973)
7	7	29–41	7–10	2.5–5.0	4.97	14:42	P. N. V	
28	28†	<28	—	3.5–12.0	2.08	9:17	P. V	Naismith and Barr (1974)
17	17†	>28	—	1.0–4.5	0.72	7:42	P. R. S. V	
23	23	24–40	1–19	0.625–5.0	1.36	17:26	P. N. V. D. S. T	Iddelkinge and Gordon (1974)
5	5	15–19	7–42	1.5–6.0	5.00	22:12	D. V. S	Roberts (1974)
3	3‡	39–40	4–21	0.25–4.0	1.47	14:00	V. S	
15	12§	24–36	1–19	0.625–5.0	1.15	11:08	D. N. V. S	Gordon and Pipe (1975)
36	32	<28	—	0.5–2.0	—	11:06	P. S. N. V. D	Murray and Clinch (1975)
26	25	>28	—		—			
13	13	18–37	—	—	7.30	11:43	D. N. V	Kunz and Schreiner (1977)
269	255							

V = Vomiting; — = Not reported; P = Pyrexia; N = Nausea; D = Diarrhoea; R = Rigors; S = Superficial phlebitis; T = Tachycardia; 0 = None

* One patient was given oxytocin infusion for 2 hours before delivery

† All patients were given simultaneous oxytocin infusion (16–2048 mU/ml)

‡ In two patients amniotomy was performed when the cervix was 2 cm dilated

§ Three patients who failed to deliver with one infusion were classified as failures with intrauterine foetal death. The former required a higher concentration of PGE_2 (1.5–6.0 µg/min) infusion and a higher mean total dose (5.0 mg) than reported by most other investigators. The interval between the start of infusion to expulsion of the foetus (22 h 12 min) was also longer in other studies. Three patients with an intrauterine foetal death required an average of 1.5 mg PGE_2 and all delivered in a mean time of 14 h.

Iddekinge and Gordon (1974) infused PGE_2 at rates varying between 0.625 and 5 µg/min in 23 patients with death *in utero* at gestation of 24–40 weeks. The authors made an interesting observation that doses of PGE_2 required for the management of deaths due to placental insufficiency were significantly lower than required in cases of death due to rhesus isoimmunization. Seven cases of deaths *in utero* due to placental insufficiency were successfully evacuated with total doses varying between 0.15 and 1.32 mg (mean 0.83 mg). The total dose required in 16 cases of deaths due to rhesus isoimmunization ranged between 0.99 and 3.5 mg (mean 1.9 mg). Three of these patients required a second infusion of PGE_2. The mean interval between the start of infusion and delivery was also significantly longer in the rhesus isoimmunization group (12½ hours for those who delivered with one infusion and 58 h 15 min for those who required a repeat infusion) than in the placental insufficiency group (9 h 6 min). The above interesting observations need to be confirmed. Gordon and Pipe (1975) have compared the efficacy of oxytocin and PGE_2 in two groups of patients. In 15 patients with death *in utero* between 24 and 36 weeks gestation PGE_2 was given at rates varying between 0.625 and 5 µg/min. Twelve patients delivered in a mean time of 11 h 4 min with a mean total dose of 1.15 mg. In the remaining three patients, delivery occurred after a second infusion of PGE_2 and were classified as failures. All 15 patients infused with intravenous oxytocin delivered at first attempt in a mean time of 21 h 25 min.

In another study, intravenous PGE_2 and oxytocin were infused simultaneously in 28 patients with a missed abortion and 17 patients with intrauterine foetal death (Naismith and Barr, 1974). The infusion rate of PGE_2 ranged between 0.5 and 12 µg/min and that of oxytocin between 1 and 884 mU/min. The treatment was successful in all patients. The average interval between the start of treatment and expulsion of the foetus in cases of missed abortion was 9 h 17 min and for intrauterine foetal death it was 7 h 42 min.

Naismith and Barr (1974) have argued that a combination of intravenous oxytocin and PGE_2 results in a higher success rate and a lower incidence of side-effects than encountered with PGE_2 alone. Even with the combination of two oxytocins, a repeat infusion was required in two patients and pyrexia occurred in one-third of the patients. With intravenous PGE_2 alone (in doses similar or even lower than used in the above study) several investigators have obtained results similar to those reported by Naismith and Barr (1974). It would therefore appear that the use of oxytocin combined with PGE_2 does not seem to offer any advantage.

Some investigators used oxytocin infusion when patients failed to deliver after several hours of prostaglandin infusion (Miller, 1973; Roberts, 1974).

Murray and Clinch used three different dose regimes of intravenous PGE_2 (1.5, 5.0 and 6.0 μg/min) in patients with a missed abortion and intrauterine foetal death. In the group of patients given 1.5 μg/min infusion, 36 out of 37 (including three cases of molar pregnancy) delivered with an average total dose of 1.9 mg in a mean time of 10 h 22 min. Twenty-three out of 26 patients (including one with a molar pregnancy) in the 5.0 μg/min group delivered in a mean time of 9 h 42 min (mean total dose 2.2 mg). Three out of four patients infused with 6.0 μg/min PGE_2 delivered with an average total dose of 4 mg in a mean time of 13 h 6 min. The overall incidence of side-effects was lower in the 1.5 μg/min group than in other groups.

Side-effects—Diarrhoea and vomiting were the most frequently reported side-effects. These appeared to be related to the dose of prostaglandin used (Murray and Clinch, 1975; Karim, 1970). In only one patient were gastro-intestinal side-effects severe enough to warrant cessation of treatment (Murray and Clinch, 1975) (see also Table 16.1). Superficial venous erythema (at the site of infusion) was encountered by some investigators (Table 16.1). This usually disappeared after stopping the infusion. Pyrexia was reported by several investigators but the temperature returned to normal after the infusion was stopped.

Filshie (1971) used PGE_2 in one patient with a missed abortion who had an elevated blood pressure before the start of treatment. Intravenous PGE_2 was given at a rate of 0.5 μg/min for 12½ hours without any complications.

16.2.1.2 $PGF_{2\alpha}$

A summary of results from 14 published papers covering a total of 174 patients with death *in utero* treated with intravenous infusion of $PGF_{2\alpha}$ is given in Table 16.2.

The duration of death *in utero* ranged from 1 to 84 days and the infusion rate between 2.5 and 200 μg/min. The treatment was successful in 166 patients (95.4%). The average time interval between the start of infusion and abortion or delivery in different studies ranged between 6 h 26 min and 48 h.

The two investigators (Karim *et al.*, 1969 and Roberts, 1974) who used infusion rates of 2.5–20 μg/min achieved the same success rate as reported by other investigators using much higher doses (Table 16.2). It is our impression that an infusion rate of $PGF_{2\alpha}$ higher than 40 μg/min is not necessary to terminate pregnancies in cases of missed abortion and intrauterine foetal death (see Tables 16.17 and 16.18).

In the first report, Karim *et al.* (1969) infused $PGF_{2\alpha}$ at 0.05 μg/(kg min) (2.5–4 μg/min) in seven patients with death *in utero* in the third trimester of pregnancy. Six patients delivered in a mean time of 8 h 7 min while the seventh patient required a second infusion the following day and delivered 28 h from

Table 16.2 Termination of pregnancy in cases of intrauterine foetal death and missed abortion with intravenous infusion of $PGF_{2\alpha}$

No. of cases	*No. successfully treated*	*Gestation (weeks)*	*Duration of death (days)*	*Infusion rate* (μg/min)	*Mean total dose* (mg)	*Mean ind.-del. interval* (h:min)	*Side-effects*	*References*
7	6	30–39	—	2.5–4.0	—	9:12	0	Karim *et al.* (1969)
6	6	28–40	3–21	62–90	36.0	8:23	N. V. D	Pedersen *et al.* (1972)
7	7	25–31	10–56	25–125	41.9	19:15	N. V. D	
8	7	19–26	14–84	25–100	42.3	9:14	V. D. Ds. S	Ruppen *et al.* (1972)
3	3	32–38	7–28		35.8	6:26		
13	13	28–34	—	25–100	25.2	7:00	N. V. D. S	Ring (1972)
5	5	<28	—	—	—	—	—	Hickl *et al.* (1973)
5	4	<28	—	25–100	37.8	12:23	—	Herrera *et al.* (1973)
2	1	30–44	—		21.0	7:15	—	
2	1	18–25	28–56	2.5–20	18.2	48:00	V. D. S	Roberts (1974)
5	5	29–34	5–56	2.5–20	8.7	19:21	V. D. S	
7	7	2nd and 3rd trimester	—	—	—	7:30	—	Soszka *et al.* (1974)
9	8	16–28	2–44	75–200	37.1	11:05	N. V. D. P	Foroohar and Behjatnia (1976)
17	17	2nd and 3rd trimester	—	5–30	—	9:36	V. D. S	Samaja *et al.* (1976)
30	29	>28	—	5–90	15.1	—	N. V. D	Secher *et al.* (1976)
16	15	>28	1–30	40–80	20.3	7:36	S	Moe (1976)
30	30	28–40	1–35	15–90	15.1	10:24	N. V. D. S	Lange *et al.* (1976)
2	2	29–32	—	—	52.3	11:42	N. V	Kunz and Schreiner (1977)
174	166							

N = Nausea; V = Vomiting; D = Diarrhoea; Ds = Dyspnoea; S = Superficial phlebitis; P = Pyrexia; 0 = None the start of first infusion. With infusion rates of 5–20 μg/min Roberts (1974) successfully managed six out of seven patients with death *in utero*. One patient with a missed abortion failed to abort and developed an upper-limb cyanosis shortly after the start of $PGF_{2\alpha}$ infusion. All 17 patients with death *in utero* treated with intravenous infusion of 5–30 μg/min $PGF_{2\alpha}$ by Samaja *et al.* (1976) also delivered in a mean time of 9 h 36 min.

The highest reported dose of $PGF_{2\alpha}$ was infused by Foroohar and Behjatnia (1976). Some of their nine patients at 16–28 weeks gestation received up to a maximum of 200 μg/min $PGF_{2\alpha}$. Eight aborted in a mean time of 11 h 5 min. In the patient who failed to abort, laparotomy was performed and an extra-uterine pregnancy was found. Foroohar and Behjatnia (1976) are of the opinion that the time required for expulsion of a dead foetus with $PGF_{2\alpha}$ is influenced mainly by the state of the cervix rather than gestation, actual uterine size or duration of foetal death.

Moe (1976) infused 40–80 μg/min $PGF_{2\alpha}$ in 16 patients with intrauterine foetal death. Fifteen delivered in a mean time of 7 h 36 min. In the patient who failed to deliver, $PGF_{2\alpha}$ was infused for 10 h without any effect on the cervix. The following day an amniotomy was performed, cervix mechanically dilated and infusion of $PGF_{2\alpha}$ given for a further period of 40 h. The patient finally delivered through a posterior cervical tear; the internal os was intact.

On the basis of their experience in 30 patients with an intrauterine foetal death (28 to 40 weeks gestation) treated with $PGF_{2\alpha}$ (5–90 μg/min), Lange *et al.* (1976) reported a negative significant correlation between the duration of infusion and gestation, i.e. the induction–delivery interval decreased with advancing gestation. This is at variance with the suggestion of Foroohar and Behjatnia (1976). However, in the latter study there were nine patients with gestation below 28 weeks.

One of the patients treated with $PGF_{2\alpha}$ by Lange *et al.* (1976) had severe hypertension with superimposed pre-eclampsia. The blood pressure decreased with $PGF_{2\alpha}$ infusion and the patient's severe headache was also alleviated. In normotensive subjects, $PGF_{2\alpha}$ did not effect blood pressure.

Side-effects—Routine laboratory analysis of physiological parameters were normal in studies where they were reported (Ruppen *et al.*, 1972; Hickl *et al.*, 1973; Foroohar and Behjatnia, 1976). These included complete blood count, clotting factors, serum creatinine, urea, bilirubin, SGOT, SGPT, alkaline phosphatase, electrolytes, glucose and urine analyses.

The most commonly encountered side-effects were vomiting, diarrhoea and superficial phlebitis. These were not serious enough to interfere with the treatment.

16.2.1.3 *PGE_1*

PGE_1 has been used to evacuate the uterus in cases of death *in utero* in only one study. Roberts (1974) treated 14 patients (11 with intrauterine foetal death and three with a missed abortion) with intravenous infusion of 1.5 to 6 μg/min PGE_1. The duration of foetal death *in utero* ranged between 3 days and 8 weeks. Amniotomy was performed in seven patients when labour was considered established and the cervix was 2 to 4 cm dilated. The treatment was successful in all. The mean infusion to delivery (or abortion) interval ranged between 4 h and 12 h 50 min with a mean of 8 h 33 min.

Side-effects—Venous erythema or phlebitis of the arm vein used for infusion was encountered in all the patients. In several patients the intravenous catheter had to be removed and inserted into another vein because of localized pain and tenderness at the site of infusion. Facial flushing was also a prominent feature associated with PGE_1 infusion. Five patients had one to five episodes of vomiting and one complained of a severe frontal headache. One patient with an anencephalic foetus complicated by polyhydramnios had an atonic post-partum haemorrhage.

16.2.1.4 *16-phenoxy-ω-17,18,19,20-tetranor-PGE_2 methyl sulphonylamide (sulprostone)*

Sulprostone given by various routes has been successfully used for the termination of pregnancy at all stages of gestation (see Karim, 1979; Karim *et al.*, 1979).

Sulprostone administered by intravenous infusion has been used in the management of death *in utero* in a total of 109 patients by four groups of investigators. This prostaglandin analogue has also been successfully used by the intramuscular route for evacuation of the uterus in cases of missed abortion and intrauterine foetal death (see Section 16.2.4.3).

Gruber (1979) treated 20 patients with death *in utero*. In 10 patients (gestation 14 to 32 weeks) sulprostone was infused at rates varying between 0.25 μg/min and 2.00 μg/min. The treatment was successful in all 10 patients with a total average dose of 845 μg in a mean time of 8 h 48 min. Another group of 10 patients (gestation 14–40 weeks) were infused with 1500 μg sulprostone in 375 ml saline over a period of 3 h (= 8 μg/min). All delivered in a mean time of 11 h 54 min.

Uterine pain requiring analgesics, meperidine 75 mg, i.m., was experienced by 85% of the patients. Vomiting occurred in two patients in the first group and in four patients in the second group. Two patients in the 8 μg/min group had 'chills' and two had pyrexia. Toppozada *et al.* (1979) reported successful treatment of seven patients with a missed abortion and two with an intrauterine foetal death with sulprostone given intravenously. Three patients similarly managed by Selander and Psytynen (1979) also delivered in a mean time of 7 h 18 min.

In the largest series reported so far, Fawzy and Basiony (1979) treated 40 cases of intrauterine foetal death and 33 cases of missed abortion with sulprostone. Patients with a missed abortion were given intravenous infusion of 500 μg sulprostone in 500 ml normal saline over a period of 6 h and those with an intrauterine foetal death received 100 μg sulprostone (in 250 ml normal saline) per hour. Including 23 cases of molar pregnancy, the mean abortion time for gestation less than 28 weeks was 8 h 35 min for nulliparous patients and 13 h 13 min for multiparae. The mean delivery time for patients with gestation over 28 weeks was 7 h 47 min for primigravidae and 12 h 17 min for multiparae. Side-effects included nausea (25%), headache (6.3%), pyrexia (6.3%), 'mesogastric spasm' (4.2%) and 'tiredness' (4.2%). No side-effects occurred in 35.4% of the patients.

16.2.2 Extra-amniotic route

Instillation of PGE_2 or $PGF_{2\alpha}$ into the space between the uterine wall and foetal membranes causes direct myometrial stimulation. Interruption of pregnancy by this route can be accomplished with a total dose 10–20 times lower than that required by the intravenous route. Side-effects can thus be considerably reduced (see Karim and Amy, 1975). In cases of death *in utero*, this technique is believed to carry less risk of infection than the intra-amniotic route.

Embrey *et al.* (1974) first advocated the use of extra-amniotic prostaglandins in the management of intrauterine foetal death. PGE_2 and $PGF_{2\alpha}$ are thought to be more effective in cases of death *in utero* than in the termination of viable pregnancies (Luengo *et al.*, 1977). This may be due to the high prostaglandin metabolizing capacity found in foetal membranes of viable intrauterine pregnancy and this capacity may be reduced once death occurs *in utero*.

The prostaglandins are usually administered via an indwelling Foley catheter retained in the extra-amniotic space by inflating the balloon. The balloon is usually expelled into the vagina prior to the expulsion of the foetus. Some investigators have used supplementary oxytocin given intravenously to maintain uterine activity if delivery fails to occur soon after the expulsion of the catheter.

16.2.2.1 *PGE_2*

Data from six publications covering a total of 115 patients with death *in utero* managed with extra-amniotic PGE_2 are summarized in Table 16.3.

In the first reported study Embrey *et al.* (1974) treated eight patients with a missed abortion and eleven with intrauterine death with PGE_2 administered extra-amniotically. Patients with a missed abortion received an initial dose of 100 μg PGE_2 followed by 200 μg every 2 h. In cases of intrauterine foetal death, PGE_2 was infused continuously into the extra-amniotic space at rates varying between 60 and 240 μg/h. All patients but one with a missed abortion expelled the products of conception in a mean time of 12 h 42 min with a mean

Table 16.3 Termination of pregnancy in cases of intrauterine foetal death and missed abortion with extra-amniotic administration of PGE_2

No. of cases	*No. successfully treated*	*Gestation (weeks)*	*Duration of death (days)*	*Dose*	*Mean total dose* (mg)	*Mean ind.-del. interval* (h:min)	*Side-effects*	*References*
8	7*	20–32	14–84	100 μg followed by 200 μg 2 hrly	1.53	12:42	V	Embrey *et al.* (1974)
11	11	30–39	7–28	60–240 μg/h infusion	0.45	7:06	V	Embrey *et al.* (1974)
26	26	31.3 (mean)	14.4 (mean)	375 μg 2 hrly	1.80	8:36	N, V, D	Secher *et al.* (1974)
2	2	28–32	—	—	—	7:00	—	Wagman and Usherwood (1974)
15 10	15 10	17–27	— —	200 μg 2 hrly 1500–2000 μg single dose gel	1.90	17:12	V, R	Calder *et al.* (1976)
22	22	29–39	—	1–4 μg/min infusion	0.70	7:48	V, R	Calder *et al.* (1976)
1	1	27	—	500 μg at 0, 4, 6, 8 h	2.00	9:00	—	Arshat (1977)
8 12	7 11	18–24 25–32	1–28	0.5–1.0 mg 3 hrly	3.80	12:00	C	Lippert and Luthi (1978)
115	112							

V = Vomiting; N = Nausea; D = Diarrhoea; C = Painful uterine contractions; R = Rigors

*Most patients were given intravenous oxytocin (80 mU/min) 4–6 h after the first dose of prostaglandin

total dose of 1.53 mg. The patient who failed to abort was given PGE_2 for 28 h. At the end of this period the 12 weeks' size uterus was surgically evacuated. Seven patients (including one who failed to abort) were given intravenous oxytocin (80 mU/min) 4–6 h after the start of prostaglandin treatment.

All the 11 patients with intrauterine foetal death delivered in a mean time of 7 h 6 min (range 2 h 30 min to 11 h 12 min). One patient was given intravenous oxytocin (4–16 mU/min) 1 h after the expulsion of the Foley catheter. The only side-effect encountered by Embrey *et al.* (1974) was vomiting which occurred occasionally.

Scher *et al.* (1974) treated 26 patients with death *in utero* with extra-amniotic PGE_2. The mean gestation was 31.3 weeks and uterine size 27.5 weeks. The initial test dose of 125 μg PGE_2 was followed by a further 250 μg 10 min later. Thereafter 375 μg PGE_2 was administered extra-amniotically every 2 h. All patients delivered in a mean time of 8 h 36 min (range 2–16 h). The average total dose of PGE_2 was 1.8 mg. Side-effects were trivial.

Twenty-five patients with a missed abortion and 22 with intrauterine foetal death were managed by Calder *et al.* (1976) with PGE_2 administered extra-amniotically. Fifteen of the patients with a missed abortion received 200 μg PGE_2 in 0.9% saline every 2 h while the remaining 10 were given a single extra-amniotic dose of 1500–2000 μg PGE_2 in 5% Tylose. All aborted in a mean time of 17 h 12 min (range 4 h 24 min to 47 h), with a total dose of 1.9 mg (mean). The 22 patients with an intrauterine foetal death received a continuous infusion of 1–4 μg/min PGE_2 into the extra-amniotic space. All delivered within 12 h (average 7 h 48 min).

The study of Lippert and Luthi (1978) differed from the above in two respects. Instead of a Foley catheter, a fine bore (intravenous) catheter was transcervically inserted about 10–15 cm into the extra-amniotic space. The tip of the catheter was located away from the placenta after determining its position by ultrasonography. PGE_2 was prepared as a viscous gel and administered through the catheter in doses of 0.5–1.0 mg every 3 h. Seven out of eight patients with a missed abortion and 11 out of 12 with an intrauterine foetal death delivered within 24 hours in a mean time of 12 h (mean total dose 3.8 mg).

Lippert and Luthi (1978) also compared the efficacy of the extra-amniotic method of terminating pregnancies in cases of death *in utero* with intravenous oxytocin, intra-amniotic hypertonic saline, intrauterine balloon catheter, extra-amniotic rivanol and intra-amniotic premarin. They concluded that extra-amniotic administration of PGE_2 gel was more effective than all other methods. The mean induction–abortion (or delivery) interval with PGE_2 was 12 h compared to 30 h with other methods.

PGE_2 given extra-amniotically has been successfully used in patients with death *in utero* and other associated complications including hypertension, diabetes mellitus, fibromyomata, previous caesarean section and pre-eclampsia, without severe complications.

Side-effects—Some investigators have reported nausea and vomiting in an occasional patient treated with extra-amniotic PGE_2 (Table 16.3).

16.2.2.2 $PGF_{2\alpha}$

Results of nine studies employing $PGF_{2\alpha}$ by the extra-amniotic route in a total of 41 patients with death *in utero* are summarized in Table 16.4. The treatment was successful in 40 patients (97.6%).

Embrey *et al.* (1974) treated two patients with a missed abortion with $PGF_{2\alpha}$. The initial dose of 300 μg was followed by 600 μg every 2 h. Both patients aborted in a mean time of 19 h 15 min with a total average dose of 4.8 mg. A patient with intrauterine foetal death was given a continuous extra-amniotic infusion of 600 μg/h $PGF_{2\alpha}$ and delivered within 12 h. Calder *et al.* (1976) have reported similar results.

One case of missed abortion at 13 weeks gestation failed to abort after extra-amniotic infusion of 10–30 μg/min $PGF_{2\alpha}$ given for 20 h 30 min. Pregnancy was terminated by curettage. Four cases of intrauterine foetal death were however, successfully delivered with a similar regimen in a mean time of 9 h 11 min. In two the treatment was supplemented with intravenous oxytocin (Samaja *et al.*, 1976).

A group of 15 patients with death *in utero* (five missed abortion, 10 intrauterine foetal death) were given an initial extra-amniotic dose of 0.5 mg $PGF_{2\alpha}$ followed by 0.25–1.0 mg every hour (Luengo *et al.*, 1977). All patients delivered in a mean time of 15 h 28 min. The total average dose of $PGF_{2\alpha}$ for the whole group was 8.9 mg.

One patient at 29 weeks gestation had idiopathic thrombocytopaenia, lupus erythematosus and hypertension. She required a total of 22.9 mg $PGF_{2\alpha}$ and delivered 36 h after the start of treatment without complication or side-effects. Another patient with severe hypertension at 31 weeks gestation also delivered 13 h after start of treatment without complications. The authors concluded that there was no relationship between induction–delivery interval and duration of foetal death. The duration of pregnancy also did not bear any relation to induction–delivery interval, total dose of $PGF_{2\alpha}$ required or the incidence of side-effects (Luengo *et al.*, 1977).

Tsalacopoulos (1978) administered 2.5 mg $PGF_{2\alpha}$ every 2 h to nine patients between 28 and 40 weeks gestation. All delivered in a mean time of 10 h 12 min (range 6½–16 h). Intravenous oxytocin (up to 6 mU/min) was given to three patients after the Foley catheter was expelled. Laboratory investigations (urinalysis, blood count, serum fibrinogen and clotting time) did not reveal any significant change.

In one study (not included in Table 16.4) $PGF_{2\alpha}$ was given intermittently in a dose of 250 μg every 1–10 min to achieve cervical dilatation (Exalto and Meuwissen, 1976). Nine out of the 10 patients were at 9 to 13 weeks gestation and one at 34 weeks with uterine size of 16 weeks. The time to achieve cervical

Table 16.4 Termination of pregnancy in cases of intrauterine foetal death and missed abortion with extra-amniotic administration of $PGF_{2\alpha}$

No. of cases	*No. successfully treated*	*Gestation (weeks)*	*Duration of death (days)*	*Dose*	*Mean total dose* (mg)	*Mean ind.-del. interval* (h:min)	*Side-effects*	*References*
2	2	18–20	28–42	300 µg initial dose, 600 µg 2 hourly	4.8	19:15	—	Embrey *et al.* (1974)
1	1	33	7	200–600 µg/h infusion	3.5	12:00	—	
1	0	13	3	10–30 µg/min infusion	—	—	—	Samaja *et al.* (1976)
4*	4	33–36	1–6		—	9:11	R	
1*	1	24	28	—	120	19:00	—	Stephens and Birnholz (1976)
5	5	18–24	1–35	0.5 mg initial dose, 0.25–1.0 mg every hour	9.0	14:56	N	Luengo *et al.* (1977)
10	10	28–39	1–19	0.5 mg initial dose, 0.25–1.0 mg every hour	8.9	15:44	N, V	
2	2	29–32	—	100 µg/min	25.0	7:25	0	Paladini *et al.* (1977)
6	6	15–18	—	5–10 mg single dose	7.5	3:18	V	Kerekes and Domokos (1977)
9	9	28–40	1–21	2.5 mg every 2 hours	8.6	10:12	—	Tsalacopoulos (1978)
41	40							

R = Rigors; N = Nausea; V = Vomiting; 0 = None
*Supplemented by intravenous oxytocin

dilatation of up to 2 cm ranged between 1 h 45 min and 9 h 30 min. Pregnancy in all cases was terminated by curettage.

16.2.3 Intra-amniotic route

The intra-amniotic route of prostaglandin administration has been successfully used for the termination of viable second trimester pregnancies in a large number of patients (see Karim and Amy, 1975). Because of a slow passage of prostaglandins from the amniotic fluid across the foetal membranes, a large single dose of prostaglandin given intra-amniotically produces uterine stimulation for several hours. It is therefore possible to terminate pregnancies with an appropriate single dose given by this route in a majority of the patients without severe systemic side-effects. Although PGE_2 and $PGF_{2\alpha}$ given intra-amniotically have been shown to be highly effective in the management of death *in utero*, this route is not widely used for the following reasons (see Thiery and Amy, 1975).

(1) The technique, although simple, requires invasion of the amniotic cavity which involves a high risk of infection in the presence of a dead foetus.

(2) There is also a possibility of leakage of thromboplastin-rich material into the maternal circulation.

(3) The altered amniotic membranes may also permit faster passage of the injected prostaglandin leading to hyperstimulation and possibly damage to the uterus and the cervix.

In the first reported study single intra-amniotic doses of 5 mg PGE_2 or 25 mg $PGF_{2\alpha}$ were administered to five patients with a missed abortion. All aborted in a mean time of 10 h 45 min. Two patients had nausea and vomiting. Six additional patients with intrauterine foetal death were treated with single intra-amniotic doses of 0.5 mg PGE_2 or 2.5 mg $PGF_{2\alpha}$. All delivered in a mean time of 9 h. There were no side-effects (Karim, 1972).

16.2.3.1 *PGE*$_2$

Apart from Karim (1972) two other investigators have used PGE_2 by the intra-amniotic route in the management of death *in utero*. Caballero *et al.* (1974) injected 1 or 2 mg PGE_2 intra-amniotically in five patients with intrauterine foetal death. All delivered in a mean time of 18 h 42 min. One patient treated with 2 mg PGE_2 suffered a ruptured uterus.

Kunz and Schreiner (1977) used 10 mg PGE_2 in nine cases and 25 mg in one with death *in utero* at 22–42 weeks gestation. All delivered in a mean time of 16 h 24 min. In spite of the massive doses of PGE_2 used, no complications were reported and only one patient had diarrhoea.

16.2.3.2 $PGF_{2\alpha}$

Results of seven studies in 86 patients with death *in utero* managed with intra-amniotic $PGF_{2\alpha}$ are summarized in Table 16.5. The treatment was successful in 85 (98.8%).

Frumar *et al.* (1974) administered an initial dose of 30 mg $PGF_{2\alpha}$ intra-amniotically followed by 15 mg 24 h later in four patients with a missed abortion and three with intrauterine foetal death. All delivered within 30 h. There was no significant difference in the injection–delivery time in the two groups. Nausea, vomiting and diarrhoea were common side-effects. Similar results were obtained by Caballero *et al.* (1974) in eight patients with a missed abortion and 14 with intrauterine foetal death given single intra-amniotic doses of 12.5 or 25 mg $PGF_{2\alpha}$.

Koning-Gans *et al.* (1975) used smaller doses of $PGF_{2\alpha}$ repeated frequently in five patients with a missed abortion. An initial dose of 125 μg was increased by 250 μg every 30 min. All five patients aborted in a mean time of 10 h 42 min with a mean total dose of 8.7 mg. There were no side-effects. The authors compared the efficacy of intra-amniotic $PGF_{2\alpha}$ with intravenous oxytocin (and ergometrine) given to five patients with a missed abortion. The patients treated with oxytocin took a significantly longer time to abort than those given $PGF_{2\alpha}$.

Thirty-six patients with a mean gestation of 27.1 weeks were treated with single intra-amniotic doses of 15–30 mg $PGF_{2\alpha}$ by Samaja *et al.* (1976). All delivered in a mean time of 10 h 57 min. There was no significant difference in the injection delivery interval between the second trimester and last trimester patients. Fifteen out of 36 patients had nausea and vomiting (1–4 episodes) and four of these also had diarrhoea. In one patient, EEG abnormalities were encountered two hours after intra-amniotic injection of 30 mg $PGF_{2\alpha}$.

A combination of 30 mg $PGF_{2\alpha}$ and 60 g urea administered intra-amniotically was used by Sher (1976) in 14 patients at 17 to 37 weeks gestation. The two compounds were injected after withdrawal of 100 ml amniotic fluid. All patients delivered in a mean time of 9 h 18 min. This compares with a mean induction–delivery interval of 9 h 17 min in Samaja's study in 36 patients given a single dose of 15–30 mg $PGF_{2\alpha}$. It would appear that addition of urea did not influence the outcome of treatment or delivery interval. Sher (1976) concluded that with urea and $PGF_{2\alpha}$ combination, delivery could be 'confidently anticipated well within 16 h of the intra-amniotic infusion'.

Intra-amniotic urea and prostaglandin combination has been successfully used for the termination of viable second trimester pregnancies (Craft, 1973; Bowen-Simpkins, 1973; Craft *et al.*, 1974). Although such a combination is more effective than either used alone, there is a high incidence of side-effects probably due to an accelerated absorption of prostaglandins into the systemic circulation (Karim, 1974; Karim and Amy, 1975). Out of the 14 patients in Sher's study seven were cases of missed abortion and only three had nausea

Table 16.5 Termination of pregnancy in cases of intrauterine foetal death and missed abortion with intra-amniotic administration of $PGF_{2\alpha}$

No. of cases	*No. successfully treated*	*Gestation (weeks)*	*Duration of death (days)*	*Dose*	*Mean total dose* (mg)	*Mean ind.-del. interval* (h:min)	*Side-effects*	*References*
4	4	15–22	7–21	30 mg starting dose, 15 mg at 24 h	33.8	11:56	N, V, D	Frumar *et al.* (1974)
3	3	31–32	7–14	45 mg starting dose, 25 mg at 6, 18 h	78.3	16:15		
8	7	16–27	7–63	12.5 mg or 25 mg single dose	21.9	8:22	V	Caballero *et al.* (1974)
14	14	28–42	7–70			10:30		
4	4	10–28	7–17	125 µg starting dose increase by 250 µg every ½ h – max 4000 µg	5.6	10:42	—	Koning-Gans *et al.* (1975)
1	1	28	2		21.25	13:00	—	
7	7	17–25	7–52	30 mg $PGF_{2\alpha}$ + 60 g urea	—	9:18	N, V, D	Sher (1976)
7	7	29–37						
36	36	27.1 (mean)	26 (mean)	15–30 mg single dose	22.9	10:57	N, V, D	Samaja *et al.* (1976)
1	1	18	21	—	40.0	14:00	—	Stephens and Birnholz (1976)
1	1	34	—	40 mg single dose	40.0	5:54	N	Kunz and Sahreiner (1977)
86	85							

N = Nausea; V = Vomiting; D = Diarrhoea; — Not reported

and vomiting while one had diarrhoea. In contrast, Craft *et al.* (1974) reported vomiting in 12 and diarrhoea in two out of 20 second trimester patients with 80 g urea and 20 mg $PGF_{2\alpha}$ injected intra-amniotically. This high incidence of side-effects may be related to higher doses of urea employed by Craft *et al.* (1974).

Post-partum haemorrhage occurred in one patient with consumption coagulopathy (Sher, 1976). It was rapidly corrected with oxytocin plus trasylol and fibrinogen.

Side-effects—These were related to the dose of $PGF_{2\alpha}$ employed. The investigators who used small single intra-amniotic doses (Karim, 1972; Caballero *et al.*, 1974; Samaja *et al.*, 1976) encountered very few side-effects. In contrast Frumar *et al.* (1974) who used 45 mg initial dose of $PGF_{2\alpha}$ and subsequent doses of 15–25 mg, 6 and 18 or 24 hours later reported side-effects in most of their patients. These included nausea, vomiting and diarrhoea. Samaja *et al.* (1976) reported EEG abnormalities suggestive of mild cerebral oedema in one patient 2 h after intra-amniotic instillation of 30 mg $PGF_{2\alpha}$.

No change in fibrinogen, thrombocytes and clotting time or other parameters for liver and renal functions were encountered before, during and after induction (Koning-Gans *et al.*, 1975). One patient with consumptive coagulopathy had post-partum haemorrhage (Sher, 1976).

16.2.3.3 *15(S)15-methyl-$PGF_{2\alpha}$*

Kinra *et al.* (1977) administered a single intra-amniotic dose of 2.5 mg 15(S)15-methyl-$PGF_{2\alpha}$ to one patient with a missed abortion at 18 weeks gestation. She aborted 5 h later. Diarrhoea was the only side-effect.

16.2.4 Intramuscular route

The efficacy of PGE_2 and $PGF_{2\alpha}$ given by the intramuscular route for induction of labour in cases of intrauterine foetal death has not been explored because these compounds produce extreme pain (lasting for several days in some cases) at the site of injection (Karim, 1972). Some synthetic analogues of natural prostaglandins do not suffer from this problem and three such compounds given intramuscularly have been used in the management of foetal death *in utero*.

16.2.4.1 *15(S)15-methyl-$PGF_{2\alpha}$*

The most important enzymes responsible for rapid metabolism and inactivation of naturally occurring PGE_2 and $PGF_{2\alpha}$ are 15-hydroxy dehydrogenase. Introduction of a methyl group in the 15 position of PGE_2 or $PGF_{2\alpha}$

gives the respective 15-methyl PGE_2 or $PGF_{2\alpha}$. These compounds are not substrates for enzyme 15-hydroxy dehydrogenase (Yankee and Bundy, 1972) and consequently are more potent and have a longer duration of action in stimulating the human uterus (see Karim and Amy, 1975).

15(S)15-methyl-$PGF_{2\alpha}$ is 20–100 times (depending upon the route of administration) more potent than $PGF_{2\alpha}$ in stimulating the pregnant human uterus (Karim and Sharma, 1972; Karim *et al.*, 1972; Wiqvist *et al.*, 1972). Unlike $PGF_{2\alpha}$ intramuscular injection of this analogue does not cause pain at the site of injection.

15(S)15-methyl-$PGF_{2\alpha}$ given intramuscularly has been successfully used by several investigators to evacuate the uterus in cases of death *in utero*. Results from six published papers covering 93 patients are summarized in Table 16.6.

Ylikorkala *et al.* (1976) used 100–250 μg 15(S)15-methyl-$PGF_{2\alpha}$ intramuscularly every 2–4 h in 11 patients with death *in utero* at 23–34 weeks gestation. The duration of death *in utero* varied from less than 7 days to 21 days. The six patients with a missed abortion aborted in a mean time of 4 h 30 min (range 15 min to 10 h). Five patients with intrauterine foetal death also delivered in a mean time of 9 h 17 min (range 4–20 h). No premedication was used. Eight patients (73%) had diarrhoea and two (18%) had vomiting.

Sharma *et al.* (1975) used 250 μg 15(S)15-methyl-$PGF_{2\alpha}$ every 3 h in six patients with a missed abortion. Intra-cervical laminaria tents (one to three) were inserted on the evening before the prostaglandin treatment. The laminaria were removed from the vagina or cervical canal 3–4 h after the first injection of 15(S)15-methyl-$PGF_{2\alpha}$. All patients aborted in a mean time of 9 h 4 min (range 4–24 h). Premedication with 5 mg Lomotil (orally) 10 and 2 h prior to the first injection of prostaglandin and compazine (intramuscular) 1 h before prostaglandin was successful in reducing the incidence of diarrhoea and vomiting respectively.

15(S)15-methyl-$PGF_{2\alpha}$ in intramuscular doses of 250 μg every 2 h has also been successfully used by Kinra *et al.* (1977) and Lange and Secher (1977).

E. M. Southern reported (in a personal correspondence, 1978) 17 cases of death *in utero* at 15–34 weeks gestation treated with 250 μg 15(S)15-methyl-$PGF_{2\alpha}$ every hour or every 2 hours. Twelve out of 13 patients with a missed abortion required a mean time of 5 h 25 min for abortion. The patient who failed to abort had also failed to do so with intravaginal administration of PGE_2. All four patients with intrauterine foetal death delivered within 24 h (mean 8 h 48 min). Nausea, vomiting and diarrhoea were frequently encountered in spite of concomitant therapy to counteract these side-effects.

Wallenburg (1978) used 15(S)15-methyl-$PGF_{2\alpha}$ in a series of 45 patients with death *in utero*. Separate data for patients with gestation below 28 weeks (missed abortion) and those above 28 weeks (intrauterine foetal death) were not given. The prostaglandin analogue was given intramuscularly in doses of 250 μg every 1–2 h. The author did not find any correlation between gestation and injection–delivery interval. The treatment was successful in 44 out of 45

Table 16.6 Termination of pregnancy in cases of intrauterine foetal death and missed abortion with intramuscular administration of 15(S)15-methyl-$PGF_{2\alpha}$

No. of cases	*No. successfully treated*	*Gestation (weeks)*	*Duration of death (days)*	*Dose*	*Mean total dose* (mg)	*Mean ind.-del. interval* (h:min)	*Side-effects*	*References*
6*	6	20–28	42–7	250 μg 3 hourly	0.71	9:04	D, V, P	Sharma *et al.* (1975)
6 5	6 5	23–27 28–34	7–21	100–250 μg every 2–4 hours	0.38 0.41	4:30 9:17	D, V	Ylikorkala *et al.* (1976)
2	2	12–16	—	300 μg every 3 hours	1.85	19:00	D, V	Kinra *et al.* (1977)
12	12	14–26	—	250 μg every 2 hours	1.35	8:12	D, V	Lange and Secher (1977)
13* 4	12 4	15–26 28–34	— —	250 μg every 1–2 hours	0.79 1.125	5:25 8:48	N, V, D V, D	Southern (1978)
45*	44	28 (mean)	1–42	250 μg every 2 hours	1.00	8:12	N, V, D	Wallenburg (1978)
93	91							

N = Nausea; V = Vomiting; D = Diarrhoea; P = Pyrexia
*Most of the patients were pre-medicated with antiemetic and antidiarrhoeal

patients in a mean time of 8 h 12 min (range 20 min to 20 h 18 min). Gastro-intestinal side-effects were recorded in most of the patients in spite of premedication with promazine, loperamide or diphenoxylate.

Side-effects—The incidence and frequency of nausea, vomiting and diarrhoea associated with intramuscular administration of 15(S)15-methyl-$PGF_{2\alpha}$ is unacceptably high. Premedication of patients with antiemetics and antidiarrhoeals reduces these side-effects to a certain extent. Sharma *et al.* (1975) are of the opinion that without premedication, gastro-intestinal side-effects would tend to limit the usefulness of 15(S)15-methyl-$PGF_{2\alpha}$ as an abortifacient in spite of its high efficacy.

Laboratory investigations were reported by Wallenburg (1978), including blood count (haematocrit, haemoglobin, white cell count and differential count, platelets), serum electrolytes, urea, creatinine, glucose, bilirubin, alkaline phosphatase, SGOT and SGPT. There was no change in mean haemoglobin level but the haematocrit showed a small but significant increase at the time of the last injection, followed by a return to pre-injection level 12 h later. The mean white blood count increased significantly at the end of treatment and was still significantly elevated at 12 h after the last injection. The mean percentage of lymphocytes decreased by 30% while neutrophils increased by about 5%. Both the serum creatinine and urea showed a significant increase at 12 h after the last injection.

16.2.4.2 *2a,2b-dihomo-15(S)15-methyl-$PGF_{2\alpha}$ methyl ester*

This analogue administered by the intramuscular route has so far been used in only one study for the management of death *in utero*. With a simple dose schedule of 0.5 mg of dihomo-15(S)15-methyl-$PGF_{2\alpha}$ injected every 8 h, Karim and Ratnam (1976) successfully induced labour in all of 26 patients

Table 16.7 Termination of abnormal intrauterine pregnancy with 2a,2b-dihomo-15(S)15-methyl-$PGF_{2\alpha}$ methyl ester*

Indication	*No. of cases*	*Uterine size (weeks)*	*Mean inj.-abortion interval (range)*	*Average no. of doses*	*Side-effects*†
Molar pregnancy	14	18–28	12½ h (4 to 22)	1.85	V(2), D(1), P(1)
Missed abortion	24†	10–24	12 h (2 to 29)	1.87	V(3), P(1)
Intrauterine foetal death	26	16–40	11 h	1.57‡	V(3)
Anencephalic foetus	8	36–42	11 h (7 to 21)	1.50	—

*0.5 mg intramuscular every 8 hours
†Loperamide 4 mg 8 hourly (oral)
‡One patient failed to abort after three doses

V = Vomiting; — = Not reported; P = Pyrexia; D = Diarrhoea
Data from Karim and Ratnam (1976)

with intrauterine foetal death in a mean time of 11 h 4 min (range 2 h 50 min to 32 h). The average number of intramuscular injections per patient was less than two. One patient was given intravenous oxytocin after the third dose because of slow progress.

Table 16.8 Termination of pregnancy in cases of missed abortion with intramuscular injections of sulprostone (0.5 mg 6 hourly)

Case no.	*Age (years)*	*Parity*	*Ut. size (weeks)*	*Amen. (weeks)*	*Abortion time* (h)	*No. of injection*	*Side-effects*
1	22	0	14	24	14	3	V × 1
2	23	2	15	20	12	2	0
3	24	1	14	14	12	2	0
4	37	2	13	20	10	2	0
5	41	8	14	14	3.75	1	0
6	28	3	12	30	6	1	Rash on hands
7	24	1	14	16	7.50	2	0
8	31	2	18	20	4	1	0
9	28	2	14	20	8	2	0
10	27	0	14	28	8.25	2	0
11	22	1	18	18	3.50	1	V × 1
12	28	0	18	22	24	4	0
13	28	1	16	30	6.50	2	0
14	30	1	14	24	15.50	3	0
15	25	0	18	28	10	2	0
16	22	1	14	20	13	3	S
17	—	0	16	26	24	4	0*
18	19	0	18	28	6.25	1	D × 1
19	29	2	14	28	9.75	2	D × 1
20	32	2	12	27	7	2	0
21	33	2	15	23	4	1	0
22	22	1	18	22	1	1	0
23	32	5	18	26	24	4	D × 4
24	22	1	14	14	20	4	0
25	23	0	18	22	1.50	1	0
26	25	1	14	16	12	2	D × 2
27	25	1	20	22	1.25	1	0
28	44	3	14	14	0.50	1	0
29	24	0	14	28	22	4	N
30	23	0	20	18	6	1	V × 1

* Vacuum aspiration foetus firmly adhered to uterine wall
Mean first injection to abortion interval (29 successful cases) = 9 h 28 min
Mean number of injections (29 cases) = 2
V = Vomiting; D = Diarrhoea; S = Shivering; N = Nausea; 0 = None
Data from Karim (1979)

A further 24 patients with a missed abortion were similarly treated. Twenty-three aborted in a mean time of 12 h 4 min (range 1 h 55 min to 29 h). One patient with a 13 weeks size uterus failed to abort with three doses. However the cervix had dilated to 3 cm and the uterus was evacuated by vacuum aspiration and curettage.

The main side-effect encountered was diarrhoea in 25% of the patients. This could be prevented by premedication with loperamide (Karim and Ratnam, 1976; see Table 16.7).

16.2.4.3 *16-phenoxy-ω-17,18,19,20-tetranor-PGE_2 methyl sulphonylamide (sulprostone)*

Two investigators have successfully used sulprostone for evacuation of the uterus in cases of death *in utero*.

Karim (1979) reported results of treatment with sulprostone in 19 patients with an intrauterine foetal death and 30 with a missed abortion. The prostaglandin analogue was injected intramuscularly in a dose of 0.5 mg every 6 h (maximum four doses).

Table 16.9 Termination of pregnancy in cases of intrauterine foetal death with intramuscular injections of sulprostone (0.5 mg 6 hourly)

Case no.	*Age (years)*	*Parity*	*Ut. size (weeks)*	*Amen. (weeks)*	*Delivery time* (h)	*No. of injections*	*Side-effects*
1	25	0	34	38	10.25	2	0
2	19	0	30	36	16	3	0
3	27	1	40	40	3	1	0
4	25	3	29	30	4	1	0
5	27	1	20	36	2	1	0
6	23	0	34	38	8.25	2	V × 2, S
7	27	1	32	32	6	1	0
8	29	0	36	36	15.75	3	0
9	28	1	26	30	8	2	0
10	31	0	42	42	8.25	2	N
11	27	0	20	30	4.75	1	0
12	26	6	22	34	8	2	0
13	27	2	14	31	4.25	1	0
14	22	1	32	38	6	1	0
15	25	1	20	30	14	3	0
16	30	3	26	34	19	4	0
17	40	0	28	37	19	3	V × 1, S
18	22	0	29	30	10	2	S
19	31	2	30	34	11	2	0

Mean first injection delivery interval = 9 h 20 min
Mean number of injections = 1.95
N = Nausea; V = Vomiting; S = Shivering; 0 = None
Data from Karim (1979)

Twenty-nine out of 30 patients with a missed abortion aborted in a mean time of 9 h 28 min (range 30 min to 24 h). An average of two (range 1–4) intramuscular injections was required by the 29 patients. One patient had failed to abort with four doses of sulprostone, 24 h after the start of treatment. At surgical evacuation the foetus was found firmly adhered to the uterine wall. Twenty-one patients (70%) experienced no side-effects. Three patients had one episode each of vomiting, four had diarrhoea and one shivering (Karim, 1979; see Table 16.8).

Treatment with sulprostone was successful in all 19 patients with an intra-uterine foetal death in a mean time of 9 h 20 min (range 2–19 h, average number of injections 1.95). There were no side-effects in 15 patients (79%). Two had vomiting and three experienced shivering (Karim, 1979; see Table 16.9).

Toppozada *et al.* (1979) treated a total of 27 patients (two in the first, 12 in the second and 13 in the third trimesters of pregnancy) with intramuscular administration of 0.5 mg sulprostone every 6 h. Treatment was considered a failure if abortion or delivery did not occur within 24 h of start of treatment. One patient (out of two) in the first trimester aborted 16 h after the first injection of sulprostone. Eleven out of 12 second trimester patients aborted in a mean time of 13½ hours and all 13 patients in the third trimester delivered within 24 hours (mean 11 h 12 min). Gastro-intestinal side-effects were encountered in 52% of the patients (mean of 1–7 episodes).

16.2.5 Oral route

Although PGE_2 given orally has been successfully used for induction of term labour (see Thiery and Amy, 1975) this route for induction of labour in cases of intrauterine foetal death has not been explored. Oral administration of 15(S)15-methyl-PGE_2 in doses of 20–40 μg every 6–8 hours was successfully used in six patients. Total dose ranged between 20 and 80 μg with a mean of 43.3 μg. The mean first dose to delivery interval was 19 h 8 min with a range of 12–15 h (Karim *et al.*, 1972).

16.2.6 Vaginal route

It has been recognized for a long time that prostaglandins administered by the vaginal route are absorbed into systemic circulation (Sandberg *et al.*, 1968). Thus the vaginal route could offer a more convenient method of prostaglandin administration than intravenous or intramuscular routes. The main disadvantage peculiar to this route of prostaglandin administration to stimulate the pregnant human uterus is that rupture of the membranes occurring early in the course of the treatment may result in leakage of amniotic fluid into the vagina and dilute or wash out the drug (Kent and Goldstein, 1976). Similarly blood from the uterus entering the vagina may interfere with drug absorption.

The vaginal route of prostaglandin administration was first employed by Karim and Sharma (1972) for the termination of viable second trimester pregnancy. By administering 20 mg PGE_2 or 50 mg $PGF_{2\alpha}$ every 2½ hours into the posterior fornix these authors successfully terminated pregnancies in 45 women. The same doses of the two prostaglandins administered every 3 h were subsequently used in the management of six patients with a missed abortion (Karim, 1972).

Several investigators have evaluated the safety and efficacy of vaginally administered prostaglandins for the termination of pregnancy in cases of

Table 16.10 Termination of pregnancy in cases of intrauterine foetal death and missed abortion with vaginal administration of PGE_2 and $PGF_{2\alpha}$

No. of cases	*No. successfully treated*	*Gestation (weeks)*	*Duration of death (days)*	*Dose*	*Mean total dose* (mg)	*Mean ind.-del. interval* (h:min)	*Side-effects*	*References*
6	6	28 (mean)	7–28	20 mg PGE_2 or 50 mg $PGF_{2\alpha}$ every 3 hours	—	9:00	N, V, P	Karim (1972)
10	10	16–26	1–42	20 mg PGE_2 every 3–8 hours	38.00	11:04	D, R, P, N, V	Bailey *et al.* (1975)
10	10	28–44	4–49		26.00	6:18	H, P, T, R, N, V, D	
17†	17	16–40	—	20 mg PGE_2 every 3–4 hours	48.15	7:54	N, V, P, H, D, T, R	Kent and Goldstein (1976)
3	2	14–28	21–42	20 mg PGE_2 every 3–5 hours	30.00	4:15	N, V, D	Stephens and Birnholz (1976)
30	29	—	—	20 mg PGE_2 every 3–6 hours	90.00	14:36	N, V, D, R, F, H	El-Damarawy *et al.* (1977)
30	30	18–41	1–56	20 mg PGE_2 every $2\frac{1}{2}$–5 hours	—	9:30	N, V, D, P	Korotkin *et al.* (1977)
20*	20	18–40	2–25	20 mg PGE_2 every 2 hours	90.00	9:48	N, V, D, R, P	Lauersen and Wilson (1977)
20	20	18–40	—	20 mg PGE_2 every 2–3 hours	52.60	7:48	N, V, R, H, D	Phelan *et al.* (1977)
50	47	10–34	—	20 mg PGE_2 every 2–3 hours	72.00	11:18	V, D, R, H, F, P	Rutland and Ballard (1977)
709	687	27 (mean)	—	20 mg PGE_2 every 3–5 hours	60.40	10:42	V, D, R, H, F	Southern *et al.* (1978)
905	878							

N = Nausea; V = Vomiting; D = Diarrhoea; P = Pyrexia; R = Rigors; H = Headache; T = Tachycardia; F = Facial flush

*Five patients received concomitant oxytocin infusion (16 mU min)

†Four patients received oxytocin because of early rupture of the membranes

death *in utero*. The results from 10 published studies involving a total of 905 patients are summarized in Table 16.10. The treatment was successful in 878 patients (97%). In most of these studies separate data for intrauterine foetal death and missed abortion are not given.

Karim and Sharma were the first to employ the vaginal route for termination of pregnancy in six patients with a missed abortion (see Karim, 1972; p. 111). Vaginal pessaries containing either 20 mg PGE_2 or 50 mg $PGF_{2\alpha}$ were administered every 3 h. All six patients aborted in a mean time of 9 h. Side-effects included nausea and vomiting in two patients and pyrexia in one.

In all other studies vaginal pessaries containing 20 mg PGE_2 were used and administered at intervals varying between 2 and 8 h. The frequency of administration was determined by the response of the uterus to PGE_2. Success rate approached 100% in most studies. In a group of 709 patients managed by several investigators and analysed by Southern *et al.* (1978) the treatment was successful in 96.9%. There was no difference in the success rate in a group of patients treated by experienced investigators and another group treated by investigators with no experience in the use of prostaglandins (Southern *et al.*, 1978).

Bailey *et al.* (1975) administered vaginal pessaries containing 20 mg of PGE_2 in 10 patients at 16–26 weeks gestation and another 10 patients between 28 and 44 weeks gestation. Treatment was successful in all. Uterine contraction was initiated 10 min to 5 h after the insertion of the first pessary. All patients with gestation below 28 weeks aborted in a mean time of 11 h 4 min (range 3 h to 20¾ h) with a mean total dose of 38 mg (range 20–60 mg). The 10 patients with gestation 28 weeks and above delivered in a mean time of 6 h 18 min (range 2 h to 12½ h) and required an average total dose of 26 mg (range 20–60 mg). Side-effects included nausea, vomiting, diarrhoea, headache, dizziness and chills. Three patients had episodes of transient hypertension and pyrexia. One patient had a blood loss of 1000 ml with blood fibrinogen level of 111 mg/100 ml at the time of haemorrhage compared to 194 mg/100 ml before the abortion. The prothrombin time before abortion was 11.8 s compared to 14.6 s at the time of haemorrhage. A curettage was performed but no placental residue was found. On discharge, 48 h after the abortion, the clotting profile was normal with fibrinogen level at 175 mg/100 ml.

Four out of 17 patients with death *in utero* (gestation 16–40 weeks) treated by Kent and Goldstein (1976) with 20 mg vaginal PGE_2 every 3–4 h had early rupture of the membranes. Prostaglandin therapy was discontinued and intravenous oxytocin given to complete the abortion process. Nausea and vomiting occurred in 83%, pyrexia in 39%, headache in 22% and diarrhoea in 16% of the patients.

One out of three patients with a missed abortion treated by Stephens and Birnholz (1976) failed to abort after 160 mg (eight pessaries) of PGE_2 had been given over a 24 h period. Dilatation and curettage was performed and there was a blood loss of 550 ml.

El-Damarawy *et al.* (1977) reported on 30 cases of missed abortion and intrauterine foetal death treated with 20 mg vaginal PGE_2, every 3–6 h. Twenty-nine aborted in a mean time of 14 h 36 min, with a mean total dose of 90.0 mg (4.5 pessaries). The patient who failed to abort was a case of missed abortion with uterine size of 14 weeks; she had an adherent conceptus at surgical evacuation after the failed trial. The authors suggested that there is a positive correlation between duration of foetal retention *in utero* and induction–expulsion time, i.e. the longer the retention of the dead foetus *in utero*, the longer the induction–expulsion time. With respect to the uterine size, the induction time was progressively shortened as the size increased (inverse relationship) up to 32 weeks after which the induction–delivery time showed a slight increase. Side-effects were common and included nausea (90%), vomiting (86.7%), diarrhoea (70%), rigors (36.7%), flushing (13.3%) and headache (6.7%). General weakness and arthralgia were also experienced by one patient each. The authors compared treatment with intravaginal PGE_2 pessaries with intravenous oxytocin, with or without intramuscular oestradiol benzoate 5 mg twice a day 3 days before the oxytocin infusion. Ten patients received intravenous oxytocin at 40–80 mU/min, while another seven had oestrogen pre-treatment. The success rates were 30% and 71.4% respectively as compared to 96.7% for PGE_2.

Korotkin *et al.* (1977) treated 30 patients between 18 and 41 weeks gestation with vaginal suppositories containing 20 mg PGE_2 every $2\frac{1}{2}$–5 h. All aborted in a mean time of 9 h 30 min. Side-effects included vomiting (70%), nausea (60%), diarrhoea (53%), transient pyrexia (46%) and severe low back pain (36%). The authors also compared the efficacy of vaginal PGE_2 pessaries with intra-amniotic hypertonic saline (oxytocin enhanced) and found that the latter treatment resulted in a longer mean induction–delivery interval. Moreover, onset of contractions with hypertonic saline occurred much later, 6 h 54 min mean, PGE_2 (19 min) and blood loss was more (average 500 ml per patient).

One out of 20 patients treated with vaginal PGE_2 pessaries by Phelan *et al.* (1977) developed a 'septic shock-like picture' with high fever, tachycardia, tachypnoea and hypotension. All bacteriological cultures were negative for growth. This 'picture' resolved within 6 h after delivery.

The largest series (709 patients) was reported by Southern *et al.* (1978), and this probably included 212 cases discussed earlier by Southern and Gutknecht (1976). The patients had a mean gestation of 27 weeks, and were given 20 mg PGE_2 vaginally every 3–5 h. Six hundred and eighty-seven patients aborted or delivered successfully (97%), in a mean time of 10 h 42 min, with a mean total dose of 60.4 mg. For those with a dead foetus retained for less than 3 weeks the mean delivery time was 9.4 h, while it was 11.1 h for those in whom the foetus had been dead for 3 weeks or more (statistically significant $p < 0.025$). The mean total dose of PGE_2 in the two groups was 54.7 mg and 65.6 mg respectively (statistically significant $p < 0.01$). Side-effects included vomiting

(56.4%), diarrhoea (42.7%), chills and shivering (21.9%), headache (11.0%), dizziness (2.0%) and flushing (2.0%). Alterations in vital signs included transient pyrexia (40.2%), tachycardia (25.2%) and tachypnoea (20.2%). A fall in diastolic blood pressure of more than 20 mmHg (2660 Pa) occurred in 12.6% and a rise in 4.2% of the patients. The mean estimated blood loss was 193.3 ml and 41.3% of the patients lost less than 100 ml. There were two serious complications. One was an acute case of myocardial infarction developing in an obese 38-year-old woman with essential hypertension of 194/97 mmHg in her fifth pregnancy. She developed severe chest pain, dyspnoea and a drop in blood pressure 2 h after the first dose of PGE_2. A dead foetus weighing 1350 g was delivered without further complication. Enzymes and ECG were indicative of acute myocardial infarction; she was discharged 3 weeks later. The second patient also experienced moderate retrosternal pain 15 min after vaginal administration of PGE_2. She became restless and had chills and tachypnoea. Her blood pressure dropped from 210/105 to 160/70 mmHg and her temperature rose from 36.8 to 38.0 °C. ECG and SGOT remained normal. The chest pain subsided within 2 h and the patient aborted a macerated foetus without further complications.

Eleven patients with death *in utero* and pre-existing medical complications have also been successfully managed with prostaglandins. Korotkin *et al.* (1977) used vaginal pessaries containing 20 mg PGE_2 in two patients with hypofibrinogenaemia, one with sickle cell disease (who had death *in utero* on two previous occasions and had been managed with PGE_2), three each with diabetes mellitus and pre-eclampsia (including one with nephrotic syndrome) and one with metabolic acidosis secondary to chronic alcoholism. There were no complications in any of these patients. Lauersen and Wilson (1977) reported one patient with a severe renal failure. Pregnancy was successfully terminated with vaginal administration of 10 mg PGE_2 (instead of the usual 20 mg) with a total of three doses.

Laboratory investigations including complete blood counts, platelet counts, serum bilirubin, SGOT, SGPT, serum alkaline phosphatase, serum creatinine, serum electrolytes, blood glucose, blood urea and blood cortisol have been done (Kent and Goldstein, 1976; Southern and Gutknecht, 1976; Phelan *et al.*, 1977; Southern *et al.*, 1978). Mean haemoglobin decreased from 12.54 g/100 ml before treatment to 12.24 g/100 ml after treatment, and haematocrit from 36.4 to 35.1% (Southern *et al.*, 1978). Leukocytosis, especially neutrophilia, was also noted (Southern and Gutknecht, 1976; Phelan *et al.*, 1977). There was no significant alteration in hepatic and renal tests. In the series, Southern *et al.* (1978) 21 out of 709 patients showed a reduction in platelet, fibrinogen, prothrombin time and partial thromboplastin time before treatment; there were no complications.

Side-effects—The incidence of side-effects associated with vaginal administration of PGE_2 has generally been high. They consisted mainly of nausea, vomiting, diarrhoea and pyrexia. In some studies the patients were pre-medicated routinely to counteract some of these side-effects (Korotkin *et al.*, 1977; Lauersen and Wilson, 1977).

The incidence of nausea varied from 60% (Korotkin *et al.*, 1977) to 90–95% (El-Damarawy *et al.*, 1977; Phelan *et al.*, 1977). Vomiting was also encountered by most investigators. The incidences were 56.4% (Southern *et al.*, 1978), 60% (Rutland and Ballard, 1977), 70% (Korotkin *et al.*, 1977), 75% (Phelan *et al.*, 1977) and 86.7% (El-Damarawy *et al.*, 1977).

Kent and Goldstein (1976) encountered diarrhoea in 16% of their patients while the incidence in other studies ranged from 50% to 70% (Phelan *et al.*, 1977; Rutland and Ballard, 1977; Korotkin *et al.*, 1977 and El-Damarawy *et al.*, 1977).

Southern *et al.* (1978) reported dizziness in 2% and an increase in diastolic blood pressure of more than 20 mmHg in 4.2% of their patients and a similar decrease in diastolic pressure in 12.6%. Hypertension occurred in two out of 10 patients in Bailey's study (Bailey *et al.*, 1975).

Flushing was encountered by several investigators and the incidence varied from 2.0% to 13.3% (Southern *et al.*, 1978; El-Damarawy *et al.*, 1977; Rutland and Ballard, 1977).

Tachypnoea of more than five breaths per minute was reported in 20.2% of patients by Southern *et al.* (1978) and in 10% by Bailey *et al.* (1975).

Pyrexia of more than 38 °C was reported by most investigators and varied between 75% (Rutland and Ballard, 1977) and 20% (Bailey *et al.*, 1975). Phelan *et al.* (1977) who reported pyrexia in 50% of their patients observed that the temperature peak was a sign of impending delivery. The temperature usually returned to pre-treatment values within a few hours after delivery.

A 'septic shock-like picture' with high fever, tachycardia, tachypnoea and hypotension was encountered by Phelan *et al.* (1977) and has already been discussed.

Shivering (chills) without pyrexia was also reported by many investigators. The incidence varied between 11% and 50% (Kent and Goldstein, 1976; Southern *et al.*, 1978; Phelan *et al.*, 1977).

Tachycardia of 30 beats per minute above baseline values in the absence of fever occurred in 11.1–53.3% of patients (Kent and Goldstein, 1976; Southern *et al.*, 1978; El-Damarawy *et al.*, 1977).

Southern *et al.* (1978) reported a blood loss of more than 500 ml in 4.4% of their patients. The corresponding figure in the series of Rutland and Ballard (1977) was 7%.

The incidence of retained products of conception ranged from a low of 3.3% (Korotkin *et al.*, 1977) to 45% (Lauersen and Wilson, 1977). This probably occurred more often in cases of missed abortion than in intrauterine foetal death though separate data are not available.

Sustained uterine contractions were reported in about 10% of the patients by Bailey *et al.* (1975) and Kent and Goldstein (1976). There was one case each of uterine rupture or cervical injury.

16.3 MOLAR PREGNANCY

Although chemotherapy in the management of non-metastatic gestational trophoblastic disease is a significant advance (Hammond *et al.*, 1967; Hertz *et al.*, 1961; Ross *et al.*, 1965), evacuation of the uterus once the diagnosis of a molar pregnancy is established is an essential part of treatment (Quigley, 1973). This is because hydatidiform mole predisposes to the development of choriocarcinoma, haemorrhage and pre-eclamptic toxaemia. The method of evacuation of uterine content in the absence of spontaneous uterine activity is dependent upon such variables as the size of the uterus, the age and parity of the patient as well as a desire for further child bearing.

Several methods of terminating molar pregnancies are available. If the uterine size is less than 16 weeks, vacuum aspiration followed by gentle curettage is widely practised. With uterine size of greater than 16 weeks, intravenous oxytocin is used to stimulate the uterus to cause expulsion of the molar tissue. This is followed by vacuum aspiration and curettage. Prior myometrial stimulation is considered necessary for uterine size of more than 16 weeks to reduce the risk of uterine perforation and haemorrhage. Suction evacuation with little blood loss has been reported by Brandes *et al.* (1966) though others have encountered unexplained sudden deaths with such a procedure (S. S. Ratnam, Singapore, and J. Honofia Medan, Indonesia, unpublished findings). Finally hysterectomy may be performed but is not the method of choice.

Since the first report on the use of PGE_2 in the termination of a molar pregnancy (Karim, 1970) several prostaglandins given by different routes have been successfully used to terminate such pregnancies.

16.3.1 Intravenous route

16.3.1.1 *PGE_2*

The results from eight publications are summarized in Table 16.11. Some investigators have given combined data for molar pregnancies and death *in utero* (Naismith and Barr, 1974; Murray and Clinch, 1975). The gestation has varied between 12 and 22 weeks. The treatment was successful in all 21 patients.

PGE_2 has been infused at rates varying between 0.3 and 12.0 μg/min. In three studies a fixed dose of 5 μg/min PGE_2 was infused until the expulsion of the molar tissue (Karim, 1970; Karim and Trussell, 1971; Filshie, 1971). Other investigators have titrated the dose according to uterine response (Roberts, 1974; Thiery *et al.*, 1975). Naismith and Barr (1974) infused PGE_2 with concomitant oxytocin given intravenously. In all studies prostaglandin infusion was continued until the expulsion of the molar tissue.

Mean total doses of PGE_2 used varied between 1.45 and 3.0 mg and mean

Table 16.11 Termination of molar pregnancy with intravenous infusion of PGE_2

No. of patients	*No. successfully treated*	*Gestation (weeks)*	*Dose of PG* (μg/min)	*Mean total dose* (mg)	*Mean abortion interval* (h:min)	*Side-effects*	*References*
1	1	20	5	3.00	10:00	0	Karim, 1970
3	3	12–20	5	2.18	7:15	—	Karim and Trussell (1971)
1	1	12	5	2.10	7:00	D, V	Filshie, 1971
1	1	22	2.5–5.0	2.50	10:45	S	Miller, 1973
5*	5	—	0.5–12.0	—	9:17†	P, V	Naismith and Barr (1974)
2	2	15–22	3–6	2.45	9:50	D, R, S	Roberts (1974)
4	4	16–19	0.1–4.0	1.53	8:31	V	Thiery *et al.* (1975)
4	4	—	0.5–2.5	—		—	Murray and Clinch (1975)
21	21						

* Simultaneous oxytocin infusion
† Mean for 28 cases of missed abortion and five cases of molar pregnancy
V = Vomiting; D = Diarrhoea; R = Rigors; S = Superficial phlebitis; — = Not reported; 0 = None

induction–abortion interval varied between 7 h and $10\frac{3}{4}$ h. Naismith and Barr (1974) who used PGE_2 and oxytocin combination have not given separate data for induction–abortion intervals in cases of molar pregnancy. It is therefore not possible to know whether such a combination has any merit over the prostaglandin alone.

Side-effects were minor. Vomiting was reported by Thiery *et al.* (1975) in two out of their four patients and by Filshie (1971) in his only patient. Other side-effects include diarrhoea, superficial phlebitis and shivering (Roberts, 1974; Filshie, 1971; Miller, 1973).

Uterine haemorrhage can be a major problem in molar pregnancy occurring spontaneously or during drug induced uterine stimulation. Excessive blood loss was not encountered by any of the above investigators. Routine curettage was done at variable intervals after the abortion (Filshie, 1971; Karim, 1970; Miller, 1973).

16.3.1.2 *$PGF_{2\alpha}$*

$PGF_{2\alpha}$ given intravenously was used in five studies to terminate molar pregnancies in 16 patients. The treatment was successful in all (Table 16.12). The gestation ranged between 10 and 25 weeks in 15 cases. In the only patient treated by Herrera *et al.* (1973), the gestation was 44 weeks. The infusion rate varied between 2.5 and 120 μg/min with total doses per patient of between 8.37 and 35 mg.

Klaush *et al.* (1976) infused $PGF_{2\alpha}$ (5–40 μg/min) until the cervix was 1–3 cm dilated. The uterus was then evacuated by vacuum aspiration and curettage. In other studies vacuum aspiration was carried out after most of the molar tissue was expelled.

In all other studies molar tissue was expelled $7\frac{1}{2}$ to 16 h after the start of infusion (Herrera and Leyton, 1973; Karim, 1972; Roberts, 1974; Thiery *et al.*, 1975).

Roberts (1974) reported vomiting, diarrhoea, rigors, pyrexia and phlebitis in his only patient. Diarrhoea and pyrexia were also reported by Thiery *et al.* (1975) in their solitary case.

16.3.1.3 *16-phenoxy-ω-17,18,19,20-tetranor-PGE_2 methyl sulphonylamide (sulprostone)*

Fowzy and Basiony (1979) have used sulprostone given by intravenous infusion (83.3 μg/min) in 23 patients with a molar pregnancy. The treatment was successful in all patients in a mean time of less than 12 h. In another study sulprostone given intravenously (500 μg over 2 h) resulted in a cervical dilatation of more than 2 cm to enable evacuation of the uterus by vacuum aspiration and curettage (Selander and Pystynen, 1979) (Table 16.13).

Table 16.12 Termination of molar pregnancy with intravenous infusion of $PGF_{2\alpha}$

No. of patients	*No. successfully treated*	*Gestation (weeks)*	*Dose of PG* (μg/min)	*Mean total dose* (mg)	*Mean abortion interval* (h:min)	*Side-effects*	*References*
1	1	14	50	37.0	12:20	N, V	Karim (1972)
1	1	44	25	35.0	10:20	—	Herrera *et al.* (1973); Herrera and Leyton (1973)
1	1	14	2.5–20	37.0	15:00	P, V, D, R, S	Roberts (1974)
1	1	13	8–120	30.0	7:30	P, D	Thiery *et al.* (1975)
12	12*	10–25	5–40	25.1	15:51	B	Klausch *et al.* (1976)
16	16						

*Criteria for success was cervical dilatation of up to 3 cm
D = Diarrhoea; V = Vomiting; S = Superficial phlebitis; R = Rigors; P = Pyrexia; B = Excessive blood loss; N = Nausea; — = Not reported

Table 16.13 Termination of molar pregnancy with prostaglandin analogues

No. of patients	*No. successfully treated*	*Gestation (weeks)*	*PG*	*Dose*	*Mean total dose*	*Route*	*Mean abortion interval (h:min)*	*Side-effects*	*References*
20	20	8–20	15(S)15-methyl-PGE_2 methyl ester	30 μg 8 hourly	37.50 μg	Intrauterine	9:04	V, D, P, R, B	Karim *et al.* (1974)
14	14	11–16	2a,2b-dihomo-15(S)15-methyl-$PGF_{2\alpha}$ methyl ester	0.5 mg 8 hourly	0.93 mg	Intramuscular	12:34	V, D, P, B	Karim and Ratnam (1976)
9	9	11–16	16-phenoxy-ω-17, 18,19,20-tetranor-PGE_2 methyl sulphonyl-amide	0.5 mg 6 hourly	1.20 mg	Intramuscular	11:05	N, V, D	Karim (1979) Karim *et al.* (1979)
23	23	—	16-phenoxy-ω-17, 18,19,20-tetranor-PGE_2 methyl sulphonyl-amide	83.3 μg/h	—	Intravenous infusion	12:00	—	Fawzy and Basiony (1979)
1	1	—	16-phenoxy-ω-17, 18,19,20-tetranor-PGE_2 methyl sulphonyl-amide	250 μg/h	0.50 mg	Intravenous infusion	2:00*	0	Selander and Pystynen (1978)

*Time from induction to 2 cm cervical dilatation
V = Vomiting; D = Diarrhoea; N = Nausea; P = Pyrexia; R = Rigors; B = Excessive blood loss; 0 = None; – = Not reported

16.3.2 Intrauterine route

Several investigators have referred to extra-amniotic and intra-amniotic routes of prostaglandin administration for termination of molar pregnancy. In such pregnancies, amniotic fluid, amniotic membranes and consequently intra-amniotic and extra-amniotic spaces do not exist. The correct description of the route of prostaglandin administration, therefore, is intrauterine or intravesicular. It is likely that when investigators talk about extra-amniotic and intra-amniotic administration, the drug is administered transcervically and transabdominally respectively into the molar tissue.

When prostaglandins are administered by the extra-amniotic route for the termination of viable second trimester pregnancy the entire dose is 'at once' in contact with the uterus which responds immediately by contractions. In contrast, after intra-amniotic administration, the amniotic fluid acts as a depot and the prostaglandins pass slowly across foetal membranes to the uterus which is gradually stimulated. Consequently in situations where the membranes are present and are intact, the intra-amniotic dose is usually much larger than the extra-amniotic dose. For the termination of molar pregnancy therefore, intrauterine (or intravesicular) doses of prostaglandins corresponding to extra-amniotic doses for termination of viable second trimester pregnancy should be employed.

16.3.2.1 $PGF_{2\alpha}$

$PGF_{2\alpha}$ given by the transcervical intrauterine route (referred to by the authors as extra-amniotic route) has been used by two investigators to terminate molar pregnancies (Table 16.14). Paladini *et al.* (1977) used a continuous infusion of 100 μg/min $PGF_{2\alpha}$ and terminated the pregnancy with a total of 25 mg in 13 h 20 min. Luengo *et al.* (1977) used 0.5 mg initial bolus dose followed by 0.25 to 1.0 mg every hour with oxytocin augmentation. the molar tissue was expelled 16 h after the start of prostaglandin treatment. Side-effects included nausea and a blood loss of 1000 ml. Caballero *et al.* (1975) treated one patient with a single 25 mg dose of $PGF_{2\alpha}$. The drug was injected transabdominally into the uterus. In spite of such a large dose the patient failed to expel the molar tissue. Details of side-effects are not given (Table 16.14).

16.3.2.2 PGE_2

In five studies involving a total of 13 patients with a molar pregnancy, PGE_2 was given by the transcervical intrauterine route either by repeated bolus doses or by continuous intrauterine infusion. The treatment was successful in all (Table 16.14).

McNicol and Gray (1977) were able to terminate a molar pregnancy within

Table 16.14 Termination of molar pregnancy with intrauterine administration of PGE_2 and $PGF_{2\alpha}$

No. of patients	*No. successfully treated*	*Gestation (weeks)*	*PG*	*Dose*	*Mean total dose (mg)*	*Mean abortion interval (h:min)*	*Side-effects*	*References*
1	1	13	E_2	60–240 μg/h infusion	0.5	20:30	DVT	Embrey *et al.* (1974)
1	1	16	E_2	0.2 mg every 2 hours	0.8	9:15	N	Thiery *et al.* (1975)
9	9	11–25	E_2	1–4 μg/min infusion	1.8	12:42	B, DVT	Calder *et al.* (1976)
1	1	16 (ut. size)	E_2	0.2 mg single dose	0.2	10:00	(see text)	McNicol and Gray (1977)
1	1	17	E_2	0.5 mg at 0, 4, 6 and 8 h bolus	2.0	8:30	—	Arshat (1977)
1	1	25	$F_{2\alpha}$	100 μg/min infusion	25.0	13:20	—	Paladini *et al.* (1977)
1	1	19	$F_{2\alpha}$	0.5 mg bolus followed by 0.25–1.00 mg every hour	3.5	16:00	N, V, B	Luengo *et al.* (1977)
1	0	16	$F_{2\alpha}$	25 mg trans-abdominally single injection	25.0	—	—	Caballero *et al.* (1975)

N = Nausea; V = Vomiting; B = Excessive blood loss; DVT = Deep vein thrombosis; — = Not reported

10 hours with a single 0.2 mg dose of PGE_2. Thiery *et al.* (1975) used 0.2 mg every 2 h in their patient who expelled the molar tissue in 9¼ h after the first dose. Arshat (1977) used 0.5 mg PGE_2 as a starting dose followed by 0.5 mg at 4, 6 and 8 h later. The patient aborted 30 min after the last dose of prostaglandin (8½ h from the first dose).

The largest series of molar pregnancy terminated with PGE_2 given by the intrauterine route was reported by Calder *et al.* (1976). In a group of nine patients PGE_2 was infused at 1–4 μg/min. All patients expelled the molar tissue in a mean time of 12 h 42 min (range 8½–20½ h). Side-effects generally were trivial and consisted of nausea and vomiting. One patient out of nine had a blood loss of 400 ml (Calder *et al.*, 1976).

Most investigators carried out curettage after the expulsion of the molar tissue. Embrey *et al.* (1974) described development of a deep vein thrombosis 2 days following a second curettage in one patient 5 days after the expulsion of molar tissue. She was treated with anticoagulants.

McNicol and Gray (1977) described a case with severe reaction to 0.2 mg PGE_2 given by the transcervical intrauterine route. The patient complained of severe abdominal pain, dizziness and difficulty in breathing. She also had a frothy blood-stained sputum, nausea and retching but no vomiting. Pulse was imperceptible and blood pressure was 90/50 mmHg. The patient was cold and clammy and had severe rigors. Intravenous pethidine 50 mg and promethazine 50 mg (i.m.) were given. The blood pressure rose to 120/70 and pulse rate was 100–120 beats per minute after 1 h. Further 40 mg promethazine (i.m.) and 100 mg hydrocortisone (i.v.) were given. The uterus remained firmly contracted and tender for 4 h after which regular contractions were felt. These were augmented with intravenous oxytocin (maximum 32 mU/min). Molar tissue was expelled 10 h after administration of PGE_2 and the uterus was evacuated under general anaesthesia. The total estimated blood loss was 1 500 ml. Two litres of blood was transfused. The patient was discharged well 2 days later. The reason for this severe reaction is not clear. Doses similar to that used by McNicol and Gray (1977) have been given by the intrauterine route by other investigators without systemic effects (see Karim and Amy, 1975).

Smith (1974) has also described a severe systemic reaction consisting of shock with hypotension, bradycardia and rigors followed by severe suprapubic pain, vomiting, tachycardia (180 mm) pyrexia and generalized flushing after 'intra-amniotic' injection of 20 mg PGE_2 in a patient with a molar pregnancy. Karim (1974), discussing this report, reiterated that intra-amniotic administration of prostaglandins is safe and practical in pregnancies not complicated by molar disease because the amniotic fluid acts as a depot for the drug which passes slowly across the foetal membranes to stimulate the myometrium. In a molar pregnancy, foetal membranes are absent and 'intra-amniotic' instillation in this case amounts to a situation similar to extra-amniotic administration in a pregnancy with intact membranes. In the latter situation, because the drug is applied directly to the uterus the dose is much smaller. To further emphasize this point, it may be worth remembering that rapid disappearance of the injected contrast material from the uterine cavity is observed when 'angiography' is employed for radiological confirmation of hydatidiform mole. Instantaneous migration of the dye through the intervesicular septa is followed by prompt absorption into the systemic circulation. The dose of 20 mg PGE_2 in the case mentioned above is 100 times higher than the usual extra-amniotic dose. It is reassuring that even such a massive dose did not prove fatal (Karim, 1974; Karim and Amy, 1975).

16.3.2.3 *15(S)15-methyl-PGE_2 methyl ester*

Karim *et al.* (1974) used 15(S)15-methyl-PGE_2 methyl ester for termination of pregnancy in 20 cases of molar pregnancy. The drug was administered by the transcervical intrauterine route in a dose of 30 μg and repeated 8 h later if necessary. Fifteen patients aborted the molar tissue with one dose and the remaining five with two doses. Mean total dose for 20 patients was 37.5 μg and mean abortion time 9 h 4 min (range $2\frac{3}{4}$–16 h).

Side-effects included vomiting in three patients and pyrexia of 1 °C in five. Three patients had shivering which lasted for 10–20 minutes. Blood loss was less than 100 ml in 17 patients and 200 ml in one. One had a blood loss of 500 ml and required a transfusion. In one patient hysterectomy was performed 4 days after prostaglandin treatment for uncontrolled haemorrhage (Table 16.13).

16.3.3 Intramuscular route

16.3.3.1 *2a,2b-dihomo-15(S)15-methyl-$PGF_{2\alpha}$ methyl ester*

Dihomo-15(S)15-methyl-$PGF_{2\alpha}$ in doses of 0.5 mg given intramuscularly every 8 h was used in 14 patients with a molar pregnancy at gestation of 11–16 weeks (Karim and Ratnam, 1976). Uterine size varied between 18 and 28 weeks. All patients expelled the molar tissue in a mean time of 12 h 34 min (range 4 to 22 h). Five aborted with a single dose, six with two doses and three required three doses. Mean dose of prostaglandin per patient was 0.93 mg. Loperamide (4 mg) was given orally 15–30 min before the prostaglandin injection to reduce the incidence of diarrhoea.

Two patients had one episode each of vomiting and one had a single episode of diarrhoea. Transient pyrexia of 101 °F (38.3 °C) was recorded in one patient. Blood loss of 250 ml and 500 ml respectively was encountered in two patients who were given a transfusion. In one patient total hysterectomy was performed for choriocarcinoma, 2 weeks after the abortion (see Tables 16.7, 16.13).

16.3.3.2 *16-phenoxy-ω-17,18,19,20-tetranor-PGE$_2$ methyl sulphonylamide (sulprostone)*

More recently sulprostone has been successfully used in the termination of molar pregnancies (Table 16.13). In a group of nine patients aged between 21 and 28 years with uterine size varying between 14 and 22 weeks, sulprostone was given intramuscularly in doses of 0.5 mg 6 hourly (Karim, 1979). All patients aborted the molar tissue in a mean time of 11 h 5 min with a range of 4–24 hours. The mean number of intramuscular injections of sulprostone per patient was 2.4 (1.2 mg). There were no side-effects in four patients (44.4%). Others had nausea, vomiting or diarrhoea. There was no excessive blood loss in any of the patients. Currettage was routinely performed in all after the expulsion of molar tissue (Table 16.13).

16.3.4 Vaginal route

Four investigators have reported on the use of PGE_2 administered vaginally for the termination of molar pregnancy. In the first reported case Karim (1972) used 10 mg PGE_2 (solution) every 2 h in a 28-year-old patient at 18 weeks gestation. The molar tissue was expelled 8 h after the start of treatment. There were no side-effects (Table 16.15).

Other investigators have used vaginal pessaries containing 20 mg PGE_2 administered at varying intervals. In Southern *et al.* (1976) a series of 27 patients, PGE_2 pessaries were administered every 2–5 h depending upon the response of the uterus. The total dose of PGE_2 varied between 20 mg and 600 mg with a mean of 78.26 mg per patient. Of the patients 14% required one pessary while 60% aborted with three pessaries or less. The first pessary to abortion interval ranged from 1½ h to 83 h 50 min with a mean of 11 h 32 min. In one patient treatment was discontinued because of bleeding while the treatment was considered a failure in three after 2–7 doses were administered. The overall success rate was 85.2% (23 out of 27 patients). All patients had curettage performed after the molar tissue was expelled. One patient was diagnosed as developing choriocarcinoma and hysterectomy was performed.

El-Damarawy *et al.* (1977) successfully aborted one patient with a molar pregnancy with a single vaginal pessary containing 20 mg PGE_2.

The incidence of side-effects was high and in Southern's series included vomiting (63%), diarrhoea (29.6%) and temperature elevation of 2 °F (1.1 °C) (22.2%). Blood loss was 500 ml or less in 12 patients who aborted (52%) and more than 500 ml in 11 (48%). Fourteen patients required a blood transfusion. Kent and Goldstein (1976) transfused 2 pints of blood in their sole patient treated with PGE_2 (Table 16.15).

Urinalyses, hepatic and renal function tests and blood electrolytes were carried out before treatment and 12 hours after initiation of therapy or when abortion occurred. All values remained within normal limits in majority of the patients (Southern *et al.*, 1976).

Table 16.15 Termination of molar pregnancy with vaginal administration of prostaglandins

No. of patients	*No. successfully treated*	*Gestation (weeks)*	*PG and dose*	*Mean total dose* (mg)	*Abortion interval* (h:min)	*Side-effects*	*References*
1	1	18	10 mg PGE_2 2 hourly solution	40.0	8:00	0	Karim (1972)
1	1	22	50 mg PGE_2 every 3 hour solution	150.0	9:00	D	Karim (1972)
27	23	6–35	20 mg PGE_2 every 2–5 hours pessaries	78.3	11:32	V, D, P, R, H, T, A, Ds	Southern *et al.* (1976)
1	1	—	20 mg PGE_2 every 3–4 hours pessaries	—	—	—	Kent and Goldstein (1976)
1	1	—	20 mg PGE_2 single pessaries	20.0	—	—	El-Damarawy *et al.* (1977)

V = Vomiting; D = Diarrhoea; P = Pyrexia; R = Rigors; H = Headache; T = Tachycardia; Ds = Dyspnoea; A = Aches; — = Not reported; 0 = None

16.4 ANENCEPHALIC PREGNANCY

The incidence of prolonged pregnancy in the presence of an anencephalic foetus is high (Myerscough, 1977). Guha-Ray (1975) reported a post-maturity rate of 21.7% in 60 anencephalic pregnancies compared with a rate of 6.3% in 6226 normal pregnancies delivered during the same period. There is on record a case of an anencephalic foetus that was alive *in utero* for 1 year and 24 days (389 days) (Higgins, 1954).

Diagnosis of anencephalic foetus early in pregnancy is preferable. The delivery of such a foetus in the third trimester of pregnancy is an emotionally traumatic experience for the parent. In addition, the associated hydramnios is a source of discomfort to the patient. There is also a risk of abrutio placenta in case of sudden release of amniotic fluid. Post-maturity with difficult induction of labour and shoulder dystocia are other possible dangers associated with anencephalic pregnancies.

With the use of ultrasonography early diagnosis of an anencephalic pregnancy is possible. Campbell *et al.* (1972) successfully diagnosed such a pregnancy by ultrasound 17 weeks after induction of ovulation with clomiphene. The pregnancy was terminated with intra-amniotic urea. In another patient, serial ultrasound suggested an anencephalic foetus at the 13th week of gestation (Chef *et al.*, 1974). This was confirmed at the 18th week of pregnancy and terminated by intra-amniotic administration of $PGF_{2\alpha}$. Serum and amniotic fluid α-fetoprotein measurements and amniotic fluid cell morphology are also useful aids in confirming anencephalic pregnancies in the second trimester (Ferguson-Smith *et al.*, 1978; Gosden and Brock, 1977).

PGE_2, $PGF_{2\alpha}$ and some synthetic analogues, given by various routes have been successfully used for the induction of labour in cases of anencephalic pregnancies. The results of various studies are summarized in Table 16.16.

16.4.1 Intravenous route

Filshie (1971) first reported the use of PGE_2 infused intravenously at 2.5 μg/min in a patient with an anencephalic foetus that had died *in utero* at 34 weeks gestation. Delivery occurred with a total dose of 1125 μg PGE_2, 7½ hours after the start of infusion. One hour after delivery the patient had vaginal bleeding and also bleeding from her gums. Fibrinogen level was 110 mg per 100 ml and a transfusion of 2500 ml blood with 5.0 mg fibrinogen was given. There were no further complications. Fibrinogen level before start of induction was not determined. Roberts (1974) used PGE_1 infused at 3.0 μg/min in a patient with an anencephalic foetus in the last trimester of pregnancy. Delivery took place 4 h after the start of infusion. Side-effects included phlebitis at the site of infusion and facial flushing (Table 16.16).

Table 16.16 Termination of anencephalic pregnancies with prostaglandins

No. of patients	*No. successfully treated*	*Gestation (weeks)*	*PG + route*	*Dose*	*Mean total dose (mg)*	*Mean delivery interval (h:min)*	*Side-effects*	*References*
1	1	35	E_2 i.v.	2.5 µg/min	1.125	7:30	(see text)	Filshie (1971)
1	1	31	E_1 i.v.	3.0 µg/min	0.72	4:00	S, F	Roberts (1974)
1	1	30	E_2 i.a.	5 mg every 6–12 hours	10.00	27:39	0	
2	2	21, 26	$F_{2\alpha}$ i.a.	25–50 mg every 6–12 hours	67.5	61:00	V, D	Thiery *et al.* (1975)
2	2	30, 31	$F_{2\alpha}$ i.a.	45 mg initial dose, 25 mg 6 hourly	137.5	33:20	N, V, D	Frumar *et al.* (1974)
2*	2	28, 36	E_2 e.a.	0.5–4.0 µg/h	0.65	10:05	0	Embrey *et al.* (1974)
13†	13	20–29	E_2 e.a.	1–4 µg/min	1.4	11:48	P	Calder *et al.* (1976)
8	8	36–43	dihomo-15-methyl $F_{2\alpha}$ i.m.	0.5 mg 8 hourly	0.75	11:07	0	Karim and Ratnam (1976)
2	2	30, 36	15-methyl $F_{2\alpha}$ i.m.	0.1 mg every 2–4 hours	0.5	8:55	V, D	Ylikorkala *et al.* (1976)
6	5	34–42	Sulprostone i.m.	0.5 mg 6 hourly	0.875	7:22	V, D	Karim (1979)
1	1	—	E_2 vaginal	20 mg every 2 hours	—	—	—	Lauersen and Wilson (1977)

N = Nausea; V = Vomiting; D = Diarrhoea; S = Superficial phlebitis; F = Facial flush; P = Pyrexia; — = Not reported; 0 = None
i.v. = intravenous infusion; e.a. = extra-amniotic infusion; i.a. = intra-amniotic infusion; i.m. = intramuscular infusion
*Supplementary oxytocin (i.v. infusion) given to one patient
†Supplementary oxytocin (i.v. infusion) given to three patients

16.4.2 Intra-amniotic route

Thiery *et al.* (1975) employed the intra-amniotic route for prostaglandin administration in three patients with an anencephalic pregnancy. Two were with a live foetus at gestations of 21 and 26 weeks respectively. There was no associated polyhydramnios. In one patient the initial intra-amniotic dose of 25–35 mg $PGF_{2\alpha}$ was followed by two similar doses at varying intervals. The foetus was expelled 72 h after the start of treatment with a total dose of 85 mg $PGF_{2\alpha}$. The second patient was given a single intra-amniotic dose of 50 μg $PGF_{2\alpha}$ and delivered 50 h later. Both patients had two episodes of vomiting and one had two episodes of diarrhoea. In a third patient at 30 weeks gestation intra-amniotic PGE_2 (10 mg in two divided doses) resulted in delivery 27 h 39 min after the first dose. There were no side-effects. In all three patients oxytocin infusion was given for a few hours before delivery. Frumar *et al.* (1974) induced two patients with an anencephalic foetus at 30 and 31 weeks gestation. One patient was given an initial dose of 45 mg $PGF_{2\alpha}$ intra-amniotically followed by 25 mg 6 h later. The second patient received an initial dose of 45 mg $PGF_{2\alpha}$ followed by 25 mg at 6, 8, 24, 30 h and another dose of 10 mg at 42 h; making a total of 205 mg $PGF_{2\alpha}$. Induction–delivery intervals were 13 h in the first patient and 53 h 40 min in the second. The second patient had gross polyhydramnios and the long induction–delivery interval may be related to this condition. In both patients the foetus was alive before the start of treatment but death preceded delivery. Both patients had nausea and vomiting and one had diarrhoea (Table 16.16).

16.4.3 Extra-amniotic route

Embrey *et al.* (1974) induced labour in two cases of anencephalic pregnancies with extra-amniotic infusion of PGE_2 administered via a Foley catheter. The initial infusion rate of 30 μg/h was increased by 15 μg/h every 15 minutes until adequate uterine stimulation was obtained. With total doses of 0.5 and 0.8 mg PGE_2 respectively, the two patients delivered 8½ h and 13 h 12 min respectively after the start of extra-amniotic infusion. In one patient the Foley catheter was expelled 5 h after the start of prostaglandin treatment. Oxytocin infusion was commenced 1 h later and continued for 7¼ h when delivery occurred. There were no complications. The largest series of anencephalic pregnancies induced by extra-amniotic administration of prostaglandins was reported by Calder *et al.* (1976). Six out of 13 pregnancies were associated with polyhydramnios. PGE_2 was administered by continuous extra-amniotic infusion at a rate of 1–4 μg/min. The total dose varied from 0.4 to 3.5 mg with a mean of 1.4 mg. The mean induction–delivery interval in the 13 patients was 11 h 48 min with a range of 4 h to 19 h 42 min. Amniotomy was performed after the Foley catheter used for extra-amniotic infusion was expelled. In three patients intravenous oxytocin (4–6 mU/min) was given 1 h after amniotomy and continued until delivery. One patient with polyhydramnios had an intrapartum haemorrhage following amniotomy and at delivery a small fresh retroplacental clot was found (Table 16.16).

16.4.4 Intramuscular route

Karim and Ratnam (1976) used 2a,2b-dihomo-15(S)15-methyl-$PGF_{2\alpha}$ methyl ester to induce labour in eight patients with anencephalic pregnancies. The gestation ranged between 36 and 43 weeks. The prostaglandin analogue was given intramuscularly in doses of 0.5 mg every 8 h. There was no case of polyhydramnios. Labour was successfully induced in all patients in a mean time of 11 h 7 min with a range of 6 h 40 min to 21½ h. Total dose per patient varied between 0.5 and 1.0 mg with a mean of 0.75 mg. Four out of the eight foetuses were born alive. There were no side-effects (Table 16.16).

15(S)15-methyl-$PGF_{2\alpha}$ given intramuscularly was used by Ylikorkala *et al.* (1976) to induce labour in two cases of anencephalic pregnancy at 30 and 36 weeks of gestation. The dose of 0.1 mg was repeated every 2–4 hours. One patient delivered 7½ hours after the start of treatment and another required 10 h 20 min. Both babies were born alive. Side-effects included diarrhoea in both and one had vomiting (Table 16.16).

16-Phenoxy-ω-17,18,19,20-tetranor-PGE_2 methyl sulphonylamide (sulprostone) given intramuscularly in doses of 0.5 mg every 6 h was used to induce labour in six patients with an anencephalic foetus. The gestation ranged between 34 and 42 weeks. Five patients delivered in a mean time of 7 h 22 min with a range of 1 h to 14½ h. One patient failed to deliver 24 h after the start of treatment (four doses). Pregnancy was successfully terminated in this patient with one intramuscular injection of 2a,2b-dihomo-15(S)15-methyl-$PGF_{2\alpha}$ methyl ester. There were no complications and the only side-effects were one episode of vomiting in each of two patients and diarrhoea (two episodes) in one (Karim, 1979) (Table 16.16).

16.4.5 Vaginal route

PGE_2 administered by the vaginal route has been used for inducing labour in one case of anencephalic pregnancy. This was included in 20 cases of intrauterine deaths and missed abortion reported by Lauersen and Wilson (1977). Separate data for the anencephalic pregnancy were not given but the treatment was successful (Table 16.16).

16.5 OTHER GROSS FOETAL ABNORMALITIES

To our knowledge prostaglandins have not been used to terminate pregnancies associated with other types of foetal abnormalities in the last trimester of pregnancy. However, it is not difficult to envisage the use of these compounds in cases of obvious foetal abnormalities such as hydrocephalus, cyclops and severe myelo-meningocele. Antenatal diagnosis of such cases is now possible with the increasing use of ultrasonography and even the fetoscope.

16.6 INEVITABLE AND THREATENED ABORTION

The process of inevitable abortion in the second trimester can be accelerated with prostaglandins. Kerekes and Domokos (1977) used $PGF_{2\alpha}$ by the extra-amniotic route to accelerate abortion in eight such cases at gestation between 16 and 20 weeks. Four patients had vaginal bleeding and in four the membranes had ruptured. Cervical dilatation varied between 2 and 4 cm. In seven patients a single extra-amniotic dose of 5–20 mg $PGF_{2\alpha}$ resulted in abortion and one patient required a second dose. The abortion time after prostaglandin administration varied from 25 min to $22\frac{2}{3}$ h (mean 6 h 23 min). One patient with ruptured membranes was given intravenous oxytocin before prostaglandin treatment but failed to abort. Side-effects included vomiting, nausea and diarrhoea (one patient each). Blood loss varied from less than 100 ml (four patients) to more than 500 ml (one patient).

Prostaglandins can be usefully employed to terminate second trimester pregnancies in women with a threatened abortion when there is no desire on the part of the patient to continue the pregnancy or attempts to preserve such a pregnancy have failed. To our knowledge no such studies have been reported. We have successfully used 2a,2b-dihomo-15(S)15-methyl-$PGF_{2\alpha}$ methyl ester or sulprostone given intramuscularly in a single dose of 0.5 mg to terminate pregnancies in cases of inevitable and threatened abortion (Karim *et al.*, unpublished results).

16.7 CONCLUSION, COMMENTS AND RECOMMENDATIONS

There is very little doubt that prostaglandins offer an attractive alternative to other methods (oxytocin, surgical procedures) in the management of abnormal intrauterine pregnancies. The efficacy of these compounds given by different routes is more predictable that that of oxytocin.

As a result of a widespread use of prostaglandins in the termination of pregnancy at different stages of gestation, it is recognized that:

(1) An abnormal intrauterine pregnancy (with the possible exception of anencephalic pregnancy) can be terminated more readily with prostaglandins than a viable pregnancy at a corresponding gestation (Karim and Amy, 1975).

(2) As with oxytocin, the sensitivity of the uterus to prostaglandin increases with the progression of pregnancy (Karim, 1972).

Many investigators have failed to take the above observations into account in determining the dose of prostaglandin for the termination of abnormal intrauterine pregnancies. In several studies no distinction is made between doses used to terminate a second and a third trimester pregnancy. Some investigators have used even higher doses to terminate abnormal intrauterine pregnancies than those required to terminate viable intrauterine pregnancies. This undoubtedly has led to an overstimulation of the uterus in several instances. High incidence of side-effects reported by some investigators, occasional damage to the uterus or the cervix and possibly increased incidence of bleeding may all be related to overdosage of patients.

Based on the analyses of results from publication reviewed in this chapter we have prepared a 'recommended dose schedule' of prostaglandins given by different routes for termination of abnormal intrauterine pregnancies (Tables 16.17, 16.18). In some instances this recommended dose schedule is based on a limited experience and may have to be revised as more information becomes available.

The choice of prostaglandin, dose and route of administration for terminating an abnormal intrauterine pregnancy would depend upon efficacy, side-effects and to a certain extent on the ease with which it can be administered.

Intravenous infusions of both PGE_2 and $PGF_{2\alpha}$ terminate abnormal intrauterine pregnancies in almost 100% of the patients. High incidence of side-effects are only encountered when doses beyond a certain range are employed.

Similarly, high efficacy and low incidence of side-effects can be obtained with prostaglandins administered by the extra-amniotic route (particularly continuous infusion). Large bolus doses of prostaglandins given extra-amniotically are likely to produce side-effects. For both the intravenous and extra-amniotic infusions, the use of a mechanical pump is preferable to ensure proper dosage. Administration of prostaglandins by the extra-amniotic route, however, does require a certain amount of technical expertise and experience particularly to avoid accidental rupture of the membranes, introduction of infection and premature expulsion of the extra-amniotic catheter. The latter occurs in a significant proportion of patients and necessitates administration of intravenous oxytocin to ensure completion of abortion or delivery.

Prostaglandins administered intra-amniotically are effective in terminating abnormal intrauterine pregnancies. However, this does not appear to be the preferred route. There is a potential risk of introducing an infection and in addition the decreasing amount of amniotic fluid with increasing duration of death *in utero* may make intra-amniotic administration of prostaglandin technically difficult.

Vaginal administration of prostaglandins is a simple procedure which does not require any expertise or prior experience. There is no doubt that PGE_2 administered by this route is very effective in terminating abnormal

Table 16.17 Recommended dose schedule of prostaglandins given by different route for the management of anencephalic pregnancy and intrauterine foetal death

Prostaglandins	*Route of administration*					
	Intravenous[1] *infusion*	*Extra-amniotic*[1] *infusion*	*Extra-amniotic*[3] *bolus*	*Intra-amniotic*[2]	*Intramuscular*	*Vaginal*
PGE_2	0.25–2.5 μg/min	0.5–25.0 μg/min	25–100 μg 2 hourly	2.5–5.0 mg every 12–24 h	NS	ND
$PGF_{2\alpha}$	2.5–20 μg/min	2.5–5.0 μg/min	125–300 μg 2 hourly	25 mg repeated 12 hourly	NS	ND
15-methyl-$PGF_{2\alpha}$	ND	ND	ND	ND	50–100 μg 3 hourly[4]	ND
dihomo-15-methyl-$PGF_{2\alpha}$	ND	ND	ND	ND	0.25–0.5 mg 8 hourly	ND
Sulprostone	ND	ND	ND	ND	0.25–0.5 mg 6 hourly	ND

[1] = Preferably given by an infusion pump
[2] = Not a preferred route; based on very limited experience
[3] = Preferably start with a small bolus 'test' dose
[4] = Based on a limited experience
ND = No data or very little data available
NS = Not suitable

Table 16.18 Recommended dose schedules of prostaglandin administration by different routes for termination of pregnancies in cases of missed abortion and hydatidiform mole

Prostaglandins	*Route of administration*					
	Intravenous[1] *infusion*	*Extra-amniotic*[1] *infusion*	*Extra-amniotic*[3] *bolus*	*Intra-amniotic*[2]	*Intramuscular*	*Vaginal*
E_2	0.5–4.0 μg/min	1–4 μg/min	50–200 μg 2 hourly	2.5 mg to be repeated at 12–24 hours	NS	20 mg every 3–6 hours
$F_{2\alpha}$	5.0–40.0 μg/min	5–10 μg/min	250–600 μg 2 hourly	25 mg to be repeated at 12–24 hours	NS	ND
15-methyl-$PGF_{2\alpha}$	ND	ND	ND	0.5 mg to be repeated at 12–24 hours	0.1–0.2 mg 3 hourly	ND
dihomo-15-methyl-$PGF_{2\alpha}$	ND	ND	ND	ND	0.5 mg 8 hourly	ND
Sulprostone	0.5–2.0 μg/min[4]	ND	ND	ND	0.5 mg 6 hourly	ND

[1] = Preferably given by an infusion pump
[2] = Not applicable to molar pregnancy: not a preferred route for missed abortion
[3] = Preferably start with a small bolus 'test' dose
[4] = Based on limited experience
ND = No data or very limited data available
NS = Not suitable

intrauterine pregnancies. However the incidence of gastrointestinal and other side-effects associated with this route has been very high. This is not surprising in view of the fact that prostaglandins administered vaginally act on the uterus after absorption into systemic circulation. An additional disadvantage is rupture of the membranes or uterine bleeding occurring early during treatment. This is likely to interfere with administration of subsequent doses of prostaglandins and their absorption from the vagina. It is possible that the dose of PGE_2 used by most investigators (20 mg every 2–3 hours) is too high. A decrease in dose may still provide a high efficacy at a reduced incidence of side-effects.

The efficacy of the three prostaglandins, 15(S)15-methyl-$PGF_{2\alpha}$, dihomo-15(S)15-methyl-$PGF_{2\alpha}$ and sulprostone, administered by the intramuscular route for termination of abnormal intrauterine pregnancies has been high. The side-effects associated with 15(S)15-methyl-$PGF_{2\alpha}$ may be further reduced by using doses lower than those used by most investigators. Both dihomo-15(S)15-methyl-$PGF_{2\alpha}$ and sulprostone given intramuscularly have proved very effective in terminating abnormal intrauterine pregnancy. The treatment is associated with a low incidence of side-effects and doses need to be given only at 6–8 hourly intervals. However, experience with these two compounds is limited and need to be confirmed in additional clinical trials.

In conclusion, the use of prostaglandins in the termination of abnormal intrauterine pregnancies is a significant advance in obstetrics and gynaecology in the last decade. With advances in the early diagnosis of abnormal intrauterine pregnancy it is now possible to terminate such pregnancies with confidence and without delay.

References

Arshat, H. (1977). Extra-amniotic prostaglandin E_2 and intravenous oxytocin in termination of mid-trimester pregnancy and in the management of missed abortion and hydatidiform mole. *Med. J. Malaysia*, **31**, 220

Bailey, C. D. H., Newman, C., Ellinas, S. P. and Anderson, G. G. (1975). Use of prostaglandin E_2 vaginal suppositories in intrauterine fetal death and missed abortion. *Obstet. Gynecol.*, **45**, 110

Beazley, J. M. and Gillespie, A. (1971). Double-blind trial of prostaglandin E_2 and oxytocin in induction of labour. *Lancet*, **i**, 152

Bowen-Simpkins, P. (1973). The induction of second trimester abortion using an intra-amniotic injection of urea and prostaglandin $F_{2\alpha}$ for therapeutic abortion. Early myometrial effects. *Am. J. Obstet. Gynecol.*, **114**, 511

Brandes, J. M., Grunstein, S. and Peretz, A. (1966). Suction evacuation of the uterine cavity in hydatidiform mole. *Obstet. Gynecol.*, **28**, 689

Briel, R. C., Kunz, S., Kidess, E. and Dieter, B. (1976). Studies on platelet function during application of prostaglandin $F_{2\alpha}$ in missed abortion and missed labour. *8th World Congress of Gynecol. and Obstet.* 7–22 October. *Excerpta Medica*. (Abstr.), p. 37

Caballero, A., Alonso-Magan, J. L., Corredera, J. and Albertos, F. G. (1975). Prostaglandins $F_{2\alpha}$, E_1 and E_2 by intra-amniotic route for the induction of partus with dead or retained fetus or with hydatiform mole. Patterns of these pregnancies. *Acta Ginecol.*, **25**, 79

Caballero, A., Garcia-Albertos, F., Corredera, J., Alonso-Magan, J. L., Guerra, J. M. and Gandara, A. (1974). Declenchement du travail a l'aide des prostaglandines E_1, E_2, $F_{1\alpha}$ et $F_{2\alpha}$. *Rev. Franc. Gynecol. Obstet.*, **69**, 75

Calder, A. A., Mackenzie, I. Z. and Embrey, M. P. (1976). Intrauterine (extra-amniotic) prostaglandins in the management of unsuccessful pregnancy. *J. Reprod. Med.*, **16**, 271

Cameron, J. M. and Dayan, A. D. (1966). Association of brain damage with therapeutic abortion induced by amniotic fluid replacement. Report of 2 cases. *Br. Med. J.*, **1**, 1010

Campbell, S., Johnstone, F. D., Holt, E. M. and May, P. (1972). Anencephaly early ultrasonic diagnosis and active management. *Lancet*, **ii**, 1226

Chef, R., Thiery, M., Van Kets, H., Yo Le Sian, A., De Hemptinne, D. and Vrijens, M. (1974). Anencéphalie: diagnostic ultrasonique précoce et interruption. *J. Gynecol. Obstet. Biol. Reprod. (Paris)*, **3**, 93

Corbett, V. H. (1958). The management of intra-uterine death of the foetus. *J. Obstet. Gynaecol. Br. Emp.*, **65**, 100

Craft, I. (1973). Intra-amniotic prostaglandin E_2 and urea for abortion. *Lancet*, **i**, 779

Craft, I., Walker, E. and Youssefnejadian, E. (1974). Intra-amniotic prostaglandin $F_{2\alpha}$ and urea for abortion. *Prostaglandins*, **5**, 397

El-Damarawy, H., El-Sahwi, S. and Toppozada, M. (1977). Management of missed abortion and fetal death *in utero*. *Prostaglandins*, **14**, 583

El-Sherbini, R. M. (1963). Retention of an 8-month foetus *in utero* for two-and-a-half years. *J. Obstet. Gynaecol. Br. Commonw.*, **70**, 154

Embrey, M. P., Calder, A. A. and Hillier, K. (1974). Extra-amniotic prostaglandins in the management of intra-uterine foetal death, anencephaly and hydatidiform mole. *J. Obstet. Gynaecol. Br. Commonw.*, **81**, 47

Exalto, N. and Meuwissen, J. H. J. M. (1976). De betekenis van prostaglandine bij de behandeling van missed abortion. *Ned. T. Geneesk.*, **120**, 1289

Fawzy, A. A. S. H. and Basiony, B. A. (1979). The use of sulprostone in the management of death *in utero* and molar pregnancy. *Singapore J. Obstet. Gynaecol.*, **10**, 39

Ferguson-Smith, M. A., Rawlinson, H. A., May, H. M., Tait, H. A., Vince, J. D., Gibson, A. A. M., Robinson, H. P. and Ratcliffe, J. G. (1978). Avoidance of anencephalic and spina-bifida births by maternal serum-alpha fetoprotein screening. *Lancet*, **i**, 1330

Filshie, G. M. (1971). The use of prostaglandin E_2 in the management of intrauterine death, missed abortion and hydatidiform mole. *J. Obstet. Gynaecol. Br. Commonw.*, **78**, 87

Foroohar, H. and Behjatnia, Y. (1976). Use of prostaglandin $F_{2\alpha}$ in the management of missed abortion. *Int. J. Gynecol. Obstet.*, **14**, 541

Frumar, A. M., Smith, I. D. and Korda, A. R. (1974). Prostaglandin $F_{2\alpha}$ for the induction of labour in pregnancies complicated by intrauterine death, anencephaly and chromosomal anomaly. *Prostaglandins*, **6**, 125

Gordon, H. and Pipe, N. G. J. (1975). Induction of labour after intrauterine foetal death. A comparison between prostaglandin E_2 and oxytocin. *Obstet. Gynecol. (NY)*, **45**, 44

Gosden, C. M. and Brock, J. H. (1977). Morphology of rapidly adhering amniotic fluid cells as an aid to the diagnosis of neural tube defects. *Lancet*, **i**, 919

Gruber, W. S. (1979). Intravenous sulprostone for induction of foetal death *in utero*. *Proceedings of International Sulprostone Symposium*, October 1978 (Vienna: Pfizer-Schering) (In press)

Guha-Ray, D. K. (1975). Obstetric problems in association with anencephaly. *Obstet. Gynecol.*, **46**, 569

Hammond, C. B., Hertz, R., Ross, G. T., Lipsett, M. B. and Odell, W. D. (1967). Primary chemotherapy for non-metastatic gestational trophoblastic neoplasms. *Am. J. Obstet. Gynecol.*, **98**, 71

Hardisty, R. M. and Ingram, G. I. C. (1965). *Bleeding Disorders. Investigations and Management.* (Oxford: Blackwell Scientific Publications)

Herrera, M. and Leyton, H. (1973). Aborto molar completo inducido con-prostaglandina $F_{2\alpha}$. *Rev. Chil. Obstet. Ginec.*, **38**, 146

Herrera, M., Wells, W. and Jil, G. (1973). Experiencia preliminar en el uso clinico de las prostaglandinas $F_{2\alpha}$ en el aborto retenido. *Rev. Chil. Obstet. Ginec.*, **38**, 187

Hertz, R., Lewis, J. and Lipsett, M. B. (1961). Five years experience with the chemotherapy of metastatic choriocarcinoma and related trophoblastic tumours in women. *Am. J. Obstet. Gynecol.*, **82,** 631

Hickl, E. J., Mickan, H. and Walther, D. (1973). Kombination von Prostaglandin $F_{2\alpha}$ und Paracervicalblock bei Missed Abortion and Intrauterinem Fruchttood. *Klin. Wochenschr.*, **51**, 140

Higgins, L. G. (1954). Prolonged pregnancy (Partus serotinus). *Lancet*, **ii**, 1154

Hodgkinson, C. P., Margolis, R. R. and Lazarde, J. H. (1954). Etiology and management of hypofibrinogenemia of pregnancy. *J. Am. Med. Assoc.*, **154**, 557

Iddelkinge, B. Van and Gordon, H. (1974). The value of intravenous prostaglandin E_2 after intra-uterine death. *S. Afr. Med. J.*, **48**, 1941

Jeffcoate, F. N. A. (1940). Missed abortion and missed labour. *Lancet*, **i**, 1045

Karim, S. M. M. (1970). Use of prostaglandin E_2 in the management of missed abortion, missed labour and hydtaidiform mole. *Br. Med. J.*, **3**, 196

Karim, S. M. M. (1972). Prostaglandins and human reproduction: Physiological roles and clinical uses of prostaglandins in relation to human reproduction. In: S. M. M. Karim (ed.), *The Prostaglandins: Progress in Research*, p. 71 (Lancaster: MTP Press)

Karim, S. M. M. (1974). Adverse reactions to intra-amniotic prostaglandin. *Br. Med. J.*, **3**, 347

Karim, S. M. M., Lim, A. L., Prasad, R. N. V., Yeo, K. C., Ng, S. C., Salmon, Y. M., Choo, H. T. and Ratnam, S. S. (1979). Termination of abnormal intra-uterine pregnancy with intramuscular administration of sulprostone. *Singapore J. Obstet. Gynecol.*, **10**, 33

Karim, S. M. M. (1979). Prostaglandins in obstetrics and gynaecology. *Proceedings of International Sulprostone Symposium*, October 1978 (Vienna: Pfizer-Schering) (In press)

Karim, S. M. M. and Amy, J. J. (1975). Interruption of pregnancy with prostaglandins. In: S. M. M. Karim (ed.), *Advances in Prostaglandin Research: Prostaglandins and Reproduction*, p. 77 (Lancaster: MTP Press)

Karim, S. M. M. and Ratnam, S. S. (1976). Termination of abnormal intra-uterine pregnancies with intramuscular administration of dihomo-15-methyl prostaglandin $F_{2\alpha}$. *Br. J. Obstet. Gynaecol.*, **83**, 885

Karim, S. M. M., Ratnam, S. S. and Choo, H. T. (1974). Intra-uterine administration of prostaglandin 15(S)15-methyl-E_2 methyl ester in the management of molar pregnancy. *J. Obstet. Gynaecol. Br. Commonw.*, **81**, 650

Karim, S. M. M. and Sharma, S. D. (1972). Termination of second trimester pregnancy with 15-methyl analogues of prostaglandin E_2 and $F_{2\alpha}$. *J. Obstet. Gynaecol. Br. Commonw.*, **79**, 737

Karim, S. M. M., Sharma, S. D. and Filshie, G. M. (1972). Termination of pregnancy with 15-methyl analogues of prostaglandin E_2 and $F_{2\alpha}$. In: E. M. Southern (ed.), *The Prostaglandins: Clinical Applications in Human Reproduction*, p. 307 (Mt. Kisco, New York: Futura)

Karim, S. M. M. and Trussell, R. R. (1971). The use of prostaglandins in obstetrics. *E. Afr. Med. J.*, **48**, 1

Karim, S. M. M., Trussell, R. R., Hillier, K. and Patel, R. C. (1969). Induction of labour with prostaglandin $F_{2\alpha}$. *J. Obstet. Gynaecol. Br. Commonw.*, **76**, 769

Keirse, M. J. N. C. (1975). Studies on prostaglandins in relation to human parturition. *D. Phil. Thesis. University of Oxford*

Kent, D. R. (1977). A modern approach to the management of intra-uterine fetal death. *West. J. Med.*, **126**, 298

Kent, D. R. and Goldstein, A. L. (1976). Prostaglandin E_2 induction of labour for fetal demise. *Obstet. Gynecol.*, **48**, 475

Kerekes, L. and Domokos, N. (1977). Termination of mid-term spontaneous and missed abortions by extra-amniotic injection of a single prostaglandin $F_{2\alpha}$ dose. *Ther. Hungar.*, **25**, 102

Kinra, G., Agarwal, N. and Hingorani, V. (1977). Use of prostaglandin for induction of second trimester abortions in high-risk pregnancy. *Contraception*, **16**, 243

Klausch, V. B., Kruse, H. J., Goretzlehner, G. and Buttner, H. H. (1976). Weheninduktion mit Prostaglandin $F_{2\alpha}$ zur behandlung derblasenmole. *Zbl. Gynak.*, **98**, 1352

Koning-Gans de, K. H. J., Martinez, A. A. V. and Eskes, T. K. A. B. (1975). Intermittent low-dose administration of prostaglandins intra-amniotically in pathological pregnancies. A comparison with oxytocin and ergometrine. *Eur. J. Obstet. Gynecol. Reprod. Biol.*, **5/6**, 307

Korotkin, J. H., Ratchford, W. J. and Blake, P. (1977). The induction of labour in intra-uterine foetal death syndrome using prostaglandin E_2 vaginal suppositories. Personal communication

Kunz, J. and Schreiner, W. E. (1977). Klinische erfahrungen mit prostaglandin E_2 und $F_{2\alpha}$ zum schwangerschaftsabbruch und zur Weheneinleitung bei intrauterinem Fruchttod. *Schweiz. Med. Wochenschr.* **107**, 757

Lange, A. P. and Secher, N. J. (1977). Mid-trimester and missed abortion treated with intramuscular 15(S)15-methyl-$PGF_{2\alpha}$. *Prostaglandins*, **14**, 389

Lange, A. P., Secher, N. J. and Westergaard, J. (1976). Termination of pregnancy in cases of fetal death *in utero* by intravenous prostaglandin $F_{2\alpha}$. *Prostaglandins*, **11**, 101

Lauersen, N. H. and Wilson, K. H. (1977). Induction of labor in patients with missed abortion and fetal death *in utero* with prostaglandin E_2 suppositories. *Am. J. Obstet. Gynecol.*, **127**, 609

Lewis, E. (1976). The management of stillbirth: coping with an unreality. *Lancet*, **ii**, 619

Liggins, G. C. (1962). The treatment of missed abortion by high dosage. Syntocinon intravenous infusion. *J. Obstet. Gynaecol. Br. Commonw.*, **69**, 277

Lippert, T. H. and Luthi, A. (1978). Induction of labour with prostaglandin E_2 gel in cases of intra-uterine fetal death. *Prostaglandins*, **15**, 533

Luengo, J., Keirse, M. J. N. C. and Bennebrock-Gravenhorst, J. (1977). Extra-amniotic prostaglandin $F_{2\alpha}$ for intra-uterine death and foetal abnormality. *Eur. J. Obstet. Gynecol. Reprod. Biol.* **7**, 325

Martin, R. H. and Menzies, D. N. (1955). Oestrogen therapy in missed abortion and labour. *J. Obstet. Gynaecol. Br. Emp.*, **62**, 256

McNicol, E. and Gray, H. (1977). Adverse reaction to extra-amniotic prostaglandin E_2. *Br. J. Obstet. Gynaecol.*, **84**, 229

Miller, A. W. F. (1973). The use of prostaglandins for missed abortion, foetal death *in utero* and hydatidiform mole. In: R. G. Jacomb and R. E. Hardy (eds.), *The Use of Prostaglandins E_2 and $F_{2\alpha}$ in Obstetrics and Gynaecology*, p. 63 (Miami: Symposia Specialists)

Moe, N. (1976). The intravenous infusion of prostaglandin $F_{2\alpha}$ in the management of intrauterine death of the fetus. *Acta Obstet. Gynecol. Scand.*, **55**, 113

Murray, C. P. and Clinch, J. (1975). Management of missed abortion, intrauterine death and hydatidiform mole using prostaglandin E_2. *J. Irish Med. Assoc.*, **68**, 133

Myerscough, P. R. (1977). *Munro Kerr's Operative Obstetrics*, p. 453 (London: E.L.B.S)

Naismith, W. C. M. K. and Barr, W. (1974). Simultaneous intravenous infusion of PGE_2 and oxytocin in the management of intra-uterine death of the foetus, missed abortion and hydatidiform mole. *J. Obstet. Gynaecol. Br. Commonw.*, **81**, 146

Paladini, A., Di Lieto, A., Martinelli, P., De Placido, G. and Di Meglio, A. (1977). Induzione del travaglio nell'aborto ritenuto, nella morte fetale e nella mola vescicolare con $PGF_{2\alpha}$ per via intracavitaria extramniotica. *Min. Gin.*, **29**, 1

Pedersen, P. H., Larsen, J. F. and Sorensen, B. (1972). Induction of labour with prostaglandin $F_{2\alpha}$ in missed abortion, fetus mortuus and anencephalia. *Prostaglandins*, **2**, 135

Peterson, E. P. and Taylor, H. B. (1970). Amniotic fluid embolism. An analysis of 40 cases. *Obstet. Gynecol. (NY)*, **35**, 787

Phelan, J. P., Matey, D., Wilder, T. L. and Newman, C. (1977). Clinical evaluation of prostaglandin E_2 vaginal suppositories for the termination of pregnancies complicated by IUFD and missed abortions. *Obstet. Gynecol. (NY)*,

Pritchard, J. A. and Ratnoff, O. D. (1955). Studies of fibrinogen and other haemostatis factors in women with intrauterine death and delayed delivery. *Surg. Gynecol. Obstet.*, **101**, 467

Quigley, M. M. (1973). Overview of gestational trophoblastic neoplasma. *NY State J. Med.*, **73**, 1869

Quinn, L. J. and Harper, J. A. (1955). Fibrinogenaemia in an iso-sensitized mother carrying a dead fetus. *J. Obstet. Gynaecol. Br. Emp.*, **62**, 280

Ring, A. (1972). Clinical experience with prostaglandin $F_{2\alpha}$ for induction of labour. In: E. M. Southern (ed.), *The Prostaglandins: Clinical Applications in Human Reproduction*, p. 129 (Mt. Kisco, New York: Futura)

Roberts, G. (1974). Induction of labour and abortion by intravenous prostaglandins in pregnancies complicated by intrauterine foetal death and hydatidiform mole. *Curr. Med. Res. Opinion*, **2** (6), 342

Robinson, A. L., Datnow, H. M. and Jeffcoate, T. N. A. (1935). Induction of abortion and labour by means of oestrin. *Br. Med. J.*, **1**, 749

Ross, G. T., Goldstein, D. P., Hertz, R. and Lipsett, M. B. (1965). Sequential use of methotrexate and actinomycin D in the treatment of metastic choriocarcinoma and related trophoblastic diseases in women. *Am. J. Obstet. Gynecol.*, **93**, 223

Ruppen, M., Keller, P. J., Schmidt, J. and Schreiner, W. E. (1972). Prostaglandine bei 'missed abortion' und bei 'missed labour'. *Schweiz Z. Gynak. Geburtsh.*, **3**, 439

Rutland, A. and Ballard, C. (1977). Vaginal prostaglandin E_2 for missed abortion and intrauterine fetal death. *Am. J. Obstet. Gynecol.*, **128**, 503

Samaja, B. A., Rigagnoli, A. and Pecorelli, S. (1976). Missed abortion and intrauterine fetal death treated with prostaglandin $F_{2\alpha}$. In: S. M. M. Karim (ed.), *Obstetric and Gynaecological Uses of Prostaglandins. 1st Inter-congress, Asian Federation of Obstetrics and Gynaecology, Singapore*, p. 241 (Lancaster: MTP Press)

Sandberg, F., Ingelman-Sundberg, A., Ryden, G. and Joeleson, L. (1968). The absorption of tritium-labelled prostaglandin E_1 from the vagina of non-pregnant women. *Acta Obstet. Gynecol. Scand.*, **47**, 22

Scher, J., Kiwi, R. and Baillie, P. (1974). Use of prostaglandin E_2 in the management of intrauterine death. *S. Afr. J. Med.* (Suppl.), **41**

Secher, N. J., Lange, A. and Westergaard, J. G. (1976). Delivery induced with prostaglandin $F_{2\alpha}$ in fetal death. *Advances in Prostaglandin and Thromboxane Research.* Meeting Abstract, **2**, 977

Selander, K. and Psytynen, P. (1979). Abortion induction in second trimester pregnancy with intravenous infusion of Sulprostone (16-phenoxy-ω-tetranor PGE_2 methylsulfonylamide). *Proceedings of International Sulprostone Symposium*, October 1978 (Vienna: Pfizer-Schering) (In press)

Sharma, S. D., Hale, R. W. and Sato, N. E. (1975). Intramuscular 15(S)15-methyl prostaglandin $F_{2\alpha}$ for mid-trimester and missed abortions. *Obstet. Gynecol.*, **46**, 468

Sher, G. (1976). Intra-amniotic use of urea and prostaglandin $F_{2\alpha}$ to induce labour in pregnancies complicated by death of the fetus. *S. Afr. J. Obstet. Gynecol.*, **50**, 510

Smith, A. M. (1974). Adverse reactions to intra-amniotic prostaglandins. *Br. Med. J.*, **2**, 382

Soszka, S., Czekanowski, R. and Litorowicz, A. (1974). Badania nad zastosowaniem prostaglandyny $F_{2\alpha}$ w indukowaniu porodu w przypadkach obumarcia plodu. *Ginekol. Polska*, **45**, 465

Southern, E. M. and Gutknecht, G. D. (1976). Management of intra-uterine fetal demise and missed abortion using prostaglandin E_2 vaginal suppositories. *Obstet. Gynecol.*, **47**, 602

Southern, E. M., Gutknecht, G. D. and Mohberg, N. R. (1976). Evacuation of the uterus in benign gestational trophoblastic disease with prostaglandins. In: S. M. M. Karim (ed.),

Obstetric and Gynecological Uses of Prostaglandins. 1st Inter-congress, Asian Federation of Obstetrics and Gynaecology, Singapore, p. 247 (Lancaster: MTP Press)

Southern, E. M., Gutknecht, G. D., Mohberg, N. R. and Edelman, D. A. (1978). Vaginal prostaglandin E_2 in the management of fetal intrauterine death. *Br. J. Obstet. Gynecol.*, **85**, 437

Stephens, J. D. and Birnholz, J. C. (1976). Modern management of fetal death *in utero* and missed abortion. In: S. M. M. Karim (ed.), *Obstetric and Gynaecological Uses of Prostaglandins. 1st Inter-congress, Asian Federation of Obstetrics and Gynaecology*, Singapore, p. 253 (Lancaster: MTP Press)

Thiery, M. and Amy, J. J. (1975). Induction of labour with prostaglandins. In: S. M. M. Karim (ed.), *Advances in Prostaglandin Research. Prostaglandins and Reproduction*, p. 149 (Lancaster: MTP Press)

Thiery, M., de Hemptinne, D., Yo Le Sian, A. and Amy, J. J. (1975). The use of prostaglandins for the termination of 'pregnancy' in cases of hydatidiform mole, intra-uterine death and anencephaly. *T. Geneesk*, **9**, 441

Toppozada, M., Warda, A., Ramadan, M. and Attar, A. E. (1979). Termination of pregnancy for medical indications by systemic administration of sulprostone. *Proceedings of International Sulprostone Symposium*, October 1978 (Vienna: Pfizer-Schering) (In press)

Tricomi, V. and Kohl, S. G. (1957). Fetal death *in utero*. *Am. J. Obstet. Gynecol.*, **74**, 1092

Tsalacopoulos, G. (1978). Intra-uterine extra-amniotic prostaglandin $F_{2\alpha}$ in the management of patients with intra-uterine fetal death. *S. Afr. Med. J.*, **53**, 848

Ursell, W. (1972). Induction of labour following fetal death. *J. Obstet. Gynaecol. Br. Commonw.*, **79**, 260

Wagatsuma, T. (1965). Intra-amniotic injection of saline for therapeutic abortion. *Am. J. Obstet. Gynecol.*, **93**, 743

Wagman, H. and Usherwood, M. (1974). Intrauterine death treated with intra-uterine extra-amniotic prostaglandin E_2. *Br. J. Clin. Pract.*, **28**, 318

Wallenburg, H. C. S. (1978). Intramuscular administration of 15(S)15-methyl-$PGF_{2\alpha}$ for induction of labour in patients with fetal death. Unpublished results

Wiqvist, N., Beguin, F., Bygdeman, M. and Toppozada, M. (1972). Recent aspects of systemic administration of prostaglandin. In: E. M. Southern (ed.), *The Prostaglandins: Clinical Applications in Human Reproduction*, p. 295 (Mt. Kisco, New York: Futura)

Yankee, E. W. and Bundy, G. L. (1972). 15(S)15-methyl prostaglandins. *J. Am. Chem. Soc.*, **94**, 3651

Ylikorkala, O., Kirkinen, P. and Jarvinen, P. A. (1976). Intramuscular administration of 15-methyl prostaglandin $F_{2\alpha}$ for induction of labour in patients with intrauterine fetal death or an anencephalic fetus. *Br. J. Obstet. Gynaecol.*, **83**, 502

17
Termination of Second Trimester Pregnancy with Prostaglandins

S. M. M. KARIM

17.1 INTRODUCTION

The subject of interruption of pregnancy with prostaglandins was reviewed in detail in the first volume in this series by Karim and Amy (1975). Termination of very early pregnancy (menstrual induction) with prostaglandins is discussed by Bygdeman in Chapter 13. In the remainder of the first trimester, prostaglandins are mainly used for cervical dilatation prior to vacuum aspiration or curettage. This aspect is covered in Chapter 14. The use of prostaglandins in the termination of abnormal intrauterine pregnancy (death *in utero*, molar and anencephalic pregnancies) is also reviewed separately in Chapter 16. The purpose of this short chapter is to discuss more recent developments in the use of prostaglandins and their analogues for the termination of second trimester pregnancy.

17.2 INTRA-AMNIOTIC ROUTE

PGF$_{2\alpha}$ given by intravenous, intra-amniotic or extra-amniotic routes for the termination of second trimester pregnancy has been used in a large number of clinical trials. The results of these studies, their efficacy and side-effects have been discussed previously (Karim and Amy, 1975). During the past few years several investigators have compared prostaglandins with other methods of terminating second trimester pregnancies.

This chapter was prepared by the editor at a very short notice after the contributor originally assigned to review the subject failed to submit his manuscript at the time of going to press.

17.2.1 Comparison between $PGF_{2\alpha}$ and hypertonic saline

In two large multicentre studies, the efficacy and safety of intra-amniotic $PGF_{2\alpha}$ and hypertonic saline were compared. The results of the first such study sponsored by the International Fertility Research Program (IFRP), North Carolina were reported by Edelman *et al.* (1976). A total of 372 patients of gestation age between 15 and 20 weeks, matched for age, parity and gestation, were randomly allocated to three treatment groups.

Group 1: $PGF_{2\alpha}$, 50 mg single dose (125 patients)
Group 2: $PGF_{2\alpha}$, 25 mg repeated at 6, 24 and 30 h if necessary (112 patients)
Group 3: 200 ml 20% sodium chloride solution

Prostaglandin and hypertonic saline were administered intra-amniotically without prior aspiration of the amniotic fluid.

Table 17.1 Complications and side-effects of two intra-amniotic $PGF_{2\alpha}$ dose schedules and intra-amniotic saline from amniocentesis to completion of the abortion*

Complications and side-effects	*$PGF_{2\alpha}$ 50 mg single dose (n = 125)*		*$PGF_{2\alpha}$ 25 mg at 0, 6, 24 and 30 h (n = 112)*		*200 ml 20% sodium chloride (n = 130)*	
	No.	*%*	*No.*	*%*	*No.*	*%*
Vomiting	36	28.8	47	42.0	6	4.6
Diarrhoea	19	15.2	25	22.3	9	6.9
Fever (>38 °C)	4	3.4	9	8.3	15	12.2
Bronchospasm	2	1.6	1	0.9	0	0.0
Convulsion	1	0.8	0	0.0	0	0.0
Pelvic infection	1	0.8	2	1.8	1	0.8
Blood loss (>500 ml)	2	1.6	2	1.8	3	2.3
Disseminated intravascular coagulation	0	0.0	0	0.0	1	0.8
Other†	9	7.2	6	5.4	4	3.1

*Data from Edelman *et al.* (1976)
†Headache (4); Dizziness (2); Profuse sweating (2); Chills (10); Hypotension (1)
n = Number of patients

Twenty-four hours after the initial instillation, 73.2% of the patients treated with the multiple 25 mg $PGF_{2\alpha}$ had expelled the foetus compared to 59.2% in the saline group. At the end of the trial period (72 h) 93.5% of the patients in the 50 mg $PGF_{2\alpha}$ group, 98.2% in the multiple 25 mg $PGF_{2\alpha}$ group and 99.2% in the saline treated group had aborted. The mean instillation to abortion time was significantly shorter in patients treated with multiple 25 mg $PGF_{2\alpha}$ doses (17.4 h) than in patients aborted with a single 50 mg $PGF_{2\alpha}$ dose (20.4 h) or hypertonic saline (26.3 h).

The rate of incomplete abortion in the 50 mg $PGF_{2\alpha}$ group was 61.7%, in the 25 mg $PGF_{2\alpha}$ 65.5% and in the saline group it was 74.4%. The difference between the two prostaglandin groups and saline group was statistically significant.

The incidence of side-effects and complications in the three groups is shown in Table 17.1.

The authors consider that intra-amniotic administration of $PGF_{2\alpha}$ or hypertonic saline resulted in a satisfactory rate of abortion with clinically acceptable rates of complications. In terms of mean instillation abortion time and cumulative abortion rate the most effective method was the multiple 25 mg $PGF_{2\alpha}$ dose schedule and the least effective was hypertonic saline. The abortion time with saline can be reduced with simultaneous intravenous infusion of oxytocin (Berger *et al.*, 1975). However, such a procedure is inconvenient and is thought to result in increased rate of uterine injury or disseminated intravascular coagulation (Cohen and Ballard, 1974).

Side-effects of vomiting and diarrhoea were more frequent with prostaglandin than with saline but it may be possible to reduce these with anti-emetic and antidiarrhoeal drugs.

One patient treated with $PGF_{2\alpha}$ had a grand mal seizure. Edelman *et al.* (1976) suggested that grand mal seizure may occur more frequently with $PGF_{2\alpha}$ than with saline.

Table 17.2 Comparative success rates with intra-amniotic $PGF_{2\alpha}$ and hypertonic saline

Treatment	*No. of patients*	*Success rates*						*Trial interrupted*	
		24 h		*36 h*		*48 h*			
		No.	*%*	*No.*	*%*	*No.*	*%*	*No.*	*%*
$PGF_{2\alpha}$*	717	439	61.2	574	80.1	614	85.6	10	1.4
NaCl†	796	161	20.2	462	58.0	641	80.5	7	0.9

*25 mg initial dose followed by 25 mg 6 h later
†200 ml 20% sodium chloride solution
From: WHO Prostaglandin Task Force Multicentre Trial (1976)

In another multicentre study sponsored by the WHO Prostaglandin Task Force (1976) the efficacy of 25 mg $PGF_{2\alpha}$ given intra-amniotically and repeated 6 h later was compared with 200 ml 20% hypertonic saline in a total of 1513 patients mainly in the 15th–20th week of gestation. Criterion for successful treatment was expulsion of the foetus within 48 h of instillation of $PGF_{2\alpha}$ or saline (cf. 72 h in IFRP Study). $PGF_{2\alpha}$ was given to 717 and saline to 796 patients. They were closely matched for state of health, age, height, weight, gravidity and parity.

In the prostaglandin group, 614 out of 717 patients (85.6%) aborted within 48 h after the first intra-amniotic injection. In the hypertonic saline group, 641 (80.57%) out of 796 patients aborted during this period. The mean instillation abortion interval in the prostaglandin group was 19.7 h compared to 30.4 h in the saline group. The proportion of complete abortion in the two groups was similar: 66.4% with $PGF_{2\alpha}$ and 68.2% with saline (Table 17.2). The incidence of side-effects and complications in the two treatment groups are listed in Table 17.3.

Table 17.3 Comparative side-effects with intra-amniotic $PGF_{2\alpha}$ and hypertonic saline

	$PGF_{2\alpha}$* (n = 717)	*Hypertonic saline*† (n = 796)
Diarrhoea	109 (15.2%)	10 (1.3%)
Vomiting	384 (53.6%)	153 (19.2%)
Dyspnoea	19 (2.6%)	3 (0.4%)
Flushing	47 (6.6%)	10 (1.3%)
Chest pain	7 (1.0%)	1 (0.1%)
Syncope	0 (0%)	2 (0.2%)
Nausea	16 (2.2%)	6 (0.7%)
Epileptic seizure	0 (0%)	1 (0.1%)
Cervicovaginal fistula	1 (0.13%)	1 (0.1%)
Heavy uterine bleeding	32 (4.5%)	12 (1.5%)
Blood transfusion	22 (3.1%)	6 (0.8%)

* 25 mg initial dose followed by 25 mg 6 h later
† 200 ml 20% sodium chloride solution
n = Number of patients
From WHO Prostaglandin Task Force Multicentre Trial (1976)

The authors consider that the main advantage of $PGF_{2\alpha}$ lies in the greater efficacy with significantly higher success rate during the first 48 h and a highly significant shorter induction–abortion interval. However, compared with hypertonic saline the treatment with $PGF_{2\alpha}$ was associated with a significantly higher incidence of vomiting, diarrhoea and heavy uterine bleeding.

Disseminated intravascular coagulation is one of the severely potentially serious complications of hypertonic saline-induced abortion. This occurred in one patient (0.8%) in the multicentre trial of Edelman *et al.* (1976). No coagulation changes consistent with disseminated intravascular coagulation have been encountered in prostaglandin-induced abortion.

Rapid intravascular absorption of hypertonic saline from the amniotic cavity or inadvertent intravascular or intraperitoneal administration of saline has resulted in hypernatraemia, necrosis of the affected tissue or more serious complications or even death. Rapid absorption of $PGF_{2\alpha}$ or inadvertent administration into the peritonium or the myometrium results in vomiting and diarrhoea and may cause bronchoconstriction. These symptoms are less severe than those occurring after inappropriate administration of hypertonic saline.

17.2.2 Comparison between $PGF_{2\alpha}$ and 15-methyl-$PGF_{2\alpha}$

The use of intra-amniotic 15(S)15-methyl-$PGF_{2\alpha}$ (15-methyl-$PGF_{2\alpha}$) for the termination of second trimester pregnancy has been previously discussed in

Table 17.4 Results of abortion with the use of intra-amniotic $PGF_{2\alpha}$ and 15-methyl $PGF_{2\alpha}$ from a multicentre study*

Compound	*Type of study*	*Dose* (mg)	*Total No. of patients*	*Success* 24 h		48 h		*Mean No. of episodes*		*Cervical injury* (%)	*Complete abortion* (%)
				No.	%	*No.*	%	*Vomiting*	*Diarrhoea*		
15-Methyl-$PGF_{2\alpha}$	Pilot study	2.5	311	238	76.4	296	95.2	1.9	0.7	NR	49.0
$PGF_{2\alpha}$	Randomized	40	251	136	54.1	205	81.7†	1.5†	0.4‡	NR	52.1
15-methyl-$PGF_{2\alpha}$	Comparison	2.5	275	198	72.0	263	95.6†	2.1†	1.3‡		51.3
$PGF_{2\alpha}$	Randomized	50	351	238	67.8	304	86.6‡	1.3	0.5‡	2.9	55.3
15-methyl-$PGF_{2\alpha}$	Comparison	2.5	333	247	74.1	309	92.8‡	1.7	1.2‡	2.9	55.3

*WHO Task Force on the Use of Prostaglandins for the Regulation of Fertility (1977a)
†$p < 0.001$
‡$p < 0.05$
NR = Not reported

detail (Karim and Amy, 1975; Karim, 1976). In this section, the results of a multicentre, multinational study involving 1521 patients treated with intra-amniotic $PGF_{2\alpha}$ or 15-methyl-$PGF_{2\alpha}$ will be reviewed. The trial was carried out in three parts (WHO Multicentre Study, 1977a).

Study 1: Pilot study to evaluate the efficacy of 2.5 mg 15-methyl-$PGF_{2\alpha}$ administered intra-amniotically in 311 patients with a mean gestational age of 17.1 weeks.

Study 2: Randomized comparison of 2.5 mg 15-methyl-$PGF_{2\alpha}$ and 40 mg intra-amniotically in a total of 526 patients divided into two groups closely matched for health, status, height, weight, gravidity and parity.

Study 3: Randomized comparison of 2.5 mg of 15-methyl-$PGF_{2\alpha}$ and 50 mg $PGF_{2\alpha}$ intra-amniotically in a total of 684 patients divided into two groups matched for physical characteristics.

The results of the trial are shown in Table 17.4. The highest success rate in the $PGF_{2\alpha}$ group at 48 h was 86.6% compared to 95.6% in the 15-methyl-$PGF_{2\alpha}$ group. The mean induction–abortion times in the three studies were similar and ranged between 18 and 20 h. In the two randomized studies the frequency of complete abortion was similar for both $PGF_{2\alpha}$ and 15-methyl-$PGF_{2\alpha}$. The frequency of heavy bleeding (>500 ml) in the 40 mg and 50 mg $PGF_{2\alpha}$ groups was 3.8% and 3.1% respectively, compared to 1.2% and 2.3% respectively, in the two 15-methyl-$PGF_{2\alpha}$ groups.

Both vomiting and diarrhoea were significantly more common following 15-methyl-$PGF_{2\alpha}$ than following 40 and 50 mg $PGF_{2\alpha}$ (Table 17.4).

In Study 3 each patient was examined vaginally immediately after the abortion. Cervical damage was found in 20 patients equally distributed between the two treatment groups and representing an overall frequency of 2.9%.

In another multicentre clinical trial carried out at 18 teaching hospitals under the sponsorship of the Indian Council for Medical Research, the efficacy and side-effects of intra-amniotic 15-methyl-$PGF_{2\alpha}$ (2.5 mg) and $PGF_{2\alpha}$ (50 mg) were evaluated in 921 women (Tejuja *et al.*, 1978). Results from 885 women of whom 430 received $PGF_{2\alpha}$ and 455 were given 15-methyl-$PGF_{2\alpha}$ are shown in Table 17.5.

The incidence of vomiting and diarrhoea was similar to that reported in the WHO Multicentre Study (1977a). There was a higher incidence of cervical injury (4.7%) in the $PGF_{2\alpha}$ group than in the 15-methyl-$PGF_{2\alpha}$ group. One death occurred in a multiparous woman at 18 weeks gestation who experienced no uterine contraction following intra-amniotic instillation of 50 mg $PGF_{2\alpha}$. Sixty-four hours after instillation of $PGF_{2\alpha}$ the patient developed tonic uterine contractions 'without additional therapy'. Six hours later she was found to have a ruptured uterus and hysterectomy was performed. She died during the operation. Another patient, also a multiparous woman at 20 weeks' gestation, aborted completely 4 h after intra-amniotic instillation of 2.5 mg 15-methyl-$PGF_{2\alpha}$. The patient was readmitted to the hospital 12 days after abortion with severe vaginal bleeding. She went into shock during hysterectomy and died.

It has been suggested previously that efficacy similar to that reported in above studies can be achieved with a smaller dose of 15-methyl-$PGF_{2\alpha}$ (Karim and Sivasamboo, 1975; Karim, 1976). Use of the lower dose results in a considerable reduction in side-effects and complications.

Table 17.5 Comparison of intra-amniotic $PGF_{2\alpha}$ (50 mg) and 15-methyl-$PGF_{2\alpha}$ (2.5 mg) for the termination of second trimester pregnancy: results of a multicentre study*

	$PGF_{2\alpha}$	15-methyl-$PGF_{2\alpha}$
Number of patients	430	455
Dose	50 mg	2.5 mg
Success rate (48 h)	88.1%	93.0%
Induction–abortion interval (h)	19.2	19.3
Complete abortion	48.8%	56.0%
Blood loss >500 ml	2.4%	1.4%
Vomiting (mean No. of episode/patient)	1.1	1.3
Diarrhoea (mean No. of episode/patient)	0.6	1.2
Cervical injury	4.7%	1.4%
Maternal death (No.)	1	1

*Data from Tejuja *et al.* (1978)

Commenting upon the higher rate of incomplete abortion and gastrointestinal side-effects in the WHO Multicentre Study discussed above, Grimes *et al.* (1978) point to a total morbidity rate of 2.77 per 100 abortions among 2500 patients who had undergone mid-trimester abortion by dilatation and evacuation. Moreover, the largest multicentre study of abortion to date has documented a rate for retained products of conception of 0.9 per 100 procedures among 6213 abortions by dilatation and evacuation in the 13 to 20 week interval of pregnancy. Grimes *et al.* (1978) suggest that 'mid-trimester abortion by dilatation and evacuation, a frequently used technique in the United States, appears to obviate most of the problems of incomplete abortion as well as the long induction–abortion times and the high rates of haemorrhage and infections associated with instillation methods of mid-trimester abortion'.

In reply to comments by Grimes *et al.* (1978), members of the WHO Prostaglandin Task Force (Borell *et al.*, 1978) have pointed out that there has not yet been conducted a randomized study systemically comparing surgical evacuation with other methods in second trimester pregnancy. 'We note the findings previously reported by Grimes and his colleagues that in weeks 13 to 20 of gestation cervical injury was twice as frequent and uterine perforation more than six times as frequent with dilatation and evacuation as compared with the saline infusion technique. It may also be mentioned that many reports cite a higher frequency of haemorrhage and infection following surgical evacuation than do Grimes and co-workers'. The dilatation and evacuation method of terminating second trimester pregnancy is now the method of choice for relatively few American gynaecologists and even fewer European gynaecologists.

17.2.3 Combination of $PGF_{2\alpha}$ and urea

In order to terminate second trimester pregnancies with a single intra-amniotic injection within 24 h, Craft *et al.* (1974) explored the use of a combination of $PGF_{2\alpha}$ (20 mg) and urea (80 g) in 20 patients. All aborted within 24 h in a mean time of 12 h 38 min (range 5 h 50 min to 20 h 45 min). However, gastro-intestinal side-effects occurred with a greater frequency than when a comparative dose of $PGF_{2\alpha}$ is given alone. Twelve patients (60%) experienced vomiting (mean of 2.83 episodes per patient) and two (10%) had diarrhoea. Unilateral cervical laceration, approximately 2 cm in length requiring suture occurred in two patients. The authors have suggested that urea probably increases the systemic absorption of $PGF_{2\alpha}$ from the amniotic cavity and causes increased incidence of gastro-intestinal side-effects and over-stimulation of the uterus.

Table 17.6 Results of termination of second trimester pregnancy with intra-amniotic urea + $PGF_{2\alpha}$ or intra-amniotic urea + intravenous oxytocin*

Treatment	*No. of cases*	*Complete abortion*		*Incomplete abortion*		*Failure*		*Instillation–abortion interval†*
		No.	*%*	*No.*	*%*	*No.*	*%*	*mean and range*
80 g urea‡ + 10 mg $PGF_{2\alpha}$	30	19	63.3	11	36.7	0	0	15.75 (2.67–31.00)
80 g urea + 332 mU per min oxytocin infusion	29	20	66.7	9	30.0	1	3.3	18.93 (6.92–42.67)
80 g urea‡ + 10 mg $PGF_{2\alpha}$	150	79	52.6	70	46.7	1	0.7	16.45 (2.50–48.33)

*Data from Burkman *et al.* (1976)
†From intra-amniotic injection to abortion of foetus
‡55.1% and 76.0% of patients respectively were given intravenous oxytocin at varying intervals after intra-amniotic instillation of urea + $PGF_{2\alpha}$

In order to reduce the side-effects and complications, Burkman *et al.* (1976) used 10 mg $PGF_{2\alpha}$ and 80 g urea in 30 second trimester patients. Those who failed to abort during the subsequent 24 h or 4 h after rupture of the membranes were given intravenous oxytocin in an effort to reduce the incidence of prolonged injection–abortion interval and prevent failure. The effectiveness of this technique was compared in a randomized study with another group of 30 patients given 80 g urea intra-amniotically and simultaneous oxytocin infusion at 332 mU/min. Following the randomized study the $PGF_{2\alpha}$–urea combination (10 mg and 80 g respectively) was used to terminate second trimester pregnancies in an additional 150 patients. The results in the three groups are shown in Table 17.6. The mean intra-amniotic instillation–abortion time in the urea + $PGF_{2\alpha}$ group was 15.75 h and in urea + intravenous oxytocin group it was 18.93 h. The difference was not statistically significant. The incidence of side-effects and complications in the three groups is shown in Table 17.7.

Table 17.7 Complications and side-effects in three groups of patients treated with intra-amniotic urea and $PGF_{2\alpha}$ or intra-amniotic urea and intravenous oxytocin*

Complications and side-effects	*Urea 80 g + $PGF_{2\alpha}$ 10 mg* (n = 30)	*Urea 80 g + oxytocin 332 mU/min* (n = 30)	*Urea 80 g + $PGF_{2\alpha}$ 10 mg* (n = 150)
Failed primary procedure	0 (0.0%)	1 (3.3%)	10 (6.6%)
Haemorrhage >500 ml	4 (13.3%)	1 (3.3%)	10 (6.6%)
Infection	0 (0.0%)	0 (0.0%)	3 (2.0%)
Vomiting	21 (70.0%)	18 (60.0%)	105 (70.0%)
Inadvertent intravascular injection of urea	0 (0.0%)	1 (3.3%)	1 (0.66%)
Cervical laceration	0 (0.0%)	0 (0.0%)	6 (4.0%)

*Data from Burkman *et al.* (1976)
n = Number of patients

More than 50% of the patients in the two urea–$PGF_{2\alpha}$ group required supplementary oxytocin infusion for failure to abort within 24 h of urea–$PGF_{2\alpha}$ instillation or 4 h following rupture of the membranes and for retained placenta or post-abortion bleeding.

Vomiting occurred in 70% of the patients in the urea–$PGF_{2\alpha}$ group and in 60% of the patients in the urea–oxytocin group. The most serious complication which occurred in the urea–$PGF_{2\alpha}$ group was cervical laceration requiring repair in six patients.

A further reduction in the dose of $PGF_{2\alpha}$ to 5 mg combined with 80 g urea has been reported to reduce the incidence of some side-effects without significantly affecting the injection–abortion interval. Results of two dose regimes (5 mg $PGF_{2\alpha}$ + 80 g urea and 10 mg $PGF_{2\alpha}$ + 80 g urea) in a total of 330 patients are compared in Table 17.8.

Wilson (1978) employed a combination of intra-amniotic urea, $PGF_{2\alpha}$, intracervical laminaria and intravenous oxytocin for termination of second trimester pregnancy. The study was carried out in three groups of patients. A laminaria was inserted into the cervical canal on the afternoon prior to admission. As much amniotic fluid as possible was withdrawn (10–200 ml) and the patients were treated with one of the following regimes:

(1) 40 mg $PGF_{2\alpha}$ intra-amniotically and simultaneous intravenous oxytocin infusion (78 patients).

(2) Urea 40 g intra-amniotically and simultaneous intravenous oxytocin (86 patients).

(3) Urea 40 g and $PGF_{2\alpha}$ 20 mg intra-amniotically and simultaneous intravenous oxytocin (113 patients).

Table 17.8 Comparison of urea and 10 mg $PGF_{2\alpha}$ with urea and 5 mg $PGF_{2\alpha}$

	*80 g urea + 10 mg $PGF_{2\alpha}$**	*80 g urea + 5 mg $PGF_{2\alpha}$†*
No. of patients	180	150
Injection–abortion interval	16.3 ± 0.07	17.5 ± 0.7
Complete abortion %	55.0	63.0
Failure %	0.6	0.7
Haemorrhage %	7.8	10.1
Infection %	6.7	2.0
Cervical laceration %	3.3	0.7
Nausea, vomiting %	70.0	63.0
Diarrhoea %	1.1	0.0

* Data from Burkman *et al.* (1976)
† Data from King *et al.* (1977)

The mean injection–abortion time in the urea + $PGF_{2\alpha}$ (with oxytocin + laminaria) group was impressively short (8 h 42 min). The criteria for success or the number of patients who aborted was not included in the publication. The author claimed that only 10% of the patients treated with this regime experienced gastro-intestinal side-effects and none suffered cervical laceration. No information on other side-effects (infection, bleeding, etc.) was given by the authors.

17.2.4 Combination of PGE_2 and urea

A combination of urea and PGE_2 administered intra-amniotically for the termination of second trimester pregnancy has been employed by several investigators. In most studies the dose of urea has been kept constant at 80 g but the dose of PGE_2 has varied between 2.5 and 10 mg.

In the first study reported by Craft (1973) the mean injection–abortion interval in 15 patients given 10 mg PGE_2 was 26 h 49 min. This was significantly longer than the mean time of 10 h 30 min in a further 15 patients given a combination of 80 g urea and 10 mg PGE_2. Three patients in the PGE_2 group had vomiting and none had diarrhoea. In contrast, 11 patients (out of 15) in the PGE_2–urea group had vomiting and three had diarrhoea. Abortion was complete in four out of 15 patients in the PGE_2 group and in nine out of 15 in the PGE_2–urea group. There was no excessive blood loss in any patient in either group.

Bowen-Simpkins (1973) used 80 g urea and 5 mg PGE_2 in 31 patients. Thirty aborted in a mean time of 10 h 30 min. Abortion was complete in 25 patients. One patient had diarrhoea, four were severely nauseated and nine patients vomited on one or more occasions. In one patient a partial annular detachment of the cervix was noted.

In order to reduce the side-effects further Craft (1975) used a smaller dose of PGE_2 (2.5 mg) in combination with 80 g urea in 110 patients. All aborted in a mean time of 10 h 41 min. In spite of the low dose of PGE_2 used, serious side-effects (cervical laceration and haemorrhage) not encountered in his previous study with 10 mg PGE_2 and 80 g urea (Craft, 1973) were present. Vomiting occurred in 46% of the patients, cervical laceration in 4.5%, pyrexia in 3%, and 2% required blood transfusion.

It would appear that although attempts to reduce the injection–abortion interval by a combination of methods have been successful, this is usually associated with a damage to the uterus or the cervix.

17.2.5 Combination of $PGF_{2\alpha}$ and hypertonic saline

Adachi *et al.* (1977) compared the efficacy of 20 mg $PGF_{2\alpha}$ combined with four different doses of hypertonic saline in 309 patients in the second trimester of pregnancy.

Group 1 100 ml 5% sodium chloride (39 cases)
Group 2 100 ml 10% sodium chloride (48 cases)
Group 3 35 ml 20% sodium chloride (167 cases)
Group 4 50 ml 20% sodium chloride (55 cases)

All patients received intravenous oxytocin at an average rate of 40 mU/min starting immediately following the $PGF_{2\alpha}$–saline injection. The patients in the four groups were matched for age and parity. All women in the four groups aborted and only two required a second intra-amniotic injection. The results are summarized in Table 17.9.

Table 17.9 Results of termination of pregnancy with intra-amniotic $PGF_{2\alpha}$, hypertonic saline and intravenous oxytocin*

Results	*100 ml 5% sodium chloride and 20 mg $PGF_{2\alpha}$ (n = 39)*	*100 ml 10% sodium chloride and 20 mg $PGF_{2\alpha}$ (n = 48)*	*25 ml 20% sodium chloride and 20 mg $PGF_{2\alpha}$ (n = 127)*	*50 ml 20% sodium chloride and 20 mg $PGF_{2\alpha}$ (n = 55)*
Injection–abortion interval (mean + SD)	22.15 ± 13.96	19.99 ± 8.75	18.55 ± 12.12	15.52 ± 7.55
Number of patients:				
Vomiting	3	1	8	6
Nausea	0	0	1	0
Diarrhoea	0	0	1	0
Fever	0	0	3	2
Chills	0	0	1	0
Fainting	0	0	1	0
Maternal deaths	0	0	1	0

Data from Adachi *et al.* (1977)
*All patients received intravenous oxytocin at 40 mU/min starting immediately after the $PGF_{2\alpha}$–saline injection

There was one maternal death in a patient treated with 20 mg $PGF_{2\alpha}$ and 25 ml 20% saline. The death occurred 34 h after drug administration and 16 h after the abortion due to intravascular haemolysis or consumption coagulopathy secondary to septicaemia. Blood transfusion was required in 3.3% of cases.

The authors consider that 20 mg $PGF_{2\alpha}$ and 25 or 50 ml 20% saline combination is better than the use of larger amounts of $PGF_{2\alpha}$ or of hypertonic saline alone.

In another study the efficacy and side-effects of intra-amniotic $PGF_{2\alpha}$ (40 mg) in combination with hypertonic saline (50 ml 20% solution) in 102 patients were compared with hypertonic saline alone in a similar number of patients (Borten, 1976). One hundred and one patients in the combination therapy group aborted within 72 h compared to 96 out of 102 in the saline group. The instillation to abortion time of 18.8 h in the combined agent group was significantly shorter than 34.0 h in the hypertonic saline group but not significantly shorter when compared to groups of patients aborted by intra-amniotic $PGF_{2\alpha}$ alone in other studies (e.g. Lauersen and Wilson, 1974). Side-effects of nausea and vomiting occurred more frequently in $PGF_{2\alpha}$–saline group. One patient in the saline group suffered a cervical laceration.

17.2.6 $PGF_{2\alpha}$ and calcium gluconate

Calcium is required for maximal contractility of uterine muscle (Carsten, 1972). Weinstein *et al.* (1976) have tested the hypothesis that the addition of calcium to intra-amniotic prostaglandin might result in 'a more efficient and/or physiologic second trimester abortion'. The authors injected 40 mg $PGF_{2\alpha}$ and one or two grams calcium gluconate intra-amniotically in a group of 10 patients in the second trimester of pregnancy. Fifty per cent of the patients were pregnant for the first time. All patients aborted within 20¼ h in a mean time of 13 h 28 min compared with a mean time of over 20 h reported by other investigators. There were no complications. The results of this pilot study remains to be confirmed in a larger group of patients.

17.3 EXTRA-AMNIOTIC ROUTE

17.3.1 PGE_2 and $PGF_{2\alpha}$ in viscous gel

Termination of pregnancy by extra-amniotic prostaglandins involves either intermittent injections at 1–2 h intervals or a continuous infusion using a mechanical pump (see Karim and Amy, 1975). In order to simplify the procedure, MacKenzie and Embrey (1976a) have explored the use of a single extra-amniotic injection of PGE_2 or $PGF_{2\alpha}$ in a highly viscous gel to induce abortion in 230 patients between 9 and 24 weeks gestation. PGE_2 in doses of

1.0, 1.5, 2.0 or 3.0 mg induced abortion within 24 h in 30%, 75%, 76% and 70% of the patients, respectively. The incidence of gastro-intestinal side-effects was dose dependent and ranged between 20% and 70%. A 10 mg dose of $PGF_{2\alpha}$ in viscous gel induced abortion within 24 h in 66% of the patients and 45% had gastro-intestinal side-effects. Abortion was complete in 75% of the patients with PGE_2 and 36% treated with $PGF_{2\alpha}$. The authors consider that the technique significantly reduced individual patient care and minimized the potential risk of intrauterine sepsis associated with extra-amniotic techniques requiring repeated or continuous prostaglandin administration.

17.3.2 Comparison between $PGF_{2\alpha}$ and rivanol

Rivanol (acridol) is a derivative of the dye acridine with antiseptic properties and has been used for the termination of first and second trimester pregnancies. Himmelman *et al.* (1975) compared the efficacy and side-effects of rivanol and $PGF_{2\alpha}$ in two groups of patients. Both drugs were administered extra-amniotically. One group of 200 second trimester patients were treated with 0.1% rivanol, 10 ml per week of gestation up to a maximum of 150 ml introduced via a Foley catheter. If contractions did not start within 24 h, an intravenous infusion of oxytocin was given. The treatment was considered

Table 17.10 Complications and side-effects in patients treated with rivanol and $PGF_{2\alpha}$

Complications and side-effects	*Rivanol group % of patients (n = 200)*	*$PGF_{2\alpha}$ group % of patients (n = 50)*
Vomiting	Not recorded	18
Diarrhoea	0	0
Bleeding	1.5	8
'Manifest infection'	1	8
'Suspected infection'	8	6
Cervical rupture	0.5	0
Uterine rupture	0	2

Data from Himmelmann *et al.* (1975)
n = Number of patients

successful if the patient aborted within 72 h after instillation of rivanol. Fifty patients received $PGF_{2\alpha}$. After an initial 250 µg test dose, 750 µg $PGF_{2\alpha}$ was administered every 2 h. This dose was reduced to 500 µg if uterine contractions were painful. $PGF_{2\alpha}$ administration was continued for 36 h and the treatment was considered a success if the patient aborted within 48 h after the first dose.

In the rivanol group, 88% of the patients aborted within 72 h in a mean time of 30 h. In the $PGF_{2\alpha}$ group, 80% of the patients aborted within 48 h.

Side-effects and complications in the $PGF_{2\alpha}$ group were higher than in the rivanol group and are shown in Table 17.10.

The authors concluded that the rivanol method is accompanied by few complications, is easy to handle and has 'few, if any contraindications, circumstances which are of considerable importance to hospital staff involved'. The essential advantage of the $PGF_{2\alpha}$ method is its more rapid abortifacient effect especially in conjunction with individual dosage.

17.3.3 Combination of $PGF_{2\alpha}$ and rivanol

In an attempt to increase the efficacy and reduce the side-effects, a combination of agents have been used to terminate second trimester pregnancies. One such combination that has been explored is rivanol and $PGF_{2\alpha}$. Such a procedure could combine the advantage of immediate uterotonic effect of $PGF_{2\alpha}$ with the delayed oxytocic response to rivanol. Martin *et al.* (1975) treated one group of 10 patients (gestation 13–18 weeks) with 130–150 ml 1% rivanol administered extra-amniotically and another group of 16 patients with a similar amount of rivanol plus a single dose of 750 μg $PGF_{2\alpha}$ immediately or 1 h after rivanol.

Five out of 10 patients in the rivanol alone group failed to abort within 48 h whereas 11 patients out of 16 in the rivanol plus $PGF_{2\alpha}$ group aborted within 31 h after instillation of the drugs.

Side-effects included vomiting which occurred twice as often in the rivanol plus $PGF_{2\alpha}$ group than in the rivanol alone group. Patients treated with rivanol required on an average 1.1 injections of analgesic compared to 3.1 injections in the combination therapy group.

On the basis of this small pilot study the authors consider that combined administration of rivanol with $PGF_{2\alpha}$ 'avoids, in many patients, inconvenient repeated administration of a primary prostaglandin compound. This modification of the extra-amniotic method has other advantages for clinical application – the procedure is simple; side-effects are acceptable; inadvertent intravascular injection is harmless and the possibility of infection is reduced since rivanol itself is an antiseptic solution'. However, experience with such a combination is limited and further clinical trials are necessary before its merit can be judged.

17.3.4 15-Methyl-$PGF_{2\alpha}$

Extra-amniotic route of PGE_2 and $PGF_{2\alpha}$ administration for pregnancy termination usually involves repeated or continuous administration via an indwelling catheter (see Karim and Amy, 1975). Because of the longer duration of uterine muscle stimulating action of 15-methyl-$PGF_{2\alpha}$, the efficacy of this compound administered extra-amniotically for pregnancy termination has been explored (MacKenzie and Embrey, 1976b). In a multicentre clinical trial sponsored by the WHO Prostaglandin Task Force (1977b), the efficacy and side-effects of 15-methyl-$PGF_{2\alpha}$ have been evaluated. A total of 660 patients at 10–20 weeks gestation were given a single extra-amniotic dose of 0.92 mg 15-methyl-$PGF_{2\alpha}$ in Hyskon (Dextran 70, 32%). Abortion of the foetus occurred within 24 h in 479 patients (72.6%) and within 36 h in 530 (80.3%). Abortion was complete in 31% of the patients. The incidence of gastro-intestinal and other side-effects was significantly lower than encountered with intramuscular administration of this compound (Table 17.11).

Table 17.11 Termination of pregnancy with a single extra-amniotic dose of 0.92 mg 15-methyl-$PGF_{2\alpha}$ in Hyskon*

	Number	*Percentage*
Patients	660	100
Primigravidae	193	29.2
Multigravidae	467	70.8
Gestation (10–20 weeks)		
Foetus expelled		
24 h	479	72.6
30 h	509	77.1
36 h	530	80.3
Side-effects:		
Diarrhoea	212	32.2
Vomiting	246	37.7
Flushing	22	3.3
Chest pain	7	1.1
Blood loss >500 ml	5	0.75
Cervical laceration	1	0.15

Data from WHO Task Force on the Use of Prostaglandins for Regulation of Fertility (1977b)
*Dextran 70, 30%

In another multicentre study a total of 1648 women with a mean gestational age between 10 and 20 weeks (mean 14.4 weeks) were treated with a single extra-amniotic dose of 1 mg 15-methyl-$PGF_{2\alpha}$ in Hyskon. Of these, 79 women were excluded from the study because of 'technical failure in instillation of the drug or because protocol procedure was not adhered to'. Out of the remaining 1569 patients 78.1% aborted during the 36 h following instillation of 15-methyl-$PGF_{2\alpha}$. Abortion was complete in 23% of the patients. The average number of episodes of vomiting and diarrhoea was 0.9 per patient. Cervical injury was reported in 0.6% of the patients. There was one death from uncontrollable post-partum vaginal bleeding in a woman who aborted 10 h after instillation of $PGF_{2\alpha}$. The overall incidence of haemorrhage (blood loss >500 ml) was low at 0.6% (Tejuja *et al*., 1978).

17.3.5 2a,2b-Dihomo-15-methyl-$PGF_{2\alpha}$ methyl ester

Karim (1976) reported on the use of another synthetic analogue administered by the extra-amniotic route for termination of late first and early second trimester pregnancies. 2a,2b-Dihomo-15(S)15-methyl-$PGF_{2\alpha}$ methyl ester given as a single 1 mg extra-amniotic dose produced abortion in 270 (85.4%)

out of 316 patients of whom 260 (82.3%) aborted within 24 h. In patients who failed to abort with a single dose, or where gestation was 14 weeks or less, the cervix was sufficiently dilated to evacuate the uterus by vacuum aspiration and curettage. The remaining subjects were given a second dose of the prostaglandin analogue (24 h after the first dose) and all aborted during the subsequent 24 h. The onset of uterine activity with this compound was slower than with 15-methyl-$PGF_{2\alpha}$. Gastro-intestinal side-effects were significantly less frequent than with 15-methyl-$PGF_{2\alpha}$. During the past 4 years this analogue has been in routine use for the termination of late first trimester and early second trimester pregnancy in several hospitals in Singapore. Results (unpublished) from over 1200 patients confirm the findings of the above study.

17.3.6 16-Phenoxy-ω-17,18,19,20-tetranor-PGE_2 methyl sulphonylamide (sulprostone)

Sulprostone given by the extra-amniotic route in a single dose of 25–50 μg has been used in the termination of second trimester pregnancies. The success rate has varied between 60% and 95% in different trials. The results are summarized by Ulbrich and Bartels (1979).

17.4 INTRAMUSCULAR ROUTE

17.4.1 15-Methyl-$PGF_{2\alpha}$

Although prostaglandins administered by intra-amniotic and extra-amniotic routes are effective in the termination of second trimester pregnancy, there is considerable interest in developing alternative routes of administration that do not involve invasion of the uterus. The efficacy of 15(S)15-methyl-$PGF_{2\alpha}$ in the termination of first and second trimester pregnancies by the intramuscular route was first reported by Karim *et al.* (1972). Since then a large number of clinical trials to evaluate the abortifacient action of this analogue have been carried out. Results from some of these studies (which include both first and second trimester patients) are summarized in Table 17.12. Success rates approaching 100% have been reported by most investigators using different dose schedules. While the efficacy of 15-methyl-$PGF_{2\alpha}$ is not in doubt, it is generally agreed that the incidence of vomiting and diarrhoea is too high (in spite of pre-medication to counteract these side-effects) to use this compound on a routine basis.

The use of laminaria tents 12–18 h before starting treatment with 15-methyl-$PGF_{2\alpha}$ results in a significant reduction in injection–abortion interval (see Table 17.12).

15-Methyl-$PGF_{2\alpha}$ given by the intramuscular route has also been successfully used for induction of second trimester abortion in high-risk pregnancy (Kinra *et al.*, 1977).

Table 17.12 Termination of pregnancy with intramuscular administration of 15(S)15-methyl-PGF$_{2\alpha}$

References	*No. of cases*	*Gestation range* (weeks)	*Dose schedule*	*Success rate* (%)	*Mean I/A interval* (h)	*Pre-medication*	*Side-effects and complications* (%)	*Complete abortion* (%)
Karim *et al.*, 1972	5	7–15	250–500 μg 8 hourly	100[1]	20	Nil	V = 60; D = 100	60
Liebman *et al.*, 1974	16	2nd trimester	250 μg 8 hourly Max. 3 doses	56.2[2]	20.2	Nil	N = 62.5; V = 68.7; D = 37.5; F = 6.25; H = 6.25	43.75
Bygdeman *et al.*, 1974	30	15.2 (mean)	200–500 μg 3 hourly	100[3]	16.1	Lomotil 5 mg orally and thiethyparazine 6.5 mg rectally ½ h before first 3 doses	V = 4.7 episodes/patient D = 0.7 episodes/patient F = 10	40
Sharma *et al.*, 1975	10	14–18	250 μg 3 hourly	90[2]	26.0	Nil	V = 95; D = 100; P = 10; H = 10; F = 25	80
Sharma *et al.*, 1975	20	14–20	250 μg 3 hourly	100[1]	9.8	1–3 laminaria evening before prostaglandin. 5 mg Lomotil 2 and 10 h before prostaglandin. Compazine 10 mg i.m. 1 h before prostaglandin	V = 26.9; D = 11.5; F = 19.2	90
Lauersen and Wilson, 1975	35	10–21	250 μg 2 hourly for 24 h; 750 μg 2 hourly until abortion	100[2]	16.0	Compazine 10 mg i.m. 6 hourly. Lomotil 10 mg oral; 5 mg 2 hourly	V = 65; D = 71.4; P = 22.8	85.7

Table 17.12—*continued*

Bolognese and Corson, 1975	80	8–22	350–500 μg 2 hourly	100[2]	15.7	Lomotil (prophylactic) chlorperazine when required	V = 89; D = 89; P = 18	65.0
Ylikorkala and Jarvinen, 1975	25	10–20	200 μg initial dose 300 μg 3 hourly Max. 30 h	80[1]	15.0	Lomotil 5 mg ½ h before first 3 doses	V = 84; D = 92; P = 4	NS
Ballard and Slaughter, 1976	50	12–20	200 μg initial dose, 300 μg 3 hourly Max. 30 h	84[1]	14.6	Lomotil 5 mg initial dose 2.5 mg ½ h before next 3 doses of prostaglandin. Chlorpromazine 50 mg 4 hourly	V = 56; D = 52; F = 26; P = 4; W = 4; R = 2	70
Lange and Secher, 1977	68	10–21	250 μg 2 hourly	97[2]	16.4	Lomotil 5 mg, 2.5 mg repeated as required. Prochlorperazine 12.5 mg i.m., 4–6 hourly	V = 79; D = 86; uterine rupture (1 case); H = 4.0	NS
WHO-multicentre study, 1977c	515	10–20	Initial dose 200 μg followed by 300 μg 3 hourly	84.9[1]	14.7	5 mg Lomotil ½ h before first 3 doses	V = 2.9 episodes/patient D = 2.8 episodes/patient F = 14.2; Cx. L = 0.6	35

N = Nausea; V = Vomiting; D = Diarrhoea; P = Pyrexia; Cx. L = Cervical laceration; R = Rigor; F = Flushing; H = Haemorrhage; NS = Not stated
[1] = Foetus expelled within 30 hours after first injection
[2] = Foetus expelled within 36 hours after first injection
[3] = Criteria for success Not defined

Table 17.13 Termination of pregnancy with intramuscular administration of 15(S)15-methyl-PGE_2

References	*No. of cases*	*Gestation range* (weeks)	*Dose schedule*	*Success rate* (%)	*Mean I/A interval* (h)	*Pre-medication*	*Side-effects and complications* (%)	*Complete abortion* (%)
Karim *et al.*, 1972	8	7–16	25–50 μg 8 hourly	100[1]	10.1	Nil	D = 12.5; R = 50; P = 12.5	50
Ballard and Quilligan, 1974	20	12–19	10 μg 2 hourly	95[1]	9.1	Chlorpromazine 25 mg ½ h before prostaglandin	V = 50; D = 85; R = 100; P = 100	75
Dillon *et al.*, 1975	32	13–20	50 μg 8 hourly or 5 μg 2 hourly or 5 μg 4 hourly	87.5[2]	15.8	Nil	V = 28.1; D = 31.2; R = 28.1; P = 28.1; H = 6.2; S = 3.1	68.7
Brenner *et al.*, 1975	21	7–20	10 μg 4 hourly	100[3]	17.6	10 mg Prochlorperazine i.m. 6 hourly and 75 mg mepederine every 2–4 h at the request of patient	V = 62; D = 86; R = 76; P = 76	67
Brenner *et al.*, 1975	21	7–20	10 μg 4 hourly	90[3]	19.5	10 mg Prochlorperazine i.m., 10 mg Lomotil, 1.3 g acetylsalicylic acid and 30 ml Maalox orally 1 h before prostaglandin: some of these drugs repeated subsequently	V = 43; D = 19; R = 52; P = 43; C = 5	74
Lauersen *et al.*, 1975	30	10–23	5 μg initial dose 10 μg 1 h later followed by 10 μg every 2 h	96.7[1]	9.52	10 mg Prochlorperazine i.m. 6 hourly, 10 mg Lomotil every 2 h	V = 16.3; D = 3.3; P = 96.7; R = 16.3	66.6
Stubblefield *et al.*, 1976	21	13–20	10 μg 2 hourly	80[1]	12.2	10 mg Prochlorperazine i.m., Lomotil oral 4 hourly	V = 66; D = 76; P = 90	50
Stubblefield *et al.*, 1976	13	13–20	10 μg 2 hourly	100[1]	9.4	1–3 laminaria tents 14–18 h before prostaglandin	V = 33; D = 33; P = 56	50

N = Nausea; V = Vomiting; D = Diarrhoea; P = Pyrexia; R = Rigor; S = Shock; H = Haemorrhage; C = Convulsion
[1] = Foetus expelled within 24 hours
[2] = Foetus expelled within 30 hours
[3] = Foetus expelled within 48 hours

17.4.2 15-Methyl-PGF$_{2\alpha}$ methyl ester

15(S)15-Methyl-PGE$_2$ methyl ester (15-methyl-PGE$_2$) has also been used to terminate first and second trimester pregnancies by the intramuscular route. The results of several clinical trials are summarized in Table 17.13. Apart from vomiting and diarrhoea, pyrexia is a common side-effect associated with the intramuscular administration of this analogue. Pre-medication of patients with anti-emetic and antidiarrhoeals reduced the incidence of side-effects (Brenner *et al.*, 1975; Lauersen *et al.*, 1975; Stubblefield *et al.*, 1976).

17.4.3 16,16-Dimethyl-PGE$_2$ *p*-benzaldehyde semicarbazone ester

16,16-Dimethyl-PGE$_2$ *p*-benzaldehyde semicarbazone ester given by the intramuscular route is also effective in the termination of second trimester pregnancy. Thirty-six patients at 14–22 weeks gestation were given intramuscular injection of 300 μg of the analogue every 5 h. All aborted in a mean time of 13.4 h (range 2–32 h). Side-effects were vomiting (20%), diarrhoea (6%) and pyrexia (15%) (Karim and Ratnam, 1977a).

17.4.4 16-Phenoxy-ω-17,18,19,20-tetranor-PGE$_2$ methyl sulphonylamide (sulprostone)

16-Phenoxy-ω-17,18,19,20-tetranor-PGE$_2$ methyl sulphonylamide (sulprostone) has been described as a 'tissue selective' prostaglandin (Hess *et al.*, 1977). When administered by the intravenous or intrauterine routes this compound is effective in terminating first and second trimester pregnancies (Karim *et al.*, 1977; Pulkkinen, 1978; Rizk *et al.*, 1978; Lichtenegger, 1977; Schmidt-Gollwitzer *et al.*, 1977). The results of a multicentre trial with this prostaglandin analogue given by different routes for the termination of pregnancy were recently reviewed at the International Sulprostone Symposium held in Vienna and details will shortly be published in the Proceedings of the Symposium (Ulbrich and Bartels, 1979). It would appear that sulprostone given by different routes produces second trimester abortion with a low incidence of side-effects. Of particular interest is the efficacy of this prostaglandin in the termination of second trimester pregnancy by the intramuscular route with a low incidence of side-effects. Results of some published studies are briefly reviewed in this section.

Karim and Ratnam (1978) and Karim *et al.* (1978) used sulprostone in 60 second trimester patients. The drug was injected intramuscularly in doses of 0.5 mg 4 hourly, 1 mg 6 hourly or 1 mg 8 hourly for a maximum of 36 h. Fifty-five patients aborted. The mean first injection to abortion time in the three groups was 18.0, 18.25 and 20.5 h, respectively (Table 17.14). The incidence of side-effects was low and is shown in Table 17.15.

Table 17.14 Results of termination of second trimester pregnancy by intramuscular injection of 16-phenoxy-ω-17,18,19,20-tetranor-PGE$_2$ methyl sulphonylamide

Group No. and dose of prostaglandin	*Foetus expelled in 36 h*						*Injection–abortion interval (h) Mean and range*		
	Nulliparae		*Multiparae*		*Total*				
	No.	*Percentage*	*No.*	*Percentage*	*No.*	*Percentage*	*Nulliparae*	*Multiparae*	*Whole group*
Group 1 0.5 mg 4 hourly	10/10	100	8/10	80	18/20	90	19.2 (8.2–26.00)	17.0 (4.5–31.00)	18.0
Group 2 1 mg 8 hourly	9/10	90	9/10	90	18/20	90	24.25 (14.75–32.25)	16.75 (9.5–31.00)	20.5
Group 3 1 mg 6 hourly	10/10	100	9/10	90	19/20	95	22.25 (12.75–30.00)	14 (6.5–23.75)	18.25

Data from Karim *et al.* (1978)

Rizk *et al.* (1978) terminated 16 out of 18 (88.9%) second trimester pregnancies with intramuscular injections of 500 μg sulprostone every 4 h (maximum six doses). The mean first injection to abortion interval was 11.9 h. The incidence of gastro-intestinal side-effects was 1.27 episodes per patient. There were no complications.

Table 17.15 Side-effects associated with intramuscular 16-phenoxy-ω-17,18,19,20-tetranor-PGE_2 methyl sulphonylamide for second trimester pregnancy termination

Dose of prostaglandin	*Nausea*	*Vomiting*		*Diarrhoea*		*Cold and shivering*	*Transient pyrexia 1 °C*
		No. of patients and %	*Mean episode per patient*	*No. of patients and %*	*Mean episode per patient*		
Group 1* 0.5 mg 4 hourly	3 (15%)	4 (20%)	0.25	1 (5%)	0.1	0	2 (10%)
Group 2 1.0 mg 8 hourly	2 (10%)	8 (40%)	0.9	2 (10%)	0.15	1 (5%)	1 (5%)
Group 3 1.0 mg 6 hourly	3 (15%)	6 (30%)	0.6	2 (10%)	0.2	1 (5%)	1 (5%)

*Each group 20 patients
Data from Karim *et al.* (1978)

Results similar to the above have been reported by Gethman *et al.* (1978) who gave 1 mg sulprostone intramuscularly every 6 h to 40 first and second trimester patients at gestation between 7 and 18 weeks. Thirty-eight out of 40 patients (95%) aborted in a mean time of 11.5 h (range 3–26 h). Side-effects included vomiting (7.5%), transient pyrexia (2.5%) and dyspnoea (2.5%). Abortion was complete in 77.5% of the patients.

Thus preliminary results with sulprostone given intramuscularly indicate that the abortifacient efficacy of this analogue is high and the incidence of side-effects low (see Ulbrich and Bartels, 1979).

17.5 VAGINAL ROUTE

17.5.1 15-Methyl-$PGF_{2\alpha}$ (suppositories)

Vaginal administration of 15(S)15-methyl-$PGF_{2\alpha}$ (free acid) was first successfully used in all of six patients for the termination of second trimester pregnancy by Karim *et al.* (1972). The drug was administered in a dose of 0.5 mg (concentrated solution) every 8 h. Five out of six patients experienced gastro-intestinal side-effects. In subsequent studies mainly the methyl ester of

Table 17.16 Termination of pregnancy with a single long-acting vaginal suppository containing 15-methyl-$PGF_{2\alpha}$ methyl ester

References	*No. of cases*	*Gestation range* (weeks)	*Dose schedule*	*Success rate* (%)	*Mean I/A interval* (h)	*Pre-medication*	*Side-effects and complications* (%)	*Complete abortion* (%)
Bygdeman *et al.*, 1977	25	12–20	3–3.5 mg single suppository	92[1]	12.4	Nil	V = 60; 1.7 episodes/patient D = 40; 0.7 episodes/patient H = 8	60.8
Ballard *et al.*, 1978	39	8–19	3 mg single suppository	87.2[2]	15.4	Anti-emetic and antidiarrhoeal 1 h before prostaglandin and repeated as necessary	V = 46.1; 1.2 episodes/patient D = 48.7; 1.9 episodes/patient P = 10.2; R = 2.5	48.7
Kinra *et al.*, 1978	58	10–14	3 mg single suppository	72.4[3]	17.9	Lomotil 5 mg at 0, 3, 6 h	V = 0.8 episodes/patient D = 1.4 episodes/patient	NS
Mandelin and Kajanoja, 1978	50	12–20	3 mg single suppository	78[1]	17.9	Lomotil 5 mg at 0, 3, 6 h	V = 3.2 episodes/patient D = 2.5 episodes/patient F = 18; R = 36; P = 16	NS

[1] = Foetus expelled within 24 hours
[2] = Foetus expelled within 27 hours
[3] = Foetus expelled within 30 hours
V = Vomiting; D = Diarrhoea; H = Haemorrhage; P = Pyrexia; F = Flushing; R = Rigors; NS = Not stated

this analogue has been used (Bygdeman *et al.*, 1976). The efficacy of vaginally administered prostaglandin is dependent upon such variables as the dose, concentration, rate of release and absorption. It is therefore difficult to compare the results obtained with different formulations. In this section only the results of WHO Prostaglandin Task Force Multicentre Trial will be discussed (WHO, 1977d).

A total of 310 patients in the 13th to 20th week of gestation (52.3% primigravidae) received one vaginal suppository containing 1.5 mg 15-methyl-$PGF_{2\alpha}$ methyl ester in Adeps solidus base every third hour until abortion or up to 24 hours. The foetus was expelled in 285 (91.9%) patients during the 30 h following the first suppository in a mean time of 14.2 h. Abortion was complete in 49.9% of the patients.

All patients were given 5 mg Lomotil simultaneously with the first three suppositories to reduce the frequency of side-effects. Diarrhoea occurred in 69.7% of the patients and vomiting in 66.8%. The mean number of episodes of each of these two side-effects per patient was 2.8. Other side-effects included dyspnoea 0.3%, flushing 6.1%, chest pain 0.3%, and pyrexia 11.3%. Cervical laceration occurred in three patients (1%). Five patients had a blood loss in excess of 500 ml.

Bygdeman *et al.* (1977) have developed long-acting vaginal suppositories containing 3 or 3.5 mg 15-methyl-$PGF_{2\alpha}$ methyl ester in Witepsol E 76 base which provides sufficient release of the drug for 12–24 hours. Preliminary clinical trials have shown acceptable success rate and low incidence of side-effects with vaginal administration of a single suppository. The results are shown in Table 17.16. The lowest success rate (72.4%) was reported by Kinra *et al.* (1978) in spite of the fact that in their trial abortion was considered successful if the patient aborted within 30 h after insertion of vaginal pessary. Bygdeman *et al.* (1977) reported a success rate of 92% within 24 h. The incidence of vomiting varied from 0.8 episodes/patient to 3.2 episodes per patient. The lowest incident of diarrhoea (0.7 episodes/patient) was reported by Bygdeman *et al.* (1977) who gave no antidiarrhoeal pre-medication and the highest incidence (2.5 episodes/patient) by Mandelin and Kajanoja (1978) who pre-medicated their patients with Lomotil. Both these investigators used suppositories from the same source and presumably were of identical formulation.

17.5.2 15-Methyl-$PGF_{2\alpha}$ (silastic device)

A silastic device impregnated with 15(S)15-methyl-$PGF_{2\alpha}$ methyl ester (15-methyl-$PGF_{2\alpha}$) has recently been developed. This device when introduced into the vagina provides a slow and sustained release of the prostaglandin. Such a device when used for pregnancy termination offers the advantage of ease of administration and removal and thus reversibility of effect in case of hypersensitivity to the drug. Clinical trials using 0.5% or 1% concentration of

15-methyl-$PGF_{2\alpha}$ methyl ester containing 10 mg of the drug in each device of surface area 20 cm^2 have been carried out. Southern (1976) has analysed the results from four investigators (Lauersen and Wilson, 1976; Dillon *et al.*, 1976; Hendricks *et al.*, 1976 and Bygdeman *et al.*, 1976, Table 17.17), who

Table 17.17 Termination of pregnancy with 0.5% and 1% vaginal silastic device containing 10 mg 15(S)15-methyl-$PGF_{2\alpha}$ methyl ester

	0.5% device		*1% device*	
	No.	%	*No.*	%
Patients	77	—	58	—
Mean gestation	13.6 weeks	—	14.9 weeks	—
Foetus expelled	70	90.9	·55	94.8
Complete abortion	60	77.9	46	79.3
Mean time to abortion	16.7 h	—	15.7 h	—
Mean estimation blood loss	140 ml	—	156 ml	—
Vomiting	26	34	32	55
Diarrhoea	31	40	30	52
Chills	0	0	7	12.1
Flushing	2	2.6	1	1.7

Data from Southern (1976)

used 0.5% device in 77 patients and 1% device in 58 cases. Seventy out of 77 patients (90.9%) in the 0.5% device group aborted in a mean time of 16.7 h. The mean gestational age of patients was 13.6 weeks. Complete abortion was reported in 78% of the patients. The success rate in the 58 patients on 1% device was 94.8%, with a complete abortion rate of 79.3%. The mean gestation of patients in this group was 14.9 weeks and mean time to abortion was 15.7 h. The difference in the efficacy and time to abortion in the two groups was not significant. Gastro-intestinal side-effects were rather high.

Fifteen out of 135 patients expelled the device prematurely on at least one occasion prior to abortion and had it re-inserted. Lauersen and Wilson (1976) sutured the device to a No. 70 diaphragm (after removing the centre portion) in an attempt to avoid unobserved expulsion. Such a procedure was effective in preventing displacement and expulsion of the device in a group of 12 patients.

Blood levels of 15-methyl-$PGF_{2\alpha}$ by radioimmunoassay at varying intervals after vaginal insertion of silastic device and measurement of the prostaglandin remaining in the device recovered after the abortion indicated that the total amount of drug (10 mg) in the device was somewhat in excess of that required for pregnancy termination (Southern, 1976; Bygdeman *et al.*, 1976).

Lauersen and Wilson (1977) used silastic device impregnated with 5 mg 15-methyl-$PGF_{2\alpha}$ weighing 0.99 g with a concentration of 0.5% prostaglandin. The device was 0.2 cm thick with a surface area of 10 cm^2. Intravaginal insertion of such a device resulted in an abortion in 27 out of 48 patients (56%)

within 24 h. Thirty-four out of 48 patients (70.8%) experienced gastro-intestinal side-effects. The device had to be removed in one patient because of 'almost constant nausea, vomiting and diarrhoea'. With another variation of the device Stubblefield (1976) successfully terminated pregnancy in all nine patients at gestation between 15 and 16 weeks. The device contained 0.25% concentration of 15-methyl-$PGF_{2\alpha}$ (the total amount of prostaglandin and the dimensions of the device were not given). All patients aborted within 22 h in a mean time of 12.7 h. All had 2–10 episodes of diarrhoea and seven out of nine patients experienced one to six episodes of vomiting. There was a blood loss of 1000 ml in one patient.

The concept of a prostaglandin-containing silastic device is attractive and would offer a non-invasive, simple method of pregnancy termination. Acceptable rate of efficacy has been achieved in the studies reported so far. However, the problems of high incidence of side-effects and premature expulsion of the device need to be resolved before such devices can be used on a large scale. Perhaps a change in the formulation (dimensions, drug concentration, total amount of drug) or the use of other prostaglandins may overcome these disadvantages.

17.5.3 16,16-Dimethyl-PGE_2 and esters

When given by the intramuscular and intravenous routes, 16,16-dimethyl-PGE_2 methyl ester is a potent oxytocic compound (Karim and Amy, 1973). However, because of a high incidence of side-effects this compound did not offer any advantage over other prostaglandins as an abortifacient (Karim and Amy, 1975). Both 16,16-dimethyl-PGE_2 and its methyl ester have also been evaluated for their usefulness as abortifacients by the oral route but the efficacy was found to be low and gastro-intestinal side-effects were encountered in a large proportion of patients (Karim *et al.*, 1974).

Martin *et al.* (1976) have successfully used 16,16-dimethyl-PGE_2 (free acid) given by the vaginal route in 30 patients in the 13th to 20th week of gestation. The dose varied between 400 and 1200μg every 3 h. All but one patient aborted during the 30 h after the first vaginal pessary in a mean time of 16.8 h. No pre-medication to counter gastro-intestinal side-effects was given. The mean number of episodes of vomiting and diarrhoea per patient was 0.73 and 0.3 respectively. Five patients had slight elevation of temperature.

16,16-Dimethyl-PGE_2 *p*-benzaldehyde semicarbazone ester was used by Karim and Ratnam (1977b) for termination of pregnancy in 54 late first trimester and second trimester patients. The drug (750 μg in gelatin glycerine pessaries) was administered every 4 h. Forty out of 42 (95%) second trimester patients aborted in a mean time of 18.7 h (range 6.5 to 36 h). Thirty-five (83%) aborted within 24 h. Out of the 12 first trimester patients, 10 aborted within 24 h of starting the treatment. In the remaining two, the cervix had dilated adequately to enable evacuation of the uterus by vacuum aspiration.

Side-effects were negligible. Five patients (9%) had one or two episodes each of vomiting and three (7%) had one episode each of diarrhoea. Two patients had a temperature of 38.3 °C which subsided after the abortion without any treatment. There was no haemorrhage or injury to the cervix.

17.6 CERVICAL TEAR AND UTERINE RUPTURE

The most serious complication of prostaglandin-induced abortion is transverse rupture of the posterior uterine wall at the level of the cervico-isthmic junction. This has been reported by several investigators and has been discussed in detail by Karim and Amy (1975). Even when recognized and repaired immediately, this type of cervical rupture may fail to heal and fistulous tract may result and interfere with reproductive performance of the patient. Extension of this type of injury into the lateral and anterior aspects of the uterus may lead to annular detachment of the cervix.

Cervical injury probably is the result of unusual cervical resistance in the face of strong uterus contractions and is therefore more likely to occur in young nulliparae in the late second trimester of pregnancy. A combination of oxytocics (e.g. prostaglandins with oxytocin, intra-amniotic saline and urea) may also contribute to cervical tear (Bradley-Watson *et al.*, 1973; Burkman *et al.*, 1976; Craft, 1973; Craft *et al.*, 1974; Kajanoja *et al.*, 1974). The incidence of cervical tear is difficult to assess but when reported it has ranged between 0.3% and 8%. The lowest incidence seems to be associated with the extra-amniotic route of prostaglandin administration but this requires confirmation.

It has been suggested that insertion of one or more laminaria tents into the cervical canal 12–18 h before prostaglandin administration may prevent cervical rupture (see Karim and Amy, 1975).

Proppoing *et al.* (1978) have reported two cases of intra-abdominal uterine rupture in older women of high parity who were given oxytocin infusion several hours after prostaglandin injection. In both patients laminaria tents were inserted into the cervical canal the night before prostaglandin administration. In both cases the uterine rupture occurred above the peritoneal reflection 'as is the usual case with uterine rupture in the third trimester'. The authors attribute the rupture to the use of oxytocin after prostaglandin administration. However, Borten and Friedman (1978) have reported a case of uterine rupture in a 42-year-old gravida five patient who was given 40 mg $PGF_{2\alpha}$ and 50 ml of 23.4% hypertonic saline for the termination of a 16-week intrauterine pregnancy. Oxytocin infusion was not given to this patient. Since such cases of intra-abdominal uterine rupture have only been reported in older women of high parity, it would seem prudent to avoid overstimulation of the uterus with combination of oxytocics in such patients.

17.7 ABORTION DEATHS ASSOCIATED WITH PROSTAGLANDINS

Gates *et al.* (1977) have described six abortion related deaths associated with the use of $PGF_{2\alpha}$ reported through the Center for Disease Control's surveillance of abortion deaths between 1972 and 1975 in the USA. In most of these cases it has not been possible to establish any causal link between prostaglandin administration and death. The authors estimate that the death to case fate for $PGF_{2\alpha}$ is 10.5 per 100 000 abortions compared with 17.7 per 100000 with hypertonic saline. Details of six cases reported by Gates *et al.* (1977) are given below.

Case 1: Pregnant chronic alcoholic with recurrent pancreatitis and central pontine myelinolysis. 'Pontine myelinolysis is frequently fatal, and death might have ensued regardless of the pregnancy termination'. The patient died of aspiration haematemesis.

Case 2: Poorly compensated cardiac patient with limited functional capacity and progressive cardiomegaly. Prostaglandin, rather than saline, was specifically selected as the abortifacient in order to avoid the increased intravascular volume and sodium load. The patient died after exhibiting symptoms suggestive of an amniotic fluid embolism but an autopsy was not permitted for confirmation.

Case 3: History of chronic hypertension and acute pre-eclampsia, necessitating pregnancy termination at 24 weeks gestation. The choice of prostaglandin over saline avoided the hypertensive risks from a sodium load. The patient died of an intracranial haemorrhage immediately after a hypertensive crisis.

Case 4: Patient apparently died from respiratory arrest secondary to the intravenous narcotic potentiated by an intravenous phenothiazine.

Case 5: Oxytocin was used as the primary abortifacient in this patient and $PGF_{2\alpha}$ was used to augment the effect of oxytocin. The patient died from overwhelming infection, complicated by coagulation defects and acute tubular necrosis.

Case 6: Microscopic pulmonary emboli and water intoxication may have contributed to death in this patient. This was the only patient who was given $PGF_{2\alpha}$ extra-amniotically (the other five patients received $PGF_{2\alpha}$ intra-amniotically). 'The presumed source of pulmonary emboli was the endometrial veins, inflamed by the presence of the adjacent extra-ovular Foley catheter'. The post-mortem finding of granulomatous pneumonitis with perivascular crystal deposit may have further undermined the patient's cardiorespiratory status.

The authors point out that it is not possible to establish any causal link between administration of $PGF_{2\alpha}$ and death. Wolf and Rubinstein (1977) commenting on the report by Gates *et al.* (1977) point out that second trimester abortion is a procedure which carries with it a certain low but definite risk of death even when performed in accordance with the currently accepted method of administration of $PGF_{2\alpha}$. 'At present however we are aware of no deaths in medically compromised patients that were the direct result of the intra-amniotic administration of $PGF_{2\alpha}$'.

Tejuja *et al.* (1978) have reported three deaths from India associated with the use of $PGF_{2\alpha}$ and its methyl analogues. A multiparous patient at 18 weeks of gestation was given 50 mg $PGF_{2\alpha}$ intra-amniotically but had no uterine contractions. Sixty-four hours later she developed tonic uterine contractions without additional therapy. Six hours later she was found to have a ruptured uterus and hysterectomy was performed. The patient died during the operation.

Another multiparous patient at 20 weeks gestation aborted completely 4 h after intra-amniotic administration 2.5 mg 15-methyl-$PGF_{2\alpha}$. She was re-admitted to the hospital on the 12th day after the abortion with severe vaginal bleeding. She went into a shock while hysterectomy was being performed and died.

The third patient was given 1 mg 15-methyl-$PGF_{2\alpha}$ extra-amniotically and aborted within 10 h. Five hours later she had uncontrollable vaginal bleeding and death occurred.

A combination of $PGF_{2\alpha}$, hypertonic saline and oxytocin given to a 33-year-old para 5 patient eventually resulted in death (Adachi *et al.*, 1977). After removal of 300 ml clear liquor the patient was given 20 mg $PGF_{2\alpha}$ and 25 ml 20% sodium chloride solution intra-amniotically and intravenous oxytocin at 40 mU/min. Fifteen hours later the patient's temperature rose to 103.6°F and the pulse to 120/min. Abortion occurred 18 h after the start of intra-amniotic administration of $PGF_{2\alpha}$ and saline. The patient experienced heavy bleeding and the placenta was manually removed and the uterus was curetted. The blood pressure was 218/127 mmHg. Blood studies gave findings consistent with intravascular haemolysis and consumption coagulopathy secondary to septicaemia.

Despite fluid replacement and diuretics the patient remained oliguric, secreting only about 5 ml/h. Subtotal hysterectomy was performed 34 h after $PGF_{2\alpha}$–saline injection. The patient died 13 h after hysterectomy. The death was reported to be caused by 'kidney failure, possibly due to a disseminated intravascular coagulopathic condition (DIC) and haemoperitoneum of 1200 g of mostly clotted blood'. There were complete fatty changes of the liver as well.

It needs to be emphasized that the low risk of death associated with second trimester termination is likely to increase in the presence of pre-existing medical condition. It is therefore essential to carefully select the method for such a procedure and terminations. Gates *et al.* (1977) consider that dilatation and evacuation may emerge as the treatment of choice for patients anticipated to tolerate labour poorly. In certain situations such a procedure or hysterectomy may carry less risk of death than use of drugs.

17.8 COMMENTS

Prostaglandins offer a valuable alternative to other methods of terminating second trimester pregnancy. With more experience their advantages and limitations are beginning to be appreciated. Attempts to reduce induction–abortion interval with a combination of prostaglandins and other methods of pregnancy termination (laminaria tents, oxytocin infusion, intra-amniotic saline or urea and extra-amniotic rivanol) have given positive results. However, with many such combinations the incidence of some immediate side-effects (vomiting and diarrhoea) and complications (cervical tear and uterine rupture) seem to be higher than with prostaglandins alone.

Although a large number of analogues of prostaglandins have been synthesized only a few have been clinically evaluated. Some of these (16,16-dimethyl-PGE_2 and esters, dihomo-15-methyl-$PGF_{2\alpha}$ methyl ester and 16-phenoxy-tetranor-PGE_2 methyl sulphonylamide) seem to offer advantages over natural prostaglandins and some of their 15-methyl analogues. Hopefully, clinical trials of other analogues will result in discovering compounds with better efficacy and a further reduction in side-effects.

Acknowledgement

The assistance of the following in the preparation of this chapter is gratefully acknowledged: Miss Lily Koh, Miss Tai Mei Yoon, Miss Leong Mei Mei, Miss Wang Gek Choo, Mr P. G. Adaikan, Dr Ashim Roy and Dr R. N. V. Prasad.

References

Adachi, A., Wilson, L. and Herzig, N. (1977). Prostaglandin $F_{2\alpha}$, hypertonic saline and oxytocin in midtrimester abortion. *N.Y. State J. Med.*, **77**, 46

Ballard, C. A., Forte, K. and Lauersen, N. H. (1978). Plasma prostaglandin concentration and abortifacient effectiveness of a single insertion of a 3 mg 15(S)15-methyl prostaglandin $F_{2\alpha}$ methyl ester vaginal suppository. *Contraception*, **17**, 383

Ballard, C. A. and Quilligan, E. J. (1974). Midtrimester abortion with intramuscular injection of 15-methyl prostaglandin E_2. *Contraception*, **9**, 523

Ballard, C. A. and Slaughter, L. (1976). Second trimester abortion with intramuscular injections of 15-methyl prostaglandin $F_{2\alpha}$. *Contraception*, **14**, 541

Berger, G. S., Edelman, D. A. and Kerenyi, T. D. (1975). Oxytocin administration, instillation–abortion time and morbidity associated with saline instillation. *Am. J. Obstet. Gynecol.*, **120**, 941

Bolognese, R. J. and Corson, S. L. (1975). Interruption of pregnancy by prostaglandin 15-methyl $F_{2\alpha}$. *Fertil. Steril.*, **26**, 695

Borell, U., Embrey, M. P., Bygdeman, M., Hendricks, C. H. and Kinch, R. (1978). Reply to Dr Grimes and Associates. *Am. J. Obstet. Gynecol.*, **131**, 232

Borten, M. (1976). Use of combination prostaglandin $F_{2\alpha}$ and hypertonic saline for midtrimester abortion. *Prostaglandins*, **12**, 625 .

Borten, M. and Friedman, E. A. (1978). Uterine rupture: a complication of midtrimester abortion. *Prostaglandins*, **15**, 187

Bowen-Simpkins, P. (1973). The induction of second trimester abortions using an intra-amniotic injection of urea and prostaglandin E_2. *J. Obstet. Gynaecol. Br. Cmnwlth.*, **80**, 824

Bradley-Watson, P. J., Beard, R. J. and Craft, I. L. (1973). Injuries of the cervix after induced midtrimester abortion. *J. Obstet. Gynaecol. Br. Cmnwlth.*, **80**, 284

Brenner, W. E., Dingfelder, J. R. and Staurovsky, L. G. (1975). The efficacy and safety of intramuscularly administered 15(S)15-methyl prostaglandin E_2 methyl ester for induction of artificial abortion. *Am. J. Obstet. Gynecol.*, **123**, 19

Burkman, R. T., Atienza, M. F., King, T. M. and Burnett, L. S. (1976). Intra-amniotic urea and prostaglandin $F_{2\alpha}$ for midtrimester abortion: a modified regimen. *Am. J. Obstet. Gynecol.*, **126**, 328

Bygdeman, M., Borell, U., Leader, A., Lundström, V., Martin, J. N., Eneroth, P. and Gréen, K. (1976). Induction of first and second trimester abortion by vaginal administration of 15-methyl $PGF_{2\alpha}$ methyl ester. In: B. Samuelsson and R. Paoletti (eds.), *Advances in Prostaglandins and Thromboxane Research*, p. 693 (New York: Raven Press)

Bygdeman, M., Ganguli, A., Kinoshita, K., Lundström, V., Gréen, K. and Bergström, S. (1977). Development of a vaginal suppository suitable for single administration for interruption of second trimester pregnancy. *Contraception*, **15**, 129

Bygdeman, M., Gréen, K., Lundström, V., Ramadan, M., Fotiou, S. and Bergström, S. (1976). Induction of abortion by vaginal administration of 15(S)15-methyl prostaglandin $F_{2\alpha}$ methyl ester. A comparison of two delivery systems. *Prostaglandins*, **12** (Suppl.), 27

Bygdeman, M., Martin, J. N., Wiqvist, N., Gréen, K. and Bergström, S. (1974). Reassessment of systemic administration of prostaglandins for induction of midtrimester abortion. *Prostaglandins*, **8**, 157

Carsten, M. E. (1972). Prostaglandin's part in regulating uterine contraction by transport of calcium. *J. Reprod. Med.*, **9**, 277

Cohen, E. and Ballard, C. A. (1974). Consumptive coagulopathy associated with intra-amniotic saline instillation and the effect of intravenous oxytocin. *Obstet. Gynecol.*, **43**, 300

Craft, I. (1973). Induction of abortion by combined intra-amniotic urea and prostaglandin E_2 or prostaglandin E_2 alone. *Lancet*, **i**, 1344

Craft, I. (1975). Intra-amniotic urea and low-dose prostaglandin E_2 for mid-trimester termination. *Lancet*, **i**, 1115

Craft, I., Walker, E. and Youssefnejadian, E. (1974). Intra-amniotic prostaglandin $F_{2\alpha}$ and urea for abortion. *Prostaglandins*, **5**, 397

Dillon, T. F., Mootabar, H., Phillips, L. L. and Rizk, A. (1976). The efficacy of intravaginal 15-methyl prostaglandin $F_{2\alpha}$ methyl ester in first and second trimester abortion. *Prostaglandins*, **12** (Suppl.), 81

Dillon, T. F., Phillips, L. L., Rizk, A., Horiguchi, T., Mootabar, H. (1975). The efficacy of intramuscular 15 methyl prostaglandin E_2 in second trimester abortion. *Am. J. Obstet. Gynecol.*, **121**, 584

Edelman, D. A , Brenner, W. E., Mehta, A. C., Phillips, F. S., Bhatt, R. V. and Bhiwandiwala, P. (1976). A comparative study of intra-amniotic saline and two prostaglandin $F_{2\alpha}$ dose schedules for midtrimester abortion. *Am. J. Obstet. Gynecol.*, **125**, 188

Gates, W., Grimes, D. A., Haber, R. J. and Tyler, C. W. (1977). Abortion deaths associated with the use of prostaglandin $F_{2\alpha}$. *Am. J. Obstet. Gynecol.*, **127**, 219

Gethmann, U., Hoppen, H. O. and Oberheuser, F. (1978). Termination of first and second trimester pregnancy with intramuscular administration of sulprostone, a new prostaglandin analogue. *IRCS Med. Sci.*, **6**, 423

Grimes, D. A., Gates, W. and Schulz, F. (1978). Midtrimester abortion by dilatation and evacuation. *Am. J. Obstet. Gynecol.*, **131**, 231

Hendricks, C. H., Dingfelder, J. R. and Gruber, W. S. (1976). Clinical observations with a prostaglandin containing silastic vaginal device for pregnancy termination. *Prostaglandins*, **12** (Suppl.), 99

Hess, H. J., Bindra, J. S., Constantine, J. W., Elger, W., Loge, O., Schillinger, E. and Losert, W. (1977). Pharmacology of 16-phenoxy-tetranor-PGE_2 methylsulfonylamide, a tissue-selective antifertility prostaglandin. *IRCS Med. Sci.*, **5**, 68

Himmelmann, A., Myhrman, P. and Svanberg, S.-G. (1975). Induction of second trimester abortion. Comparison between Rivanol and prostaglandin $F_{2\alpha}$ regarding time factors and complications. *Contraception*, **12**, 645

Kajanoja, P., Jungner, G., Widholm, O., Karjalainen, O. and Seppälä, M. (1974). Rupture of the cervix in prostaglandin abortions. *J. Obstet. Gynaecol. Br. Cmnwlth.*, **81**, 242

Karim, S. M. M. (1976). Singapore experience with prostaglandins—routine use and recent advances. In: S. M. M. Karim (ed.), *Obstetric and Gynaecological Uses of Prostaglandins*, p. 127. Proc. Asian Federation of Obstet. Gynaecol. Intercongress (Lancaster: MTP Press)

Karim, S. M. M. and Amy, J. J. (1973). Effect of prostaglandin 16,16-dimethyl E_2 methyl ester on the pregnant human uterus. *Prostaglandins*, **4**, 581

Karim, S. M. M. and Amy, J. J. (1975). Interruption of pregnancy with prostaglandins. In: S. M. M. Karim (ed.), *Advances in Prostaglandin Research: Prostaglandins and Reproduction*, p. 23 (Lancaster: MTP Press)

Karim, S. M. M., Choo, H. T., Lim, A. L., Yeo, K. C. and Ratnam, S. S. (1978). Termination of second trimester pregnancy with intramuscular administration of 16-phenoxy-ω-17,18,19,20-tetranor-PGE_2 methylsulfonylamide. *Prostaglandins*, **15**, 1063

Karim, S. M. M., Rao, B., Ratnam, S. S., Prasad, R. N. V., Wong, Y. M. and Illancheran, A. (1977). Termination of early pregnancy (menstrual induction) with 16-phenoxy-ω-tetranor-PGE_2 methylsulfonylamide. *Contraception*, **16**, 377

Karim, S. M. M. and Ratnam, S. S. (1977a). Newer aspects of practical applications of prostaglandins in obstetrics and gynaecology. In: N. Kharasch and J. Fried (eds.), *Biochemical Aspects of Prostaglandins and Thromboxanes*, p. 115 (New York: Academic Press)

Karim, S. M. M. and Ratnam, S. S. (1977b). Termination of pregnancy with vaginal administration of 16,16-dimethyl prostaglandin E_2 *p*-benzaldehyde semicarbazone ester. *Br. J. Obstet. Gynaecol.*, **84**, 135

Karim, S. M. M. and Ratnam, S. S. (1978). Termination of second trimester pregnancy with intramuscular administration of 16-phenoxy-ω-tetranor-PGE_2 methylsulfonylamide (SHB 286). *IRCS Med. Sci.*, **6**, 146

Karim, S. M. M., Sharma, S. D. and Filshie, G. M. (1972). Termination of pregnancy with 15-methyl analogues of prostaglandins E_2 and $F_{2\alpha}$. In: E. M. Southern (ed.), *The Prostaglandins: Clinical Applications in Human Reproduction*, p. 307 (Mount Kisco, N.Y.: Futura Publishing Co.)

Karim, S. M. M. and Sivasamboo, R. (1975). Termination of second trimester pregnancy with intra-amniotic 15(S)15-methyl prostaglandin $F_{2\alpha}$–A two dose schedule study. *Prostaglandins*, **9**, 487

Karim, S. M. M., Sivasamboo, R. and Ratnam, S. S. (1974). Abortifacient action of orally administered 16,16-dimethyl prostaglandin E_2 and its methyl ester. *Prostaglandins*, **6**, 349

King, T. M., Dubin, N. H., Atienza, M. F., Burkman, R. T., Blake, D. A and Baros, N. A. (1977). Intra-amniotic urea and prostaglandin $F_{2\alpha}$ for midtrimester abortion: Clinical and laboratory evaluation. *Am. J. Obstet. Gynecol.*, **129**, 817

Kinra, G., Agarwal, N. and Hingorani, V. (1977). Use of prostaglandin for induction of second trimester abortions in high risk pregnancy. *Contraception*, **16**, 243

Kinra, G., Agarwal, N., Jagannath, K. T. and Hingorani, V. (1978). Evaluation of a single dose schedule of 15(S)15-methyl $PGF_{2\alpha}$ methyl ester suppository for the termination of 10–14 weeks of pregnancy. *Contraception*, **17**, 455

Lange, A. P. and Secher, N. J. (1977). Midtrimester and missed abortion treated with intramuscular 15(S)15-methyl $PGF_{2\alpha}$. *Prostaglandins*, **14**, 389

Lauersen, N. H., Secher, N. J. and Wilson, K. H. (1975). Midtrimester abortion induced by serial intramuscular injections of 15(S)15-methyl prostaglandin E_2 methyl ester. *Am. J. Obstet. Gynecol.*, **123**, 665

Lauersen, N. H. and Wilson, K. H. (1974). Midtrimester abortion induced with a single intra-amniotic instillation of prostaglandin $F_{2\alpha}$. *Am. J. Obstet. Gynecol.*, **118**, 210

Lauersen, N. H. and Wilson, K. H. (1975). Midtrimester abortion induced by serial intramuscular injections of 15(S)15-methyl prostaglandin $F_{2\alpha}$. *Am. J. Obstet. Gynecol.*, **121**, 273

Lauersen, N. H. and Wilson, K. H. (1976). Hormone release and abortifacient effectiveness of a newly developed silastic device containing 15-me-$PGF_{2\alpha}$ methyl ester in concentrations of 0.5% and 1.0%. *Prostaglandins*, **12** (Suppl.), 63

Lauersen, N. H. and Wilson, K. H. (1977). The effect of a 10 cm^2, 0.5% 15-me-$PGF_{2\alpha}$ methyl ester intravaginal silastic device on abortion and plasma prostaglandin concentration. *Prostaglandins*, **13**, 755

Lichtenegger von W. (1977). Abortinduktion mit prostaglandin $F_{2\alpha}$ und einem neuen prostaglandin E_2 Derivat. *Wien. Med. Wochenschr.*, **127**, 536

Liebman, T., Saldana, L., Schulman, H., Cunningham, M. A. and Randolph, G. (1974). Midtrimester abortion with 15(S) methyl prostaglandin $F_{2\alpha}$. *Prostaglandins*, **7**, 443

Mackenzie, I. Z. and Embrey, M. P. (1976a). Single extra-amniotic injection of prostaglandins in viscous gel to induce abortion. *Br. J. Obstet. Gynaecol.*, **83**, 505

Mackenzie, I. Z. and Embrey, M. P. (1976b). Extra-amniotic 15(S)15-methyl $PGF_{2\alpha}$ to induce abortion. A study of three administration schedules. *Prostaglandins*, **12**, 443

Mandelin, M. and Kajanoja, P. (1978). Induction of second trimester abortion. Comparison between vaginal 15-methyl $PGF_{2\alpha}$ methyl ester and intra-amniotic $PGF_{2\alpha}$. *Prostaglandins*, **16**, 995

Martin, J. N., Bygdeman, M., Leader, A. and Wiqvist, N. (1975). Early second trimester abortion by the extra-amniotic instillation of rivanol solution and a single $PGF_{2\alpha}$ dose. *Contraception*, **11**, 523

Martin, J. N., Bygdeman, M., Ramadan, M., Gréen, K., Leader, A., Lundström, V. and Wiqvist, N. (1976). Vaginally administered 16,16-dimethyl PGE_2 for the induction of midtrimester abortion. *Prostaglandins*, **11**, 123

Propping, D., Stubblefield, P. G., Golub, J. and Zuckerman, J. (1977). Uterine rupture following midtrimester abortion by laminaria, prostaglandin $F_{2\alpha}$ and oxytocin. Report of two cases. *Am. J. Obstet. Gynecol.*, **128**, 689

Pulkkinen, M. O. (1978). Pregnancy termination with the PGE_2-analogue SHB 286. *Prostaglandins*, **15**, 161

Rizk, M. A., Sallam, A. N., Nayel, S. A., El-Damarawy, H. and Toppozada, M. K. (1978). Therapeutic abortion with a prostaglandin suitable for systemic use. *Singapore J. Obstet. Gynaecol.*, **9**, 57

Schmidt-Gollwitzer, M., Schmidt-Gollwitzer, K., Schüssler, B., Koch, R. and Nevinny-Stickel, J. (1977). Erste Erfahrungen mit rinem neuen Prostaglandin-E_2-Derivat. *Geburtsh. Frauenheilk.*, **37**, 1030

Sharma, S. D., Hale, R. W. and Sato, N. E. (1975). Intramuscular (15S)-15-methyl prostaglandin $F_{2\alpha}$ for midtrimester and missed abortions. *Obstet. Gynaecol.*, **46**, 468

Southern, E. M. (1976). Preliminary trials of vaginal silastic devices containing (15S)-15 methyl prostaglandin $F_{2\alpha}$ methyl ester for the induction of menses and for pregnancy termination. *Prostaglandins*, **12** (Suppl.), 147

Stubblefield, P. G. (1977). Vaginal silastic device containing 0.25% 15(S)15 methyl prostaglandin $F_{2\alpha}$ methyl ester for early second trimester abortion. *Contraception*, **15**, 175

Stubblefield, P. G., Naftolin, F., Lee, E. Y., Frigoletto, F. D. and Ryan, K. J. (1976). Combination therapy for midtrimester abortion. Laminaria and analogues of prostaglandins. *Contraception*, **13**, 723

Tejuja, S., Choudhury, S. D. and Manchanda, P. K. (1978). Use of intra and extra-amniotic prostaglandins for the termination of pregnancies—Report of multicentric trial in India. *Contraception*, **18**, 641

Ulbrich, I. and Bartels, H. (1979). Clinical results with sulprostone: In *Proceedings of International Sulprostone Symposium*. Vienna 1978. (To be published)

Weinstein, L., Droegemuellar, W. and Greer, B. (1976). The synergistic effect of calcium and prostaglandin $F_{2\alpha}$ in second trimester abortion. A pilot study. *Obstet. Gynecol.*, **48**, 469

WHO Prostaglandin Task Force Multicentre Trial (1976). Comparison of intra-amniotic prostaglandin $F_{2\alpha}$ and hypertonic saline for induction of second trimester abortion. *Br. Med. J.*, **1**, 1373

WHO Task Force on the use of Prostaglandins for the Regulation of Fertility (1977a). Prostaglandins and abortion. III. Comparison of single intra-amniotic injections of 15-methyl prostaglandin $F_{2\alpha}$ and prostaglandin $F_{2\alpha}$ for termination of second trimester pregnancy: An International Multicentric Study. *Am. J. Obstet. Gynecol.*, **129**, 601

WHO Task Force on the use of Prostaglandins for the Regulation of Fertility (1977b). Prostaglandin and abortion. II. Single extra-amniotic administration of 0.92 mg of 15-methyl prostaglandin $F_{2\alpha}$ in Hyskon for termination of pregnancies in weeks 10 to 20 of gestation: An International Multicentric Study. *Am. J. Obstet. Gynecol.*, **129**, 593

WHO Task Force on the use of Prostaglandins for the Regulation of Fertility (1977c). Prostaglandin and abortion. I. Intramuscular administration of 15-methyl prostaglandin $F_{2\alpha}$ for induction of abortion in weeks 10 to 20 of pregnancy. *Am. J. Obstet. Gynecol.*, **129**, 597

WHO Task Force on the use of Prostaglandin for the Regulation of Fertility (1977d). Repeated vaginal administration of 15-methyl $PGF_{2\alpha}$ methyl ester for termination of pregnancy in the 13th–20th week of gestation. *Contraception*, **16**, 175

Wilson, W. B. (1978). Midtrimester abortion with urea. Prostaglandin $F_{2\alpha}$, laminaria and oxytocin. A new regimen. *Obstet. Gynecol.*, **51**, 699

Wolf, J. A. and Rubinstein, L. M. (1977). Safety of prostaglandin $F_{2\alpha}$ and abortion. *Am. J. Obstet. Gynecol.*, **129**, 928

Ylikorkala, O. and Järvinen, P. A. (1975). Induction of abortion with intra-amniotic or intramuscular 15(S)15-methyl prostaglandin $F_{2\alpha}$. *Prostaglandins*, **10**, 423

18
Prostaglandins and their Inhibitors in Premature Labour

H. ZUCKERMAN and S. HARPAZ-KERPEL

18.1 INTRODUCTION

Premature labour is a leading cause of perinatal mortality and morbidity. Any measure found effective in combating premature labour could have a beneficial effect on perinatal outcome.

Many drugs have been tried to inhibit uterine activity during premature labour (Johnson *et al.*, 1975; Fuchs and Stakemann, 1960; Brenner and Hendricks, 1962; Fuchs, F., 1965b; Lauersen *et al.*, 1977; Brucke *et al.*, 1956; Fuller, 1978; Baillie *et al.*, 1970; Tyack *et al.*, 1971; Baumgarten *et al.*, 1971; Barden, 1972; Andersson *et al.*, 1973; Korda *et al.*, 1974; Lipshitz, 1977; Zuckerman *et al.*, 1974).

The exact cause and mechanism of the onset of labour are unknown but several theories have been put forward.

Prostaglandin (PG) levels in amniotic fluid are higher at term than in mid-pregnancy and are also higher during labour than before its onset (Karim and Devlin, 1967; Gréen *et al.*, 1974; Sharma *et al.*, 1973; Keirse and Turnbull, 1973; Salmon and Amy, 1973; Hillier *et al.*, 1974; Keirse *et al.*, 1974; Dray and Frydman, 1976; Karim, 1968; Zuckerman *et al.*, 1978a; see also review by Karim and Hillier, 1975). There is good evidence that prostaglandins play an important role in the pathogenesis of premature labour (see review by Karim, 1978).

Aspirin and indomethacin are potent inhibitors of prostaglandin biosynthesis in the body. They inhibit the formation of prostaglandins in the uterus and reduce uterine motility in animals (Chester *et al.*, 1972; Aiken, 1972; Fuchs *et al.*, 1974; Novy *et al.*, 1974; Vane, 1972; Lau *et al.*, 1975) and in women (Waltman *et al.*, 1973b; Reiss *et al.*, 1976; Zuckerman *et al.*, 1974; Zuckerman *et al.*, 1975). Indomethacin is the most potent of the available inhibitors of prostaglandin synthesis and may prove useful in the treatment of premature labour.

18.2 PHARMACOLOGICAL INHIBITION OF PREMATURE LABOUR

The four main groups of drugs used to inhibit premature labour are: (1) progestogens, (2) ethanol, (3) β-mimetics, and (4) inhibitors of prostaglandin synthesis. In a recent study Steer and Petrie (1977) have shown that magnesium sulphate is effective in the inhibition of labour, probably through a direct effect on the myometrium. Among agents currently in use for the therapy of premature labour, none have achieved uniform success.

18.2.1 Progestogens

Since its discovery by Corner and Allen (1929), progesterone has been regarded as an important substance in the maintenance of pregnancy. The human placenta synthesizes large amounts of progesterone from the precursor cholesterol, derived from maternal plasma (Hellig *et al.*, 1970). During pregnancy plasma progesterone levels gradually increase to a plateau at around 32 weeks of gestation (Johansson, 1969). Knauss (1934) and Csapo (1969) have postulated that parturition in the human is preceded by a withdrawal of progesterone. Although a drop in progesterone may precede labour in some animal species, there is no good evidence for this in humans (Llauro *et al.*, 1968; Neher and Zarrow, 1954; Short, 1960; Zarrow and Neher, 1955). Recently, Turnbull *et al.* (1973) have produced evidence in support of the progesterone withdrawal hypothesis. However, there was no decrease in plasma progesterone levels in several of their patients prior to the onset of labour. Csapo *et al.* (1974) have reported low values of plasma progesterone in patients in premature labour.

Several studies on the efficacy of progesterone and other progestogens in preventing premature labour have been undertaken. Results from some of these studies are encouraging (Reiffenstein, 1958; Le Vine, 1964; Shearman and Garrett, 1963) but they came under criticism because of lack of substantiation by valid statistical analyses. Johnson *et al.* (1975) reported postponement of premature labour in 18 out of 21 patients treated with 17α-hydroxy-progesterone caproate; nine out of 22 patients receiving placebo delivered prematurely. However Fuchs and Stakemann (1960) using progesterone, Ovlisen and Inversen (1963) using 6a-methyl 17a-acetoxy-progesterone, Brenner and Hendricks (1962) using medroxy-progesterone acetate and Hill *et al.* (1975) using 17a-hydroxy-progesterone caproate failed to show any influence of these progestogens in inhibiting uterine contractions. In addition recent evidence indicates that administration of progestational compounds during the early stages of pregnancy may induce congenital abnormalities (Nora *et al.*, 1976).

18.2.2 Inhibition of oxytocin with ethanol

In 1951 van Dyke and Ames (1951) demonstrated that ethanol inhibits the release of vasopressin from the posterior pituitary. Since oxytocin was thought to play a role in the initiation of labour (Fuchs, A. R., 1965), ethanol has been used to prevent uterine contractions (presumably caused by oxytocin), in threatened premature labour (Fuchs, F., 1965). The first major clinical study by Fuchs *et al.* (1967) demonstrated that administration of alcohol delayed labour for a minimum of 72 h in 65% of patients with intact membranes. This treatment was thereafter widely used (Luukkainen *et al.*, 1967; Lynn, 1970; Zlatnik and Fuchs, 1972; Fuchs, 1976; Lauersen *et al.*, 1977).

Some doubts have arisen about the role of ethanol as an inhibitor of oxytocin release in parturition. Observations of labour in hypophysectomized women and in women with diabetes insipidus imply that oxytocin is not essential in the onset of normal labour (Caldeyro-Barcia *et al.*, 1971). In addition, some results of studies indicate that insufficient oxytocin is released during labour to cause uterine activity (Cobo, 1968), or that maternal plasma oxytocin levels during labour were not different from those before the onset of labour (Gazarek, 1976). However, results of more recent studies (Dawood *et al.*, 1978; Zuckerman *et al.*, 1978b) indicate that there is a substantial increase in oxytocin levels during parturition.

Ethanol probably also acts directly on the myometrium (Bueno-Montano *et al.*, 1966; Mantell and Liggins, 1970). Sandholm (1971) demonstrated that alcohol fails to inhibit the pumping stimulation of the lactiferous ducts by oxytocin in puerperal women. However Gibbens and Chard (1976) have shown that administration of ethanol during labour reduces circulating levels of oxytocin. Karim and Sharma (1971) reported that ethanol inhibits uterine activity in spontaneous labour and uterine activity induced by PGE_2 and $PGF_{2\alpha}$ but not that induced by oxytocin.

There are also practical objections to the use of ethanol in the prevention of premature labour. Graff (1971) found no difference between ethanol and 5% glucose in the inhibition of labour. Aspiration pneumonia (Greenhouse *et al.*, 1969) and severe lactic acidosis (Ott *et al.*, 1976) have also been associated with the use of ethanol. In addition there are reports of adverse effects of ethanol on infants, including metabolic acidosis and central nervous system depression (Mann *et al.*, 1975a, 1975b).

18.2.3 β-Mimetic drugs

Langley (1905) provided the basis for current concepts of adrenergic receptors. He suggested that effector cells contain excitatory and inhibitory substances, The response to adrenalin being dependent upon the type of substance predominant in a particular structure. Dale (1906) was the first to use the receptor concept. He suggested that the sympathetic neuromuscular junction was the receptive mechanism for adrenaline.

Ahlquist (1948, 1966) defined the adrenergic receptor as an entity in or on effector cells which interacts with adrenergic agonists to elicit the response characteristic of the cell. The α-adrenergic-receptor increases uterine contractility and the inhibition of the uterine musculature is mediated by an action on the β-receptors.

The introduction of the β-receptor blockers dichloro-iso-prenaline and propranolol led to a more specific study of the β-receptors (Powell and Slater, 1958; Black *et al.*, 1964). β-Receptor activity was further clarified by Lands *et al.* (1967). They subdivided these receptors into β_1-receptors, which have a marked cardiac influence with an increased heart rate and cardiac output, and β_2-receptors, which are more specific for reducing myometrial activity and decreasing smooth muscle tone in arteriolar vessels and bronchioles.

The effects of adrenergic agonists upon the uterus vary with species and with endocrine status of the animal (Pauerstein and Zander, 1970). The human myometrium at term displays both (α and β) receptor activity, but appears to be β dominated. Adrenaline decreases spontaneous and oxytocin-induced activity of the uterus (Barden and Stander, 1968; Zuspan *et al.*, 1962). Noredrenaline increases uterine activity (Althabe *et al.*, 1968; Barden and Stander, 1968; Cibils and Hendricks, 1961; Nakanishi *et al.*, 1969; Zuspan *et al.*, 1962). Several analogues of these amines reduce spontaneous and oxytocin-induced activity of the pregnant human uterus (Barden and Stander, 1968; Hendricks *et al.*, 1961; Lanman, 1968; Stolte *et al.*, 1965).

In order to inhibit the uterine activity, drugs with effects mainly on the β-receptors of the uterus should be used. Konzett (1940) introduced isoprenaline, which acted almost exclusively on β-receptors. However, infusion of isoprenaline, while causing inhibition of uterine activity at term (Mahon *et al.*, 1967) also causes cardioacceleration and hypotension. Eskes *et al.* (1965) found that administration of *p*-hydroxyphenylisopropylarterenol (Cc-25) after pronethalol depressed uterine activity without causing significant changes in heart rate or blood pressure. Others did not find such a dissociation between uterine and cardiovascular effects (Mahon *et al.*, 1967; Barden and Stander, 1968).

Efforts to use the uterine-relaxant properties of the β-mimetic drugs while avoiding their cardiac effects have led to clinical trials of a number of such drugs. Some of these, including ritodrine, salbutamol and fenoterol have been claimed to be effective in the management of pre-term labour.

18.2.4 Prostaglandin antagonists

It is well recognized that prostaglandin levels increase during labour (Hillier *et al.*, 1974; Dray and Frydman, 1976; Willman and Collins, 1976; Coats *et al.*, 1977; Willman *et al.*, 1977; Keirse *et al.*, 1977; Shaikh *et al.*, 1977; Whalen *et al.*, 1978; Mitchell *et al.*, 1978a, 1978b; Haning *et al.*, 1978; Zuckerman *et al.*, 1978a, 1978b), and the possibility that they are involved in labour as natural uterine stimulants has been suggested (Karim, 1972; Karim and Hillier, 1975). It has therefore been proposed that prostaglandin antagonists could prove useful in preventing premature labour (Bodin, 1971; Lippert, 1972; Scher and Baillie, 1973).

There are many non-steroidal anti-inflammatory drugs which inhibit the synthesis and some of the actions of prostaglandins. Meclofenamate and flufenamate inhibit contractions of human isolated smooth muscles produced by $PGF_{2\alpha}$ (Collier and Sweatman, 1968). Phenylbutazone and aspirin are equally effective against $PGF_{2\alpha}$ in this respect. Meclofenamic acid has also been shown to selectively block the vasodepressor effect of $PGF_{2\alpha}$ in anaesthetized rabbits (Levy and Lindner, 1971). Aspirin inhibits the production and release of prostaglandins *in vitro* in guinea-pig lung (Vane, 1971), human platelets (Smith and Willis, 1971) and dog spleen (Ferreira *et al.*, 1971).

Sorrentino *et al.* (1972) reported that indomethacin inhibits contractions of the isolated rat uterus and guinea-pig ileum produced by serotonin, bradykinin and PGE_2. On the other hand Eckenfels and Vane (1972) found that indomethacin potentiated the effect of PGE_2 on rat stomach strips *in vitro*.

Amongst the non-steroidal anti-inflammatory drugs only aspirin and indomethacin have been used in the prevention of premature labour. Lewis and Schulman (1973) were able to demonstrate that long-term intake of aspirin during pregnancy prolongs gestation and duration of labour. This was confirmed by Collins and Turner (1975) and Turner and Collins (1975), who also showed that the use of salicylates during pregnancy is associated with serious maternal and foetal complications.

18.3 PLASMA $PGF_{2\alpha}$ VALUES IN PREMATURE AND TERM LABOUR

The exact mechanism of action of prostaglandins in initiating and maintaining the progress of labour has not been elucidated. Studies of the dynamic function of endogenous prostaglandins and their levels in the peripheral blood in various stages of labour and during and between contractions are conflicting (Gréen *et al.*, 1974; Sharma *et al.*, 1973; Brummer and Craft, 1973; Hillier *et al.*, 1974; Karim, 1968). Previous studies on peripheral blood have shown an increase in PGE or PGF concentrations during labour (Brummer, 1972; Caldwell *et al.*, 1971; Hertelendy *et al.*, 1973; Mitchell *et al.*, 1978b; Zuckerman *et al.*, 1978a). Most investigators have also found an increase in amniotic fluid levels of prostaglandins during premature (Tamby Raja, 1977) and term labour (Salmon and Amy, 1973; Hibbard *et al.*, 1974; Keirse *et al.*, 1974; Hillier *et al.*, 1974; Keirse and Turnbull, 1973; Kinoshita *et al.*, 1977; Karim, 1966; Karim and Devlin, 1967). Karim (1968) reported that levels of $PGF_{2\alpha}$ in maternal venous blood increased just prior to a contraction of the uterus during labour, reaching a peak concentration at the height of contraction, followed by a decrease during the phase of uterine relaxation and finally an absence after the contraction has subsided. This pattern was repeated with each contraction until delivery was accomplished. He suggested that $PGF_{2\alpha}$ is not released as a result of contraction. Karim also found that in the majority of these women there was more $PGF_{2\alpha}$ in blood taken during the second stage of labour than in the first stage. The blood taken during expulsion of the placenta contained less prostaglandins than the second-stage samples in seven out of 10 women. The other three contained more. Only two out of 10 samples taken 3 hours post-partum contained detectable concentrations of $PGF_{2\alpha}$.

Brummer and Craft (1973) and Brummer (1972) found the highest levels of $PGF_{2\alpha}$ at the time of maximum uterine activity during the late first stage of labour. They found that the change in serum $PGF_{2\alpha}$ levels appears to be related to the stage of cervical dilatation. After full cervical dilatation was reached, the mean level fell and remained low during the second stage, delivery and post-partum. Brummer's study however did not take into consideration rapid fluctuations in plasma levels of prostaglandins.

Sharma *et al.* (1973) in a timed study reported that concentration of $PGF_{2\alpha}$ in blood from the antecubital vein usually reached a peak in samples obtained 15–45 s after the height of uterine contraction, yet in two of 10 patients the peak of $PGF_{2\alpha}$ was obtained 45–60 and 60–70 s after the contraction. Sharma's emphasis that the circulation time from the uterus to antecubital vein is 30–55 s, is compatible with the suggestion that prostaglandin is released into the circulation after the onset of uterine contraction.

Gréen *et al.* (1974) found that the levels of $PGF_{2\alpha}$ in peripheral plasma did not show any correlation with cervical dilatation either in normal or oxytocin-induced labour and reached a peak immediately before parturition and decreased to 20–75% of the values 1 hour after birth. The authors however, found that the levels of 15-keto-13,14-dihydro-$PGF_{2\alpha}$ increased in four out of five patients with increasing dilation of the cervix. Gréen *et al.* examined a total of 11 blood samples from two patients, during five contractions with a wide time gap between and did not find any variation in the level of $PGF_{2\alpha}$ in the peripheral plasma in relation to contractions.

Hillier *et al.* (1974) studied three groups of women during labour (spontaneous; induced with oxytocin; induced with prostaglandin) and found no significant difference in the plasma levels of $PGF_{2\alpha}$ between these groups. In addition they found no difference in the prostaglandin levels during the various stages of labour. Mitchell *et al.* (1978b) found a small increase in plasma levels of PGE in early term labour, and a marked increase in PGF and its metabolites in early- and late-term labour. Challis *et al.* (1974) found that maternal plasma PGF levels were higher at vaginal delivery than at caesarean section, but this difference was not statistically significant. They reported that maternal plasma PGF levels in samples taken 45–60 s after the peak of a uterine contraction were always higher than in samples taken 45 or 30 s later, or at the peak itself. They also found that the concentration of PGF in cord plasma was significantly elevated in spontaneous or oxytocin-induced vaginal delivery as compared to elective caesarean section. In all groups of patients the PGF concentration in the cord plasma was significantly greater than in maternal plasma.

Lackritz *et al.* (1978) found that during spontaneous labour there were no significant minute-to-minute fluctuations in plasma PGE_2 and $PGF_{2\alpha}$ metabolites and the concentrations at peak uterine contractions were not different from those following or preceding the contractions. The authors also found that the concentrations of PGF_2 and $PGF_{2\alpha}$ metabolites did not appear to be related to the degree of cervical dilatation, to the strength or timing of uterine contractions or to whether the labour was spontaneous or induced. They concluded that the increase in levels of prostaglandin metabolites in

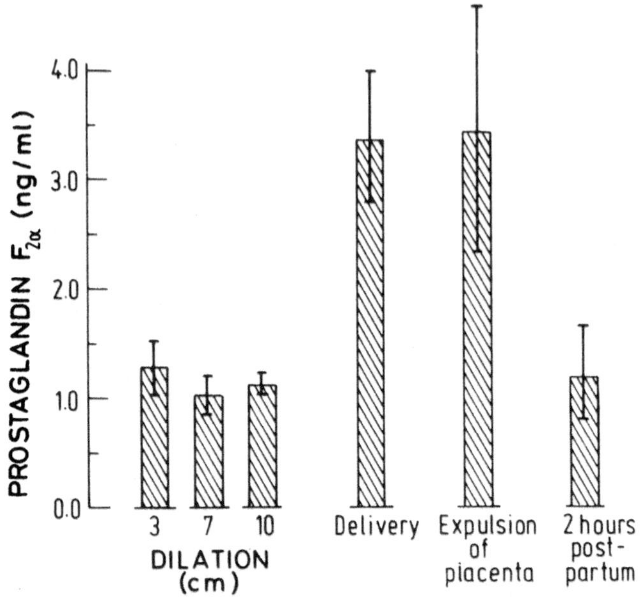

Figure 18.1 Concentrations of $PGF_{2\alpha}$ in maternal blood at different stages of labour (mean values $\pm$SD)

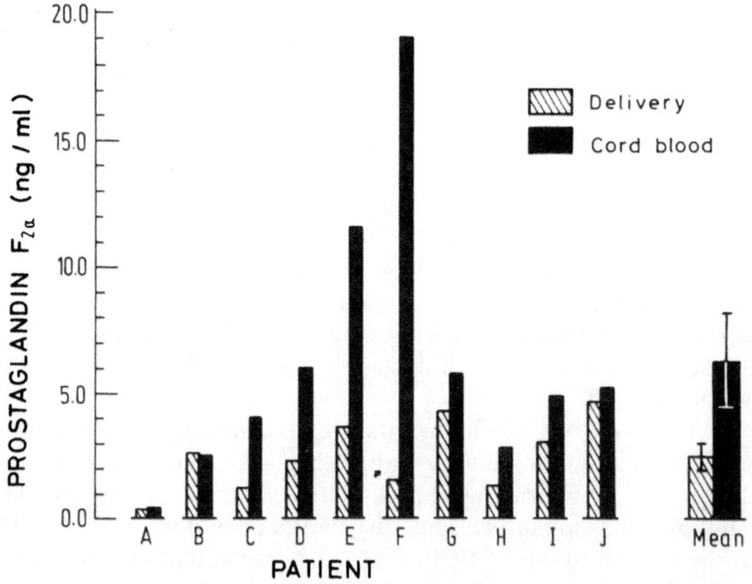

Figure 18.2 $PGF_{2\alpha}$ levels in maternal blood during delivery and in foetal cord blood. (The last columns represent mean values $\pm$SD)

peripheral plasma is secondary to the initiation of uterine contractions in term pregnancy.

Zuckerman *et al.* (1978a) reported that $PGF_{2\alpha}$ levels during labour showed two peaks, one at the time of foetal expulsion and one at the time of placental expulsion (Figure 18.1). $PGF_{2\alpha}$ levels were much lower during the first stage of labour compared to the second and third stages. Two hours after delivery the concentrations of $PGF_{2\alpha}$ had returned to the levels found in the first-stage labour. The authors have suggested that $PGF_{2\alpha}$ plays a role in the expulsion of the placenta and the involution of the uterus. Zuckerman *et al.* (1978a) reported that $PGF_{2\alpha}$ levels in cord blood were higher than those in blood taken during delivery (Figure 18.2). The mean value of $PGF_{2\alpha}$ in peripheral blood during delivery was 2.5 ng/ml, while the mean cord blood levels were

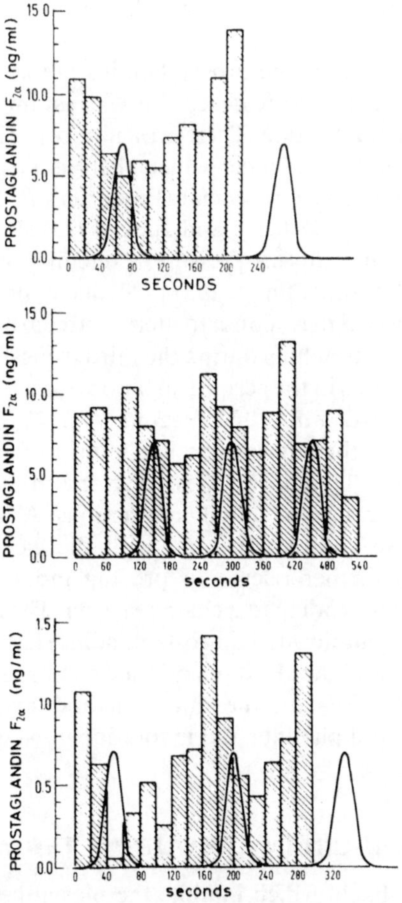

Figure 18.3 $PGF_{2\alpha}$ concentrations in maternal blood in relation to contraction. Serial sampling every 20–30 s

6.3 ng/ml. The possibility arises that in addition to the decidual contribution (Karim, 1968; Singh and Zuspan, 1974), there may also be a foetal source of prostaglandins (Yoffee *et al.*, 1971; Keirse and Turnbull, 1973) and this may explain the high levels of prostaglandin in the amniotic fluid (Hillier *et al.*, 1974; Hibbard *et al.*, 1974). Zuckerman *et al.* (1978a) demonstrated that $PGF_{2\alpha}$ values of the maternal blood obtained over a 20–30 s interval during pre-term and term labour showed fluctuations and the peak levels appeared approximately 100–120 s after the peak of uterine contractions, or 40–60 s before the peak of the next contraction (Figure 18.3). In their opinion investigators evaluating the levels of prostaglandin during various stages of labour must take into consideration the rapid fluctuation of $PGF_{2\alpha}$ during and between contractions. The authors have pointed out that the fluctuations in $PGF_{2\alpha}$ levels are more closely correlated with the rhythm of contractions, without there being a correlation between the absolute levels and the progress of labour.

The question of whether the prostaglandins are a cause or the result of uterine contractions could be resolved if it was assumed that the process of labour is part of a chain reaction. There are a number of studies which indicate the physiological conditions under which there is production or release of prostaglandins. Evidence from animal (Poyser *et al.*, 1971; Caldwell *et al.*, 1972) and human studies (Kloeck and Jung, 1973) show that the release of $PGF_{2\alpha}$ is a result of intrauterine pressure, stretching or manipulation of the uterus. Csapo (1973) and Flint *et al.* (1973) have also shown that prostaglandins may be released in response to uterine stretch and vaginal distension. The increased uterine stretching during the third trimester causes an increased release of prostaglandins in the peripheral blood (Gréen *et al.*, 1974) and in the amniotic fluid (Hibbard *et al.*, 1974; Beguin *et al.*, 1973).

One may speculate that during the 9th month of pregnancy the uterine tension in the individual patient reaches a level that results in sufficient release of prostaglandins to cause the initial contractions. As a result of the muscle activity during these contractions and with the elevation of intrauterine pressure there is a further release of prostaglandins which enhances the following contractions leading to a chain reaction. The immediate contractile effect of exogenously administered prostaglandins (Karim *et al.*, 1969; Roth-Brandel *et al.*, 1970) and the above-mentioned results of various studies stress the importance of $PGF_{2\alpha}$ in the initiation and maintenance of labour, expulsion of foetus and placenta and involutionary stage after delivery.

18.4 INDOMETHACIN IN LABOUR AT TERM

The use of indomethacin which inhibits the biosynthesis of prostaglandins (Vane, 1971; Smith and Willis, 1971) and thus suppresses their release both *in vivo* (Ferreira *et al.*, 1971) and *in vitro* (Vane, 1971) should help to evaluate the functional role of prostaglandins in labour. Indomethacin prolongs pseudopregnancy (O'Grady *et al.*, 1972) and delays parturition in rats (Chester *et al.*, 1972; Aiken, 1972), mice, hamsters (Lau *et al.*, 1975) and primates (Novy *et al.*, 1974).

For a better understanding of the role of prostaglandins in the initiation of term labour and in the second and third stage of labour, the authors (Reiss *et al.*, 1976) administered indomethacin as a single 100 mg suppository to 16 women in labour at term and recorded uterine activity (Figure 18.4). All the

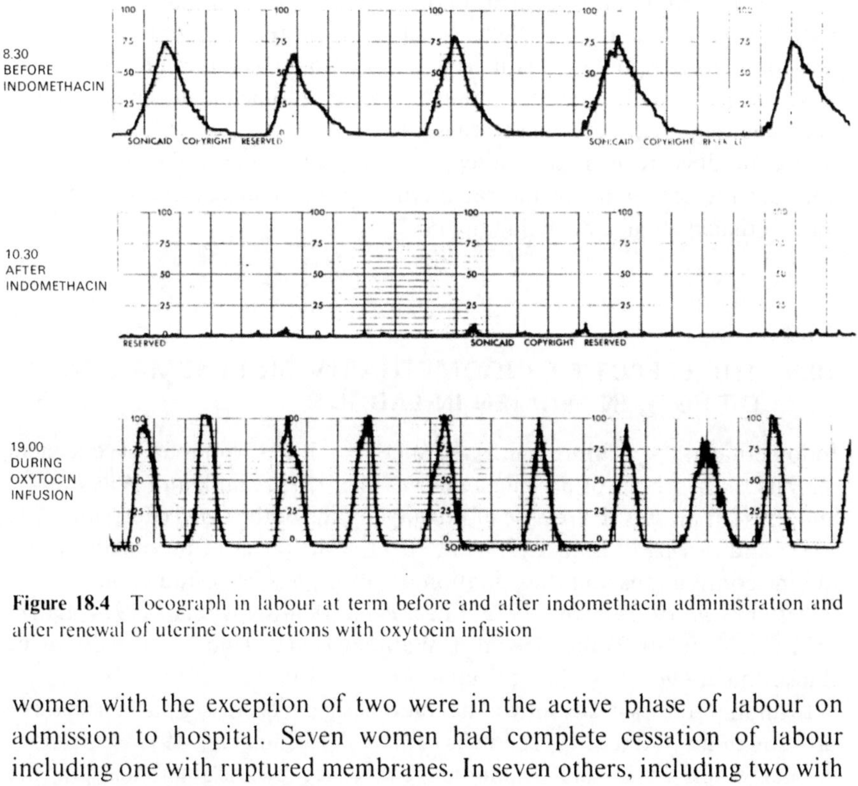

Figure 18.4 Tocograph in labour at term before and after indomethacin administration and after renewal of uterine contractions with oxytocin infusion

women with the exception of two were in the active phase of labour on admission to hospital. Seven women had complete cessation of labour including one with ruptured membranes. In seven others, including two with ruptured membranes, the duration of labour was markedly prolonged. Two patients did not respond to indomethacin.

In the group with complete cessation of labour cervical dilatation (which ranged between 2–5 cm) did not change from the time of administration of indomethacin until the beginning of spontaneous contractions or the administration of intravenous oxytocin. The delay in labour, induced by indomethacin, varied from $2\frac{1}{2}$ to 192 h. In two patients labour terminated spontaneously and five patients received intravenous oxytocin to augment contractions (Figure 18.4). All seven were multiparas and delivered spontaneously and all infants had an (Apgar) score of 10.

In the group where labour was protracted, the active phase was prolonged by 3–17 h and the cervical dilation increased by 1–5 cm. Three births terminated spontaneously and in four cases it was necessary to administer oxytocin intravenously. This group contained two primiparas and five multiparas.

Two women did not respond to indomethacin and delivered within 1 hour following its administration. All neonates were in good condition at birth. All 16 patients were monitored carefully and no changes in the maternal blood pressure or foetal heart rate were noted. Within the group of 16 patients the authors did not find any correlation between the effect of indomethacin and initial cervical dilatations or effacement or rupture of membranes and the development of spontaneous uterine contractions. The uterine response to oxytocin was not affected by administration of indomethacin. These findings are consistent with the report that uterotonic activities of oxytocin and prostaglandins are mediated via separate receptor sites (Soloff *et al.*, 1973). In contrast the sensitivity of the rat uterus to oxytocin was diminished after indomethacin (Vane and Williams, 1972).

18.5 THE EFFECT OF INDOMETHACIN ON PLASMA LEVELS OF $PGF_{2\alpha}$ IN WOMEN IN LABOUR

Indomethacin 1-(*p*-chlorobenzoyl)-5-methoxy-2-methylindole-3-acetic acid inhibits the synthesis of prostaglandins (Vane, 1971; Smith and Willis, 1971) and thus suppresses the release of prostaglandins both *in vivo* (Ferreira *et al.*, 1971) and *in vitro* (Smith and Willis, 1971). The effect of indomethacin on uterine contractions and the initiation of labour has been studied in animals (Chester *et al.*, 1972; Aiken, 1972; Fuchs *et al.*, 1974; Novy *et al.*, 1974; Lau *et al.*, 1975; Vane, 1972) and in women (Waltman *et al.*, 1973b; Reiss *et al.*, 1976; Zuckerman *et al.*, 1974, 1975; Wiqvist *et al.*, 1975).

In animal studies it was shown that indomethacin decreases plasma levels of prostaglandins (Aiken, 1972; Fuchs *et al.*, 1974; Lau *et al.*, 1975).

Zuckerman *et al.* (1977) studied the effect of indomethacin on the fluctuations in levels of $PGF_{2\alpha}$ in maternal plasma during uterine contractions in labour. The samples of maternal blood were collected every 20 or 30 s during contractions before and 30–60 s after rectal administration of 100 mg indomethacin. The uterine activity was recorded by cardiograph. There was a significant decrease in the plasma level of $PGF_{2\alpha}$ 30–60 min after indomethacin administration (see Figure 18.5). Indomethacin did not alter the pattern of rapid short-term fluctuations in prostaglandin levels.

Wiqvist *et al.* (1975) found a marked decrease in plasma levels of 15-keto-13,14-dihydro-$PGF_{2\alpha}$ in three out of four women in labour treated with indomethacin.

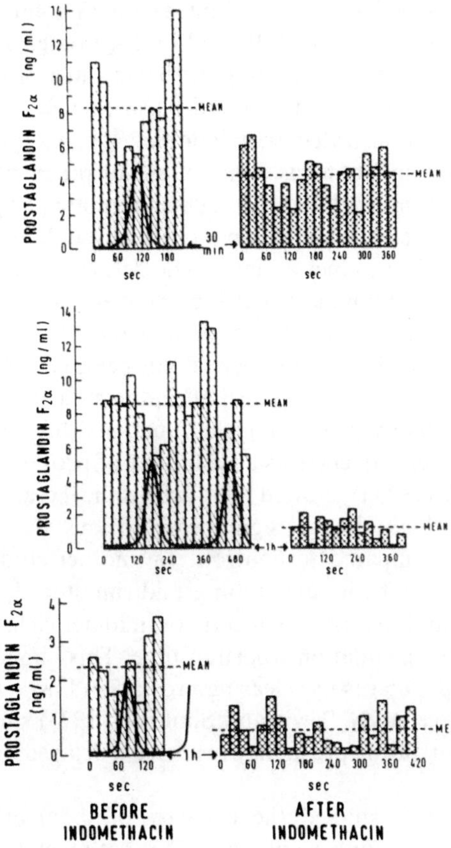

Figure 18.5 Effect of indomethacin on $PGF_{2\alpha}$ levels in peripheral blood of a woman in labour

18.6 PROSTAGLANDINS AND THEIR INHIBITORS IN PREMATURE LABOUR

18.6.1 Historical review

Vane (1971) demonstrated that aspirin and indomethacin inhibit the synthesis of prostaglandins in rabbit lung. The concentrations of aspirin and indomethacin needed to block 50% of the synthesis of prostaglandin were 6.3 and 0.27 μg/ml respectively, which are within the plasma levels achieved with therapeutic doses of these drugs. The potency ratio on a weight basis for indomethacin and aspirin for inhibition of prostaglandin synthesis is reported as 25 to 1. Indomethacin has been shown to inhibit prostaglandin synthesis in human skin (Greaves and McDonald-Gibson, 1973) and in inflammatory exudate (Barbieri *et al.*, 1977). Ferreira *et al.* (1971) showed that indomethacin prevents the release of $PGF_{2\alpha}$ from the perfused spleen of the dog. Collier and

Flower (1971) showed that human volunteers taking soluble aspirin orally for 1 week had reduced values of PGE_2 and $PGF_{2\alpha}$ in their semen. Orczyk and Behrman (1972) found that in rats indomethacin and aspirin caused a marked decrease in hypothalamic, pituitary and plasma levels of $PGF_{2\alpha}$. Vane and Williams (1972) demonstrated that indomethacin inhibited the release of prostaglandins and spontaneous contractions of pregnant rat uteri *in vitro*. Chester *et al.* (1972) showed that indomethacin prolonged parturition in rats.

Aiken (1972) treated Harlam pregnant rats with indomethacin and aspirin at different stages of pregnancy and found no delay in the onset of parturition. However, once parturition has started, prostaglandin antagonists prolong it significantly. These data suggest that prostaglandins are required for expulsion of the foetus. The last results were confirmed by Fuchs *et al.* (1974).

O'Grady *et al.* (1972) showed that indomethacin lengthens pseudopregnancy in rabbits by prolonging the functional life span of the corpora lutea indicating its effectiveness as an inhibitor of prostaglandin synthesis.

Waltman *et al.* (1973a) showed that acetylsalicylic acid administered to pregnant rats in high dosage significantly delays the time of onset of parturition when compared to controls. In another study Waltman *et al.* (1973b) found that patients undergoing midtrimester abortion induced by hypertonic saline and treated with aspirin or indomethacin show a significant prolongation of the instillation–abortion time. This implies that hypertonic saline stimulates the uterus by releasing prostaglandins.

In a retrospective study Lewis and Shulman (1973) showed that regular ingestion of aspirin during pregnancy results in a delayed onset of labour and prolonged labour.

Novy *et al.* (1974) studied the capacity of indomethacin to prolong gestation in the rhesus monkey and found that both foetal and placental units continued to develop beyond term. Pregnancy was terminated electively by caesarean section at 185 and 183 days of gestation (normal 165). At surgery no evidence of spontaneous uterine contraction was noted. These studies explain neither the rather precise timing of parturition within the species, nor the foetal or maternal trigger to labour but they do indicate that prostaglandins are a necessary prerequisite for its physiological onset.

Gyory *et al.* (1974) reported that administration of 2.0–2.5 g of sodium salicylate (not mg as erroneously printed in the original article: personal communication) to patients at term could suspend uterine activity for 8 hours. Lau *et al.* (1975) showed that indomethacin decreases uterine production of prostaglandins and prolongs parturition in mice.

18.6.2 Inhibition of human premature labour by indomethacin

Prematurity still remains one of the unsolved problems in obstetrics. A high foetal wastage occurs in spite of the many methods used to stop early labour. Interruption of the onset of premature labour could reduce perinatal deaths and improve neonatal prospects. Therefore it is not surprising that various compounds (Fuchs, F., 1965b; Cibils, 1966; Pose *et al.*, 1962; Barden, 1971; Baillie *et al.*, 1970; Bishop *et al.*, 1966) have been investigated to determine their ability to inhibit uterine contractions.

The functional role for endogenous prostaglandin in parturition is suggested by the increase in concentration of prostaglandins in human blood (Gréen *et al.*, 1974; Sharma *et al.*, 1973; Karim, 1968; Zuckerman *et al.*, 1978a) and amniotic fluid (Hillier *et al.*, 1974; Karim and Devlin, 1967) during labour and there is good evidence that prostaglandins may play an important role in the pathogenesis of premature labour (see Karim, 1978 for review).

Indomethacin is a potent inhibitor of prostaglandin synthesis and is completely absorbed after oral and rectal administration though the absorption is slower by the rectal route (Alvan *et al.*, 1975). Peak serum levels are reached in 1 or 2 hours, after oral administration (Traeger *et al.*, 1973; Alvan *et al.*, 1975). In late pregnancy and in labour absorption of indomethacin is slightly slower and the peak concentration is lower than in non-pregnant women, though its excretion is unchanged (Traeger *et al.*, 1973). Indomethacin crosses the placenta easily, the level in the umbilical artery equilibrating with that in the maternal blood within 5 h after oral administration. However the half-life of the drug in the newborn is significantly longer (14.7 h) compared to the adult (2.2 h) (Niebyl *et al.*, 1978).

A trial of indomethacin was conducted by Zuckerman (1978) in 300 women with clinical evidence of premature labour by studying the effect on uterine activity and in preventing premature labour. The patients were 16–44 years of age. There were 120 primiparas and 180 multiparas between the 24th–36th week of gestation. Cervical dilatation at the time of initial administration averaged 2.5 cm ranging from 0 to 5 cm. There were 45 patients with premature rupture of membranes. Labour was considered active when contractions were regular, frequent, mild to strong and continuous over a 30 min period. Uterine contractility was recorded by an external cardiotocagraph. Every patient received 100 mg of indomethacin in suppository form, followed by 25 mg orally every 6 h up to 24 h after contractions ceased. If uterine contractions continued after 100 mg indomethacin the patient received an additional 100 mg suppository after 1 h and then the treatment was followed orally. The total daily dose needed for successful treatment was between 200 and 300 mg indomethacin. The effect was classified as satisfactory when the contractions ceased completely for more than 1 week and the foetus reached maturity. The effect of the drug was considered as mild if uterine contractions stopped and the labour was arrested for 48 h to 7 days. The result was considered unsuccessful if the uterine contractions could not be stopped or if they were arrested for less than 48 h and delivery took place within 48 h. The criterion for prematurity was a birth weight less than 2500 g.

After administration of indomethacin uterine contractions stopped completely for 1–12 weeks in 82% of the patients. In 11% there was a mild effect, that is the labour was arrested for 48 h to 7 days. This period is also very important for foetal lung maturity by treatment with betametazone. In 8% of patients there was no effect and delivery took place within 48 h.

Among the patients with cervical dilatation of up to 3 cm, the contractions were arrested completely in 89% of the cases. When the dilatation was more than 3 cm, the contractions were stopped in 58% of the cases. The effect of indomethacin on uterine contractions and on the delay of delivery decreased with the progress of cervical dilatation. In most cases the delay in delivery ranged from 5–9 weeks although in some patients delivery was delayed for 11 and 12 weeks. Better results were noted in patients with intact membranes. Forty-eight patients had more than one course of treatment because of reappearance of contractions after a minimum of 2 weeks interval. Thirty minutes after indomethacin administration, uterine contractions decreased in frequency and intensity and complete uterine relaxation was noted within 2–13 h (Figure 18.6).

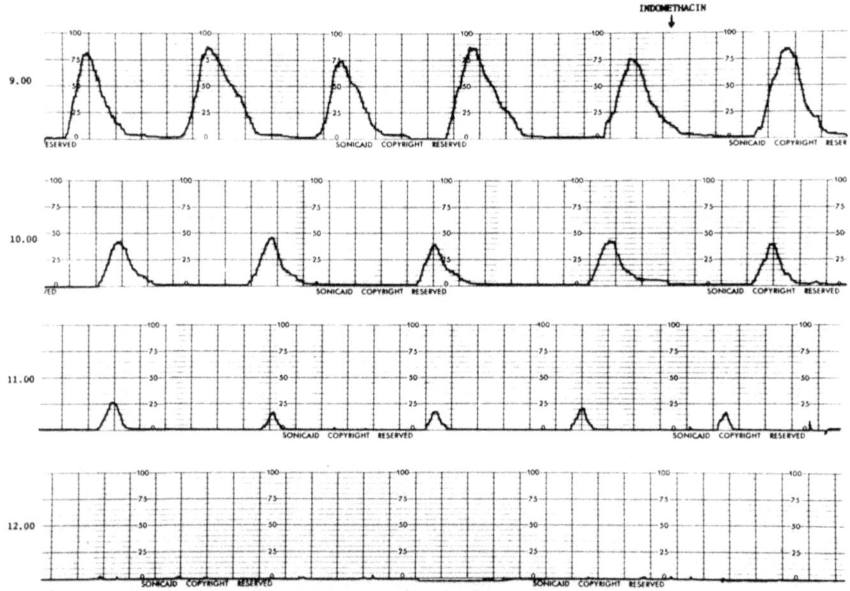

Figure 18.6 Tocograph showing effects of indomethacin administration in premature labour

In all 300 patients there was no change in blood pressure, pulse or foetal heart tones during the treatment. In this series there were mild gastro-intestinal disturbances – nausea, vomiting and dyspepsia in eight patients, maculopapular eruption in two patients and in one patient there was epistaxis. All symptoms disappeared a few hours after the treatment was discontinued. Fifty-four babies were born in spite of therapy. In the last group three infants were dead *in utero* before the start of treatment and 15 with birth weights of 700–1500 g suffered from respiratory distress syndrome and died. All the rest, 39 premature and 246 mature infants were examined carefully by the paediatrician and no ill effects related to the treatment were observed. The follow-up of development of these children was satisfactory. The results show that indomethacin has a marked inhibitory effect on uterine contractions in premature labour and this probably results from the inhibition of prostaglandin synthesis or its release.

Manchester *et al.* (1976) have described a possible association between maternal indomethacin therapy and primary pulmonary hypertension in two newborns. In one of them the delivery was associated with intrauterine infections requiring antibiotics and the second infant was born by breech extraction after administration of 10 mg of morphine and 200 mg secobarbitol. As pulmonary hypertension was associated with sepsis and foetal asphyxia in these two newborns, it is difficult to attribute this effect to indomethacin treatment. The two infants were discharged from hospital and have suffered no further complications. Congenital closure of the ductus arteriosus is a rare event (Kohler, 1967). The only published case claiming to demonstrate a correlation between aspirin and congenital ductus arteriosus (DA) closure is an infant whose mother received chronically large doses of aspirin (Arcilla *et al.*, 1969). The closure of the ductus after birth occurs in two stages. Initially closure is brought about by contraction of the smooth muscle in the wall of the ductus. The second stage of closure is permanent and may be delayed for 2–3 weeks in human infants (Heymann and Rudolph, 1975). The effect of indomethacin is on the first stage which is physiological rather than on the stage of anatomical constriction (Sharpe *et al.*, 1974; Sharpe *et al.*, 1975; Heymann and Rudolph, 1976). In rats indomethacin causes narrowing of the foetal ductus arteriosus only at oral doses 15 times greater than those used in humans (Sharpe *et al.*, 1974). A gestational variation in sensitivity of DA towards indomethacin was clearly demonstrated by Sharpe *et al.* (1975). Even this occurred only if the drug was given near delivery (12–18 h). The earlier in pregnancy the drug was given, the lower its effect on ductal diameter. While the 18-day (premature) rat foetus showed no reactivity, the 20-day rat foetus displayed about half the sensitivity of that seen in the full-term 22-day foetus. The conclusion from this study is that during the premature period the possibility of any effect of indomethacin on DA is very unlikely. The lack of influence on indomethacin in early pregnancy could explain the lack of deleterious effects by this drug in premature labour (Zuckerman, 1978; Wiqvist *et al.*, 1975; Cabellero *et al.*, 1977).

In the author's series of 300 infants whose mothers were treated with indomethacin for premature labour the children were examined cardially and haemodynamically and no side-effects were noted. There were no cases exhibiting signs of pulmonary hypertension. Also in the group 14 women at term (Reiss *et al.*, 1976) who were treated with indomethacin and subsequently induced with oxytocin delivered within 24 h without any complications.

Wiqvist *et al.* (1975) treated nine women in premature labour with oral indomethacin (25 mg every 6 h for 5 days), and reported a significant decrease in the frequency of contractions in all and a complete arrest of contractions in some women. Paediatric examination of the infants did not reveal any circulatory disturbances or other abnormalities. They concluded that indomethacin is a potent and useful drug in the treatment of premature labour.

Cabellero *et al.* (1977) treated 50 women in premature labour with 100 mg indomethacin in suppository form followed by 25 mg every 6 h for 48 h. Complete inhibition of uterine activity for 1½ to 30 h in 45 cases. There were practically no side-effects. No adverse foetal effects attributable to indomethacin were noted in any of the above studies.

Acknowledgements

The authors thank Dr U. Reiss, Dr J. Atad, Dr G. Gilad, Dr E. Shalev for help in these studies and to Mrs Cherry Wendel for secretarial assistance.

References

Ahlquist, R. P. (1948). A study of the adrenotropic receptors. *Am. J. Physiol.*, **153**, 586

Ahlquist, R. P. (1966). The adrenergic receptor. *J. Pharmacol. Sci.*, **55**, 359

Aiken, J. W. (1972). Aspirin and indomethacin prolong parturition in rats. *Nature*, **240**, 21

Allen, H. H., Short, H. and Fraleigh, D. M. (1965). The use of isoxuprine in the management of premature labour. *Appl. Ther.*, **7**, 544

Althabe, O., Jr., Schwarcz, R. L. Jr., Sala, N. L. and Fisch, L. (1968). Effect of phentolamine methanesulfonate upon uterine contractility induced by l-norepinephrine in pregnancy. *Am. J. Obstet. Gynecol.*, **101**, 1083

Alvan, G., Orme, M. and Bertilsson, L. (1975). Pharmacokinetics of indomethacin. *Clin. Pharm. Ther.*, **18**, 364

Andersson, K. E., Ingemarsson, I. and Persson, C. G. A. (1973). Relaxing effects of β-receptor stimulators in isolated gravid human myometrium. *Life Sci.*, **13**, 335

Arcilla, R. A., Thilenius, O. G. and Ranniger, K. (1969). Congestive heart failure from suspected ductal closure *in utero*. *J. Pediatr.*, **75**, 74

Baillie, P., Meehan, F. P. and Tyack, A. J. (1970). Treatment of premature labour with orciprenaline. *Br. Med. J.*, **4**, 154

Barbieri, E. J., Orzechowski, R. F. and Rossi, G. V. (1977). Measurement of prostaglandin E_2 in an inflammatory exudate: effects of nonsteroidal anti-inflammatory agents. *J. Pharmacol. Exp. Ther.*, **201**, 769

Barden, T. P. and Stander, R. W. (1968). Myometrial and cardiovascular effects of an adrenergic blocking drug in human pregnancy. *Am. J. Obstet. Gynecol.*, **101**, 91

Barden, T. P. (1971). Inhibition of human premature labour by mesuprine hydrochloride. *Obstet. Gynecol.*, **37**, 98

Barden, T. P. (1972). Effect of ritodrine on human uterine motility and cardiovascular responses in term labour and the early postpartum state. *Am. J. Obstet. Gynecol.*, **112**, 645

Baumgarten, K., Fröhlich, H., Seidl, A., Sokol, K., Lim-Rachmat, F. and Hager, R. (1971). A new β sympathomimetic preparation for intravenous and oral inhibition of uterine contractions. *Eur. J. Obstet. Gynecol.*, **2**, 69

Beguin, F., Bygdeman, M., Gréen, K., Samuelsson, B., Toppozada, M. and Wiqvist, N. (1973). Analysis of prostaglandin F_2 and metabolites in blood during constant intravenous infusion of prostaglandin F_2 in the human female. *Acta Physiol. Scand.*, **86**, 430

Bishop, E. H., Bolognese, R. J. and Piver, M. S. (1966). Effect of methanesulfonamide on uterine contractions. *Obstet. Gynecol.*, **28**, 784

Black, J. W., Crowther, A. F., Shanks, R. G., Smith, L. H. and Dornost, A. C. (1964). A new adrenergic beta-receptor antagonist. *Lancet*, **i**, 1080

Bodin, M. (1971). Prostaglandins and habitual abortion. *Br. Med. J.*, **2**, 587

Brenner, W. E. and Hendricks, C. H. (1962). Effect of medroxyprogesterone acetate upon duration and characteristics of human gestation and labour. *Am. J. Obstet. Gynecol.*, **82**, 1094

Brücke, F., Hertting, G., Lindner, A. and Loudon, M. (1956). Zur pharmakologie einer neuen gefässerweiternden Substanz aus der p-Oxy-Ephedrin-Reihe. *Wein. Klin. Wochenschr.*, **68**, 183

Brummer, H. C. (1972). Serum $PGF_{2\alpha}$ levels during late pregnancy, labour and the puerperium. *Prostaglandins*, **2**, 185

Brummer, H. C. and Craft, I. L. (1973). Prostaglandin $F_{2\alpha}$ and labour. *Acta Obstet. Gynecol. Scand.*, **52**, 273

Bueno-Montano, M., McGaughey, H. S. Jr., Harbert, J. M. Jr., and Thornton, W. N. Jr. (1966). Drug preservatives and uterine contractility. *Am. J. Obstet. Gynecol.*, **94**, 1

Caballero, A., Tejerina, A. and Dominguez, Y. A. (1977). The prevention of premature labour by indomethacin. *Hosp. Gen.*, **17**, 199

Caldeyro-Barcia, R., Melander, S. and Coch, J. A. (1971). Neurohypophyseal hormones. In: F. Fuchs and A. Klopper (eds.), *Endocrinology of Pregnancy*, p. 235 (New York: Harper and Row)

Caldwell, B. V., Burnstein, S., Brock, W. A. and Speroff, L. (1971). Radioimmunoassay of the F prostaglandins. *J. Clin. Endocrinol.*, **33**, 171

Caldwell, B. V., Auletta, F. J., Gordon, J. W. and Speroff, L. (1972). In: S. Bergström, K. Gréen and B. Samuelsson (eds.), *Prostaglandins in Fertility Control 2*, p. 217 (Stockholm: WHO, Karolinska Institute)

Challis, J. R. G., Osathanondh, R., Ryan, J. K. and Tulchinsky, D. (1974). Maternal and fetal plasma prostaglandin levels at vaginal delivery and cesarean section. *Prostaglandins*, **6**, 281

Chester, R. M., Dukes, M., Slater, S. R. and Walpole, A. L. (1972). Delays of parturition in rat by anti-inflammatory agents, which inhibit the biosynthesis of prostaglandins. *Nature (New Biol.)*, **240**, 37

Cibils, L. A. and Hendricks, C. H. (1961). Efecto de la isoxuprina sobre la contractilidad del utero humano gravido. *Mem. X. Nac. Ginec. Obstet. Merida, Mexico*, **1**, 418

Cibils, L. A. (1966). Inhibitory effect of isoxuprine on uterine contractility. *Am. J. Obstet. Gynecol.*, **94**, 762

Coats, P., Walker, E., Youssefnejadian, E. and Craft, I. L. (1977). Variations in plasma steroid and prostaglandin concentrations during human pregnancy. *Acta Obstet. Gynecol. Scand.*, **56**, 453

Cobo, E. (1968). Uterine and milk-ejection activities during human labor. *J. Appl. Physiol.*, **24**, 317

Collier, H. O. J. and Sweatman, W. J. F. (1968). Antagonism by fenamates of prostaglandin $F_{2\alpha}$ and of slow reacting substance on human bronchial muscle. *Nature*, **219**, 864

Collier, J. G. and Flower, R. J. (1971). Effect of aspirin on human seminal prostaglandins. *Lancet*, **ii**, 852

Collins, E. and Turner, G. (1975). Maternal effects of regular salicylate ingestion in pregnancy. *Lancet*, **ii**, 335

Corner, G. W. and Allen, W. M. (1929). Physiology of corpus luteum: production of special uterine reaction by extracts of corpus luteum. *Am. J. Physiol.*, **88**, 326

Csapo, A. I. (1969). The four direct regulatory factors in myometrial function. In: G. E. W.

Wolstenholme and J. Knight (eds.), *Progesterone: Its Regulatory Effect on the Myometrium*, p. 13 (London: J. and A. Churchill, Ltd)
Csapo, A. I. (1973). The prospects of prostaglandins postconceptual therapy. *Prostaglandins*, **3**, 245
Csapo, A. I., Pohanka, O. and Kaihola, H. L. (1974). Progesterone deficiency and premature labour. *Br. Med. J.*, **1**, 137
Dale, H. H. (1906). On some physiological actions of ergot. *J. Physiol.*, **34**, 163
Dawood, M. Y., Raghavan, K. S., Pociask, C. and Fuchs, F. (1978). Oxytocin in human pregnancy and parturition. *Obstet. Gynecol.*, **51**, 138
Dray, F. and Frydman, R. (1976). Primary prostaglandins in amniotic fluid in pregnancy and spontaneous labour. *Am. J. Obstet. Gynecol.*, **126**, 13
Eckenfels, A. and Vane, J. R. (1972). Prostaglandins, oxygen tension and smooth muscle tone. *Br. J. Pharmacol.*, **45**, 451
Eskes, T., Stolte, L., Seelen, H. D., Moed, C. and Vogelsang, C. (1965). Epinephrine derivates and the activity of the human uterus. *Am. J. Obstet. Gynecol.*, **92**, 871
Ferreira, S. H., Moncado, S. and Vane, J. R. (1971). Indomethacin and aspirin abolish prostaglandin release from the spleen. *Nature (New Biol.)*, **231**, 237
Flint, A. P. F., Anderson, A. B. M. and Patten, P. T. (1973). In: *Proceedings of the 134th Meeting of the Society for Endocrinology*. September, 1973, p. 73
Fuchs, A. R. (1965). The role of oxytocin in the initiation of labor. *Excerpta Med. Int. Congr. Sr.*, **83**, 753
Fuchs, A. R., Smitasiri, Y. and Chantharaksri, U. (1974). Prostaglandins and the onset of parturition in rats. *Gynecol. Invest.*, **5**, 30
Fuchs, F. (1965). Treatment of threatened premature labour with alcohol. *J. Obstet. Gynaecol. Br. Cmnwlth.*, **72**, 1011
Fuchs, F. (1976). Prevention of prematurity. *Am. J. Obstet. Gynecol.*, **126**, 809
Fuchs, F., Fuchs, A. R., Poblete, V. F. Jr. and Risk, A. (1967). Effect of alcohol on threatened premature labor. *Am. J. Obstet. Gynecol.*, **99**, 627
Fuchs, F. and Stakemann, G. (1960). Treatment of threatened premature labor with large doses of progesterone. *Am. J. Obstet. Gynecol.*, **79**, 172
Fuller, W. E. (1978). Management of premature labor. *Clin. Obstet. Gynecol.*, **21**, 533
Gazarek, F., Pohauka, J., Talas, M., Fingerova, H., Januskova, M., Krikal, Z. and Hamal, Z. (1976). *Endocrinol. Experium.*, **10**, 283
Gibbens, G. L. D. and Chard, T. (1976). Observations on maternal oxytocin release during human labor and the effect of intravenous alcohol administration. *Am. J. Obstet. Gynecol.*, **126**, 243
Graff, G. (1971). Failure to prevent premature labor with ethanol. *Am. J. Obstet. Gynecol.*, **110**, 878
Greaves, M. W. and McDonald-Gibson, W. (1973). Effect of non-steroid anti-inflammatory and antipyretic drugs on prostaglandin biosynthesis by human skin. *J. Invest. Dermatol.*, **61**, 127
Gréen, K., Bygdeman, M., Toppozada, M. and Wiqvist, N. (1974). The role of prostaglandin $F_{2\alpha}$ in human parturition. *Am. J. Obstet. Gynecol.*, **120**, 25
Greenhouse, B. S., Hook, B. and Hehre, F. W. (1969). Aspiration pneumonia following intravenous administration of alcohol during labor. *J. Am. Med. Assoc.*, **210**, 2393
Györy, G., Kiss, C., Benyo, T., Bagdany, S., Szalay, J., Kurcz, M. and Virag, S. (1974). Inhibition of labour by prostaglandin antagonists in impending abortion and preterm and term labour. *Lancet*, **ii**, 293
Haning, R. V., Barett, D. A., Albertino, S. P., Linskey, M. T., Donabedian, R. and Speroff, L. (1978). Interrelationships between maternal and cord prolactin, progesterone, estradiol, 13,14-dihydro-15-beta prostaglandin F and cord cortisol at delivery with respect to initiation of parturition. *Am. J. Obstet. Gynecol.*, **130**, 204
Hellig, H., Gattereau, D., Lefebure, Y. and Balte, E. (1970). Steroid production from plasma

cholesterol. I. Conversion of plasma cholesterol to placental progesterone in humans. *J. Clin. Endocrinol.*, **30**, 624

Hendricks, C. H., Cibils, L. A., Pose, S. V. and Eskes, T. K. (1961). The pharmacological control of excessive uterine activity with isoxuprine. *Am. J. Obstet. Gynecol.*, **82**, 1064

Hendricks, C. H. (1964). The use of isoxsuprine for the arrest of premature labor. *Clin. Obstet. Gynecol.*, **7**, 687

Hertelendy, F., Woods, R. and Jaffe, B. M. (1973). Prostaglandin E levels in peripheral blood during labor. *Prostaglandins*, **3**, 223

Heymann, M. A. and Rudolph, A. M. (1975). Control of the ductus arteriosus. *Physiol. Rev.*, **55**, 62

Heymann, M. A. and Rudolph, A. M. (1976). Effects of acetylsalicylic acid on the ductus arteriosus and circulation in fetal lambs *in utero*. *Circ. Res.*, **38**, 418

Hibbard, B. M., Sharma, S. C., Fitzpatrick, R. J. and Hamlett, J. D. (1974). Prostaglandin $F_{2\alpha}$ concentrations in amniotic fluid in late pregnancy. *J. Obstet. Gynaecol. Br. Cmnwlth.*, **81**, 35

Hill, L. M., Johnson, C. E. and Lee, R. A. (1975). Prophylactic use of hydroxy-progesterone caproate in abdominal surgery during pregnancy. *Obstet. Gynecol.*, **46**, 287

Hillier, K., Calder, A. A. and Embrey, M. P. (1974). Concentrations of prostaglandin $F_{2\alpha}$ in amniotic fluid and plasma in spontaneous and induced labours. *J. Obstet. Gynaecol. Br. Cmnwlth.*, **81**, 257

Johansson, E. (1969). Plasma levels of progesterone in pregnancy measured by a rapid competitive protein binding technique. *Acta Endocrinol.*, **61**, 607

Johnson, J. W. C., Austin, K. L., Jones, G. S., Davis, G. H. and King, T. M. (1975). Efficacy of 17α-hydroxy-progesterone caproate in the prevention of premature labor. *N. Engl. J. Med.*, **293**, 675

Karim, S. M. M. (1966). Identification of prostaglandins in human amniotic fluid. *J. Obstet. Gynaecol. Br. Cmnwlth.*, **73**, 903

Karim, S. M. M. and Devlin, J. (1967). Prostaglandin content of amniotic fluid during pregnancy and labour. *J. Obstet. Gynaecol. Br. Cmnwlth.*, **74**, 230

Karim, S. M. M. (1968). Appearance of prostaglandin $F_{2\alpha}$ in human blood during labour. *Br. Med. J.*, **4**, 618

Karim, S. M. M., Trussel, R. R., Hillier, K. and Patel, R. C. (1969). Induction of labour with prostaglandin $F_{2\alpha}$. *J. Obstet. Gynaecol. Br. Cmnwlth.*, **76**, 769

Karim, S. M. M. and Sharma, S. D. (1971). The effect of alcohol on prostaglandins E_2 and $F_{2\alpha}$ induced uterine activity in pregnant women. *J. Obstet. Gynaecol. Br. Cmnwlth.*, **78**, 251

Karim, S. M. M. (1972). Prostaglandins and human reproduction: physiological roles and clinical uses of prostaglandins in relation to human reproduction. In: S. M. M. Karim (ed.), *The Prostaglandins: Progress in Research*, pp. 71–164 (New York: Wiley-Interscience)

Karim, S. M. M. and Hillier, K. (1975). Physiological roles and pharmacological actions of prostaglandins in relation to human reproduction. In: S. M. M. Karim (ed.), *Advances in Prostaglandin Research, Prostaglandins and Reproduction*, p. 23 (Lancaster: MTP Press)

Karim, S. M. M. (1978). On the use of blockers of prostaglandin synthesis in the control of labor. In: F. Coceani and P. M. Olley (eds.), *Advances in Prostaglandin and Thromboxane Research*, Vol. IV, p. 301 (New York: Raven Press)

Keirse, M. J. N. C. and Turnbull, A. C. (1973). E prostaglandins in amniotic fluid during late pregnancy and labour. *J. Obstet. Gynaecol. Br. Cmnwlth.*, **80**, 970

Keirse, M. J. N. C., Flint, A. P. F. and Turnbull, A. C. (1974). F prostaglandins in amniotic fluid during pregnancy and labour. *J. Obstet. Gynaecol. Br. Cmnwlth.*, **81**, 131

Keirse, M. J. N. C., Mitchell, M. D. and Turnbull, A. C. (1977). Changes in prostaglandin F and 13,14-dihydro-15-keto-prostaglandin F concentrations in amniotic fluid at the onset of and during labour. *Br. J. Obstet. Gynaecol.*, **84**, 743

Kinoshita, K., Satoh, K. and Sakamoto, S. (1977). Prostaglandin ($F_{2\alpha}$ and E_2) in plasma and amniotic fluid during human pregnancy and labor. *Endocrinol. Jap.*, **24**, 155

Kloeck, F. K. and Jung, H. (1973). *In vitro* release of prostaglandin from the human myometrium under the influence of stretching. *Am. J. Obstet. Gynecol.*, **115**, 1066

Knauss, H. H. (1934). Ueber die Ursachen der Geburtsauslösung. *Med. Klin.*, p. 1694

Kohler, H. G. (1967). Intrauterine cardiac failure associated with premature closure of the ductus arteriosus. *Arch. Dis. Child.*, **42**, 335

Konzett, H. (1940). Neue bronkolytisch hochwirksame Körper der Adreanalinreihe. *Naunyn-Schmiedebergs Arch. Pharmakol. Exper. Pathol.*, **197**, 27

Korda, A. R., Lyneham, R. C. and Warren, R. J. (1974). The treatment of premature labour with intravenously administered salbutamol. *Med. J. Aust.*, **1**, 744

Lackritz, R., Tulchinsky, D., Ryan, K. J. and Levine, L. (1978). Plasma prostaglandin metabolites in human labor. *Am. J. Obstet. Gynecol.*, **131**, 484

Lands, A. M., Arnold, A., McAuliff, J., Luduena, F. P. and Brown, T. G. (1967). Differentiation of receptor systems activated by sympathomimetic amines. *Nature*, **214**, 597

Langley, J. N. (1905). On the reactions of cells and of nerve-endings to certain poisons, chiefly as regards the reaction of striated muscle to nicotine and to curare. *J. Physiol.*, **33**, 374

Lanman, J. T. (1968). Delays during reproduction and their effects on the embryo and fetus. *N. Engl. J. Med.*, **278**, 993

Lau, I. F., Saksena, S. K. and Chang, M. C. (1975). Effects of indomethacin and prostaglandin $F_{2\alpha}$ on parturition in the hamster. *Prostaglandins*, **10**, 1011

Lauersen, N. H., Merkatz, I. R., Tejani, N., Wilson, K. H., Robertson, A., Mann, L. I. and Fuchs, F. (1977). Inhibition of premature labor: A multicenter comparison of ritrodrine and ethanol. *Am. J. Obstet. Gynecol.*, **127**, 837

Le Vine, L. (1964). Habitual abortion: a controlled study of progestational therapy. *W. J. Surg.*, **72**, 30

Levy, B. and Lindner, H. R. (1971). Selective blockade of the vasodepressor response to prostaglandin $F_{2\alpha}$ in the anesthetized rabbit. *Br. J. Pharmacol.*, **43**, 236

Lewis, R. B. and Schulman, J. D. (1973). Influence of acetylsalicylic acid, an inhibitor of prostaglandin synthesis, on the duration of human gestation and labour. *Lancet*, **ii**, 1159

Lippert, T. H. (1972). Therapeutische Aspekte der Prostaglandinforschung in der Frauenheilkunde. *Geburtshilfe Frauenheilkd.*, **32**, 13

Lipshitz, J. (1977). The uterine and cardiovascular effects of oral fenoterol hydrobromide. *Br. J. Obstet. Gynaecol.*, **84**, 737

Llauro, J. L., Runnebaum, B. and Zander, J. (1968). Progesterone in human peripheral blood before, during and after labor. *Am. J. Obstet. Gynecol.*, **101**, 867

Luukkainen, T., Väistö, L. and Järvinen, P. A. (1967). The effect of oral intake of ethyl alcohol on the activity of the pregnant human uterus. *Acta Obstet. Gynecol. Scand.*, **46**, 486

Lynn, J. M. (1970). Intravenous alcohol infusion for premature labor. *J. Am. Osteopath. Assoc.*, **70**, 1

Mahon, W. A., Reid, D. W. J. and Day, R. A. (1967). The *in vivo* effects of beta-adrenergic stimulation and blockade on the human uterus at term. *J. Pharmacol. Exp. Ther.*, **156**, 178

Manchester, D., Margolis, H. S. and Sheldon, R. E. (1976). Possible association between maternal indomethacin therapy and primary pulmonary hypertension of the newborn. *Am. J. Obstet. Gynecol.*, **126**, 467

Mann, L. I., Bhakthavathsalan, A., Liu, M. and Makowski, P. (1975a). Placental transport of alcohol and its effects on maternal and fetal acid base balance. *Am. J. Obstet. Gynecol.*, **122**, 837

Mann, L. I., Bhakthavathsalan, A., Liu, M. and Makowski, P. (1975b). Effect of alcohol on fetal cerebral function and metabolism. *Am. J. Obstet. Gynecol.*, **122**, 845

Mantell, C. D. and Liggins, G. C. (1970). The effect of ethanol on the myometrial response to oxytocin in women at term. *J. Obstet. Gynaecol. Br. Cmnwlth.*, **77**, 976

Mitchell, M. D., Brunt, J. B., Bibby, J., Flint, A. P. F., Anderson, A. B. M. and Turnbull, A. C. (1978a). Prostaglandins in the human umbilical circulation at birth. *Br. J. Obstet. Gynaecol.*, **85**, 114

Mitchell, M. D., Flint, A. P., Bibby, J., Brunt, J., Arnold, J. M., Anderson, A. B. M. and Turnbull, A. C. (1978b). Plasma concentrations of prostaglandins during late human pregnancy: influence of normal and preterm labor. *J. Clin. Endocrinol. Metabol.*, **46**, 947

Nakanishi, H., McLean, J., Wood, C. and Burnstock, G. (1969). The role of sympathetic nerves in control of the non-pregnant and pregnant human uterus. *J. Reprod. Med.*, **2**, 20

Neher, G. M. and Zarrow, M. X. (1954). Concentration of progestin in serum of non-pregnant, pregnant, and post-partum ewe. *J. Endocrinol.*, **11**, 323

Niebyl, J. R., Blacke, D. A., Johnson, W. C. and King, T. M. (1978). The pharmacologic inhibition of premature labor. *Obstet. Gynecol. Surv.*, **33**, 507

Nora, J. J., Nora, A. H., Perinchief, A. G., Ingram, J. W., Fountain, A. K. and Peterson, M. J. (1976). Congenital abnormalities and first trimester exposure to progestagen/oestrogen. *Lancet*, **i**, 313

Novy, M. J., Cook, M. J. and Manaugh, L. (1974). Indomethacin block of normal onset of parturition in primates. *Am. J. Obstet. Gynecol.*, **118**, 412

O'Grady, J. P., Caldwell, B. V., Auletta, F. J. and Speroff, L. (1972). The effects of an inhibitor of prostaglandin synthesis on ovulation, pregnancy and pseudo-pregnancy in the rabbit. *Prostaglandins*, **1**, 97

Orczyk, G. P. and Behrman, H. R. (1972). Ovulation blockade by aspirin or indomethacin: *In vivo* evidence for a role of prostaglandin in gonadotropin secretion. *Prostaglandins*, **1**, 3

Ott, A., Hayes, I. and Polin, J. (1976). Severe lactic acidosis associated with intravenous alcohol for premature labor. *Obstet. Gynecol.*, **48**, 362

Ovlisen, B. and Iversen, J. (1963). Treatment of threatened premature labor with a 6a-methyl-17a-acetoxy-progesterone. *Am. J. Obstet. Gynecol.*, **86**, 291

Pauerstein, C. J. and Zander, H. L. (1970). Autonomic innervation, sex steroids and uterine contractility. *Obstet. Gynecol. Surv.*, **25**, 617

Pose, Sv., Cibils, L. A. and Zuspan, F. P. (1962). Effect of l-epinephrine infusion on uterine contractility and cardiovascular system. *Am. J. Obstet. Gynecol.*, **84**, 297

Powell, C. E. and Slater, I. H. (1958). Blocking of inhibitory adrenergic receptors by a dichloroanalog of isoproterenol. *J. Pharmacol. Exp. Ther.*, **122**, 480

Poyser, N. L., Horton, E. W., Thompson, C. J. and Los, M. (1971). Identification of $F_{2\alpha}$ by distension of guinea-pig uterus *in vitro*. *Nature*, **230**, 526

Reiffenstein, E. C. (1958). Clinical use of 17a-hydroxy-progesterone 17-*n*-caproate in habitual abortion. *Ann. N.Y. Acad. Sci.*, **71**, 762

Reiss, U., Atad, J., Rubinstein, I. and Zuckerman, H. (1976). The effect of indomethacin in labor at term. *Int. J. Obstet. Gynecol.*, **14**, 369

Roth-Brandel, U., Bygdeman, M., Wiqvist, N. and Bergström, S. (1970). Prostaglandin for induction of therapeutic abortion. *Lancet*, **i**, 190

Salmon, J. A. and Amy, J. J. (1973). Levels of prostaglandin $F_{2\alpha}$ in amniotic fluid during pregnancy and labour. *Prostaglandins*, **4**, 523

Sandholm, L. H. (1971). Effect of alcohol on oxytocin in pueperal women. *Acta Obstet. Gynecol. Scand.* (Suppl.), **41**, 36

Scher, J. and Baillie, P. (1973). The effect of a β-adrenergic agent on prostaglandin stimulated labor. *Adv. Biosci.*, **9**, 743

Shaikh, A. A., Nakvi, R. H. and Saksena, S. K. (1977). Prostaglandins E and F in uterine venous plasma in relation to peripheral plasma levels of progesterone and 20_a-hydroxyprogesterone in the rat throughout pregnancy and parturition. *Prostaglandins*, **13**, 311

Sharma, S. C., Hibbard, B. M., Hamlett, J. D. and Fitzpatrick, R. J. (1973). Prostaglandin $F_{2\alpha}$ concentrations in peripheral blood during the first stage of normal labour. *Br. Med. J.*, **1**, 709

Sharpe, G. L., Thalme, B. and Larsson, S. (1974). Studies on closure of the ductus arteriosus. *Prostaglandins*, **8**, 363

Sharpe, G. L., Larsson, K. S. and Thalme, B. (1975). Studies on closure of the ductus arteriosus. *Prostaglandins*, **9**, 585

Shearman, R. P. and Garrett, W. J. (1963). Double blind study of effect of 17a-hydroxyprogesterone caproate on abortion rate. *Br. Med. J.*, **1**, 292

Short, R. V. (1960). Blood progesterone levels in relation to parturition. *J. Reprod. Fertil.*, **1**, 61

Singh, E. J. and Zuspan, F. P. (1974). Content of amniotic fluid prostaglandins in normal diabetic and drug-abuse human pregnancy. *Am. J. Obstet. Gynecol.*, **118**, 358

Smith, J. B. and Willis, A. L. (1971). Aspirin selectivity inhibits prostaglandin production in human platelets. *Nature (New Biol.)*, **231**, 235

Soloff, M., Swartz, T., Morrison, M. and Saffron, M. (1973). Oxytocin receptors: oxytocin analogs, but not prostaglandins, complete with 3H-oxytocin for uptake by rat uterus. *Endocrinology*, **92**, 104

Sorrentino, L., Capasso, F. and di Rosa, M. (1972). Indomethacin and prostaglandins. *Eur. J. Pharmacol.*, **17**, 306

Steer, C. M. and Petrie, R. H. (1977). A comparison of magnesium sulfate and alcohol for the prevention of premature labor. *Am. J. Obstet. Gynecol.*, **129**, 1

Stolte, L., Eskes, T., Seelen, J., Moed, H. D. and Vogelsang, C. (1965). Epinephrine derivates and the activity of the human uterus. Part I. *Am. J. Obstet. Gynecol.*, **92**, 865

Tamby Raja, R. L., Salmon, J. A., Karim, S. M. M. and Ratnam, S. S. (1977). F prostaglandin levels in amniotic fluid in premature labour. *Prostaglandins*, **13**, 339

Traeger, A., Noschel, H. and Zaumseil, J. (1973). The pharmocokinetics of indomethacin in pregnant and parturient women and in their newborn infants. *Zentral. Gynäk.*, **95**, 635

Turnbull, A. C., Patten, P. T., Fling, A. P. D., Keirse, M. J. N. C., Jeremy, J. Y. and Anderson, A. B. M. (1973). Significant fall in progesterone and rise in oestradiol levels in human peripheral plasma at the approach of labour. *J. Obstet. Gynaecol. Br. Cmnwlth.*, **80**, 210

Turner, G. and Collins, E. (1975). Fetal effects of regular salicylate ingestion in pregnancy. *Lancet*, **ii**, 338

Tyack, A. J., Baillie, P. and Meehan, F. P. (1971). *In vivo* response of the human uterus to orciprenaline in early labour. *Br. Med. J.*, **2**, 741

Van Dyke, H. B. and Ames, R. G. (1951). Alcohol diuresis. *Acta Endocrinol.*, **7**, 110

Vane, J. R. (1971). Inhibition of prostaglandin synthesis as a mechanism of action for aspirin-like drugs. *Nature (New Biol.)*, **231**, 232

Vane, J. R. (1972). Prostaglandins and aspirin-like drugs. *Hosp. Pract.*, **7**, 61

Vane, J. R. and Willians, K. I. (1972). Prostaglandin production contributes to the contractions of the rat isolated uterus. *Br. J. Pharmacol.*, **45**, 146P

Waltman, R., Tricomi, V. and Palav, A. (1973a). Aspirin and indomethacin: Effect on instillation/abortion time of midtrimester hypertonic saline induced abortion. *Prostaglandins*, **3**, 47

Waltman, R., Tricomi, V. and Shabanah, E. H. (1973b). The effect of anti-inflammatory drugs on parturition parameters in the rat. *Prostaglandins*, **4**, 93

Whalen, J. B., Clancey, C. J., Farley, D. B. and van Orden, D. E. (1978). Plasma prostaglandins in pregnancy. *Obstet. Gynecol.*, **51**, 52

Willman, E. A. and Collins, W. P. (1976). The concentrations of prostaglandin E_2 and prostaglandin $F_{2\alpha}$ in tissues within the fetoplacental unit after spontaneous or induced labour. *Br. J. Obstet. Gynaecol.*, **83**, 786

Willman, E. A., Rodeck, C. H., Collins, W. P. and Clayton, S. G. (1977). The relation between umbilical cord tissue prostaglandin E_2 levels, mode of onset of labour, fetal distress and method of delivery. *Br. J. Obstet. Gynaecol.*, **84**, 605

Wiqvist, N., Lundström, V. and Gréen, K. (1975). Premature labour and indomethacin. *Prostaglandins*, **10**, 515

Yoffee, B. M., Smith, J. W. and Newton, W. T. (1971). Radioimmunoassay for prostaglandins. *Science*, **171**, 494

Zarrow, M. X. and Neher, G. M. (1955). Concentration of progestin in serum of rabbit during pregnancy, puerperium, and following castration. *Endocrinology*, **56**, 1

Zlatnik, F. and Fuchs, F. (1972). A controlled study of ethanol in threatened premature labor. *Am. J. Obstet. Gynecol.*, **112**, 610

Zuckerman, H., Reiss, U. and Rubinstein, I. (1974). Inhibition of human premature labor by indomethacin. *Obstet. Gynecol.*, **44**, 787

Zuckerman, H., Reiss, U., Atad, J. and Rubinstein, I. (1975). Indomethacin as an inhibitor of premature labor. *Harefuah*, **89**, 201

Zuckerman, H., Reiss, U., Atad, J., Lampert, I., Ben Ezra, S. and Sklan, D. (1977). The effect of indomethacin on plasma levels of $PGF_{2\alpha}$ in women in labour. *Br. J. Obstet. Gynaecol.*, **84**, 339

Zuckerman, H., Reiss, U., Atad, J., Lampert, I., Ben Ezra, S. and Sklan, D. (1978a). Prostaglandin $F_{2\alpha}$ in human blood during labor. *Obstet. Gynecol.*, **51**, 311

Zuckerman, H., Harpaz-Kerpel, S., Gilad, G. and Shalev, E. (1978b). Oxytocin and prostaglandins during labor. (Submitted for publication)

Zuckerman, H. (1978). Indomethacin and human premature labor. (Submitted for publication)

Zuspan, F. P., Cibils, L. A. and Pose, S. V. (1962). Myometrial and cardiovascular responses to alterations in plasma epinephrine and nonepinephrine. *Am. J. Obstet. Gynecol.*, **84**, 841

19
Induction of Labour with Prostaglandins

J.-J. AMY and M. THIERY

19.1 INTRODUCTION: PRINCIPLES OF LABOUR INDUCTION

'Induction' means the artificial initiation of labour at or beyond 28 weeks gestation. Women already 'in labour' and having uterine contractions which result in cervical dilatation or rupture of the membranes may receive oxytocics (or have amniotomy performed) for 'augmentation' ('stimulation', 'acceleration') of labour. Depending on the length of gestation, labour is induced 'before term', 'at term' (38–42 weeks) or 'after term'. Induction is 'elective' when performed at term in a clinically normal patient with favourable induction prospects. All other inductions are called 'therapeutic'. In most of these, labour is being induced because of some foetal or maternal complication, and the cervix is often unfavourable. This considerably affects the ease and the safety of induction. The selection of a proper method in therapeutic induction is therefore of great importance.

Current clinical methods of induction of labour are mainly limited to amniotomy ('surgical induction') and the administration of oxytocin or a prostaglandin ('chemical induction'). When both surgical and chemical methods are used together, one speaks of 'combined induction', which is more effective than either one used alone (see Amy *et al.*, 1976; Amy and Thiery, 1979, for references).

The lower uterine segment forms towards the end of pregnancy and the cervix becomes more anterior, softer, shorter and starts to dilate. Once this process is completed, the cervix is said to be 'ripe' or 'favourable' and a limited amount of residual work is required to achieve complete dilatation. In the presence of a favourable cervix spontaneous labour is usually imminent and induction of labour, if attempted, is most likely to be successful.

Of the different methods of assessing inducibility, the pelvic scoring system described by Bishop (1964) has gained the widest acceptance. A numerical value (from 0 to a maximum of 3) is given for each of four characteristics of the cervix and for the station of the presenting part (Table 19.1). The sum (Bishop score, maximum 13) is an index of inducibility. When the score is less than six, the cervix is said to be 'unfavourable' and protracted labour may follow attempted induction.

Table 19.1 The Bishop scoring system

Score	*0*	*1*	*2*	*3*
Station presenting part	−3	−2	−1/0	+1/+2
Dilatation (cm)	0	1–2	3–4	⩾5
Effacement (cm)	⩾2, 5	2	1	⩽0.5
Consistency	firm	medium	weak	
Position of os	posterior	central	anterior	

As defined here, elective induction only applies to the normal foetus after 38 weeks of gestation. Gestational length, calculated from the first day of the last menstrual period (LMP) must therefore be known with certainty. Labour should not be induced electively in women with a history of irregular cycles, uncertain LMP, decidual bleeding or those who become pregnant soon after stopping the use of hormonal contraceptives.

Therapeutic (non-elective) induction of labour is often performed in patients with a low Bishop score, relative foetal immaturity, post-maturity and for a number of other foetal or maternal problems. Usually, more than one of these factors are involved. Typical examples of cases requiring therapeutic induction of labour are patients with hypertensive and other cardiovascular diseases, diabetes, rhesus iso-immunization, intrauterine growth retardation, prolonged gestation and premature rupture of the membranes. The combination of an unfavourable cervix and a diminished foetal reserve makes therapeutic induction more difficult and hazardous than in elective cases. An oxytocin challenge test (Freeman, 1975) may be helpful in determining whether the foetus is capable of sustaining the stress of labour.

Induction should not be attempted when uterine activity *per se* or vaginal delivery are contraindicated. Such contraindications include certain types of malpresentation (e.g. transverse lie; breech presentation with deflexed head), a history of previous uterine surgery (e.g. myomectomy; Strassman procedure; classical caesarean section; second trimester hysterotomy); the finding of an active herpes infection of the genital tract, of severe pelvic contraction or of a tumour praevia. Acute respiratory tract infection markedly increases the maternal risk should operative delivery and inhalation anaesthesia become necessary. Finally, after removal of a Shirodkar circlage of the cervix, one often may notice some fibrosis of the previous suture tract. This should be allowed to soften spontaneously, before induction is attempted.

Continuous electronic monitoring of myometrial activity and foetal heart rate (FHR) must be an inherent feature of labour induction; facilities for determining the foetal acid–base equilibrium must also be available.

19.2 ELECTIVE INDUCTION OF LABOUR WITH PROSTAGLANDINS

The first report on the clinical application of a prostaglandin goes back a mere 10 years and it actually concerned labour induction (Karim *et al.*, 1968). This book is proof of the extraordinary amount of research done since 1968 on the therapeutic potential of prostaglandins and their synthesis inhibitors.

Extensive reviews of the literature pertaining to the induction of labour with prostaglandins have been published elsewhere (Thiery and Amy, 1975, 1977). The purpose of this shorter chapter is to highlight some practical aspects of the procedure.

PGE_2 and $PGF_{2\alpha}$ have mainly been used. Depending on the route of administration, PGE_2 is about three to 10 times more potent than $PGF_{2\alpha}$ (Table 19.2), but when given in proportionate doses, these drugs are equally effective. Less than 100 cases of labour induction with PGE_1 have been reported and only two with $PGF_{1\alpha}$. Toppozada *et al.* (1976) reported on the successful use of PGA_1 given by intravenous infusions, 0.25–1.0 ug/kg/min for the induction of labour in 10 patients. This compound, with its known vasodilator property, lowered the blood pressure in some toxaemic subjects. However, episodes of uterine hypertonus and abnormal FHR patterns were noted in several instances. Additional data are needed in order to assess the value of PGA_1 as an oxytocic agent. Synthetic analogues, because of their longer biological half-life are considered to be more difficult to titrate during induction of labour. Little is known concerning placental inactivation of these compounds and it is conceivable that they cross unaltered into the foetal compartment. Their use, therefore, has been restricted to cases of foetal death or anomaly, in which they have proved extremely effective (Karim, Ng and Ratnam, Chapter 16).

Table 19.2 Intravenous infusion of natural prostaglandins: Dose levels

Dose ratio	PGE_2†	$PGF_{2\alpha}$†
Induction at term*	0.5 μg/min	5.0 μg/min
Termination of early pregnancy	5.0 μg/min	50 μg/min

* Dose level determined by the titration method
† 1 μg PGE_2 ~ 10 μg $PGF_{2\alpha}$

Prostaglandins can be given by a variety of routes (see Chapter 17) but, for the induction of labour, only the intravenous, oral, buccal and extra-amniotic routes are currently used. As with oxytocin, uterine hyperstimulation may follow intramuscular or subcutaneous administration; and natural prostaglandins can cause an intense pain at the site of injection. Absorption by the vaginal route is unpredictable and this route therefore is used only for the termination of abnormal intrauterine pregnancies (see Karim, Ng and Ratnam, Chapter 16).

19.2.1 Intravenous route

As with oxytocin, the best results are obtained when prostaglandins are used in combination with amniotomy. The prostaglandin is infused by means of a pump, the flow of which may be automatically regulated by the cardiotocographic unit (Calder and Embrey, 1975). Dose levels (initial dose level: 0.1 μg/min PGE_2 or 1.0 μg/min $PGF_{2\alpha}$) are progressively stepped up by a constant increment or by 30–100% at 20–30 min interval until there is adequate myometrial stimulation. The infusion rate is then maintained until delivery unless uterine hyperactivity, abnormal FHR patterns or maternal side-effects occur, in which case the infusion is slowed down or stopped altogether until recovery (Table 19.3).

Induction combining amniotomy with the intravenous infusion of PGE_2 or $PGF_{2\alpha}$ effects delivery within 24 h in nearly 100% of women treated. Nausea and vomiting have been reported in 0–20% of the cases, depending on the series, diarrhoea on 0–6% and a transient venous erythema in 0–12%. All of these are usually of minor severity and do not require interruption of drug administration. In case of uterine hypertonus, the intravenous injection of a β-mimetic compound (e.g. ritodrine) causes the uterus to relax promptly. A single case of maternal mortality has been reported following intravenous infusion of $PGF_{2\alpha}$ for the induction of labour, but the death was not related to the use of this specific oxytocic (Johnson *et al.*, 1974).

Table 19.3 Induction of labour. Recommended doses

Method	*Initial dose*	*Dose increment**	*Maximum dose*
I.V. oxytocin	2 mU/min	dose doubled at 15–30 min intervals	32 (64) mU/min Restrict fluid intake Consider other method
I.V. PGE_2	0.2 µg/min	dose increased by 30–100% at 30 min intervals	—
I.V. $PGF_{2\alpha}$	2 µg/min	dose increased by 30–100% at 30 min intervals	—
Oral PGE_2	0.5 mg	2nd dose: 1.0 mg; 3rd dose: 2.0 mg; then 3.0 mg at 30–60 min intervals	3.0 mg/30 min
Buccal PGE_2	0.5 mg	dose increased by 0.5 mg at 60 min intervals	3.0 mg/60 min
Extra-amniotic PGE_2	0.4 µg/min	dose increased by 0.2 µg/min at 15 min intervals	—

*Dependent on patient's response (myometrial activity, side-effects)

19.2.2 Oral route

The oral route of prostaglandin administration appeals to patients and nurses alike as it avoids a venepuncture and an intravenous infusion. By increasing the comfort of the patient being induced, it contributes to a more relaxed atmosphere.

$PGF_{2\alpha}$ causes an unacceptably high rate of gastro-intestinal side-effects when given orally (see Seng and Salmon, 1976) and hence only PGE_2 is used by this route. Its administration in incremental doses (e.g. 0.5 mg, doubled every 30 min, until adequate uterine activity or a maximum single dose of 3.0 mg) has proven more effective than fixed dose regimens (e.g. 0.5 mg at intervals of 30–60 min). The best results have been reported in parous women with favourable cervix and in combination with artificial rupture of the membranes. In these cases, oral PGE_2 has an efficacy similar to that of oxytocin or a prostaglandin given intravenously. It is less effective in nulliparae and in other patients with unfavourable inducibility prospects (Craft, 1973; Lauersen and Wilson, 1975; Miller *et al.*, 1975).

Side-effects observed during oral administration of PGE_2 for labour induction are limited to the gastro-intestinal tract. Vomiting occurs in 5–34%

of the cases and diarrhoea in 0–6%, depending on the series. In most instances the disturbance is not severe and discontinuation of drug administration is rarely required. One case of uterine rupture complicated by amniotic fluid embolus and maternal death has been reported. The woman, however, had previously been subjected to a myomectomy and she should not have been allowed to go into labour, much less be stimulated with an oxytocic (Karim and Sharma, 1972).

Despite the fact that the myometrial activation following oral administration of each dose of PGE_2 may last for 1 hour or more, titration of the drug is usually readily achieved. Hyperstimulation, mostly short-lived, was seen in less than 1% of the cases.

19.2.3 Buccal (oromucosal) route

Scher *et al.* (1976) first reported the successful use of PGE_2 by the buccal route for the induction of labour. In this regimen, commercially available tablets of PGE_2 are kept under the tongue or in the cheek instead of being swallowed. We (Thiery *et al.*, 1977) have compared the oral and buccal administration of PGE_2 using a similar protocol. The initial dose of 0.5 mg was increased by 0.5 mg at hourly intervals up to a maximum single dose of 3.0 mg. No difference was found between the two methods in terms of efficacy or maternal and foetal tolerance. Buccal administration of the drug does not seem to offer any advantage over the oral route (Scott and Craft, 1976).

19.2.4 Extra-amniotic route

Calder *et al.* (1976) extended the extra-amniotic method, formerly used solely for interruption of second trimester pregnancy (see Chapter 17), to the induction of labour. A PGE_2 solution is infused (0.33 μg/min, increased if necessary by 0.17 μg/min, every 15 min) by a pump via a Nelaton catheter (16 French) transcervically inserted into the extra-amniotic space of the lower uterine segment. As soon as feasible low amniotomy is performed, without the catheter being displaced, and drug administration is continued.

The method is highly efficacious (even in subjects with poor inducibility features), very safe and causes negligible side-effects (Miller and Mack, 1974). The foetal membranes can be kept intact until the cervix has dilated and the presenting part has descended sufficiently, thereby reducing the risk of intrauterine infection and cord prolapse. This technique may be particularly indicated for induction in women with an unfavourable cervix, breech or unengaged cephalic presentation.

Kennedy *et al.* (1978) have applied a technique originally described for pre-induction ripening of the cervix (Calder, Chapter 15) to the elective induction of labour in women with favourable induction prospects. The extra-amniotic injection of a single dose of 400 μg PGE_2 suspended in 5 ml of a 5% methyl-hydroxyethyl cellulose gel (Tylose MH 300 (R), Hoechst), followed 3 hours later by amniotomy, was sufficient to induce and maintain uterine activity in 23 out of 30 patients. The other seven subjects required uterine stimulation with intravenous oxytocin. The method was particularly effective in parous women: all of them had delivered vaginally within 9 h of treatment in a mean time of 5.4 ± 0.9 h. The authors stressed the simplicity and the high acceptability of the technique among patients.

19.2.5 Foetal and neonatal effects

While hypertonus may occur somewhat more frequently with intravenous prostaglandin than with intravenous oxytocin, it is less frequent with oral PGE_2. In the absence of or after prompt correction of hypertonus, the perinatal outcome is comparable to that with spontaneous or oxytocin-induced labour. Maternal blood gases, acid–base equilibrium, and usual blood and urine laboratory values, utero-placental blood flow and placental function are unimpaired during labour induction with a prostaglandin. No difference is found in FHR patterns, foetal and neonatal acid–base and lactate–pyruvate equilibria (Apgar) scores, neonatal course (Thiery and Amy, 1978) and psychomotor development of the child up to 2½ years of age (Decoster *et al.*, 1976). The incidence of neonatal hyperbilirubinaemia in patients induced with PGE_2 is not higher than in those induced by other methods (Beazley and Weekes, 1976; Sivasuriya *et al.*, 1978).

19.3 THERAPEUTIC INDUCTION OF LABOUR WITH PROSTAGLANDINS

Therapeutic induction of labour differs from elective induction in two respects: (1) the cervix is frequently unripe, and (2) the foetus is more prone to oxygen deprivation. The use of oxytocin in these complicated pregnancies has not proved entirely satisfactory. Adequate uterine stimulation may require high doses of this hormone, occasionally causing: (1) cardiovascular side-effects including peripheral vasodilatation and transient hypotension with compensatory tachycardia and increased cardiac output (Weiss *et al.*, 1975) or (2) antidiuresis culminating in water intoxication (Liggins, 1962). Prostaglandins, on the contrary, are capable of stimulating the myometrium and of interrupting pregnancy at any stage of gestation and they accomplish this within a narrow dose range. They lack the antidiuretic action of oxytocin and their side-effects are mostly trivial.

We prefer the intravenous and extra-amniotic routes which permit accurate titration of the prostaglandin. In patients with favourable induction features, oxytocin may be used (in combination with amniotomy) with good chances of success. In difficult cases, prostaglandins are superior to oxytocin in terms of absence of antidiuretic effect, overall success rate and shorter duration of labour. PGE_2 is given via the intravenous or extra-amniotic route, amniotomy being performed as soon as practicable. If the cervix is extremely unfavourable, the induction can be preceded by cervical ripening (Calder, Chapter 15).

19.4 ACCELERATION OF LABOUR WITH PROSTAGLANDINS

Prostaglandins (i.v. PGE_2) and oxytocin are equally effective for the stimulation of desultory labour (Weekes et al., 1976). PGE_2, however, offers no further advantages and is more expensive than oxytocin.

19.5 CONCLUSION

Prostaglandins are more than a mere alternative to oxytocin. The latter, because of its lesser cost and its excellent tolerance at the usual doses, remains the drug of choice for the induction of labour in gravidae with favourable inducibility features, and for the acceleration of desultory labour. On the other hand, prostaglandins, given by the intravenous or the extra-amniotic route, should be preferred in difficult cases of induction and in patients with cardiovascular or renal pathology. The oral (or buccal) administration of PGE_2, in combination with early amniotomy, is a simple and well-accepted means of inducing labour in women with a ripe cervix (Table 19.4).

Table 19.4 Induction of labour. Selection of method.

Inducibility	*Method*		
Good	amniotomy at once	+	i.v. oxytocin or oral (or buccal) PGE_2
Poor	i.v. PGE_2 or $PGF_{2\alpha}$ or extra-amniotic PGE_2	+	amniotomy as soon as practicable

Acknowledgements

The authors wish to thank Mrs Sonja Pieters for her expert secretarial assistance.

References

Amy, J. J. and Thiery, M. (1979). Labour, spontaneous and induced. In: S. Aladjem, A. K. Brown and C. Sureau (eds.), *Clinical Perinatology*, 2nd Ed. (St Louis: C. V. Mosby) (In press)

Amy, J. J., Thiery, M., Crawford, J. S., Kerenyi, T. D., Bygdeman, M. and Karim, S. M. M. (1976). A suggested set of working definitions and criteria applicable to induction of labour. *Int. J. Gynecol. Obstet.*, **14**, 379

Beazley, J. M. and Weekes, A. R. L. (1976). Neonatal hyperbilirubinaemia following the use of prostaglandin E_2 in labour. *Br. J. Obstet. Gynaecol.*, **83**, 62

Bishop, E. H. (1964). Pelvic scoring for elective induction. *Obstet. Gynecol.*, **24**, 266

Calder, A. A. and Embrey, M. P. (1975). Comparison of intravenous oxytocin and prostaglandin E_2 for induction of labour using automatic and non-automatic infusion techniques. *Br. J. Obstet. Gynaecol.*, **82**, 728

Calder, A. A., Hillier, K. and Embrey, M. P. (1976). Induction of labor with extra-amniotic prostaglandin E_2. In: B. Samuelsson and R. Paoletti (eds.), *Advances in Prostaglandin and Thromboxane Research*, Vol. II, p. 994 (New York: Raven Press)

Craft, I. (1973). Oral prostaglandin E_2 and amniotomy for induction of labor. *Adv. Biosci.*, **9**, 593

Decoster, W., Goethals, A., Vandierendonck, A., Thiery, M. and Derom, R. (1976). Labor induction with prostaglandin $F_{2\alpha}$. Influence on psychomotor evolution of the child in the first 30 months. *Prostaglandins*, **12**, 559

Freeman, R. (1975). The use of the oxytocin challenge test for ante-partum clinical evaluation of uteroplacental respiratory function. *Am. J. Obstet. Gynecol.*, **121**, 481

Johnson, A., Hyatt, D., Newton, J. and Phillips, L. (1974). Experience with prostaglandin $F_{2\alpha}$ (free acid) for the induction of labor. *Prostaglandins*, **7**, 487

Karim, S. M. M. and Sharma, S. D. (1972). Oral administration of prostaglandin E_2 for the induction and acceleration of labor. *J. Reprod. Med.*, **9**, 346

Karim, S. M. M., Trussell, R. R., Patel, R. C. and Hillier, K. (1968). Response of pregnant human uterus to prostaglandin $F_{2\alpha}$. Induction of labour. *Br. Med. J.*, **4**, 621

Kennedy, J. H., Quinn, M. A., Howie, P. W. and Calder, A. A. (1978). Single shot prostaglandin gel for labor induction. *Prostaglandins*, **15**, 169

Lauersen, N. H. and Wilson, K. H. (1975). Induction of labour with oral prostaglandin E_2. *Obstet. Gynecol.*, **44**, 793

Liggins, G. C. (1962). The treatment of missed abortion by high dosage Syntocinon intravenous infusion. *J. Obstet. Gynaecol. Br. Cmnwlth.*, **69**, 277

Miller, A. W. F. and Mack, D. S. (1974). Induction of labour by extra-amniotic prostaglandins. *J. Obstet. Gynaecol. Br. Cmnwlth.*, **81**, 706

Miller, J. F., Welply, G. A. and Elstein, M. (1975). Prostaglandin E_2 tablets compared with intravenous oxytocin in induction of labour. *Br. Med. J.*, **1**, 14

Scher, J., Dryden, P. and Davey, D. A. (1976). Induction of labour with buccal prostaglandin E_2. *Br. Med. J.*, **1**, 812

Scott, J. W. and Craft, I. (1976). Labor induction using buccal prostaglandin E_2. *Prostaglandins*, **11**, 853

Seng, K. M. and Salmon, Y. M. (1976). A comparative study on the use of oral prostaglandins E_2 and $F_{2\alpha}$ in the induction of labour. In: S. M. M. Karim (ed.), *Obstetric and Gynaecological Uses of Prostaglandins*, pp. 165–169 (Lancaster: MTP Press)

Sivasuriya, M., Tan, K. L., Salmon, Y. M. and Karim, S. M. M. (1978). Neonatal serum bilirubin levels in spontaneous and induced labour. *Br. J. Obstet. Gynaecol.*, **85**, 619

Thiery, M. and Amy, J. J. (1975). Induction of labour with prostaglandins. In: S. M. M. Karim (ed.), *Advances in Prostaglandin Research: Prostaglandins and Reproduction*, pp. 149–228 (Lancaster: MTP Press)

Thiery, M. and Amy, J. J. (1977). Spontaneous and induced labor: two roles for the prostaglandins. In: R. M. Wynn (ed.), *Obstetrics and Gynecology Annual*, Vol. VI, pp. 127–171 (New York: Appleton-Century-Crofts)

Thiery, M. and Amy, J. J. (1978). Perinatal effects of natural prostaglandins used for labor induction. In: F. Coceani and P. M. Olley (eds.), *Advances in Prostaglandin and Thromboxane Research*. Vol. IV, *Prostaglandins and Perinatal Medicine*, pp. 307–324 (New York: Raven Press)

Thiery, M., Benijts, G., Martens, G., Yo Le Sian, A., Amy, J. J. and Derom, R. (1977). A comparison of buccal (oromucosal) and oral prostaglandin E_2 for the elective induction of labor. *Prostaglandins*, **14**, 371

Toppozada, M., El-Damarawy, H. and Kamel, M. (1976). Renal prostaglandins for induction of labor. A dual clinical advantage in toxemia of pregnancy. *Prostaglandins*, **12**, 581

Weekes, A. R. L., Makanji, H. H. and West, C. R. (1976). Comparison of intravenous oxytocin and prostaglandin E_2 for accelerating labour. *Br. Med. J.*, **1**, 987

Weiss, R., Markello, R., Mo, B. and Bochiechio, P. (1975). Cardiovascular effects of oxytocin. *Obstet. Gynecol.*, **46**, 211

Index

GPSR Compliance

The European Union's (EU) General Product Safety Regulation (GPSR) is a set of rules that requires consumer products to be safe and our obligations to ensure this.

If you have any concerns about our products, you can contact us on ProductSafety@springernature.com

In case Publisher is established outside the EU, the EU authorized representative is:

Springer Nature Customer Service Center GmbH
Europaplatz 3
69115 Heidelberg, Germany

Batch number: 10823811

Printed by Printforce, the Netherlands